Healing with Flowers

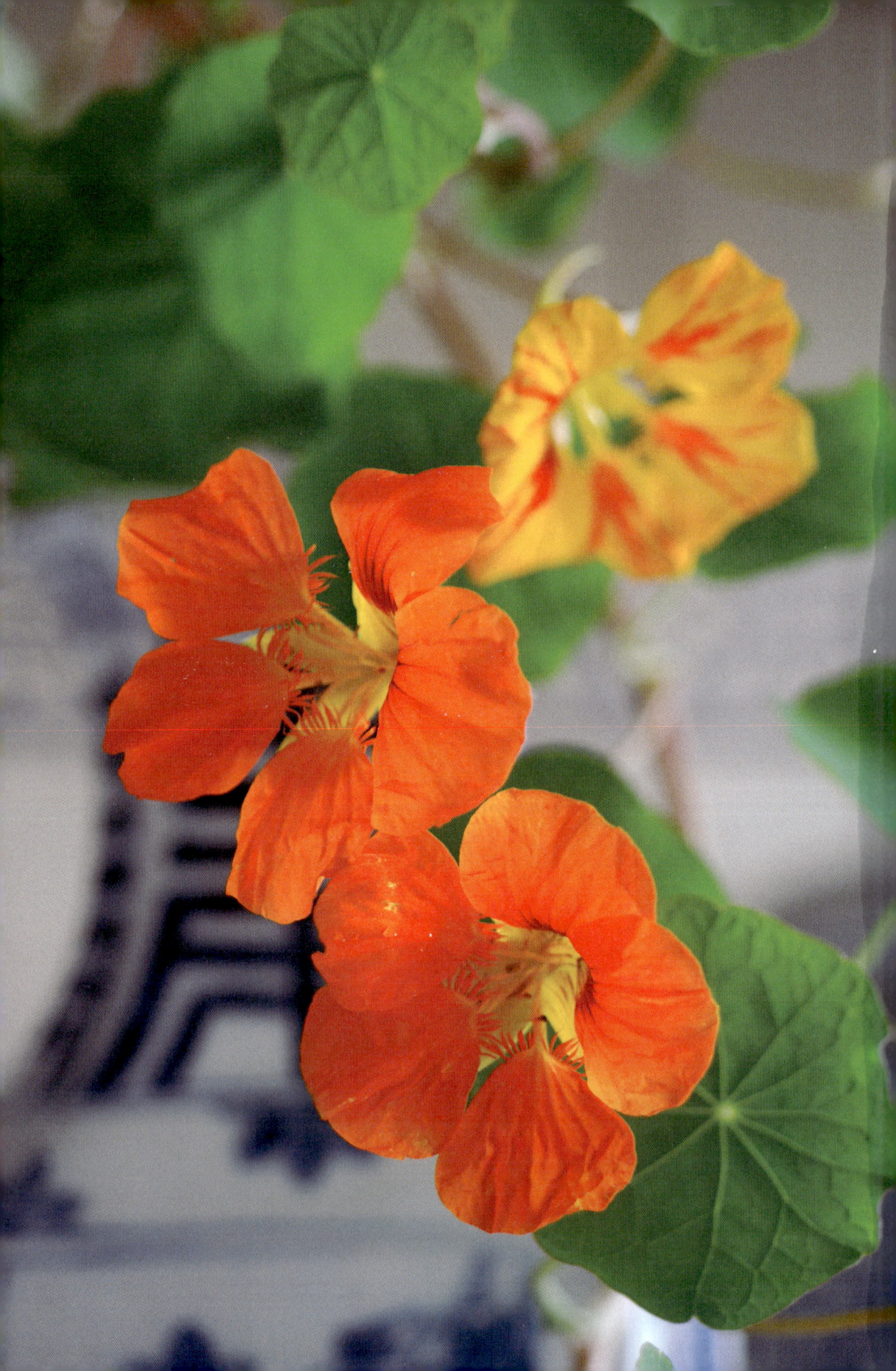

Healing with Flowers

The Power of Floral Medicine

Anne McIntyre
FNIMH, MCPP, MAPA

photographs by
Julie Bruton-Seal & Anne McIntyre

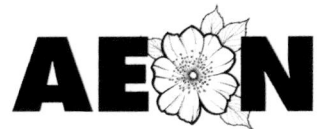

First published in 2022 by Aeon Books Ltd

Copyright © 2022 by Anne McIntyre

The right of Anne McIntyre to be identifed as the author of this work has been asserted in accordance with §§ 77 and 78 of the Copyright Design and Patents Act 1988.

All rights reserved. No part of this publication may be reproduced, stored in a retrieval system, or transmitted, in any form or by any means, electronic, mechanical, photocopying, recording, or otherwise, without the prior written permission of the publisher.

British Library Cataloguing in Publication Data

A C.I.P. for this book is available from the British Library

ISBN-13: 978-1-91350-479-3

Typesetting & design by Julie Bruton-Seal

www.aeonbooks.co.uk

Please note:
The information in this book is compiled from a blend of historical and modern sources, from folklore and personal experience. It is not intended to replace the professional advice and care of a qualified herbal or medical practitioner. Do not attempt to self-diagnose or self-prescribe for serious long-term problems without first consulting a qualified professional. Heed the cautions given, and if already taking prescribed medicines or if you are pregnant, seek professional advice before using herbal remedies.

Contents

7   Introduction

11   The Significance of Flowers in our Lives

27   Healing with Flowers

59   The Healing Flowers

393   Growing and Gathering Flowers

421   The Still Room

441   The Amazing World of Edible Flowers

475   Index

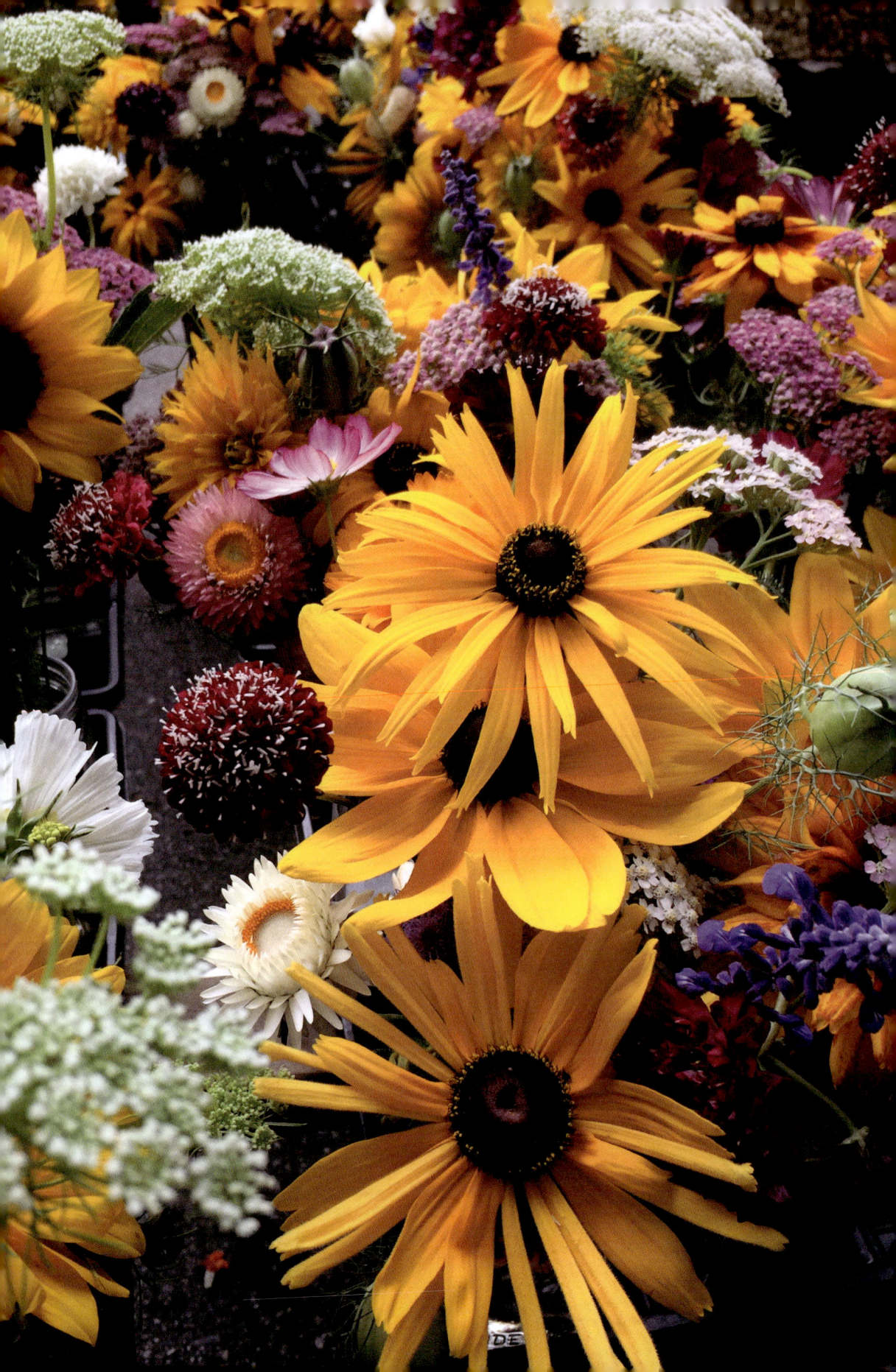

Introduction

The rose that with your earthly eyes you see
Has flowered in god from all eternity
  – Angelus Silesius (1624–1677)

Exuberant red peonies, sweet-smelling primroses, exotic lilies, cheerful calendulas, delicate anemones and wonderfully perfumed roses – just some of the flowers that we all know and cannot help but love. All over the world such flowers are part of human life, marking every important occasion, every change and ritual from the cradle to the grave. Today, as thousands of years ago, flowers are able to express what we often cannot find the words to say. As Wordsworth so aptly wrote, inspired by flowers as many a poet before and after him, "*To me the meanest flower that blows can give, thoughts that do often lie too deep for tears.*"

Flowers are given to express joy at the birth of a child and they adorn all ceremonies in every religion. They are exchanged between men and women as tokens of love, they are presented on birthdays and given to family and friends, hosts and honoured guests as gestures of appreciation. It is hard to imagine visiting a sad or unwell relative or friend without bearing flowers to lift their spirits and speed them to health or picture a wedding without flowers woven into bridal crowns and bouquets to enhance the beauty and romance of the occasion. Flowers grace our tables at celebratory meals and banquets, they brighten the house through every season and warm the heart, even on cold winter days when the rest of nature apparently sleeps. Flowers in garlands and wreaths at funerals comfort the bereaved and pay respect to the departed. They give universal pleasure, inspiring us to grow them to delight us in our gardens, pots and window-boxes. Similarly, they have inspired artists and poets through the ages. Our soft furnishings, cosmetics, soaps and perfumes invariably incorporate floral motifs or flowers, as do many of our medicines, for since the beginning of time we have used flowering plants to heal our ills.

Clearly there exists a deep bond between flowers and humankind and yet we may be unaware how they came to play such an important part in our lives. We appreciate their aesthetic beauty, their perfect form and often heavenly smell, but may not know the history and significance of the flowers we see around us today which dates back to antiquity. Flowers have featured in the beliefs, art and medicine of our ancestors for thousands of years. All over the world flowers have been part of myth and legend, worship and religion. They have become symbols of a whole range of human and spiritual experience, including love and remembrance, purity and fidelity, fertility and abundance, joy and sorrow, death and rebirth, mortality and immortality. They are an integral part of our everyday existence and it would be hard to imagine life without them!

This book is about the healing power of flowers that permeates every dimension of our lives. It tells the story of the mythological and historical origins of flowers in healing and medicine and is a reminder of the significance, even magnitude, of flowers that is still with us today as it was thousands of years ago. Since earliest times, when people lived so much closer to nature than we do now, flowers have been endowed with magical, supernatural or divine properties, and often with natures and temperaments much like our own. Just as human life was imbued with the divine spirit, so too flowers were seen to possess an in-dwelling spirit or soul which determined each flower's shape and form, its way of growth, its taste and smell and its purpose in the world in relation to human life.

In the ancient wisdom traditions of the world, healing plants have long been seen as manifestations of the conscious intelligence of the universe. The 'life force,' 'qi' or 'prana' of each plant is understood to be a dynamic manifestation of the divine or consciousness and every plant has its own subtle intelligence or unique wisdom, its life force and attributes which give it 'energetic' qualities as well as its array of medically active constituents and its potential ability to heal.

Herbs and flowers from all over the globe can impart their wisdom or intelligence to us and help us to balance energetic disruptions that create imbalances and health problems in mind and body. They have the power to reconnect or realign us with the conscious intelligence of nature that we a part of and in this way bring about healing. They are an extraordinary gift. Whether we live in town or country, we can benefit from the incredible healing ability of the flowers around us and use them to care for ourselves and others.

In these pages you will read about myths and legends that tell meaningful stories about flowers, the historical and folkloric importance of flowers in healing and other aspects of life, and the symbolism and language of each flower as you go through the repertory of healing flowers. You will also read about how each of the 64 flowers described here can be used in healing and the different modes of preparation used; as a herbal maceration of the flower, a distilled oil of the flower, a potentised homeopathic remedy from the flower and as a flower essence. As each flower is described you will hopefully find a thread that runs through the stories and myths about that flower, its historical and folkloric use, the details of its modern medicinal use as a herbal remedy relating to its biochemical constituents and its use in aromatherapy, homoeopathy and as a flower essence. This thread portrays each flower as having its own particular energy and vibration, its unique healing attributes, almost with its own personality as a healer. The healing power of each flower exists in whichever way it is used and I hope that this book will convey to you that it is the story of the flower itself which binds its use in healing together and that as you spend time getting to know each flowering plant, you will gain a deeper understanding of its unique character that can be of help to you as you journey through life.

> *What a desolate place would be a world without a flower!*
> *It would be a face without a smile, a feast without a welcome.*
> *Are not flowers the stars of the earth, and are not our stars the*
> *flowers of the heaven*
> – Clara Lucas Balfour (1808–1878)

Introduction

*They are autographs of angels, penned
In Nature's green-leaved book, in blended tints,
Borrowed from rainbows and the sunset skies,
And written everywhere–on plain and hill,
In lonely dells, 'mid crowded haunts of men;
On the broad prairies, where no eye save God's
May read their silent, sacred mysteries. Thank God for flowers!
They gladden human hearts; Seraphic breathings part their fragrant lips
With whisperings of Heaven.*
– Albert Laighton (1829–1887)

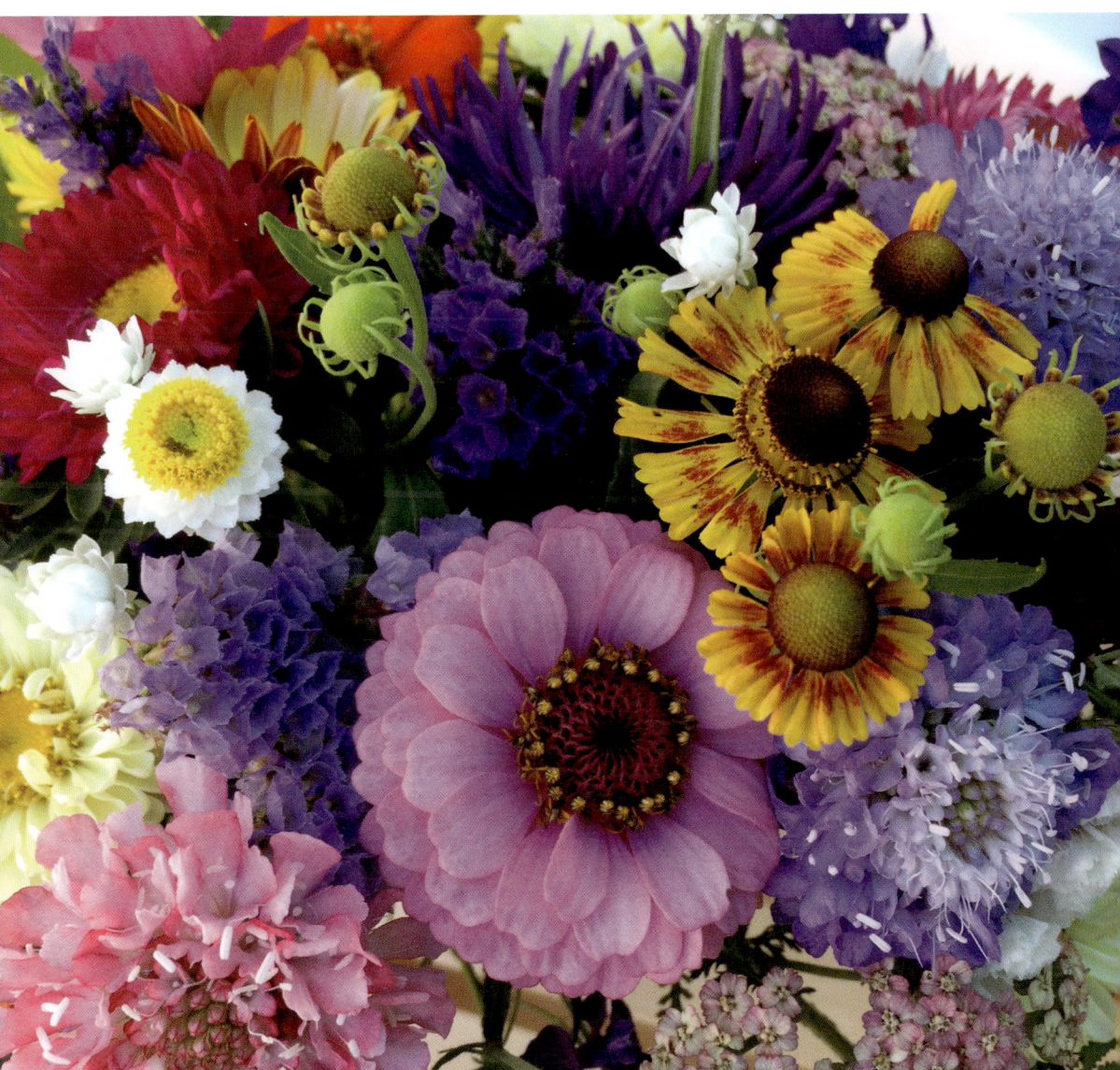

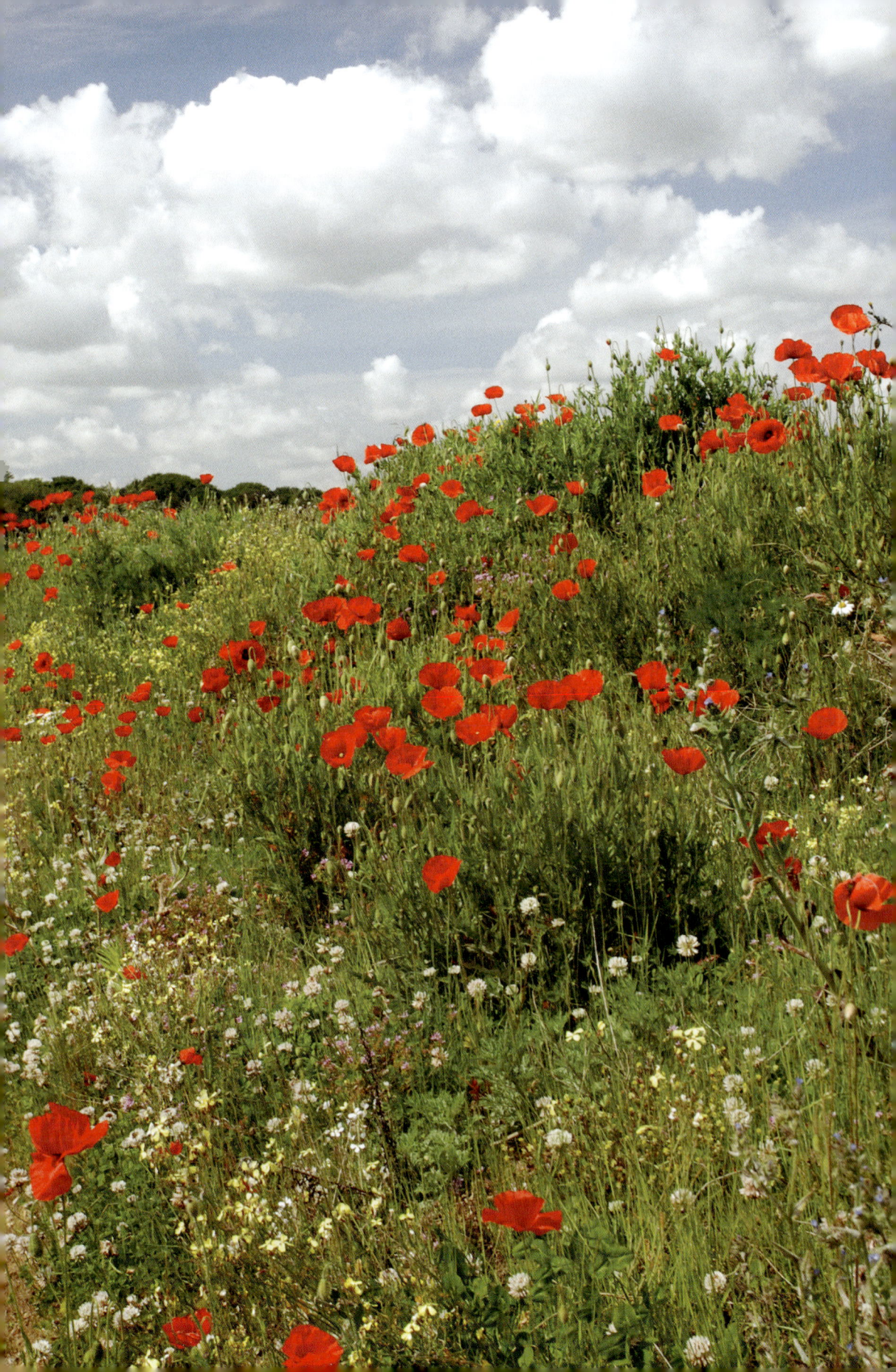

The Significance of Flowers in our Lives

As Aphrodite bore her lover's body out of the woods, crimson anemones sprung up where each drop of blood and nectar fell onto the earth. It is said that that the wind which blows the blossoms open, will soon afterwards blow the petals away; so it is called the Anemone, or Wind Flower, for that which brings forth its life, ends it.

The Greek Myths
Many of the flowers used for thousands of years for their medicinal virtues featured in the Greek legends, each story providing insight into their wonderful healing powers. Some of these legends are retold in the profiles of individual flowers. The ancient Greek myths are a vast storehouse of flower legend and symbolism and we can look to them for the origin of many of our own floral customs and traditions. Classical Greece of about 2000 to 3000 years ago was the intellectual and literary centre of Europe and the land richest in flowers. The ancient Greeks were also responsible for the origins of western medicine, the inspiration of which has survived in the writings of great physicians such as Hippocrates and Dioscorides and those of their followers.

Anyone visiting the Greek countryside in spring today will witness the extraordinary wealth of native flowers. It is not hard to imagine the days when the mythical gods and goddesses played on Mount Olympus and flowers were born into creation. The diversity and beauty of flowers and trees was an integral part of the spiritual lives of the ancient Greeks. Their heroes, nymphs and deities were created alongside them as expressions of human archetypes and spiritual truths. To the Greeks nature itself was a religious symbol. The healing power of plants was a gift from the gods, and their beauty an inspiration to art. The innate character of specific plants leant meaning to and understanding of the reality of human and divine life. Temples and sacred places to worship and sacrifice to their gods were built in places of outstanding beauty, as ancient remains will testify. Flowers gave expression to a great deal of unconscious human and spiritual experience which would otherwise be difficult to communicate. In those ancient days the Greeks would *'say it with flowers'* and ever since those times flowers have been used to convey secret meanings, love and intimate messages, healing powers and religious significance.

A closer look at Greek mythology will reveal the symbolic meaning of some of the plants with which we are familiar today. Chloris (from *chloe* meaning *first green shoot* and equivalent to the Latin *flora*) was the goddess of flowers and personified spring. She carried out the wishes of Hera and made plants grow with the help of Horae, the daughters of Zeus and Themis who reigned over the seasons and the cycle of growth. Chloris' lover was Zephyr, the god of the West wind who reawakened nature each spring. The nymphs of the springs took care of the plants and made sure they received vitalising moisture from Oceanus the father of streams and rivers. Artemis the moon goddess revived the flowers each night with her refreshing dew, and her twin brother Apollo the sun god, sent the sun's rays to make the plants live and grow in the daytime.

The fields and crops were the responsibility of Demeter whose daughter Persephone was carried off by Hades, god of the underworld, to be his queen. She was imprisoned under the ground for half the year throughout the winter and returned to earth each spring. When Persephone was first captured, Demeter was inconsolable and searched for her daughter high and low until exhausted, she sat down on a stone where she stayed for nine days and nights.

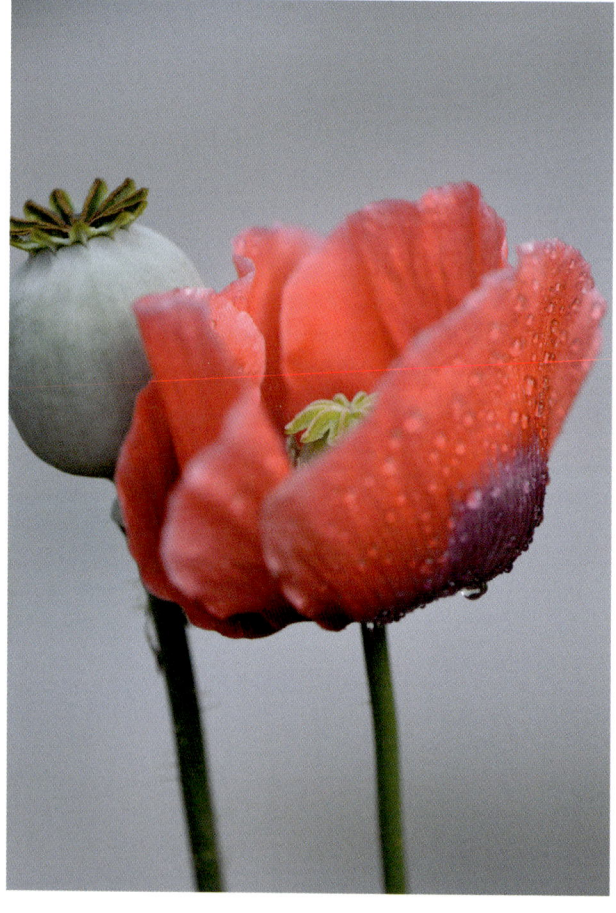

During that time the gods caused poppies to grow up around her feet and Demeter breathed their heady scent and ate their narcotic seeds until she forgot her pain in the oblivion of sleep. Persephone symbolises the corn seed hidden underground or in the earth during winter, germinating in the spring, and then disappearing again with the coming of winter. She is sought by Demeter, goddess of harvest and agriculture. The poppies represent winter and sleep and their seeds represent fertility. When we eat bread decorated with poppy seeds, we might bring to mind the allegorical story of Persephone and Demeter and the continual cycles of the seasons in earthly life.

Another story tells of the narcissus which Gaia made grow to please Hades so that its sweet scent would entice Persephone into the underworld. Since the underworld symbolises death, this relates to the custom of decorating graves with the bright daffodil in modern times. The name Narcissus comes from the story of the son of Cephisus the river god and Liriope a forest nymph, who was called Narcissus. He was so beautiful that many a nymph fell in love with him, but he loved only himself. Aphrodite decided to punish him for this and made him fall in love with his reflection in a spring. He either slipped in and drowned or pined away and died by the side of the water. Narcissus remained as a sweet-smelling spring flower crowned with gold which still leans over streams and rivers in search of its reflection in the water.

Daphne was a beautiful shy young nymph, the daughter of Ladon the river god. Apollo the sun god was in love with her and amorously pursued her. To escape him Daphne fled to her mother Gaia, who changed her into a laurel tree (*Laurus nobilis*). From then onward, the laurel was sacred to Apollo. When he killed the dragon Python, he went into Delphi crowned as the conqueror with laurel branches and thus the laurel became a symbol of respect, victory and fame, from which story originated the term *'laureate'* we commonly use today as in *'poet laureate'* to describe a celebrated poet.

But since thou canst not be my wife, at least thou shalt be my tree; my hair, my lyre, my quiver shall always have thee, oh laurel!

The elegant white myrtle flower (right) with its lovely perfume and evergreen leaves was sacred to Aphrodite the goddess of love, who hid her naked beauty behind a myrtle when she rose from the sea near Paphos in Cyprus. Myrtle thus became a symbol of beauty and youth and is still commonly used today in wreaths and crowns to adorn brides.

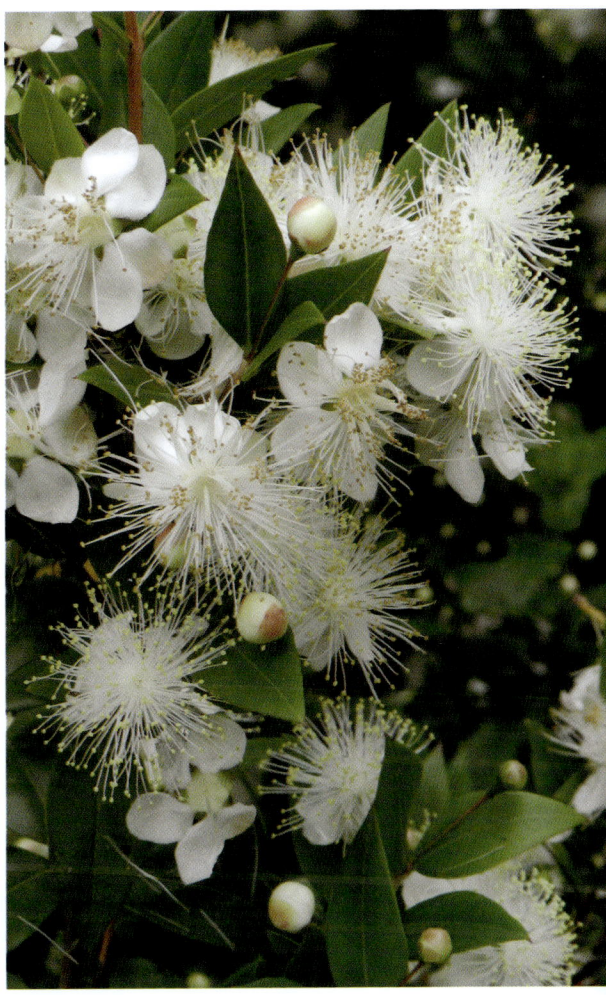

Flowers and the Cycle of Life

Flowers were also closely intertwined with the ancient concepts of life after death. In the gloomy regions of the Elysian fields presided over by Hades, the vast plains were covered with asphodels. These were planted on graves by the Greeks and Romans to symbolise eternal life. Flowers were believed in many cultures to grow in profusion in paradise or heaven; being spiritual in nature they were impervious to the destructive workings of time. Flowers were planted on tombs to aid the journey of the departed to the afterlife and symbolised the victory of the soul over earthly life. The dead were often buried in groves of sacred trees as the Greeks believed the souls delighted to walk amongst them. We still pay tribute to the dead with floral wreaths in the shape of a circle, designed originally to enclose the soul of the dead.

The ancient Egyptians crowned their dead with chaplets of flowers as a farewell gift and to ensure a safe journey. Graves of loved ones were also strewed with flowers such as myrtle, polyanthus and amaranth. Spring and summer flowers were placed on graves of those who had died in the bloom of youth and ancient trees and aromatic herbs were grown by graves of the elderly. White roses were planted on virgins' graves, while red roses were placed on graves of those who had led untarnished lives. Favourite funereal flowers included hyssop, sweet William, carnations and rosemary, as well as evergreens such as laurel and bay to signify eternal life.

Today mourners still favour rosemary as well as roses, winter-flowering heather and aubretia. The snowdrop is an emblem of death, derived from the fact it appears to wear a shroud or burial robe. However, the snowdrop has also been seen as a symbol of life and hope. A story goes that when Adam and Eve were banished from the Garden of Eden, Eve stood sorrowfully looking at the flowerless earth around her covered with snow. An angel appeared and catching a falling snowflake, blew on it and it was transformed into a snowdrop. As the angel handed the flower to Eve, he told her to have hope as the summer was on its way, and as he left a ring of snowdrops appeared on the ground. Certainly, as the first flowers to appear after the cold and apparent death of winter, the snowdrop is a very welcome sight.

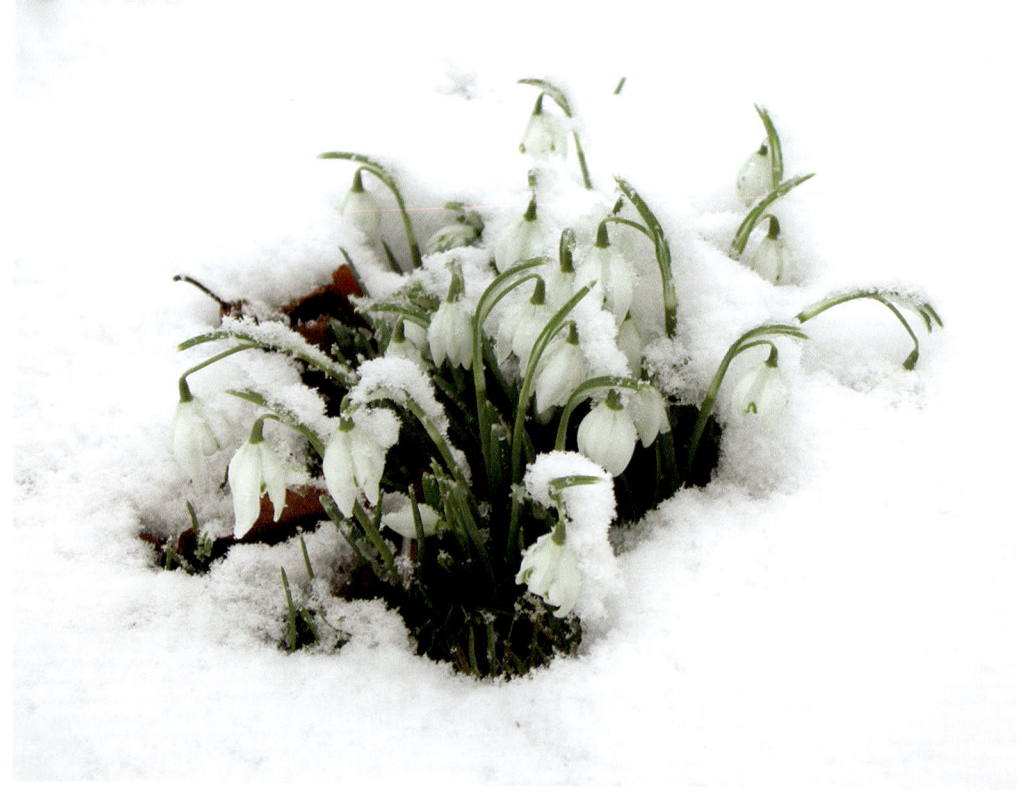

I've brought some snowdrops; only just a few
But quite enough to prove the world awake,
Cheerful and hopeful in the frosty dew
And for the pale sun's sake
– Christina Rosetti (1830–1894)

Despite their apparent frailty and ephemeral nature, the beauty of flowers imparts a lasting happiness. For a brief moment they seem to bring a touch of eternity, of joy that lies beyond the cares of the physical, mortal world.

> *The world's senseless beauty mirrors God's delight,*
> *That rapture's smile is secret everywhere;*
> *It flows in the wind's breath, in the tree's sap,*
> *Its hued magnificence blooms in leaves and flower*
> – Aurobindo Ghose (1872–1950)

The poignancy of the brief life of the flower has influenced poets and artists alike and has been used as a symbol of the transience of physical life, with a wider message to seize the hour before it passes. As the poet Robert Herrick said, "*Gather ye rosebuds while ye may, Old Time is still a-flying.*" At the same time flowers have represented a sense of eternity to others who have been inspired by this message from the flower world.

> *Though storms may break the Primrose on its stalk,*
> *Though frosts may blight the freshness of its bloom,*
> *Yet spring's awakening breath will woo the earth*
> *To feed with kindliest dews its favourite flower*
> *That blooms in mossy banks and darksome glens,*
> *Lighting the greenwood with its sunny smile;*
> *Fear not then, spirit, Death's disrobing hand*
> – Percy Shelley (1792–1822)

This is also expressed by Aurobindo Ghose, "*Earth's flowers spring up and laugh at time and death.*"

To the ancient Greeks, the continual renewal of life in nature was seen as a manifestation of the mystery of the gods or the divine, and this gave sacred meaning to many plants and trees. The oak, the most majestic of all trees, was sacred to Zeus whose wisdom was consulted at Dodona beneath a sacred oak. When the prayers of the believers were heard by Zeus, the tree was said to acknowledge this by rustling its leaves. The white poplar or aspen with its two-coloured leaves, was seen to symbolise the two worlds of the underworld and the living. Evergreens such as privet, laurel and olive were used in offerings to the Greek gods as symbols of the permanence of the divine order.

Flowers and the Life of the Spirit
Since these classical times, flowers have provided a perfect vehicle for the expression of religious ideas, concepts so intangible as to escape verbal communication. Throughout history they have expressed religious truths hidden within the great mysteries and hinted at the divine nature of God. In the days of Christian persecution, floral emblems were used in art, literature or architecture as a secret form of communication.

In ancient Egypt the lotus was a symbol of new life, while in Europe it represented the mystical centre of things. In the East the lotus was depicted springing from the navel of

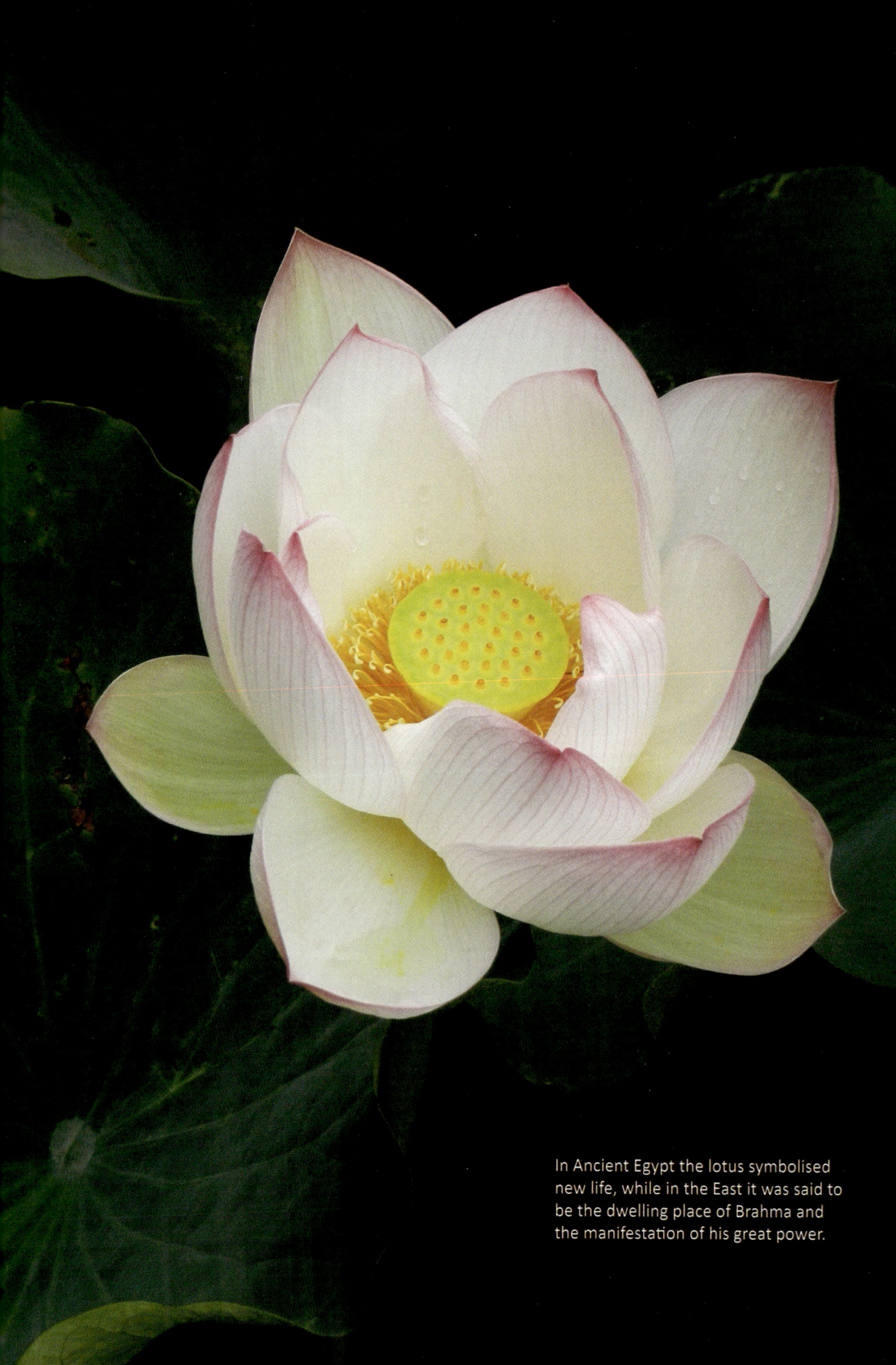

In Ancient Egypt the lotus symbolised new life, while in the East it was said to be the dwelling place of Brahma and the manifestation of his great power.

Vishnu, representing the universe evolving from a central sun. The lotus was the dwelling place of Brahma and the manifestation of his great power. With the coming of Christianity, flowers originally dedicated to Greek or Roman gods were assigned to saints, and churches were often built on the sites of pagan worship. Many flowers originally said to be ruled by Aphrodite or Venus became emblems of the Virgin Mary, the Christian symbol of female divinity or the goddess within.

The Madonna lily is the flower most famously used in religious symbolism. It was originally used to illustrate the marvels of paradise; later it was frequently depicted in paintings in the hands of the Virgin Mary, where it signified purity and chastity and still does to this day. An angel carrying an olive branch in his hand represented a peacemaker; the rose originally and still is a symbol of earthly love and was also an emblem of heavenly delight and the heart or mystic centre of being.

> *The rose was not searching for the sunrise*
> *almost eternal on its branch,*
> *it was searching for something else.*
> *The rose was not searching for darkness or science:*
> *borderline of flesh and dream,*
> *it was searching for something else*
> – Federico Garcia Lorca (1899–1936)

The trefoil or shamrock represented the Holy Trinity and was used by St Patrick to illustrate the meaning of the true Godhead to the pagan Irish. The iris was a symbol of purity and majesty, the pink a flower of holy love, while jasmine, also known as *'the star of divine hope,'* was an emblem of the Virgin Mary. In a similar way flowers were used to represent evil and the forces of darkness and were used by witches and magicians in their spells.

The mystery of the flowers' growth and ephemeral yet continuous existence meant that flowers were believed to have many magical and supernatural qualities. Flowers such as hawthorn, clover, St John's wort, lavender and heather were believed, as they are still today, to bring luck. Others including anemone, peony, lily and St John's wort were used to protect against evil and the forces of darkness. Dandelions, daisies and calendulas, still a delight to children, were used not only as floral clocks as their petals opened and closed at certain times each day, but also as love oracles. They revealed whether 'she loves me' or 'she loves me not' in a tradition that remains in many places today.

Flowers have been closely associated with the world of dreams. The ancients believed that dreams were communication from the world of spirits or indications of God's divine will, and their symbolic meaning was interpreted by magicians and diviners. The ancient Egyptians believed that dreams were inspired by the goddess Isis. To dream of lavender, for example, meant 'a reunion', while calendula meant 'you will do well'. Jasmine signified 'romance', daisy 'a birth' and cowslip meant 'unexpected love'.

Flowers are Love in Search of a Word

And what of flowers and love? Today as ever, flowers express what we may not find the words to convey to the ones we love. The beautiful rose springs to mind as the flower most closely associated with love in most minds, artist, poet or lover. "*My luve is like a red red rose*" said Robert Burns, and Yeats wrote:

> *With the earth and the sky and the water*
> *remade like a casket of gold*
> *For my dreams of your image that blossoms*
> *a rose in the depths of my heart.*

When a medieval lady was called a 'rose' by her knight, it was to convey that he considered her an exotically perfumed goddess of love, a delight to the eye and heart. The rose was the symbol of love, beauty and perfection, an emblem of the mystic heart of things. It was adopted by poets and artists to symbolise the perfect world – an ideal or paradise. To ancient magicians a rose had other special meanings. If seven-petalled, it represented the seven degrees of absolute perfection and if eight-petalled, it meant regeneration or rebirth.

The rose, the most beautiful symbol of love, was created when Chloris the Greek goddess of flowers, found the body of a beautiful nymph one day and asked the Three Graces to help her to make a special flower in honour of his beauty and her love.

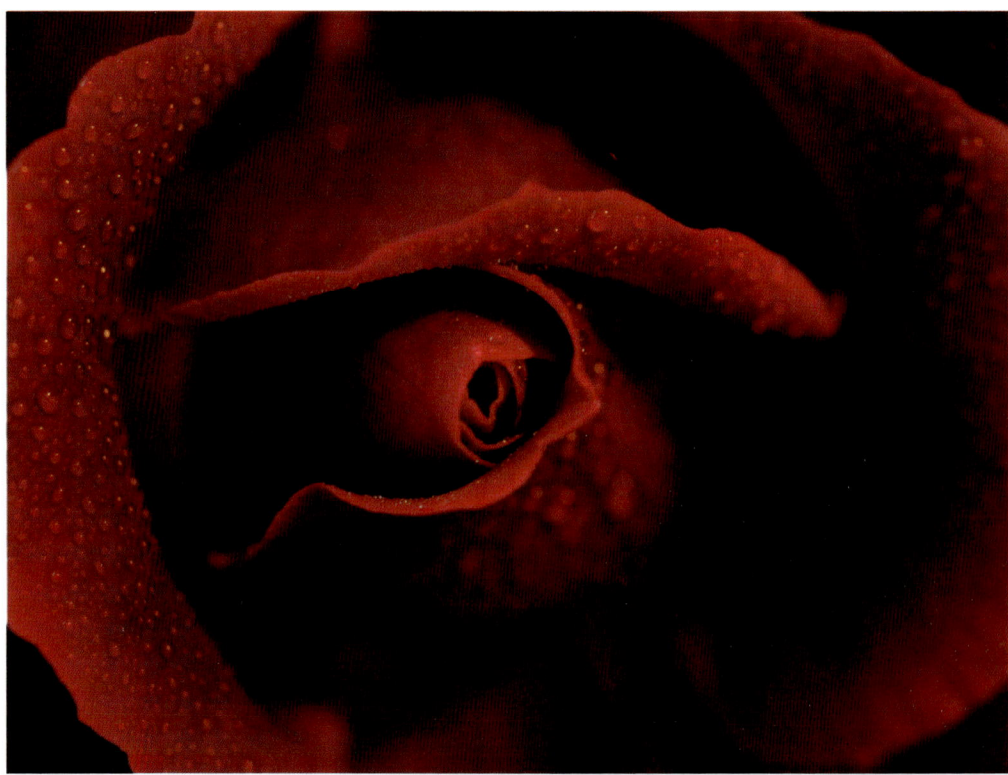

The tulip was once a young Dalmatian girl who was turned into a flower to avoid the advances of Vertuminus, the Roman god of the seasons. The forget-me-not, long an emblem of love and remembrance, derives its name from the German legend which tells of a knight and his lady walking along the banks of the river Danube. The lady caught sight of the pretty blue flower and as the knight leant by the water to pick it, he lost his footing and fell into the river. As he drifted away to his death he was heard to say, 'forget me not'.

A posy was originally the name given to a poem which accompanied a bouquet of flowers given as a token of love. Several of the flowers commonly found in such bouquets were traditionally associated with love, since their mythical origins derived from love stories. Some flowers were said to grow from the blood or teardrops of sad lovers, or from beautiful girls fleeing from advances of over-amorous lovers. Apollo fell in love with Hyacinthus thereby arousing the jealousy of Zephyr, the wind god. One day when Apollo and Hyacinthus were playing quoits, Zephyr in a jealous rage threw one of the quoits and killed Hyacinthus. From his blood arose the flower that bears his name.

Flowers associated with courtship and marriage are designed to win the favour of the desired person and to symbolise the joy of their union. These were often plants associated with fertility and aphrodisiacs for 'stirring up the passions'. Orchids for example, were dedicated to Venus the goddess of love and ruled

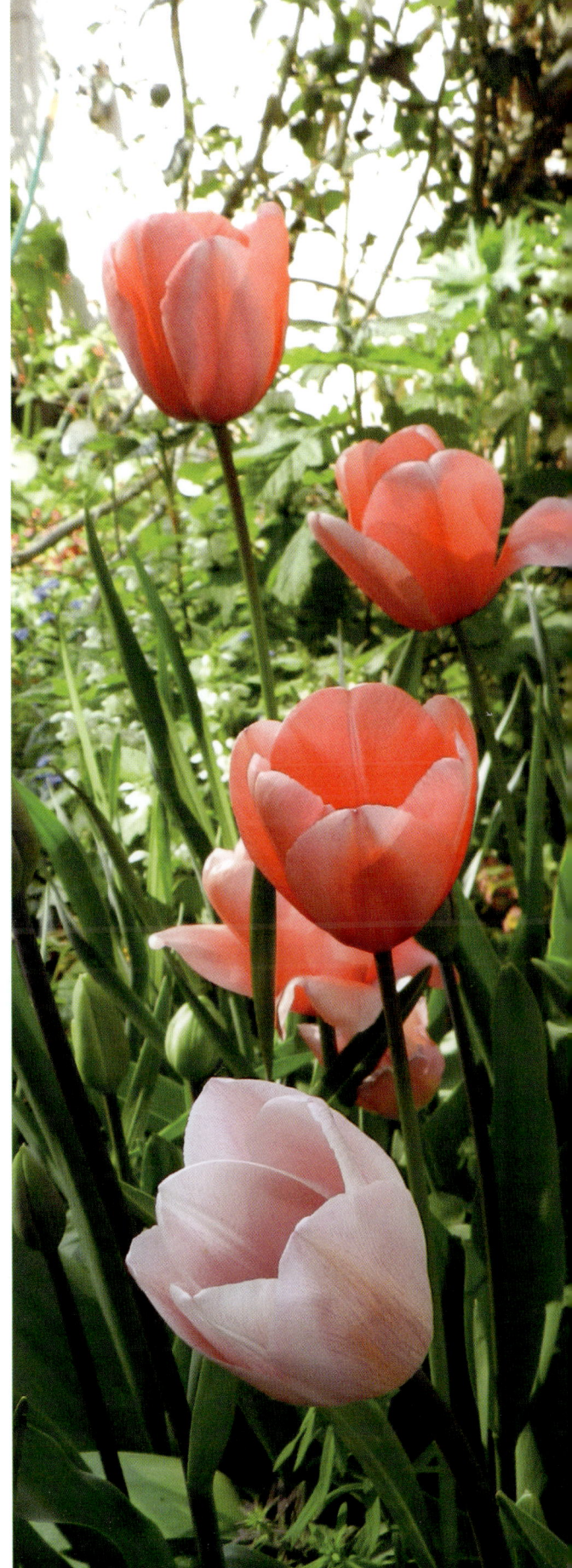

by her. Satyrs of classical mythology were said to gorge themselves on the roots of orchids to excite the passions. In fact, one of the old names for orchids is *satyrion*. Such flowers were traditionally used in love potions or philtres to conquer the hearts of the desired man or woman. Pansies were a favourite; often they would be placed over the eyes of the loved one while asleep, to make him fall for the first person he saw on waking, as we know well from Shakespeare's Midsummer Night's Dream.

Vervain was given by young girls to their lovers to keep their affections. Jasmine, roses and orange flowers were symbols of love and fertility and often used in garlands for a bride's head. Marjoram, basil, carnations, myrtle and rosemary were similarly associated with love, weddings and fidelity. Many of the flowers associated with marital union were climbing plants like jasmine, honeysuckle, clematis and ivy, which entwine themselves like lovers in each other's arms.

The Language of Flowers

The use of flower meanings or the language of flowers was a common form of communication in old China, Egypt and India. It further developed in the harems of Turkey for illicit communication between lovers and to idle away the hours. By the Elizabethan era, Shakespeare was well versed in the significance of floral messages and obviously most of his audiences would have been familiar with his references and hidden meanings. In *A Midsummer Night's Dream* Oberon describes where Titania sleeps, using the symbolism of flowers to describe more than just a place of natural beauty:

> *I know a bank where the wild thyme blows,*
> *where oxslips and the nodding violet grows,*
> *Quite over-canopied with luscious woodbine,*
> *with sweet musk roses and with eglantine.*

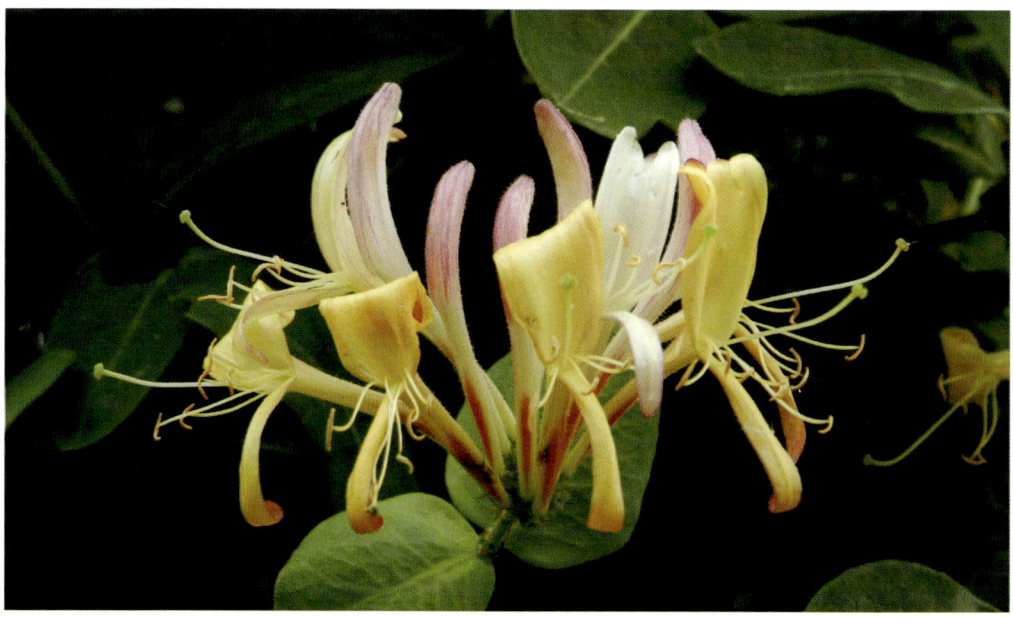

Thyme symbolised 'sweetness,' oxslips meant 'comeliness', the violet meant 'love in idleness'; the rose represented 'love' and eglantine (honeysuckle) meant 'united in love'. In Hamlet Ophelia says, *"There's rosemary, that's for remembrance; pray love remember; and there's pansies, that's for thoughts."*

The language of flowers was further developed in England by Lady Mary Wortley Montagu, an 18th century writer who during her extensive travels in Asia discovered some of the secrets of the harem. Around the same time Aubrey de la Mottraie who accompanied Charles XII of Sweden during his exile in Turkey, popularised flower language in France. He wrote, *"fruit, flowers, and gold and silver thread ... have each of them their particular meaning explained by certain Turkish verses, which young girls learn by tradition of one another."* Writings in France were translated into German and the language of flowers gradually found its way to other parts of the world.

It was developed into a popular art by the Victorians in Great Britain who expressed meaning in the colour and arrangement of the flowers as well as the choice of species. This was a source of great amusement and relief to many in the days when codes of courtship were extremely rigid and their reticence almost contrived. According to the rules, a gentleman was supposed to make the first move, although in reality this was prompted by a subtle indication of interest from the lady. Certain gestures accompanying floral gifts further detailed their messages. If the romantic young man wanted to convey thoughts about himself, he would pass the plant inclined to the left. If he wished to say something about her, he would incline the flower to the right. The answer to a floral question depended on the hand used. A flower presented with the right was positive, while if given with the left it meant a refusal. A flower worn in the hair meant 'caution', but if worn across the heart it meant 'love'. The language of flowers was beautifully expressed in Valentine cards fashionable in the Victorian era, which were a wonderful means of secret communication between sweethearts.

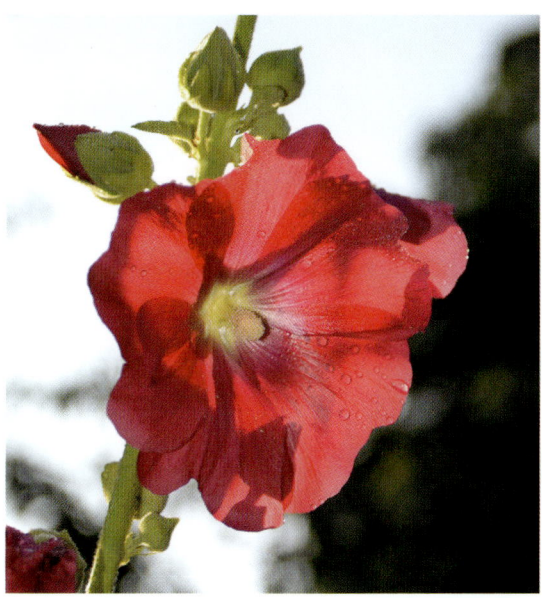

The Victorian Language of Flowers
Camellia: *perfect loveliness*
Candytuft: *indifference*
Gentian: *you are unjust*
Daffodil: *regard*
Passionflower: *faith*
Wallflower: *fidelity in adversity*
Hawthorn: *hope*
Broom: *ardour*
Clover: *happiness*
Carnation: *pure love*
Geranium: *comfort*
Hollyhock: *ambition*

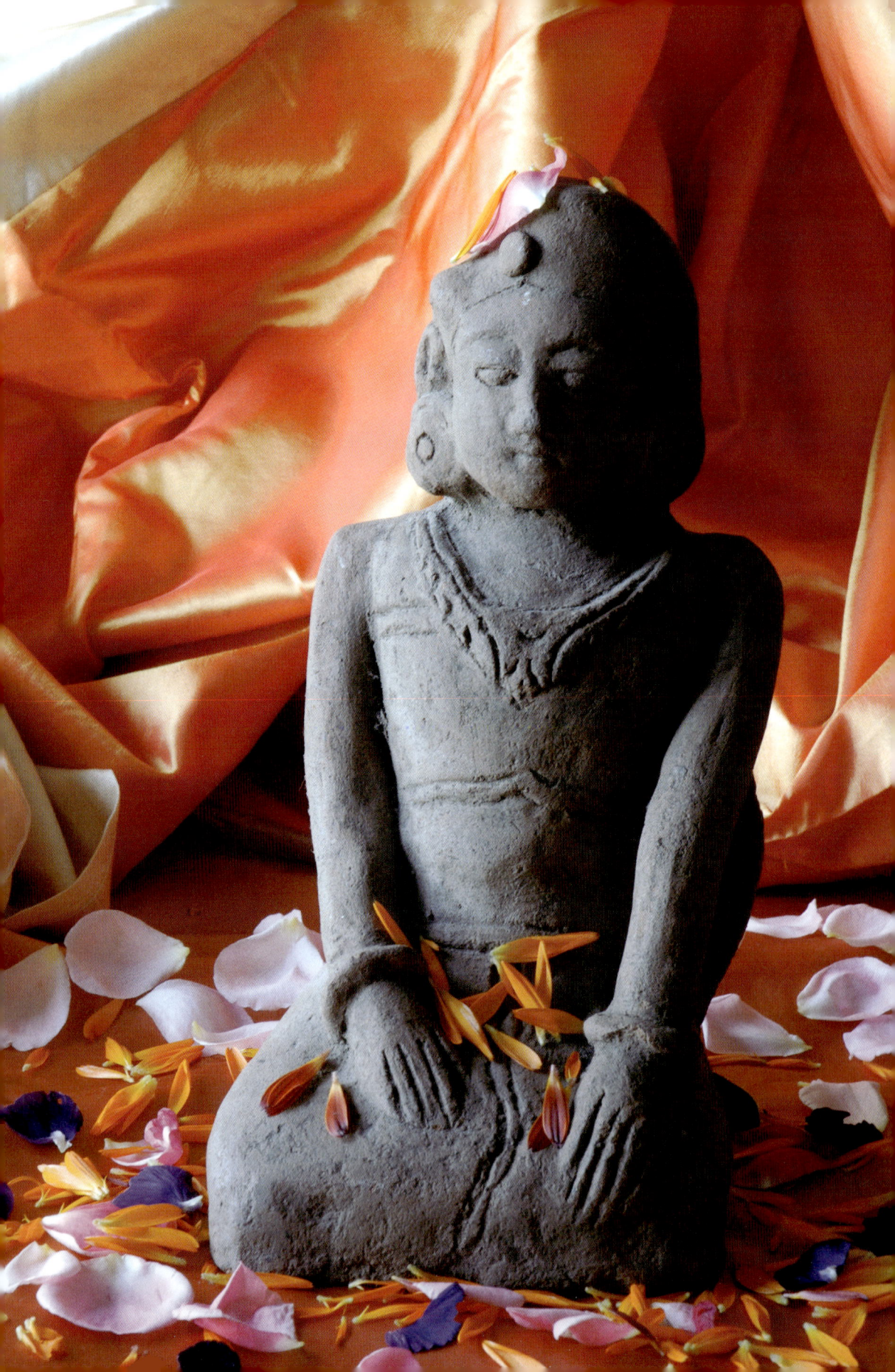

Flowers and the Soul

There is something very healing about being with flowers which may explain the worldwide love of growing flowers in gardens. A garden represents an enclosure, separate from the wildness of nature, a place of peace and a sanctuary. It was a symbol of the feminine reflected in nature, a specially devised womb for the conception and growth of living forces. Some might say it contains the secret of life itself. Many flowers were depicted in religious art in representations of the Garden of Eden, including the rose, the lily and the pink. Gardens in such art often represented sacred enclosures and feminine secrets.

Our ancestors planted certain flowers and trees to ward off intrusion by inharmonious spirits that threatened the garden's safety and tranquillity. Elder, apple, medlar and almond trees served such purposes, while flowers such as St John's wort, yarrow and angelica would protect against evil. To the psychologist the garden has represented a sanctuary. It is a symbol of the unconscious mind, a sanctified enclosure, while a forest represents the primordial instinct struggling to overtake our efforts to be in control of our destiny. Those who enjoy their gardens will know a serenity that is hard to describe, a sense of joy and peace, a release from the trials and tensions of the working day or everyday life. The garden can give us a glimpse of paradise. In fact, the notion of paradise or the Garden of Delight is to be found in nearly all ancient cultures. The Garden of Eden was in Judaism the first abode of the parents of mankind; Mount Olympus was the home of the Greek gods; while paradise or heaven is the place of peace in Christianity for the spirits of the blessed dead. The Garden of Indra is where Indian gods relaxed among miraculous trees, bright-coloured flowers and fruits that conferred immortality.

Paradise is a word in ancient Persian meaning 'garden' or 'park', and poets and artists have made use of this image to conjure up a sense of heaven, supreme bliss and the divine. In China and Japan, from the times of ancient civilisations to the present day, gardens have been developed to great heights of artistic creation and tranquillity. The Chinese and Japanese are famous for their planting of exotic flowers, gardens of quiet pools and

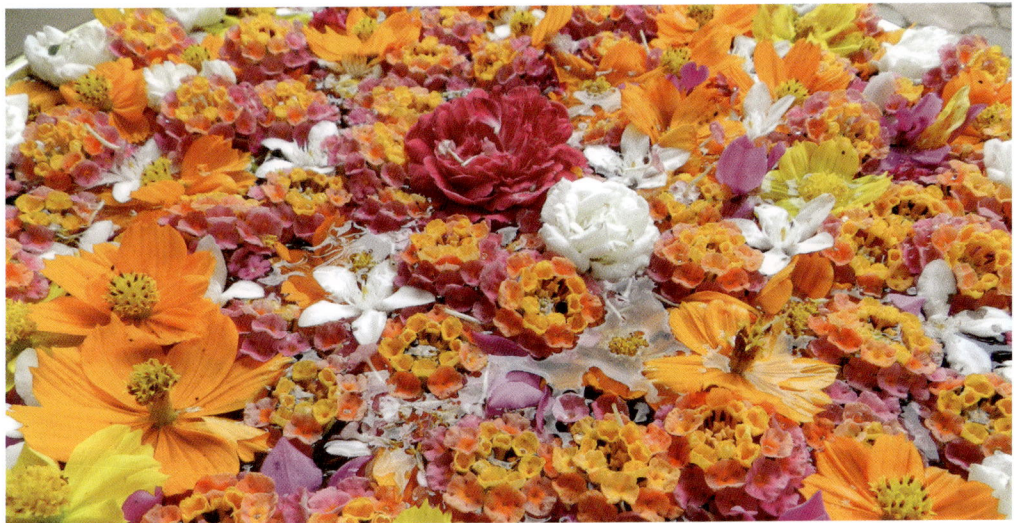

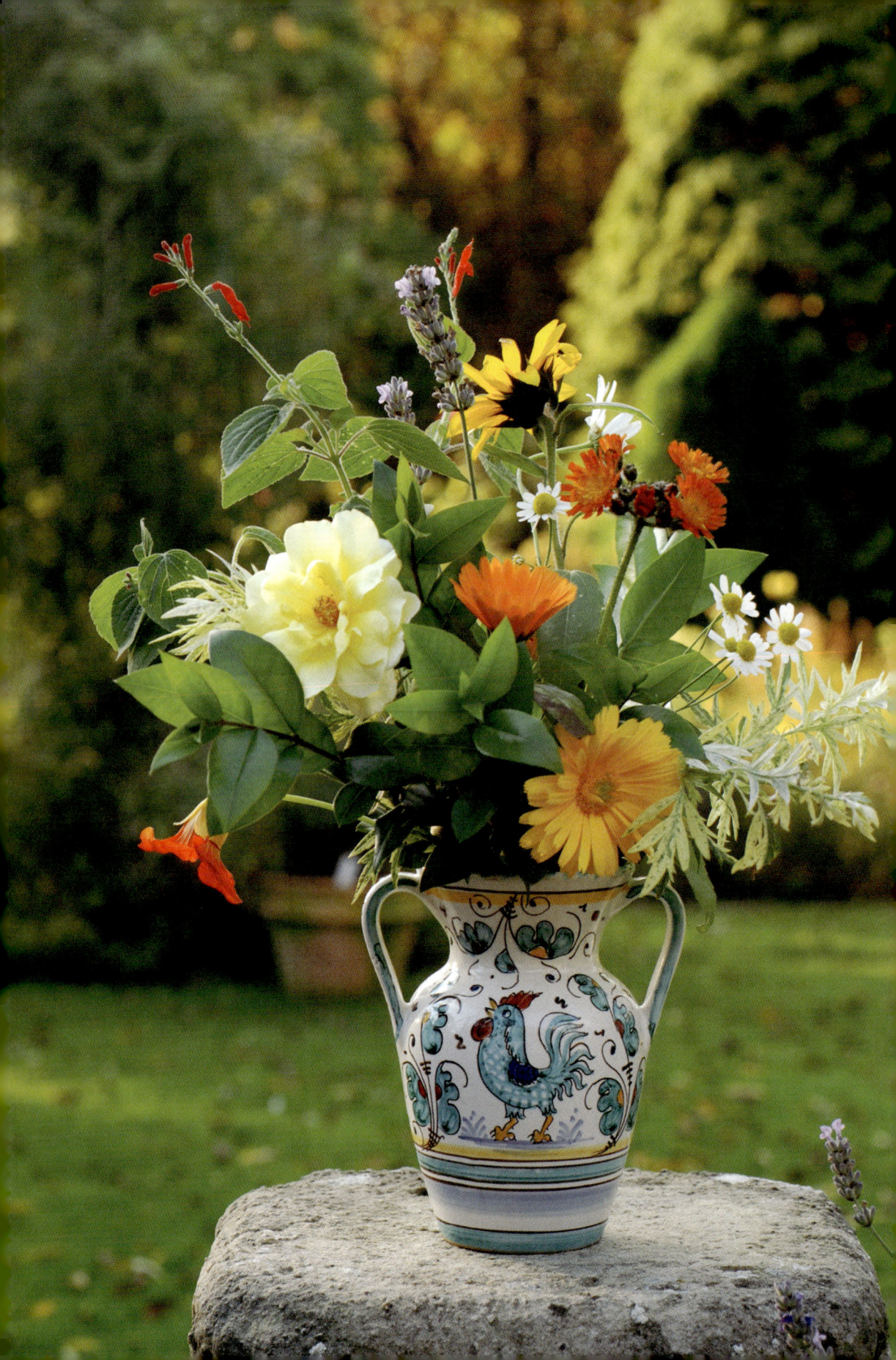

streams, bridges, fountains and pagodas to provide refreshment and inspiration. Enjoyed today by young and old, *hanami* or flower-viewing is an integral part of Japanese people's appreciation of beauty in nature, as well as being an important aspect of their social life. Cherry blossom time is the most favoured by the Japanese, but they also find symbolic beauty in many other flowers and trees, such as the pine, maple, bamboo, plum, narcissus, willow, peony and iris. By their exquisite painting and flower arranging, the Japanese capture the essence of nature at a particular time of year with a few seasonal blossoms and bring into their homes the flavour of beauty outside that is not always possible to see in its natural habitat. In this way their everyday life is enhanced by living with the spirit of the season and depending on the flowers used, flower arrangement is a mystical rite which confers upon the arranger special powers and virtues.

> *Flowers have I seen, and honey have I tasted*
> *and heard the cuckoo's song through to the end.*
> *Now in this world or in the next, dear friend,*
> *I shall forever know life was not wasted*
> – 17th century Japanese poem

In Japan, a bride is given the name 'flower daughter' by her husband's family. In other traditions, gardens and flower lore have deeply influenced our language and thinking. We talk about the 'seeds' of love, the 'budding' of romances, a family 'tree', the blossoming of a child into adulthood or of a girl into a woman. The word 'flower' has frequently been used to describe places - the ancient Middle Kingdom of China was called 'the flowery kingdom', while great historical figures have also been referred to in floral language. The legendary King Arthur of England was 'the flower of kings', Geoffrey Chaucer was the 'flower of poets'. Flowers are also used to describe personalities: the 'wallflower,' the 'shrinking violet', or someone who is 'narcissistic' - all epithets springing from the ancient symbolism of flowers.

Flowers touch our lives in ways that bring healing of infinite and indefinable measure. Imbued with philosophical, religious and symbolic meaning, they unite us with the rest of humanity, which has gazed upon the same flowers from which we derive meaning and pleasure today. They connect us to true beauty, which is infinite, and enable us to become part of this infinitude through our connection with flowers in everyday life. A flower contains all the elements of nature: ether, air, water, fire and earth. It has form, colour, texture and fragrance and still something more - an indefinable and mysterious quality, the vibrations of something that is abstract, pure and perfect. It is the form behind which is pure consciousness, the sound, the all-powerful creative mantra, the word, the womb of creation. It is for these almost inexplicable reasons that flowers are loved by men, women and children alike, and have the power to heal us on all levels of our being.

> *Little flower — but if I could understand*
> *What you are, root and all, and all in all,*
> *I should know what God is and man is*
> – Alfred, Lord Tennyson (1809–1892)

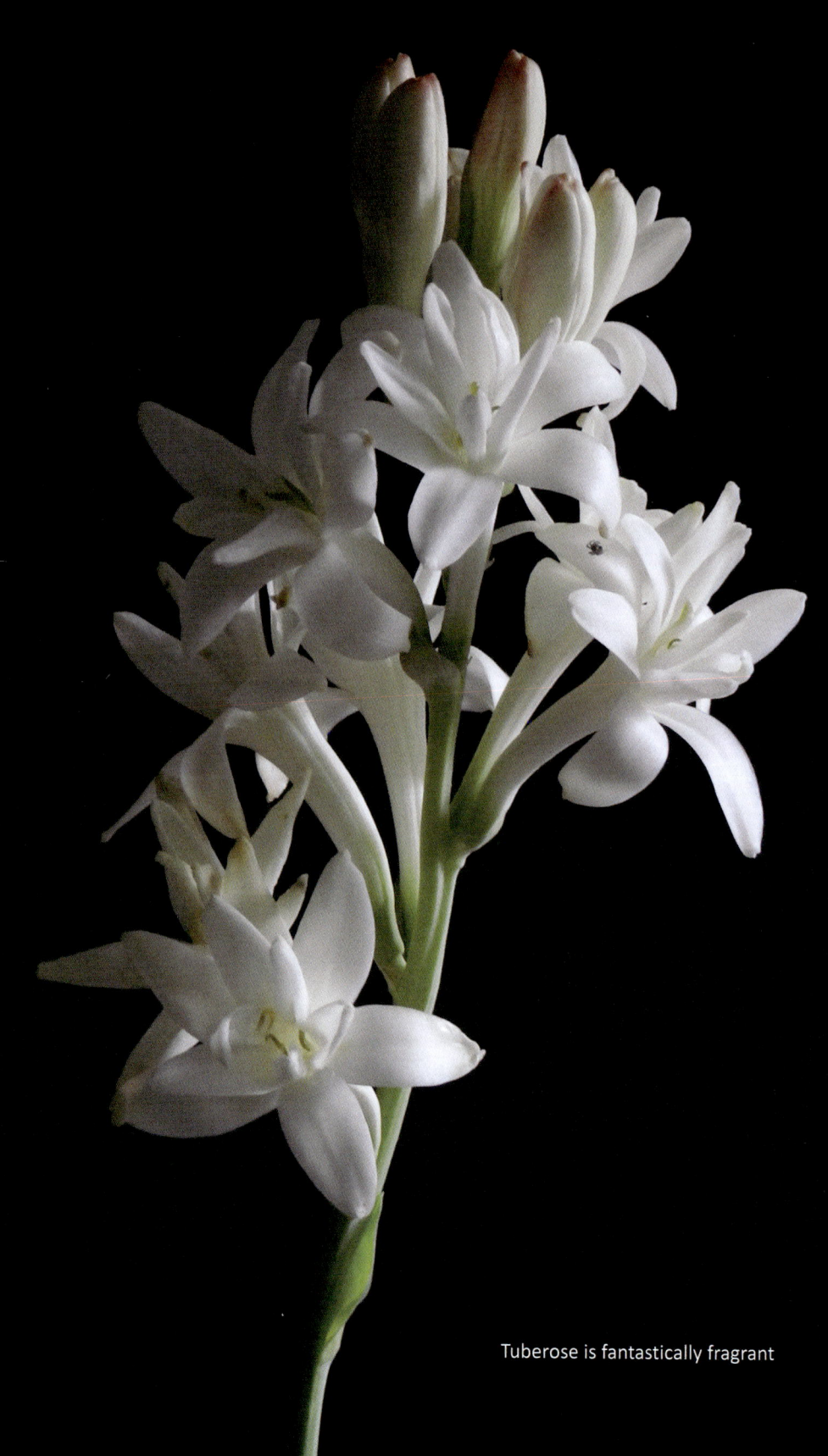
Tuberose is fantastically fragrant

Healing with Flowers

If a man would pass through Paradise in a dream
and have a flower presented to him as a pledge
that his soul had really been there, if he
found that flower in his hand when he awoke.
Aye, and what then?
– Samuel Taylor Coleridge (1772–1834)

The world of flowers with its extraordinary repertoire of vibrant colour, beautiful intricate patterns and alluring scent brings more than a touch of paradise to our earthly lives. It also brings the possibility of incredible healing on both physical and non-physical levels of our existence. True health depends on the elusive harmony of body, mind and spirit, and is (as defined by the World Health Organisation) *'the condition of perfect bodily, spiritual and social wellbeing and not solely the absence of illness and injury'*.

Plants and flowers have long been associated with healing, not only for our physical ills but also imbalances in the realms of the mind and the spirit that may give rise to our bodily symptoms. As Dr Bach said, "*disease of the body itself is nothing but the result of the disharmony between the soul and mind...health is therefore the true realisation of what we are; we are perfect; we are children of God.*"

The Unity of All Things
People throughout the world have always associated flowers with spirituality, irrespective of their religion. Mystics have referred to the spiritual forces of flowers and trees and often described them as 'angels,' 'beings of light' or 'devas' and along with the creator, responsible for human existence and continued growth. May day celebrations with dancing round the maypole are pagan rituals performed yearly in honour of the spirit of trees and the fertile blooming of nature in spring. Native Americans have always believed in the spirit of the earth and the world of plants. In 1855, Young Chief of the Cayuses said, "*the Ground says, it is the Great Spirit that placed me here. The Great Spirit tells me to take care of the Indians, to feed them aright.*" Chief Luther Standing Bear said, "*the man who sat on the ground in his tipi meditating on life and its meaning, accepting the kinship of all creatures and acknowledging unity with the universe of things, was infusing into his being the true essence of civilisation.*" Likewise, the holistic approach to healing is based on the concept of this perfect unity of all things.

The Earth as Gaia
The idea that nature was alive, animated by the same spirit or vital force as humans and everything in creation, was in fact the standard accepted view until the scientific revolution in the 17th century. It was only after that time that people began to regard nature as inanimate and unconscious, composed solely of matter in motion. In the last thirty years or so, *'new'* hypotheses and perceptions from the scientific world are seeing

nature as alive and animate, even conscious. James Lovelock in his Gaia hypothesis perceives the earth as an infinitely complex living and evolving entity, *"involving the earth's biosphere, oceans and soils, the totality constituting a feedback or cybernetic system, which seeks an optimal physical or chemical environment for life on this planet."* Just like the human organism, the earth possesses an inherent power to protect, regulate, adjust and heal itself and thereby maintain 'homeostasis'. Gaia was the Greek goddess of the earth, who created the universe and gave birth to the race of gods and the first human beings.

Modern theories of quantum physics are now recognising that all forms of existence have the same nature and that although they may appear solid and separate from each other, they are in fact simply energy vibrating at different frequencies. The energy vibrations of the mind may not be entirely different from the subtle vibrations of a flower or a tree, or even those things that appear as solid as a stone or a rock may actually be vibrating but so slowly that we may not feel or know it, except that we are aware of the healing power of gemstones.

This unified realm of existence may go some way to explaining the deep connection we feel to the plant world. It is hardly to be wondered at, for we have lived side by side with plants since the dawning of human life, we have been fed and clothed by them, sheltered and housed by them. They provide the oxygen we breathe, the food we eat, fuel to keep us warm and for thousands of years have given us medicines for almost every ill. By trapping the sun's energy through photosynthesis, plants enable solar or life energy on which all life depends, to be accessible to every inhabitant of the earth.

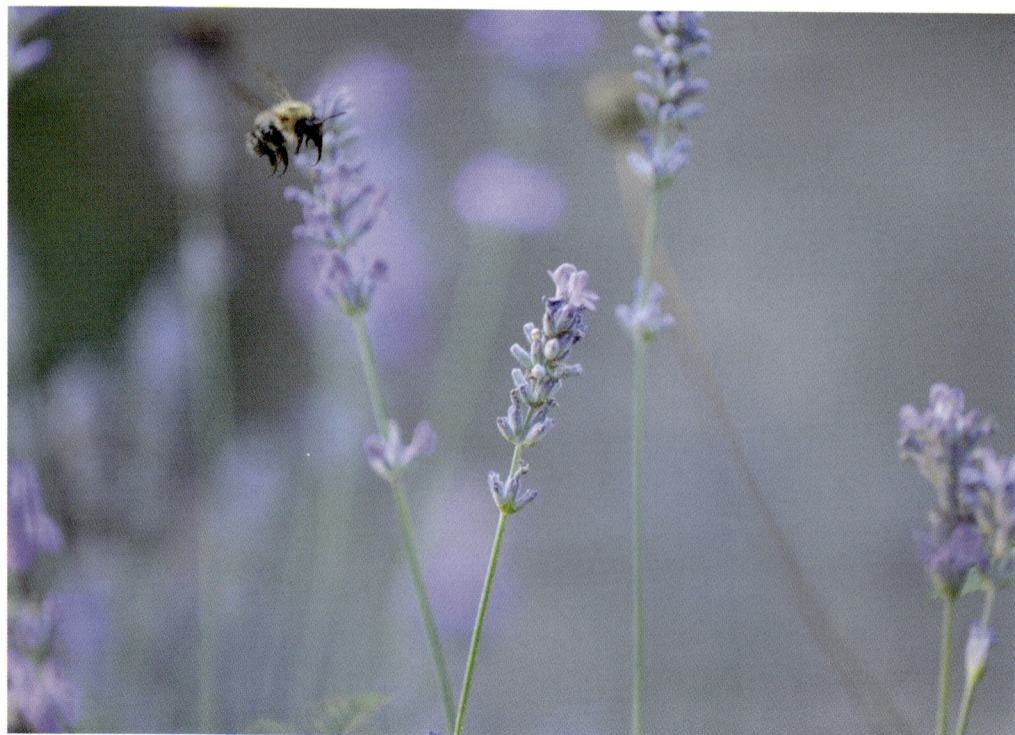

The Role of Flowering Plants

By resonating with us at all speeds of vibration, from the spiritual to the material, plants have the potential to heal us on every level of our being. Yet this is not all; something about flowers is particularly special, as if they express the essential nature of all flowering plants and convey their messages to us in all their variation of purpose. They are vital to the plant's survival and represent the peak of plants' evolution.

The first organisms were single-celled bacteria living in the sea. Then came algae, which are believed to be the ancestors of all other plants, followed by fungi, mosses and lichens. Ferns, taller plants and then trees such as giant horsetails came next, followed about 200 million years ago by plants bearing seeds known as gymnosperms – of which the wonderful ginkgo tree is a living example, as are conifers.

Flowering plants, botanically known as angiosperms, evolved about 140 million years ago, the earliest of them probably resembling a magnolia tree. In botanical terms, a flower represents a reproductive structure made up of modified leaves which attract insects and a variety of other small creatures in order to ensure their cross-fertilisation and reproduction and hence their survival. This was a far more sophisticated means of reproduction than had gone before. The cones of conifers have sperm cells packed tightly in pollen grains relying on the wind to blow them to the ovules of female cones. Spores of fungi and mosses are also vulnerable to the vagaries of the wind. More than 80 per cent of all green plants are flowering plants and every flower has the same purpose, to ensure that male pollen grains from the stamens of one flower come into contact with the stigma of a female pistil.

The intricacies of nature are amazing in their perfection. The stigma produces special secretions making sure that no pollen from other species than its own germinates, and once the right pollen has germinated, it extends a tube into the stigma down its style and makes contact with the ovary below, where two male pollen cells fertilise three female cells. An embryo is thereby produced with a food store wrapped up neatly in a seed capsule and primed to spark into life once it is in favourable conditions.

The beautiful colours and shades of flowers, their enormous variety of shape, size and pattern, as well as their wonderful perfumes, are all developed to attract specific pollinators – insects, birds, moths, beetles, even snails. The evolutionary links between the form, colour, nectar and scent of flowers and the sensory perceptions of their pollinators is truly fascinating. One of the earliest pollinators was the beetle, which crawled into primitive flowers to eat pollen, distributing grains around the area and enabling self-pollination. More evolved species of flowers developed nectar-secreting glands to attract flying insects that would brush against the pollen and so carry it to other flowers.

Flowers with tubular shapes developed simultaneously with those insects and birds with a sucking proboscis or beak sufficiently long to reach the nectar. Some flowers, such as antirrhinums, will only open when the right size pollinator lands on its lower lip. In some flowers, patterns such as lines or spots on the petals, as seen in horse chestnut and eyebright, point the way to the nectar to a hungry insect. Scents wafting through the air will attract pollinating insects from huge distances, as will bright colours to those insects with good sight. Some flowers only emit their scents at night when their colour fades; many, including evening primrose, open only at night to attract night-flying moths.

It is clear that one of the vital roles of flowers is to ensure the continuation of their species and therefore their survival. Flowering plants make up 80 per cent of all plants on the planet, and we as human beings also depend on plants for our survival. Flowers are absolutely essential to all human life. Not only do flowers convey messages to their pollinators, but the early herbalists believed that flowering plants embodied messages regarding their healing virtues in their shape, colour, form and pattern. The delicate drooping blooms of the purple Pasque flower certainly do intimate the sad drooping head of the nymph Anemone, forsaken by her lover, Zephyr the Greek god of the West wind. This points towards the flower's famous healing powers for women feeling similarly forsaken and forlorn when taken as a homeopathic remedy.

By contrast, the bright blue, purple and yellow heart-shaped flowers of heartsease have a much more uplifting nature, with their ability to heal the heart and lift the spirits. Heartsease has been used by healers for thousands of years as a love potion and to bring comfort to those feeling hurt, rejected, lonely or broken hearted as Shakespeare well knew,

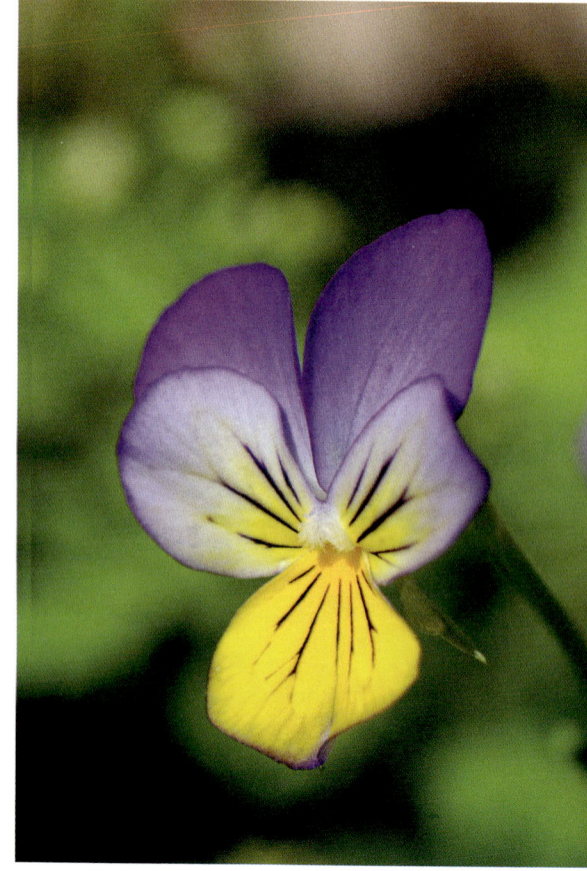

Yet mark'd I where the bolt of Cupid fell:
It fell upon a little western flower,
Before, milk-white, now purple with love's wound,
And maidens call it love-in-idleness
– Midsummers Night's Dream

The healing potential of flowering plants is an integral part of the deep bond that exists between humans and nature. That flowers have the ability to heal us, not only physically but also emotionally and spiritually, is something that has been recognised and utilised as far back as we know. Now in the 21st century with evidence of the healing role of flowers going back 60,000 years, we are still striving to understand the totality of their significance in our lives.

Flowers have been used in many different ways for healing, in a variety of herbal preparations, as essential oils, homeopathic remedies and flower essences. Each system of medicine claims a certain mode of action or vibrational level of healing for its own. One thing is clear to me from the flowers' history of healing set out in the pages to come: the essence of the flower that permeates every remedy has the same healing potential that permeates the essence of our being.

The History of Floral Healing

A brief journey through the history of the use of flowering plants in healing will help to clarify our debt to nature and the circle which this evolutionary journey is forming. It is hard to know exactly how the ancients used flowers for healing in prehistoric times before the time of writing and keeping records, but the recorded use of medicinal plants in the great civilisations including China, Egypt, Mesopotamia, Greece and India shows remarkable similarities, indicating considerable exchange of plants at this time. There was also a cross-fertilisation of ideas, as the early herbalists sought answers to questions about the workings of the human body and the mysteries of the universe.

The first herbalists of every culture are known as shamans – men or women who had a particular gift for healing, whose instincts were raised to a highly intuitive level through years of training to develop their inner eye. This deeper perception enabled them to communicate directly with the plant world and the world of the spirit, which may explain some of the personification of plants or vice versa in Greek mythology and other ancient cults. These healers were also called priest physicians, since health of the body was not separated from that of mind and spirit as it was much later in the history of medicine.

Hallucinatory and mind-altering plants were traditionally used by the priest physicians. Incense and aromatic plants were also burned at religious rituals as tools of transformation to help transport the minds of the participants to another dimension - this was perhaps the origin of modern aromatherapy. The gods on whom all human life was considered to depend, were honoured in temples with incense and aromatic plants, since the gods were deemed particularly partial to fragrant smokes. In the cult of Asclepius, priest physicians used recipes of therapeutic perfumes and incense to enhance the psychological and physical wellbeing of their patients. They used aromatic herbs such as rosemary, pine and thyme for fumigation to ward off infection and negative influences such as sorcery and evil.

We can trace the link between human life and healing herbs and flowers to Neanderthal man. In 1963 archaeologists opened a 60,00 year old grave in a cave in Iraq. The man had been buried along with many flowers. Grains of flower pollen there were analysed and found to include the distinctive pollen of cornflower, horsetail, hollyhock, St Barnaby's thistle, yarrow, grape hyacinth and ephedra. These flowers were no doubt present at the burial not only for their aesthetic value but also for their symbolic and healing virtues. Amongst these flowers there were diuretics, emetics, astringents, stimulants and pain relievers.

As long ago as 3000 BC schools of herbal medicine existed in Egypt. Imhotep was the first known physician there and he served Zoser, a 3rd dynasty pharaoh in around 2980 BC. Imhotep was renowned as an astrologer, magician and healer and was elevated in the minds of people as the god of healing. Like the Greek gods, the Egyptian gods played an important role in early Egyptian medicine. Osiris was the god of vegetation and both his twin sister Isis and his mother were ascribed the power to renew life and believed to have given their secrets of healing to mankind. The Ebers Papyrus written around 2000 BC describes symptoms and their treatments using 85 herbs including castor oil, dill, lettuce, senna, mint, gentian and poppy. Aromatic plants such as myrrh, cumin, coriander and balm of Gilead were used for fumigation. The Egyptians placed flower wreaths in the tombs of mummies and planted flower gardens near the tombs.

Meanwhile in China, the *Pen T'sao* by Shan Xiang dating from 2800 BC lists 366 plant medicines used at the time including Ephedra. In Babylon around 1800 BC, King Hammurabi recorded on stone tablets information about flowering plants used for healing, which included henbane, mint and liquorice. Merodach Baladin, King of Babylon around 720 BC, was known to have grown 70 different medicinal plants in his garden including thyme, coriander and saffron. Tablets from the library of Ashurbanipal, King of Assyria 668–626 BC, show that 250 herbs were used for healing including turmeric, myrrh, poppy, almond, sesame and cumin.

Ancient Greek and Roman Medicine

The Greek myths tell stories from long ago when the Greek gods played on Mount Olympus among the vegetation that was the green canopy of the world, creating flowers and trees to be of service to both the gods and living mortals.

Asclepius was the god of healing symbolised by the image of the serpent, which itself represents the renewal of energy and renovation. The serpent had the power to discover healing plants as it slid along the undergrowth. Asclepius was the son of Apollo the sun god and had learnt his healing arts from Chiron the centaur in his cave. Chiron was the wise teacher of other famous Greek heroes, including Jason the Argonaut and Peleus, Achilles' father; so say the myths of classical Greece – when people believed that healing was a gift of the gods who alone understood the nature of plants.

The ancient Greeks had many other delightful stories in their

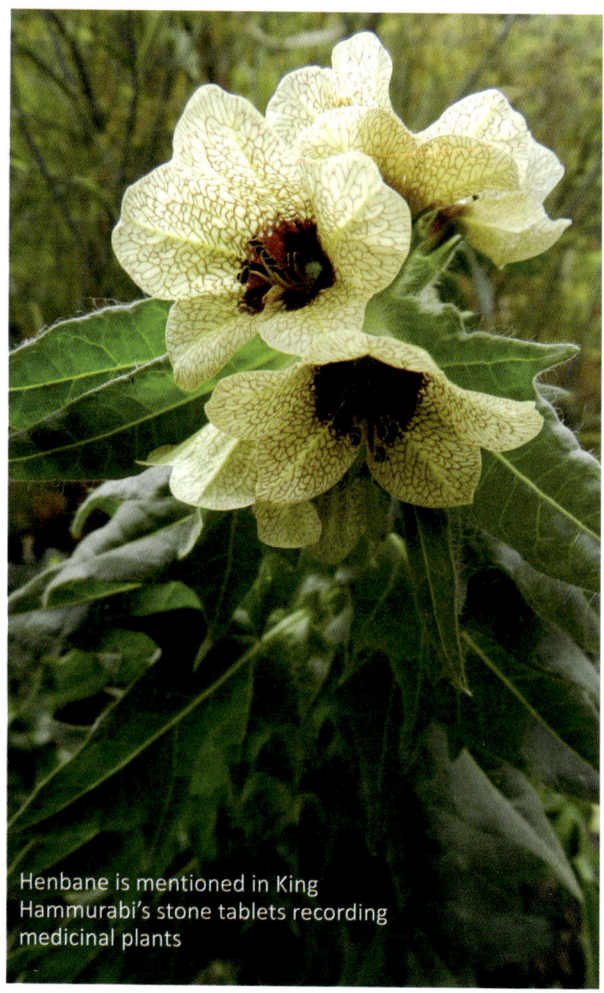

Henbane is mentioned in King Hammurabi's stone tablets recording medicinal plants

mythology which explained how their healing plants came into being and gave clear pointers to how they could be used. These undoubtedly illustrate the close relationship that has always existed between plants and human life and the great respect the ancients had for the plant world, so much so that many plants were held sacred and worshiped as attributes of the gods.

The celebrated Hippocrates (468–377BC) was the first important medical thinker that we know about and is known as the 'father of medicine' of the western tradition. In Greece, Hippocrates began to establish a scientific and yet holistic basis for medicine, relying less on magic and ritual and basing his treatments on results. He is recorded as using around 400 herbs as well as advocating the importance of fresh air, exercise and good diet. He saw that all matter could be explained by the five basic elements: ether, air, fire, water and earth. The individuality of people was explained by the four *'humours'* arising from these elements: blood, phlegm, choler and melancholy. The proportions of these humours in each person would determine his or her personality and body type.

- The element water corresponded to phlegm and a phlegmatic temperament. Phlegm had a cold and damp nature, epitomised by the season of winter, and it gave rise to illnesses such as catarrh, respiratory infections, overweight and fluid retention. Warming and drying herbs such as thyme, hyssop and ginger were used to clear cold and damp symptoms and thereby restore the balance of the humours.

- Earth corresponded to the melancholic humour or temperament, black bile and the season of autumn. It had a cold and dry nature, giving rise to symptoms such as constipation, arthritis, depression or anxiety. Warming herbs such as ginger and senna would be used to clear black bile and restore balance.

- The element air corresponded to blood and the sanguine temperament, epitomised by the season of spring. A sanguine type would be easy-going and good humoured, but prone to excesses and over-indulgence, giving rise to problems such as gout and diarrhoea. Cool, dry herbs such as burdock or figwort were used to balance the humours.

- Lastly, fire corresponded to choler or yellow bile, related to summer. A choleric type would be hot-tempered and prone to liver and digestive problems. Cooling and moistening herbs such as dandelion, violets and lettuce would help to balance the excess heat and dryness of the choleric temperament.

Hippocrates perceived that illness was not a punishment of the gods, as was believed by his forefathers, but that it arose from imbalances of the elements that composed everything in nature. His humoral theory was paralleled in both China which has a similar five-element theory, and in India's Ayurvedic medicine.

In Ayurveda, the five elements of all matter relate directly to the three basic constitutional types or *doshas*. These are *vata* (air and ether), *pitta* (water and fire) and *kapha* (earth and water). In each system the foods and herbs used in treatments would be dictated by the predominant humour, element or *dosha*, so they became subject to the same classifications.

From ancient times until about the 6th century AD, practicing medicine was a privilege reserved only for men; they practiced either privately or publicly and held positions as doctors. It is fairly clear that women were largely excluded from medicine during antiquity from the absence of writings about medicines and any mention of their existence in current literary sources. However, information has come to light about the medical education and training of certain women, which went beyond the normal field of gynaecology and obstetrics that most women were restricted to. In ancient Greece there are rare cases where women were called doctors and may have had similar professional rights as their male colleagues, as well as the same 'scientific education'. Pantheia of Pergamon was the wife of professional physician Glycon, who lived around the 2nd century AD. On her death her husband's famous tribute to her was, " *you raised high our common fame in the art of medicine, and even though a woman, you did not fall short of my skill*" - a statement clearly interwoven with reservations that were classic of the times, since this would have threatened the norms of hierarchical gender structures. Nonetheless it serves to indicate that Pantheia's practice in the medical profession was worthy of great respect.

Metrodora, a Greek physician who lived sometime between 200–400 AD, wrote *On the Diseases and Cures of Woman* which is thought to be the oldest surviving medical text written by a woman. Today, the book exists in two volumes and contains 63 chapters. In it Metrodora wrote about a wide range of medical problems including gynaecological issues but not obstetrics as was commonly found in the works of most other female physicians at that time. She was greatly influenced by the works of Hippocrates and approached her writing in a similar way to her male counterparts, placing particular emphasis on the discussion of pathology.

Another famous Greek male physician was Theophrastus (372–286BC), who was both a friend and pupil of Aristotle. Theophrastus inherited Aristotle's garden and library and wrote *Enquiry into Plants,* the first important herbal to survive until today. He listed 500 healing plants and described the properties of oils and spices, basing much of his work on Aristotle's botanical writings which expanded much of Hippocrates' work. He established himself as a scientific botanist and his work has been referred to throughout history and remains an interesting and valuable source of information. We know from him, for example, that bay-laurel was used to produce a trance-like state and that roses, coriander and myrtle were used as aphrodisiacs.

A further great source of herbal knowledge comes from the Alexandrian school, the first Christian institution of higher learning, founded in the middle of the 2nd century AD in Alexandria, Egypt. Alexandria was named in honour of the Greek Emperor, Alexander the Great. The school enabled Greek medicine to flourish – it drew on Greek knowledge as well as Egyptian, Sumerian and Assyrian healing traditions and included learning brought back from the emperor's campaigns in Asia. The strong traditions developed here survived into medieval Europe through the writers and scholars of the Arab world.

Galen (131–201 AD) was another notable Greek physician. He studied at the Alexandrian school and became renowned as surgeon to the gladiators in Rome and personal physician to Emperor Marcus Aurelius (121-180 AD). In his herbal *De Simplicíbus* he expanded on Hippocrates' philosophy and his classification of medicinal plants into the four humours.

His works became the standard medical text of Rome and later of Arab physicians and medieval monks. His theories are still clearly to be found in Unani medicine today.

Pedanius Dioscorides from Anazarb in Cilicia was a Greek physician serving with the Roman Emperor Nero's army, which allowed him to travel extensively in Asia Minor. Around 60 AD he set himself the enormous task of collating all the current knowledge on medicinal plants and healing substances in one work: *De Materia Medica*. It included discussion of the components of perfumes and their medicinal properties; aromatic herbs used for these included balm, basil, coriander, fennel, garlic, hyssop, marjoram, mint, myrtle, rosemary and violet. The famous herbal written by Dioscorides provided the major source of herbal knowledge for the next 1500 years. It has been copied and quoted in all the herbals that followed right up to the present day.

The Roman armies were responsible for the spread of herbal traditions and medicinal plants around Europe – the Madonna lily, for example, was taken from camp to camp and used as a wound herb. Garlic was similarly valued for its antiseptic and strengthening properties. The Romans also developed the use of aromatic flowers and herbs for perfumes

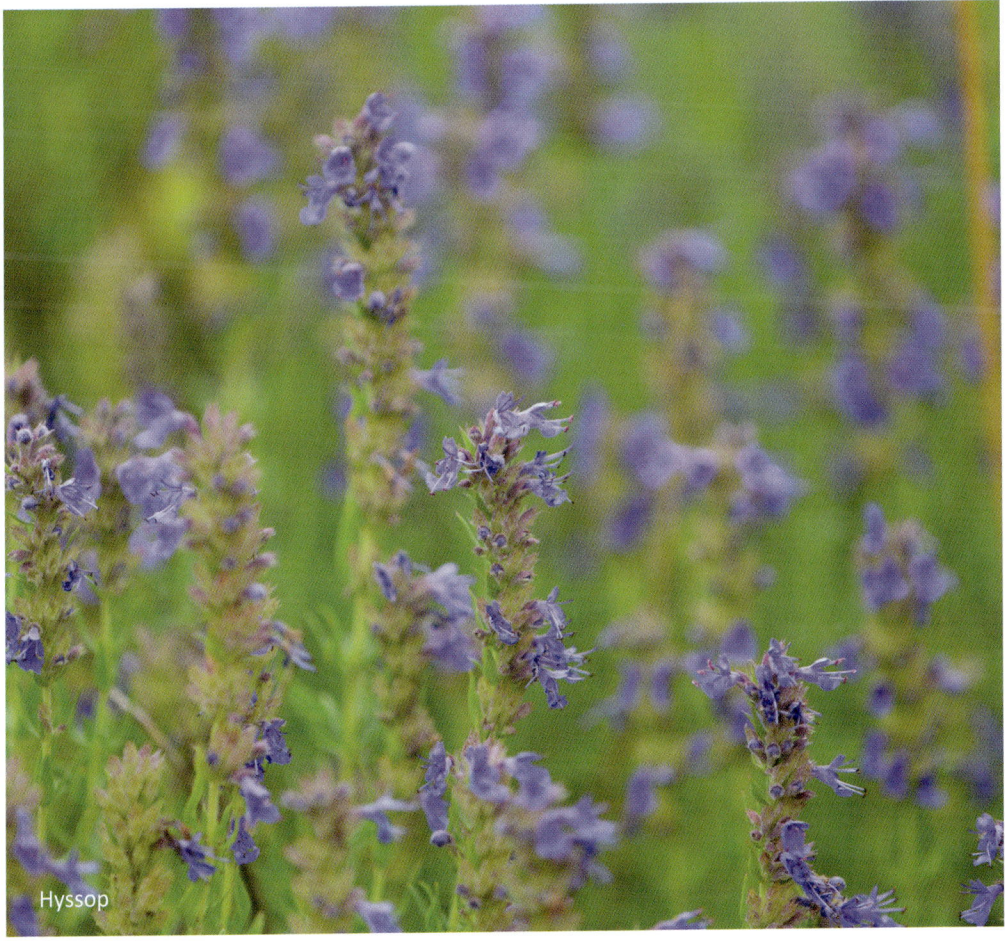

Hyssop

and fragrant oils which played a central role in their bathing rituals - almonds, quinces and roses were among their favourites. As in Greece and Egypt, such perfumes and oils were commonly used for basic hygiene, to oil the skin and hair to keep it healthy and to mask unpleasant odours when water was scarce and washing infrequent.

Pliny the Elder, also known as the 'worthy Pliny' (23–79 AD), was a Roman naturalist who collected together herbal knowledge, often unreliably, for a sort of universal encyclopaedia known as the *Naturalis Historia.* This appeared in Rome in 77AD. Under the Romans however, the attitude to medicinal plants began to change. The Catholic papacy grew more powerful and the early Christians, feeling that the church rather than the physicians should be responsible for health of mind and soul, started to repress the use of many 'pagan' herbs. In 529 AD Pope Gregory the Great ruled that learning which was not in accordance with the political ambitions of the papacy should be forbidden. Because of this during the Dark Ages (roughly 200–800 AD) knowledge of healing plants and the use of the great herbals was pushed underground and medical research and writing in Europe came to a halt.

Greek and Arab Traditions
Luckily however, the highly sophisticated Arab culture of the time maintained and developed the healing legacy of the Greeks, merging it with their ancient folk medicine and what had survived of the Egyptian tradition. By 900 AD all surviving Greek herbal and botanical texts were translated into Arabic in the cultural centres of Cairo, Damascus and Baghdad. When Arab armies invaded North Africa and Spain, they took with them their knowledge of healing plants and medicine. A succession of renowned Arab physicians including Albucasis, Razis and Avicenna were particularly responsible for the development of medicine at this time, adding their own inventions and discoveries to the sum of herbal and botanical knowledge.

Avicenna (980–1037 AD) brought together all that was available on the nature of disease, plant medicine, aromatics and medical theories in his *Canon Medicinae.* It was Avicenna who developed the process of distillation which had originated in the Alexandrian school in the 3rd century. He invented the apparatus and method of alembic distillation to extract essential oils from aromatic plants - a great landmark in the history of aromatherapy. Fragrant oils were used particularly for their purifying and restorative properties at this time and were thought to make destructive emotions such as grief and fear have less of an impact on the health of the body.

The Greek and Arabic traditions were revived in medieval Europe through two major routes. In Toledo in Spain (Christian since 1085) a body of translators established a school and translated herbal texts from Arabic to Romance (old French) and then into Latin. In Italy, Constantine 'the African' (1020–1087) became a Benedictine monk and spent many of the last years of his life translating Arabic texts into Latin. The great medical schools of the Middle Ages blossomed from this time on. The famous school at Salerno, for example, made great use of Constantine's translations. The school at Montpelier was founded by Gerald of Cremona (1114–87) who had translated Avicenna's work which was used as a standard text for the students at the school. Crusaders returning from the Middle East also brought back ancient knowledge that had been lost to Europe during the Dark Ages.

Medieval Monasteries

Throughout medieval Europe, the teachings of Hippocrates and Dioscorides in particular were kept safe and alive in Christian monasteries. Monks copied and recopied manuscripts in many languages, translating them from other languages including Arabic and exchanging their works with other monasteries and countries. However, throughout the medieval period observation and empirical knowledge and techniques were very limited. As in the days of the early Greeks, healing involved as much prayer as medicine, which was often administered with incantations and supplications.

Outside the monasteries, Anglo-Saxon healers such as the renowned physicians of Myddfai in Wales, were still using herbs in traditional ways and some manuscripts from those times have survived, the best known being the *Leech Book of Bald*. This was compiled around 950 by a scribe named Cild under the direction of Bald, who apparently was a friend of King Alfred, and it was one of the few texts not to be based on the Greek herbals. Flowering herbs such as vervain, plantain, lungwort, wood betony and yarrow were popular in Anglo-Saxon times to remedy physical illnesses and to ward off the evil eye.

The *perfumes of Arabia* as essential oils were known, were popular both for their aesthetic pleasure and to use in fragrant rubs for aches and pains and for fumigation to protect against disease, particularly the plague. Pomanders, scent boxes and *tussie mussies* (herb posies) were carried for this purpose. Fragrant herbs were strewn in halls of dwellings and castles, wherein, it must be remembered, as many animals as people lived.

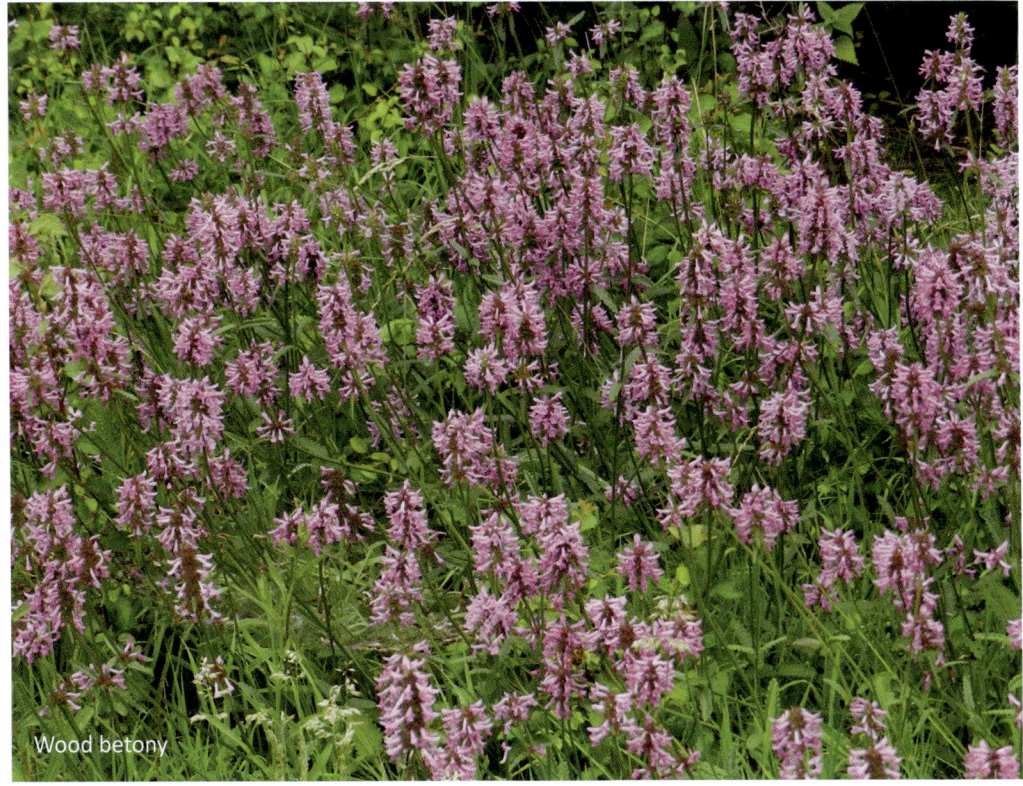
Wood betony

Herb and flower gardens came into their own in the grounds of European abbeys and monasteries in the Middle Ages. Particularly memorable is the beautiful poem written by a monk called Walafrid Strabo around 840. He was tutor to Charles, the son of Charlemagne's successor Louis the Pious and later Bishop of Richenau (the home of another famous medical school). His poem *Hortulus* meaning 'the little garden', tells of the changing seasons and serenity of the monastery garden and its herbs and flowers, *"Who can describe the exceeding whiteness of the lily? The rose, it should be crowned with pearls of Arabia and Lydian gold. Better and sweeter are these flowers than all other plants and rightly called the flower of flowers."*

Hildegard von Bingen, a 12th century German Benedictine nun and then abbess, is still to this day one of the most renowned women in herbal history. As well as being a saint, a composer, a scholar, a philosopher, a scientist and a mystic, Hildegard spent much of her life doing ground-breaking work in natural medicine. She took a great interest in reading the works of great herbalists who came before her. She tended the herb garden

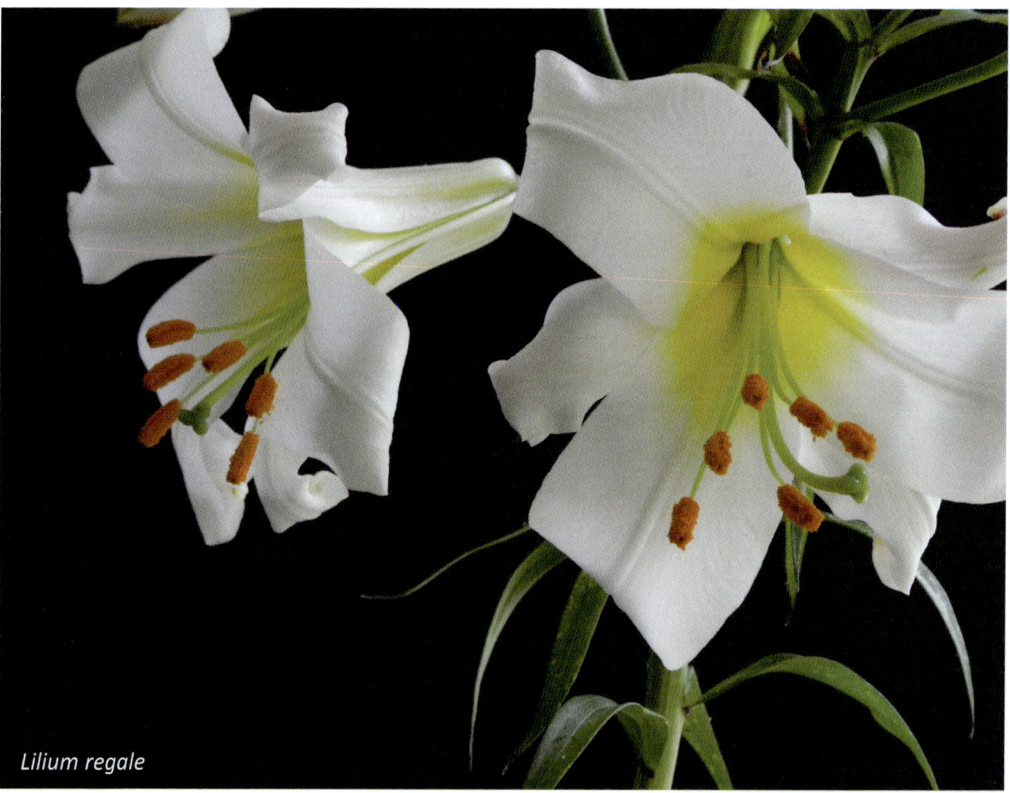
Lilium regale

of the monastery and gained experience in the practical applications of medicinal plants and preparations made from them through helping in and then leading the infirmary. In this way she became known for her healing powers. Bringing together her knowledge and love of spirituality, science and nature, Hildegard coined the term 'viriditas' which roughly translates 'vital green energy' meaning the divine healing power of nature that can be transferred from plant to human. Her revolutionary ideas paved the way for what became traditional European herbal medicine, and many of these can still be found in her renowned herbal texts *Liber Simplicis Medicine*, *Causae et Curae* and *Physica*.

With the dawning of the Renaissance, the Golden Age of Herbals began originally with translations and adaptations of former great works, culminating in beautiful herbals adorned with botanical drawings. An increasing number of exotic herbs and spices were arriving from the East and the Americas. The arrival of William Caxton's printing press further revolutionised and spread the thinking of the time and increased the number of herbals available. Many new herbals were compiled, reflecting the theories not only of Hippocrates and Galen, but also of Paracelsus. These included theories of planetary influence, current magic and superstition and the doctrine of signatures.

The Doctrine of Signatures

The Doctrine of Signatures was first elucidated by a German called Theophrastus Bombastus von Hohenheim who was born in 1493 and better known by his alchemical name, Paracelsus. The theory probably originated much before this as is indicated in early literature. It was based on the premise that the Creator had provided guidance for humans looking for remedies for their ills by imprinting on herbs certain outward signs.

The spotted leaves of lungwort, resembling the lungs, was therefore indicated for pulmonary ailments; walnuts looked like the head and the brain and were considered good for enhancing mental activity; hepatica with leaves resembling the three lobes of the liver acquired a wide reputation for curing liver problems. Pilewort or lesser celandine has root tubers looking rather like haemorrhoids and was used to treat them; flowers with milky juice were considered to promote copious supply of breast milk in feeding mothers and plants containing red juice were used to purify the blood. The leaves of beetroot with their branching red veins signified a cure for the heart and circulation. Plants with yellow juice resembling bile were used to treat complaints of the liver.

In the late Middle Ages and early Renaissance, herbalists searching for meaning and unifying threads between nature and humans delighted in reading great significance into such resemblances. Paracelsus, despite his obscure way of writing, developed a large following. If any herb valued for its medicinal virtues was not imprinted with a clear sign from God, it would be considered the will of God intent on testing the skill of the herbalist in matching the plant to the complaint!

Some of these apparently quaint ideas actually contained more than a grain of truth and have remained applicable to the present day. Many herbs with yellow juice, such as greater celandine and dock, make valuable remedies for the liver and gallbladder. St John's wort, with little oil glands on the leaves that resemble tiny perforations and signify its use for cuts and wounds, is in fact a wonderful remedy for healing the skin and stopping bleeding.

In the 16th and 17th centuries, several herbalists supported the Doctrine of Signatures, notably William Cole who was born in 1626 in Oxfordshire and educated at New College, Oxford. He took up the study of botany and became the most celebrated herbalist of his day. His books, *The Art of Simpling* and particularly *Adam in Eden or Nature's Paradise*, indicate his independent character and originality and his repudiation of beliefs in any planetary influence. Another renowned work was that of Mattiolus, *Commentaries on the six books of Dioscorides* in 1565. Mattiolus was a flamboyant Italian scholar and physician who attended several European courts.

The classic century of herbals was really established with William Turner's A *New Herball* in 1551 and included the works of John Gerard, a barber-surgeon, John Parkinson and Nicolas Culpeper. Turner was the first Englishman to study and classify plants scientifically and, like Theophrastus centuries before, he was known as *'the father of botany'*. He is memorable for having written in English so that his work was available to the apothecaries and women of the household who gathered herbs for the still room, and not simply the physicians who were educated in Latin.

More popular however, is John Gerard's *The Herball* printed in 1597. Although much of his knowledge and writing derived from the Dutch physician to Maximilian II and Rudolf II, Rembert Dodoens (1517–1585), it is a large repository of knowledge of the time and is quoted time and again in herbals of the 20th century. Gerard loved herbs and flowers and apparently grew 1000 varieties in his riverside garden in Holborn, London.

John Parkinson was also a great enthusiast and produced a vast and lovingly illustrated 'flower book' called *Paradisi in sole Paradisus Terrestris* in 1629. The title is a pun on his own name: 'Park-in-sun's Earthly Paradise'. He had his own garden at Long Acre and was the first appointed royal herbalist in England and later wrote a less flowery book, an extensive herbal called *Theatrum Botanicum* (1640) which described 3800 plants.

Nicolas Culpeper, born in 1616, the famous and controversial apothecary and herbalist, based much of his herbal treatment and classification of medicinal plants on the laws of astrology. This was nothing new – since the time of Hippocrates physicians had studied astronomy and the influence of the stars. He was a colourful and revolutionary character, full of scorn for the money-grabbing tendencies of many contemporary doctors. He was daring enough to translate the Latin pharmacopeia into English and provide free treatment for the poor. Even in his own time, Culpeper was severely criticised by more orthodox writers such as Cole, but it will gratify many that Culpeper's *Herbal* has run and run since the 17th century and still appears in bookstores to this day.

Not forgetting the women of the time, Elizabeth Grey, Countess of Kent, was a medical and culinary recipe collector who lived between the late 1500s and early 1600s. Following her death, a collection of her most practiced recipes was published in *A Choice Manual, or, Rare Secrets in Physick and Chirurgery* which became hugely popular at the time. Her book was revised and republished about twenty-two times throughout the 17th century. Though presented as a single work, the collection was divided into two parts – the first with medical recipes while the second contained culinary recipes.

The Dawning of the Scientific Age
After this period of medical history things began to change. Paracelsus was one of those responsible for sowing the seeds of this transformation. He publicly burned the books of Hippocrates and Galen, rejecting their ideas of humoral medicine and planetary influence.

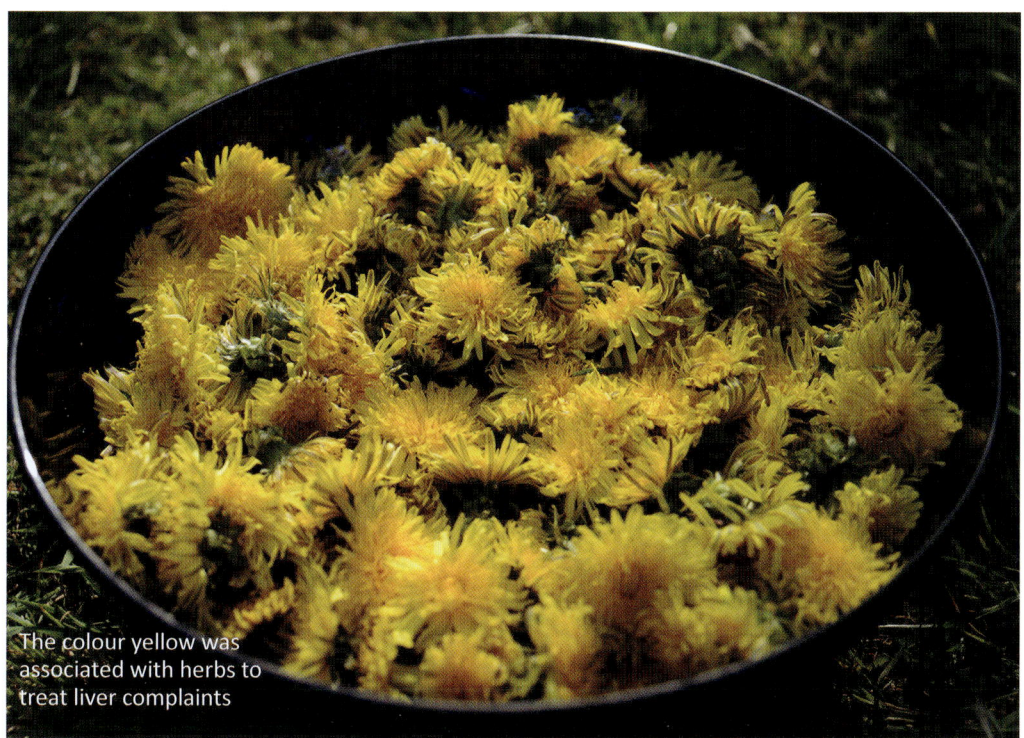
The colour yellow was associated with herbs to treat liver complaints

He preferred to use individual preparations, including small doses of metals, to treat specific diseases. Paracelsus then propounded the 'like curing like' method of healing, proposing that a poison that caused a disease could, in minute doses, become its cure. Together with Hippocrates many centuries earlier, who had also written about healing by 'similars' as well as by 'contraries', he founded the basis of homeopathy which was to be developed 200 years later by Hahnemann.

Paracelsus' vast pharmacopeia included almost every animal, vegetable and mineral medicine known at the time. Unfortunately, physicians following in his footsteps used metals and other substances in far larger doses than he ever advised, and medicines were sometimes more dangerous than the diseases for which they were prescribed. Paracelsus had also advocated that the active ingredients should be extracted from plant medicines and used in isolation, giving a much more potent medicine while, he purported, remaining as safe as in its whole form. In this way, the holistic approach to treatment of disease began to disintegrate. It was the start of allopathic medicine, which focussed on treating the disease rather than the patient, using powerful medicines that brought with them an array of side-effects. This approach was supported by great discoveries in the plant world. Peruvian bark (*Cinchona*) was found to be an excellent cure for malaria and sarsaparilla (*Smilax ornata*) a specific for syphilis.

At the same time, the ideas of Rene Descartes (1596-1650) with his division of mind and body, nature and ideas, were taking hold and the dawn of the scientific age was bringing to light all kinds of exciting advances in medicine, botany and chemistry. For example, in 1628 William Harvey discovered the way the blood circulated around the body and the old idea of 'humours' became obsolete. The body was beginning to be seen more as a machine and disease as a breakdown in its mechanics. The sciences of anatomy and physiology, as separate disciplines from psychology and religion, were fast developing.

Homeopathy

Against this backdrop emerged a doctor who was sorely disillusioned by the limits of the orthodox medical approach and by the cruel and often unsuccessful treatments of his day. These treatments included bloodletting, purging and the use of poisonous drugs with terrible side-effects. His name was Samuel Hahnemann and he was born in Saxony in 1755. He abandoned his practice, preferring to spend his time studying, writing and translating to support him during his research.

While translating Dr William Cullen's *A Treatise on Materia Medica*, Hahnemann felt sceptical of Cullen's explanation of the effectiveness of Peruvian bark for treating malaria and decided to test small amounts on himself. His experiments revealed that it produced the same symptoms in a healthy person as it was used to cure. This discovery was the instigator of the development of homeopathic medicine. Further experimentation proved that other substances produced the same symptoms in a healthy person that they were able to cure when used therapeutically.

The system of healing that grew up as a result of this was named 'homoeopathy', from the Greek word 'homoios' meaning 'similar' and 'pathos' meaning 'suffering' or 'disease', to differentiate it from orthodox medicine known as 'allopathy' meaning 'opposite

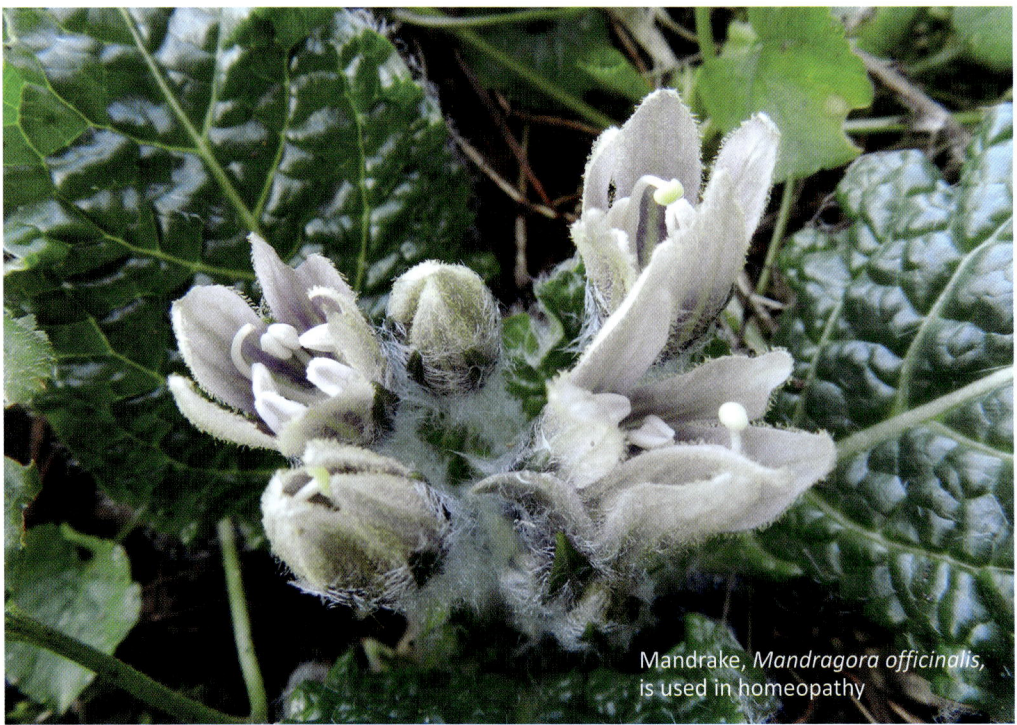

Mandrake, *Mandragora officinalis*, is used in homeopathy

suffering'. Up to this time any symptom, such as constipation, would have been treated with an opposite medicine or antidote, a laxative. During the next six years Hahnemann carried out more 'provings' of a whole range of substances and eventually set up his medical practice again, armed with this new knowledge.

To prescribe the right remedy, Hahnemann needed to take an accurate case history and establish a 'symptom picture' which he could use to match the symptoms caused by one of the remedies in his dispensary. In this way he could match the symptoms to the treatment, and despite the disbelief he witnessed from his contemporaries, he began to achieve remarkable results. He also incurred the wrath of his local pharmacists, not only by prescribing only one remedy at a time, but also in smaller and smaller doses to minimise the risk of side-effects.

Hahnemann found that when diluting the strength of his remedies, if he shook the remedy in between each dilution (this process is known as *'succussion'*) it had the effect of potentising the infinitesimal amounts of the remedy prescribed. Even more interesting, the more the remedy was diluted and *'succussed'* the more powerful and effective it became. He believed this was because the shaking released the energy of the healing substance and so made it more active. Remedies were numbered according to the number of times they were diluted, so one diluted six times would be called 6c and one diluted thirty times would be 30c.

In 1810, Hahnemann published *The Organon of Rational Medicine* which clearly described his homeopathic system, and between 1811 and 1821 he published six volumes of *Materia Medica Pura* containing his proving of 66 remedies. In 1828, he published *Chronic Diseases and their Homeopathic Cure* containing more of his provings, his use of remedies up to the 30th dilution and his theory of 'miasms' to explain why some patients failed to respond to their indicated remedies. From his experience he saw that a history of diseases such as syphilis, gonorrhoea or tuberculosis were linked to certain conditions and that specific homeopathic remedies could remove these, often inherited, blocks to health which he called 'miasms'.

After Hahnemann's death in 1843, homeopathy continued to survive and flourish both in Europe and North America, developed by many notable homeopaths who followed in his footsteps. Constantine Hering (1800-80) continued to prove remedies and to take further Hahnemann's theories, such as that of miasms. James Kent (1849-1916) was an American who advocated the use of much higher potencies and published his famous *Repertory*, his *Philosophy* and *Materia Medica*. He further developed Hahnemann's and Hering's symptom pictures into 'constitutional types', describing more fully the emotional and mental tendencies of each type. In 1844, a Dr Frederick Quin with a highly successful homeopathic practice established the British Homoeopathic Society (later to become the Faculty of Homeopathy) and founded the London Homoeopathic Hospital in 1849.

Towards the end of the 19th century, however, allopathic medicine was going from strength to strength. The existence of microbes had been established, and the dangerous drugs detested by the herbalists and homeopaths alike were being replaced by powerful new ones with less apparent side-effects. Gradually, with the emergence of pharmacology and biochemistry, the value of homeopathy and plant remedies diminished in the public and scientific mind. Herbal remedies began to be lumped together with old wives' tales and homeopathy was considered too unscientific, while scientists developed the means to isolate and then synthesise constituents of certain plants. The famous heart medicine digitalis (foxglove) later yielded digoxin, the poppy produced morphine (1803), the wild yam provided steroids and willow bark provided the chemical base for aspirin.

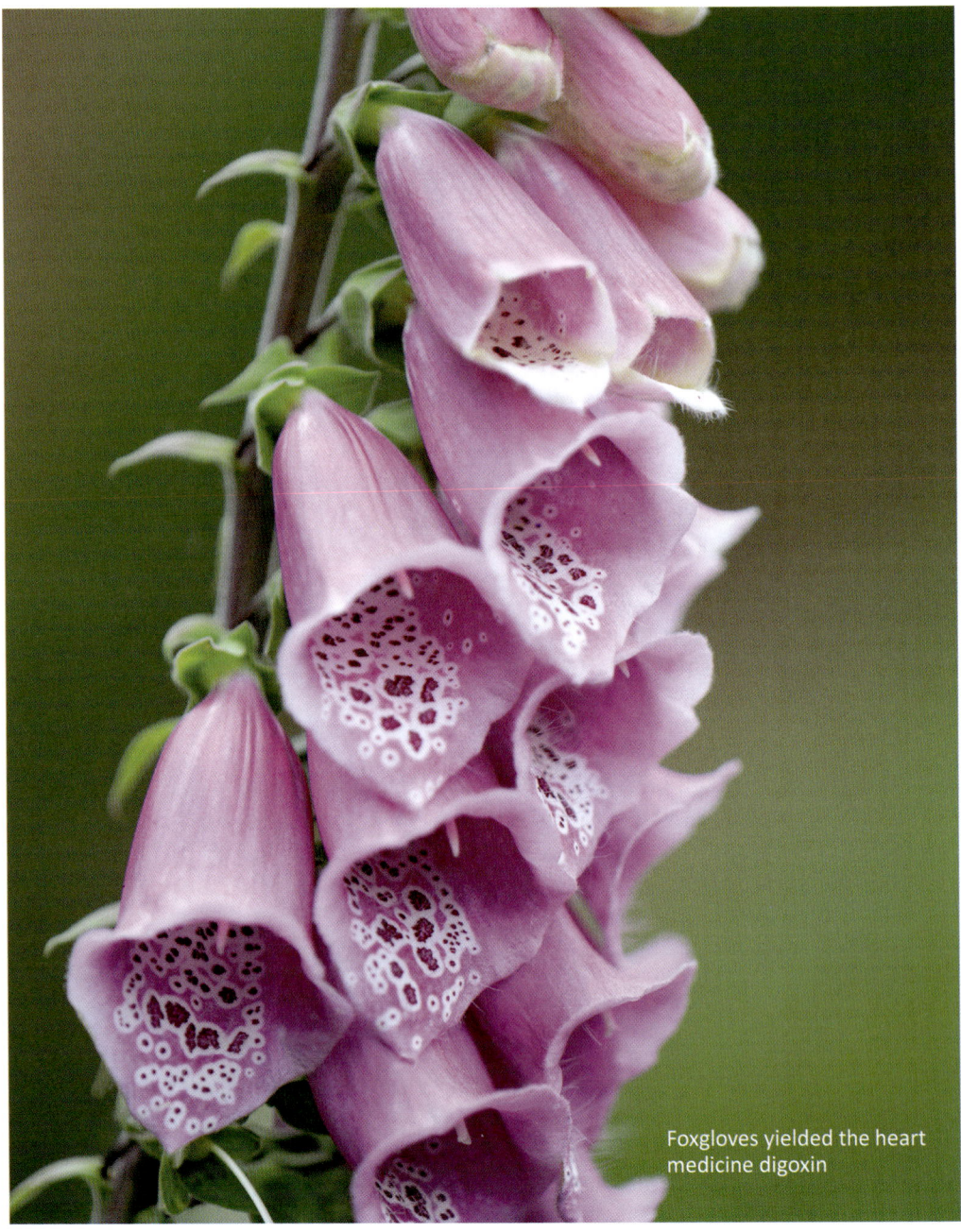

Foxgloves yielded the heart medicine digoxin

The Healing Tradition in America

A handful of traditional herbalists remained, maintaining their holistic outlook and basing their treatments on the person rather than the disease and the use of whole plant medicines as opposed to the more potent isolated or synthetically made chemical compounds with their accompanying risk of side-effects.

In the mid-19th century, the National Association of Medical Herbalists (now the National Institute of Medical Herbalists) was set up in the UK to represent the small body of professional herbalists. This was inspired by a similar small body of herbalists in North America known as Physiomedicalists who blended together the traditions of European herbalism brought to America by the Pilgrim Fathers with the herbal wisdom of the people then called the North American Indians.

Native American medicine, like South American plant medicine, was a shamanic tradition. Ritualistic dances, playing of drums and rattles and mind-altering plants such as peyote and datura were used to enable the shaman or medicine man or woman to enter a trance-like visionary state. This enabled communication with the plant world and the soul of the ill person to bring about healing. Plants were revered not only for their ability to cure

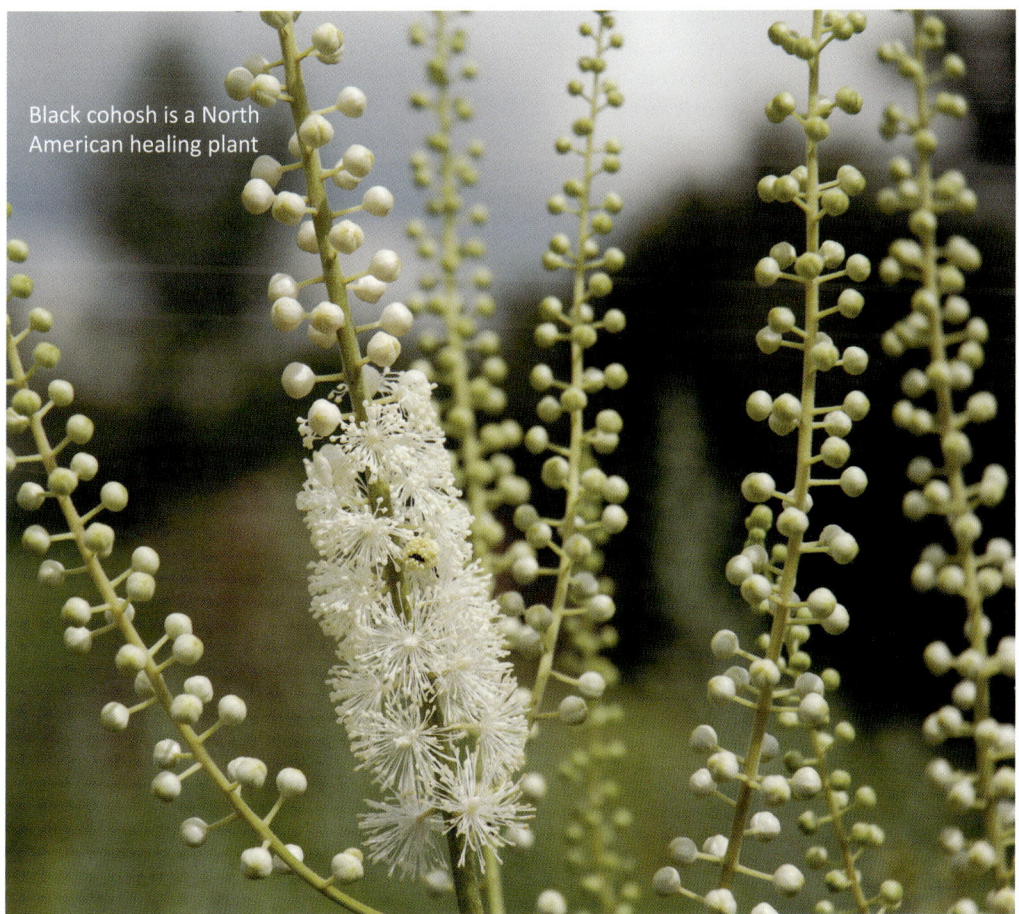

Black cohosh is a North American healing plant

diseases of the body, but also imbalances in the mind, emotions and spirit. They were an inextricable part of native religion and mythology and used in ceremonies and rituals. Disease was seen to be caused by either human, supernatural or natural causes and the medicine man or woman was called upon to administer medicinal plants for anything from wounds and broken bones to unfulfilled dreams, spiritual intrusion and soul loss.

Everything that the native North American healer did was in a circle, and according to Black Elk of the Teton Dakota, the 'Power of the World' always worked in circles. "*All our power came to us from the sacred loop of the nation*" he said, and his people flourished as long as the circle was unbroken. "*The flowering circle of the four quarters nourished it. The east gave peace and light, the south gave warmth, the west gave rain and the north with its cold and mighty wind gave strength and endurance.*"

The renowned physiomedicalist Dr Samuel Thomson (1769-1843), was the first to bring the Indian remedy lobelia to the attention of the medical world. He kept alive traditional ideas such as that of allowing the body to heal itself and helping to create the ideal conditions for this with the use of medicinal plants. He mixed these traditions with knowledge he had gained by observation of the North American native medicine men, such as the value of sweating for clearing toxins from the body. Thomson, like ancient as well as modern herbalists, recognised the presence of 'the vital force', the energy which flows throughout nature and animates all in existence. The same energy described as the 'spirit' in plants by the ancient Greeks and American cultures, the *qi* of China's medicine and philosophy, and *prana* of Ayurveda, is our innate healing ability that manifests itself daily in the amazing feats of the body. The cough to clear the airways of phlegm, the sneeze to shift irritants from the nose, vomiting to clear the stomach of infection, diarrhoea to remove toxins from the bowel, are all examples. This self-healing mechanism is known as 'homoeostasis'.

Thomson also held that all bodies were composed of the four elements: earth, air, fire and water, and that health derived from their harmonious interplay. Healing plants were used primarily to maintain or correct this balance and prescriptions were designed to do one of four things: astringe (tone) or relax, stimulate or sedate. Toning plants include shepherd's purse, agrimony and beth root, relaxing herbs include cramp bark and lemon balm. Ginger and cayenne are stimulating while chamomile and yellow jasmine are sedating.

Thomson's model led to the founding of Physiomedicalism by physicians such as Dr Curtis and Dr Cook. It was followed in America by other botanic schools, notably the Eclectics founded by Dr Wooster Beech in the 1830s. The Eclectics were the dominant group in both numbers and their legacy today. Beech also used native American traditions mixed with European knowledge as well as orthodox practices. Physiomedicalism was brought to England in 1838 by Dr Albert Coffin, and Wooster Beech arrived in the 1850s to bring Eclectic medicine to Europe.

Flower Healing in Modern Times
Despite the enormous advances in modern scientific medicine, the emergence of powerful drugs and the miracles of microsurgery, there is something that still draws many of us to these more ancient and holistic systems of medicine. Herbal medicine is again enjoying enormously popular benefit from the marriage of ancient wisdom and

modern scientific development and discovery. The latter have served not to bring herbal medicine into disrepute after all, but rather to prove, through pharmacological analysis of the constituents involved, a scientific explanation of their ability to heal.

So much has herbal medicine earned respect and recognition, that several degree courses in the subject was established in British universities during the 1990's and this was followed in the USA. With the enormous interchange of cultural ideas possible nowadays, the old systems of the East, whose ancient medical traditions have never been broken as they have here in the West, are beginning to become more integrated into modern healing methods.

Ayurvedic Medicine

The name Ayurveda derives from two Indian words, 'ayur' meaning 'life' and 'veda' meaning 'knowledge' or 'science'. Ayurveda is the knowledge or science of life; more than a system of healing, it is a way of life, encompassing science, religion and philosophy, and intended to enhance wellbeing and enable the achievement of longevity and eventually self-realisation. It is said that Ayurveda evolved in India over 5000 years ago from the deep understanding of creation by spiritually enlightened beings known as 'rishis' in the far reaches of the Himalayas. It has survived largely as an oral tradition until the present day, one of its greatest values being its timelessness and its application to every facet of daily living, now as it was all those centuries ago.

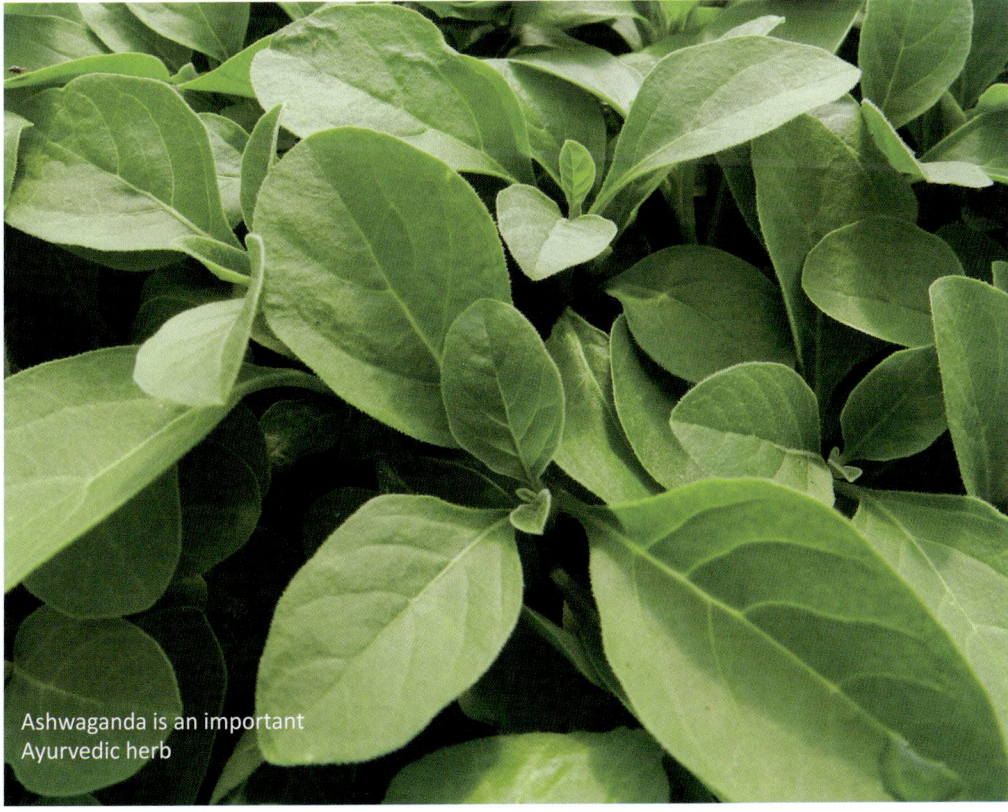

Ashwaganda is an important Ayurvedic herb

According to Ayurveda, the origin of all aspects of existence is the field of pure intellect or consciousness. This appeals to those influenced by the theories of modem quantum physics which locate the basis of the physical universe in a single unified field that directs and orchestrates the continuous flow of matter. Energy and matter are one. Ayurveda does not separate the external world from the inner world. Everything that exists in the macrocosm has its counterpart in the microcosm of the inner universe of a human being. Cosmic energy manifests in the five elements that are the basis of all matter: ether, air, fire, water and earth.

- In the body ether is present in the spaces such as the mouth, the abdomen, the thorax, the capillaries and cells.
- Movement of space is air, manifest in movements of, for example, muscles, the pulsation of the heart, peristalsis of the digestive tract and nervous impulses.
- Fire is present in the digestive system, governing enzyme systems and metabolism, as well as body temperature, vision and the light of the mind, intelligence.
- Water is present in secretions like the digestive juices, saliva, mucous membranes, plasma and cytoplasm.
- Earth is responsible for the solid structures holding the body together, bones, cartilage, muscles and tendons and skin.

The five elements manifest also in the functioning of the five senses: hearing, touch, vision, taste and smell, so they are closely related to our ability to perceive and interact with our environment. From the five elements derive three basic forces called the *tridoshas*, that exist in everything and influence all mental and physical processes. From ether and air, *vata*, the air principle is created, from fire and water comes *pitta*, the fire principle, and from earth and water derives the water principle, *kapha*.

The balance of the *doshas* in each person will promote health and wellbeing, while imbalance leads to ill-health and disease. We are all born with a certain balance of *doshas* bought about mainly by the *dosha* balance in our parents at the time of conception. This is our basic constitution (our *prakruti*) that remains unchanged throughout our lives. The dominant *dosha* determines our body type, temperament and those illnesses to which we may be susceptible. Our *vikruti*, which is our present *dosha* balance, reflects the effect that lifestyle has had on our *prakruti* to cause further imbalances that predispose to ill-health.

Both *prakruti* and *vikruti* can be ascertained by careful diagnosis which includes taking a detailed case history, observation of the body, tongue and pulse diagnosis. Once a person's *dosha* balance has been correctly diagnosed, then the correct treatment and lifestyle advice may be given. Initial treatment consists usually of cleansing methods to eliminate toxins that have contributed to imbalance. Then medicines from plant or mineral sources will be prescribed and diet and lifestyle advised, which is appropriate to the individual and their *dosha* balance.

Chinese Medicine

Traditional Chinese medicine is an equally ancient system of healing that can be traced back to around 2500 BC. As in Ayurveda, the early texts such as the *Yellow Emperor's Canon of Internal Medicine* dated around 1000 BC are still studied, and their precepts adhered to

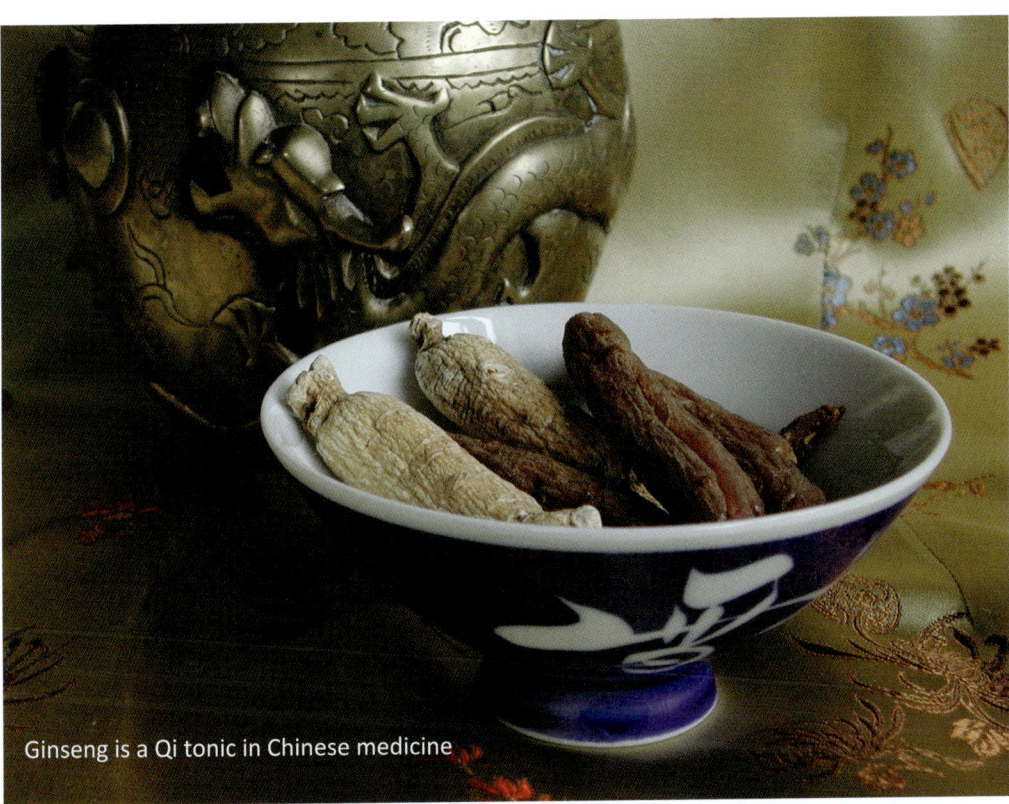
Ginseng is a Qi tonic in Chinese medicine

by modern practitioners. The Chinese, like the Indians, regard the human body and all its functions as a microcosm of the macrocosm. All forms of life are seen to be animated by the same essential life force called 'qi'. By breathing we take in 'qi' from the air and pass it into the lungs, and by digesting we extract 'qi' from food and drink and pass it into the body. When these 'qis' meet in the bloodstream, they become what is known as 'Human Qi' which circulates around the body as vital energy. The quality, quantity and balance of 'qi' in each person influences their state of health and lifespan and this in turn is affected by factors such as the season, climate, lifestyle, diet and air breathed. 'Qi' flows in a network of channels or meridians throughout the body and can be stimulated and balanced using acupuncture, acupressure, diet and herbal medicine.

The principles of Chinese medicine originated in traditional Taoist philosophy, China's most ancient school of thought. Central to this philosophy is the idea of fluctuation and mutability, explaining natural phenomena in terms of the constant ebb and flow of cosmic forces. 'Yin' and 'yang', the two primordial cosmic forces, are concepts that are familiar to many. 'Yin' symbolises passive yielding force that is cold, dark, negative, contractive and female, and represented by water. 'Yang' is active, positive, hot, light, expansive and male, and symbolised by fire. The constant interplay between these opposite and mutually dependent forces produces all the change and movement in the universe. Different parts of the body are described as being predominantly 'yin' or 'yang'. 'Yin' is found in the internal, lower and front part of the body, in the body fluids and blood, and governs

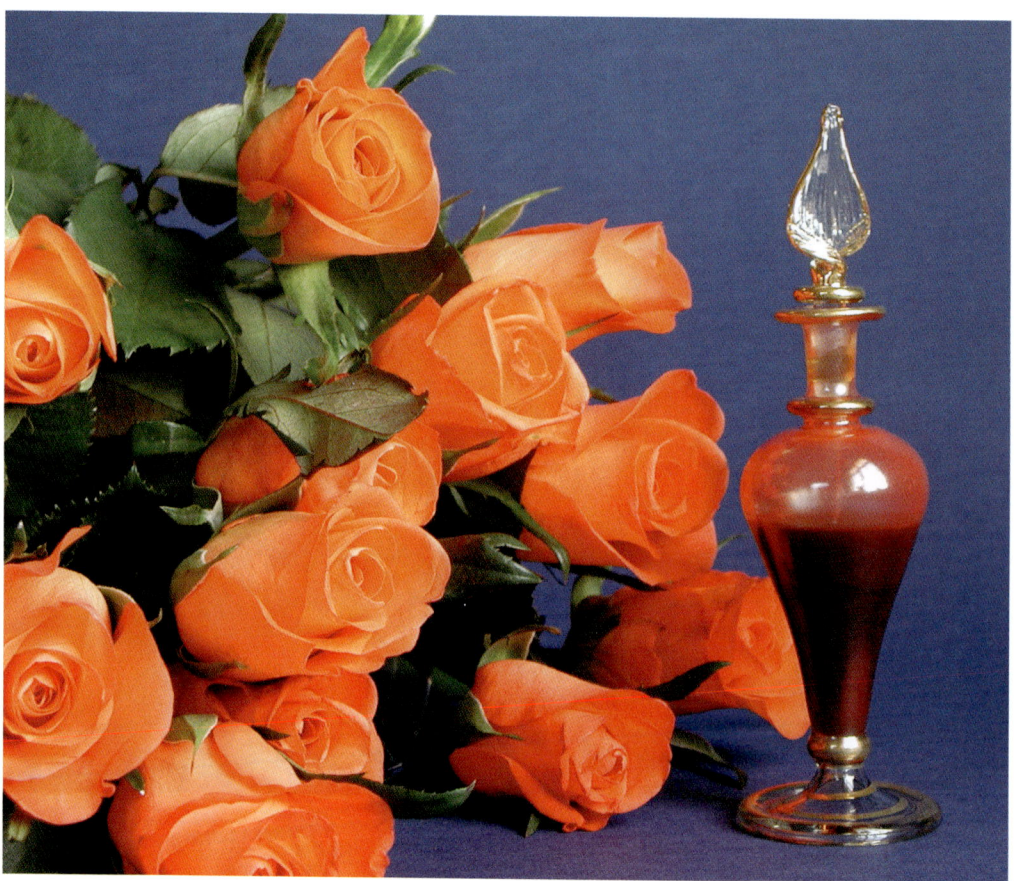

innate instincts. 'Yang' governs 'qi', vital energy and learned skills, and presides in the upper, external and back parts of the body. To maintain health, 'yin' and 'yang' need to be in balance.

As in Ayurveda, the theory of five elements is vital to the Chinese understanding of life in all its variety. Wood, fire, earth, metal and water are the elements that compose and relate to all aspects of life, including parts of the body, vital organs, emotions, seasons, colours and tastes. To illustrate, wood relates to spring, the colour green, the liver and gallbladder, anger and the sour taste. Fire corresponds to summer, the heart and small intestine, joy and the bitter taste. The constant interplay of the five elements along with that of '*yin*' and '*yang*' sparks off all change and activity in nature. The fundamental relationships among the five elements are the key to understanding how our bodies and the environment interact and influence each other. To maintain good health, the elements need to be in harmony – if one element becomes over-dominant, imbalance and illness can result.

Using diet, medicinal plants and acupuncture, it is possible to manipulate these natural relationships to adjust energy imbalances caused by excess or deficiency of these forces in the body. Before this is possible, a clear diagnosis needs to be made which involves reading of the basic indicators of health and disease such as the complexion, lustre of the eyes and hair, colour and texture of the tongue and its coating and the pulse. Neither diagnosis nor treatment remain static; the practitioner regularly reviews the situation throughout a course of treatment.

Aromatherapy

Today, amid the flurry of natural healing methods that have grown up as alternative or complementary to orthodox medicine, the use of essential oils distilled from flowers as well as herbs and trees is enormously popular. This is only natural, given that people have enjoyed the perfumes of plants as far back as we can remember. What could feel more luxurious than soaking in a warm bath breathing in the delicate fragrance of orange blossom or being massaged with that most sensuous of fragrances, rose?

Most ancient civilisations have used fragrant oils and plants; herbs, flowers and aromatic woods were burned in temples to purify the atmosphere and to please the gods. Their perfumes were believed to rise higher than the temple ceilings to the heavens where they scented the realms of paradise. In Biblical times, aromatic oils were used for anointing and as temple incense – we read of the smell of spikenard, and smoke suffused with myrrh and frankincense, camphor and cinnamon to perfume rooms. Myrrh and frankincense were obviously so highly valued that they were considered by the Magi as worthy gifts for the infant Jesus.

The ancient Egyptians used aromatic oils skilfully in their healing ointments and in the mummification process and enjoyed perfumes in courtship just as we do today. Queen Cleopatra's royal barge apparently emitted the most exotic perfumes as it sailed down the Nile to meet Mark Anthony. Cleopatra is said to have bathed several times daily with essence of rose and orange blossom. The Romans loved aromatic oils, favouring rose above all for wine making, perfumes and their famous baths. Roman emperors used to fill their swimming baths and fountains with rose water and sat on carpets of rose petals for their feasts and orgies. When the fashion for bathing died out or when water was short, aromatic oils would be applied to skin and clothes to mask more unpleasant smells – they were particularly popular in Tudor and Elizabethan times in England. In Queen Elizabeth I's reign, perfumed gloves were the height of fashion, and in fact the queen possessed her own still room for distilling oils for the making of the royal floral perfumes.

So powerful was the effect of scent with its sensual, often mind-altering properties, that when the Crusaders returned from the Holy Land laden with perfumes of the Orient, the medieval clergy were greatly alarmed and associated it with the forces of evil. Later in the 18th century, the British parliament considered applying the laws of witchcraft against women who tried to seduce any of His Majesty's subjects into marriage with the aid of scent! Certainly, the fragrances of plants have always been associated with the supernatural, used in magical or religious ceremonies to heighten perception, for divination and love potions.

Fragrant oils have long been associated with healing too. From Hippocrates onwards we know that aromatic baths, massages and inhalations have been employed to remedy all kinds of health problems. Throughout history aromatic plants have been used to combat disease during epidemics, even of the plague. Herbs such as rosemary, pine and juniper were burned, and pomanders were worn to keep contagion away.

With the development of scientific analysis of plants and their constituents, more has become known about the amazing range of biochemical constituents that make up the volatile oils producing such wonderful aromas. In the 1920s, a French chemist called Rene Gattefosse brought the healing benefits of oils to the attention of the orthodox scientific world. By this time much of the benefit to be derived from the plant world was ignored, and preference given to the synthesis of more powerful drugs in the laboratory. Gattefosse had a family perfume business, and while experimenting in his laboratory he burned his arm badly and plunged it into a vat of lavender oil. The result was, to his great delight, that the arm healed quickly with no scarring.

Gattefosse was thereby inspired to devote much time researching essential oils and their medical application, particularly in relation to their benefit on the skin. In 1937 he published a book entitled *Aromatherapy* - the name he coined for describing the healing benefits of essential oils, used to this day. Gattefosse's research papers were read by a French army doctor, Jean Valnet, who was so interested in the subject he began his own clinical research. He used oils on soldiers as antiseptics and wound healers and was greatly impressed by their efficacy. He then began to experiment with treating the emotional or psychological problems of war veterans, and to write extensively about aromatherapy. Valnet's *Practice of Aromatherapy*, published in 1964, is a standard text now for all professional aromatherapists.

The practice of aromatherapy as it exists today, using essential oils with massage for health and wellbeing, was popularised by an Austrian biochemist, Marguerite Maury, who was married to a homeopath. Dr Maury was particularly interested in the healing and rejuvenating properties of essential oils and carried out an extensive research programme on the effectiveness of oils when absorbed through the skin. She went on to write about essential oils and published *La Capital Jeunesse* in 1961 which has been reprinted and translated into English as *The Secret of Life and Youth*. Dr Maury opened several clinics for aromatherapy as have many practitioners since, offering massage using essential oils to treat a wide range of physical problems. At the same time, she viewed the use of oils in a holistic way, using them to address many underlying emotional and mental imbalances. Massage gives the benefit of the comfort of touch, which is of great therapeutic value, as well as the great versatility of the effects of the essential oils.

Flower Remedies and Essences

Homeopathy regained much of its popularity with ups and downs, throughout Europe, North and South America, Australia and New Zealand and over much of Asia. Meanwhile, further developments in the realm of 'vibrational' medicine have taken place, that is in healing methods which act on a subtle or vibrational level as opposed to the purely physiological level perceived by orthodox medicine. The story of flower remedies really begins with Dr Bach.

Dr Edward Bach (1886–1936) had a deep compassion for all living things, particularly those suffering pain or distress. He was led to train in medicine at which he excelled

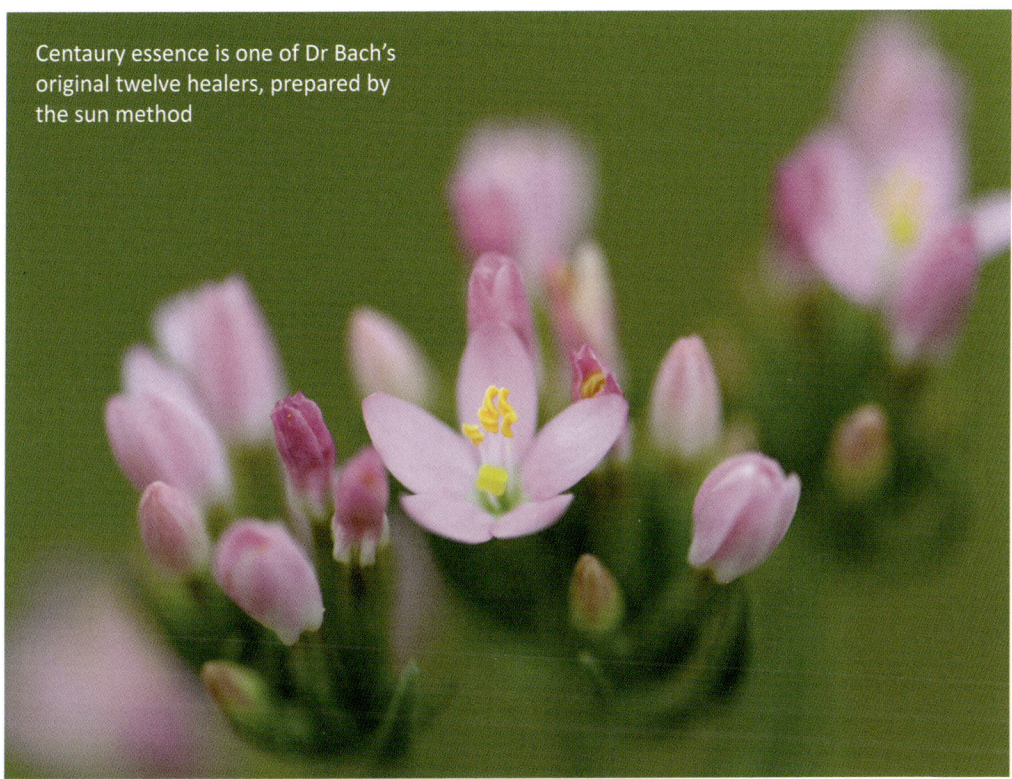

Centaury essence is one of Dr Bach's original twelve healers, prepared by the sun method

and in the first years of his practice he was a respected immunologist, pathologist and bacteriologist. Dissatisfied however with medicine's palliative rather than curative effect on illness, he was driven to continue his studies. He knew like Hippocrates, Paracelsus and Hahnemann before him that true health and wellbeing come from within and depend on harmony of body, mind, emotion and spirit. His research as a bacteriologist led to his discovery of the relationship between the bacterial population of the gut and chronic illness and the use of vaccines from these bacteria.

In 1919, working in the London Homeopathic Hospital, he discovered the work and philosophy of Dr Samuel Hahnemann which echoed much of his own approach to medicine – the treatment of the person not the disease. He began to prepare his vaccines homoeopathically and used them, now referred to as '*nosodes*', with great success but still felt that he was working in the area of physical disease and not addressing the underlying causes. His understanding was that disease resulted from inner disharmony, negative thoughts and feelings, which were frequently manifested on a physical level. He saw that stresses arising from fear, anxiety, panic, anger, intolerance and impatience put a strain on an individual, depleting their general vitality and resistance to disease.

Dr Bach had a great love of nature and intuitively understood, like so many before him, that remedies to unhappy thoughts and feelings were to be found among flowers, herbs and trees. At the height of his medical career he left to spend the rest of his life travelling in Wales and southern England in search of such remedies to restore peace of mind and happiness which he believed to be the essential nature of our being. During this time, he discovered 38 remedies which he felt provided answers to the many sufferings of people, derived (with the exception of one) from flowering trees and plants.

Among nature Dr Bach's intuition developed and his senses became more refined. The intense physical and mental disharmony he experienced led him to find the right flower in the fields or hills around him within a few days of the onset of the symptoms, for he could touch a flower with his hand or place it on his tongue and experience its healing effect on both mind and body. He also discovered that the early morning dew on plants exposed to sunlight had absorbed the properties of that plant far better than on those growing in the shade. He then devised a method of extracting the properties of the plants that anybody could employ, and which would not damage the plant.

The sun method involves placing the picked flower heads in a glass bowl to float on top of the spring water that fills it. The bowl is placed on the ground near the parent plants and exposed to sunlight for a few hours, after which time the flowers are removed carefully with a twig or leaf. The essence is then poured into bottles half full of brandy as a preservative. The alternative boiling method involves placing the plant in an enamel pan of spring water and simmering it for half an hour. Once cool the essence is filtered and preserved in equal parts of brandy.

Dr Bach said it was *"our fears, our cares, our anxieties and such like that open the path to the invasion of illness."* By using the flower remedies that he discovered, he said we could treat our cares and our worries and thereby *"not only free ourselves from our illness, but the Herbs given unto us by the Grace of the creator of all, in addition take away our fears and worries and leave us happier and better in ourselves."*

He published his discoveries in the main homeopathic journals and produced several booklets for lay people so that his remedies would be accessible to everyone. These included *Heal Thyself, Free Thyself* and the *12 Healers*.

As they gained in popularity, flower remedies soon became associated with Dr Bach in people's minds, but they had

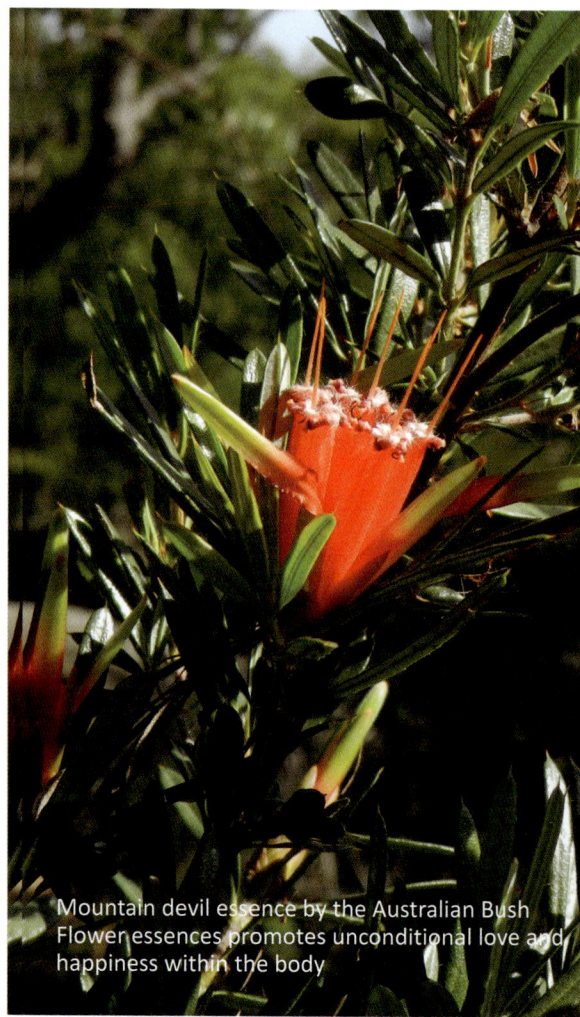

Mountain devil essence by the Australian Bush Flower essences promotes unconditional love and happiness within the body

actually been described in the 1500s by Paracelsus. He had prepared remedies from dew collected from flowers to treat his patients' emotional problems. In the early 1970s *'flower power'* were the words on many people's lips, particularly in California, and such people would refer to 'good vibrations', the wisdom of the East, the power of love and meditation. Flowers were in vogue, and not surprisingly various people in the healing and psychic world began to discover intuitively a cornucopia of new flower essences.

Within the context of mind-altering substances and popular New Age concepts, the profusion of flower remedies led to doubts about their healing abilities. Richard Katz and Patricia Kaminski were among those who were developing flower essences, having worked with the Bach Flower Remedies for many years. They were concerned that charlatans in the area would bring flower healing into disrepute. In 1979, they set up the Flower Essence Society to separate the sound from the speculative, to gather case studies from practitioners around the world, and to confirm the genuine effects of flower essences. They also ran training courses for students and seminars for practitioners.

After extensive testing of their remedies on health practitioners, the Flower Essence Society (FES) produced a range of flower essences called Quintessentials, made from organically grown flowers cultivated around the Californian Sierra Nevada. While Dr Bach's remedies reflected the spirit of his era, during the Depression, with flowers for negative emotions such as fear, anger, resentment, depression and discouragement, the Californian Flower Essences were affected by California in the 1970s. Their remedies include flowers for enhancing spiritual development, for sexual inhibitions, blocks to creativity and problems in relationships. From that time onward the world of flower essences has continued to blossom with ranges of flower essences originating from many parts of the world – New Zealand, Hawaii, Alaska, Scotland, the Himalayas, Africa, the Amazon and Australia.

The Australian Bush Flower Essences were evolved by a naturopath, Ian White, who had used the Bach remedies and wanted to explore the healing potential of flowers closer to home. As a boy he had grown up in the Australian bush and there his appreciation and respect for nature developed as he accompanied his herbalist grandmother on walks searching for medicinal herbs. As an adult, information about bush essences, a picture of the flower, where it could be found and often its name, was channelled to Ian White during meditation. Working with other practitioners who were excited by this new discovery, he set about verifying the effects of the remedies, not only by working with patients but also testing them with Kirlian photography, kinesiology and vega machines, and with other mediums. His book *Bush Flower Essences* describes 50 Australian essences and their applications; since its publication twelve more remedies have been discovered and researched.

Since then many more companies including Alaskan Flower Essences, Saskia's Flower Essences, Lotus Wei, Perelandra Essences and Healing Herbs have established themselves and spread the popularity of flower essences further.

Flower remedies are highly dilute from a physical or chemical perspective, effective not because of their chemical constituents but for the life force derived from the flower contained within the water-based fluid. Like homeopathic remedies, their presence is more subtle than physical. They address profound issues of spiritual wellbeing, emotional and mental harmony, and the healing of emotional and mental difficulties that have created blocks to spiritual development and the realisation of our full potential. They can provide catalysts for helping people to heal themselves, to understand their purpose and direction in life, and free themselves from mental or emotional suffering that may be hindering them on their path.

The Deeper Significance of Flowers

Dr Bach said that flower essences *"raise our vibrations and open up our channels for the reception of our spiritual self. They are able, like beautiful music or any gloriously uplifting thing which gives us inspiration, to raise our very natures and bring us nearer to ourselves and by that very act to bring us peace and relieve our suffering."* These words echo the words and experience of so many others who have glimpsed the deeper significance of the world of flowers. The essential nature of flowers inspires healing of every dimension in us simply by being in their presence. The world of writing and poetry offers many illustrations of this.

> *Yes! in the poor man's garden grow*
> *far more than herbs and flowers*
> *kind thoughts, contentment, peace of mind*
> *And joy for wary hours*
> – Mary Howitt (1799–1888)

> *Flowers ... have a mysterious and subtle influence*
> *upon the feelings, not unlike some strains of music.*
> *They relax the tenseness of the mind*
> – Henry Ward Beecher (1813–1887)

> *O, see a world in a grain of sand,*
> *and heaven in a wildflower*
> – William Blake (1757–1827)

> *The kiss of the sun for pardon,*
> *The song of the birds for mirth,*
> *One is nearer God's Heart in the garden*
> *Then anywhere else on earth*
> – Dorothy Frances Gurney (1858–1932)

That vital force of subtle energy that was recognised as the 'spirit of the flower' by the ancient Greeks, as 'qi' in China and 'prana' in India, is central to the story of medicine since its ancient beginnings. Just as human life has always been understood to be imbued with the divine spirit, so too flowers have been seen to possess a soul or essence which determined the shape and form of each flower, the ways it grows, its taste and smell, and its purpose in the world in relation to human life. The healing power that exists in a flower becomes clearer as one looks closer at individual flowers and their healing potential, whether they are eaten as the flower itself, taken as a herbal remedy, used in an aromatherapy oil, taken as a potentised homeopathic remedy or in a flower essence. In Chapter Three: The Healing Flowers, each flower's healing properties are described according to the different ways it is used, but it is the story of the flower itself which brings its message for healing.

Take yarrow, for example, the famous wound remedy of the Greek warrior Achilles. It is a great astringent and healing herb with its main influence observed on the blood and circulation, an essential oil with astringent properties and to enhance the circulation, a homeopathic remedy for venous haemorrhages, and a flower remedy to astringe the boundaries around a person and prevent their energy from bleeding into their environment.

Mugwort, whose Latin name *Artemisia* comes from the Greek moon goddess Artemis, the patron and protector of women, is an excellent female herb for enhancing their inner strength and their receptive quality and was used by the ancients in dream pillows to help gain important spiritual insights. As a homeopathic remedy, mugwort is an excellent female remedy for menstrual problems and threatened miscarriage as well as for spasms and epilepsy brought on by extremes of emotion. As a flower essence, mugwort also enhances the moon-like receptive quality of the psyche, allowing greater awareness of the dream world, and is predominantly a women's remedy, useful for a whole range of physical imbalances of the cycle, as well as in pregnancy and childbirth.

It may be believed by some that herbs and essential oils have an impact on the physical and emotional world, while homeopathy and flower remedies affect the subtler emotional and spiritual realms. However, one only has to look at the flower in all its simplicity to know that its very presence is healing. Certainly, flowers as herbal remedies and essential oils have their powerful physical effects partly explained by their amazing range of biochemical constituents. However, their more subtle attributes live within their physical forms, just as our soul animates us in our human bodies.

In the various healing methods, different parts of a flowering plant may be employed – sometimes the root, other times the stem, or the bark or the seed, but these are only parts of the whole, of which the flower is its vital expression. It is the flower that displays itself in all its magnificence, not only to attract pollinating insects, but also to bring its healing nature to the attention of mankind who has such need of its gifts. Flowers, their beauty, their scent, said Pope,

> *All are but parts of one stupendous whole*
> *whose body Nature is, and God the soul:*
> *look around our World, behold the chain of love*
> *combining all below and all above.*

Night-flying moths and hungry insects, as well as the whole of mankind, continue to gaze on their beauty in wonder.

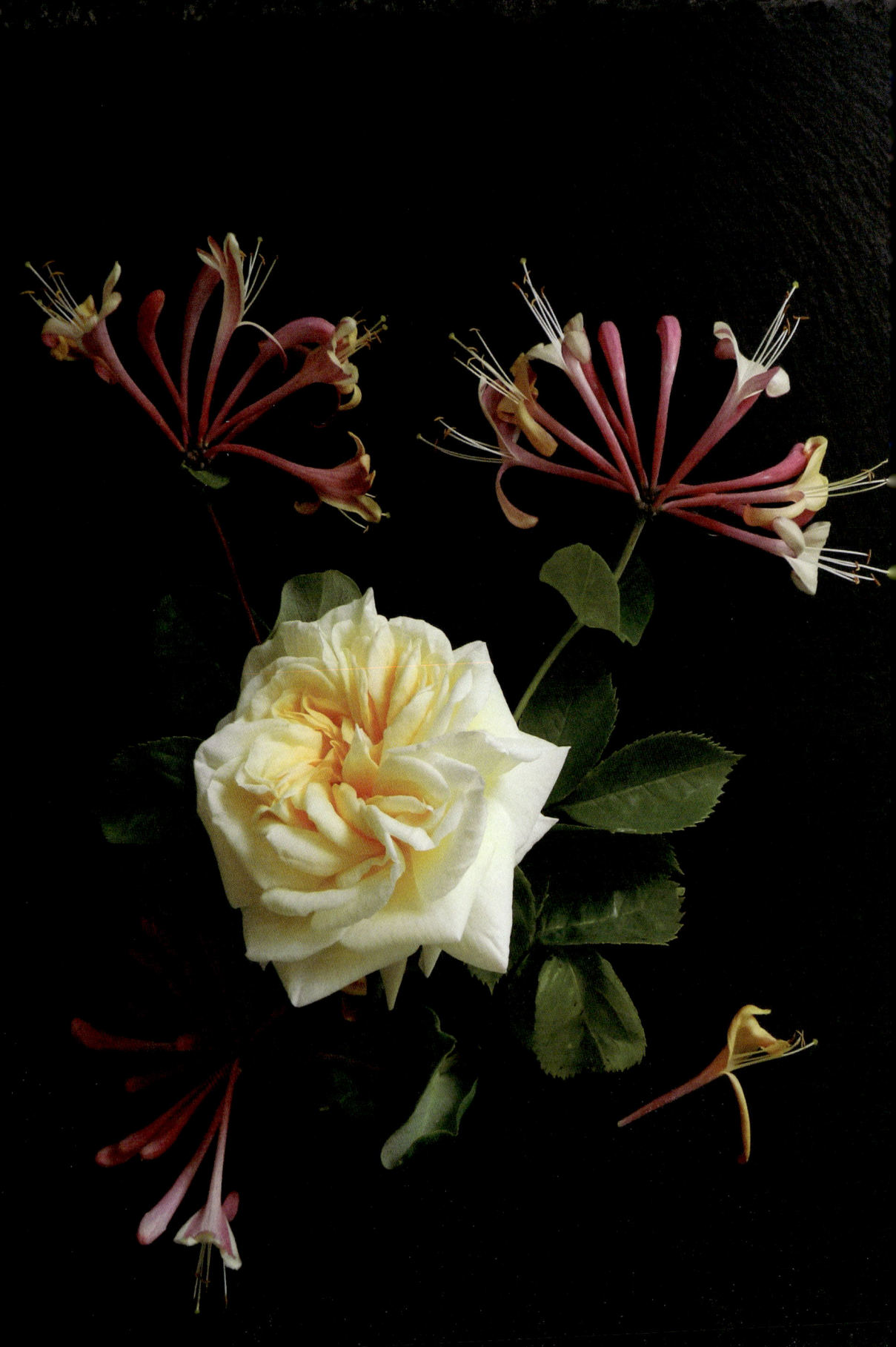

The Healing Flowers

That pleasure which is at once the most pure, the most elevating and the most intense, is derived, I maintain, from the contemplation of the beautiful.
– Edgar Alan Poe (1809–1849)

The amazing natural world gives us incredible healing plants which could be seen as manifestations of the conscious intelligence of the universe. The 'life force,' 'qi' or 'prana' of each plant is a dynamic manifestation of consciousness and every plant has its own subtle intelligence or unique wisdom, life force and attributes which give it *'energetic'* effects as well as its array of medically active constituents and its potential ability to heal. Herbs and flowers from all over the globe can impart their wisdom or intelligence to us and help us to balance energetic disturbances that create imbalances and health problems in mind and body, reconnect or realign us with consciousness and in this way bring about healing. They are an extraordinary gift. Whether we live in town or country, we can benefit from the incredible healing ability of the flowers around us and use them to care for ourselves and others.

In the pages that follow you will be introduced to sixty-four healing flowers. You will read about the myths and legends that tell stories about the flowers, their historical and folkloric use and the symbolism and language of each flower, all contributing to your knowledge and understanding of the healing attributes of each flower and the rich and colourful tapestry of floral healing. You will read about how each flower can be used to bring about healing and the different modes of preparation; as a herbal remedy, as an aromatherapy oil, a homeopathic remedy and as a flower essence. You will hopefully find a thread that runs through the stories and myths, the historical and folkloric use, the details of the modern medicinal use of the flowers as a herbal remedy relating to their biochemical constituents and their use in aromatherapy, in homeopathy and as flower essences. This thread describes each flower with its own particular energy and vibration, its unique healing attributes, almost with its own personality as a healer.

Every flower has its own exclusive blend of many different attributes. It has myriad biochemical constituents and physiological actions; it has its qualities and properties, being either heating or cooling, drying or moistening, heavy or light. It has its own texture and appearance, its own combination of tastes and smells and with time and experience it is possible to become acquainted with each individual herb almost like a different character. Since earliest times when people lived much closer to nature than we do now, flowers were believed to have natures and temperaments much like our own. Just as human life was suffused with the divine, so too each flower was envisaged as having a spirit or soul which determined its shape and form, the way it grew, its taste and smell and its meaning and purpose in the world in relation to human life. Taking all this into consideration, we can consider a healing flower as a whole and not assess its healing potential based solely on its active constituents or even its different qualities.

Every plant has its way of communicating its properties to us so that we can understand it and make the best use of its healing benefits. Before the days of microscopes and thin layer chromatography, we had only our senses to rely on and understandably the classification of plant medicines according to their effect on the senses was the foundation of the 'energetics' of the ancient wisdom traditions of medicine. The ancient Western herbalists believed that the Creator had provided relief from every ill, and for guidance to humankind had imprinted on each herb certain visual signs. This plant language became popular in the 17th century and was based on the recognition of the unity of all things in nature. It is thought to have originated from the vision of the design of God's creation experienced by a young German shoemaker, Jakob Böhme. The alchemist Paracelsus expanded this vision by advocating that close observation of the colour and form of plants could give vital indications of their medical use. He called the secret signs of plants the *Doctrine of Signatures* and published a book describing many plants, their signatures, and possible medicinal uses.

One of the best-known examples of the doctrine was the red beet with its branching red veins through the green leaf signifying a cure for heart and circulation problems. The form of the red beetroot corresponds to the shape of the heart, and the veins in the leaf branch as ours do. Similarly, lungwort has speckled leaves which were said to resemble the shape and pattern of the lungs, and the plant is still used today for lung problems. Many of the remedies used for the liver are yellowish. Yellow is the colour of bile, a secretion associated with the function of the liver and the colour of jaundice, an illness associated with disturbances of liver function such as hepatitis. The yellow of the remedy comes from the root of the plant, in the case of the yellow dock or from the juice, as with the greater celandine. Pilewort or lesser celandine has root tubers that rather resemble haemorrhoids and is used to treat them.

Even now our senses can still serve us very well in this respect, but we need to spend time with plants to develop a real sense of their healing potential. We have taste, smell, sight and touch to interpret the messages from plants, and maybe even hearing as the wonders of the plant world may even speak to us in a subtle way. Certainly, we can hear the different notes of plants as they rustle in the breeze. And of course, we have the mind. There is now a well-used scientific term 'organoleptics' for the use of the senses to detect the shape, colour, taste and smell of each plant and evaluate the presence, concentration and quality of its constituents. Most big herb companies are using specialists in 'organoleptics' as part of quality control, so that they can be assured of their identity and quality and this may go hand in hand with scientific analysis such as thin layer chromatography. When we devote time and attention to a flower, we can taste and smell it, note its form and colour and in so doing observe its energetic effects in mind and body (how it makes us feel) and in this way gain a sense of its role in healing based on these observations. This is a skill that animals possess. Even our domesticated companions will still sniff the ground and taste the plants out on their daily walks. Wild animals have the ability to understand whether a plant is food, medicine or poison through deep and ancient instinct combined with sensory perception developed by constant practice as well as necessity for their survival in the wild.

The best way to learn about a herb is to become intimately acquainted with it: we need to know its natural habitat, growing tendencies, climatic likes and dislikes, its shape, colour, taste, smell, the best harvest times and most importantly the herb must be experienced personally. Through contemplation and quiet time outside in nature, we can re-connect with our ancient skills to reawaken and develop our senses for better understanding of the healing properties of the plants around us. The qualities experienced by the senses can give us a deep sense of knowing but at the same time they are to some extent subjective and perhaps not to be relied upon totally. They can be combined with reason and experience.

It is important to understand a plant though our left brain also; its traditional use, dosage range, appropriate method of administration, modern pharmacology, contraindications as well as its potential and known drug-herb interactions. A pharmacological approach means remembering which constituents are present in each herb and what its actions and indications are, while an 'energetic' approach is experiential and so is more easily incorporated into our being. Through a combination of reading and study and a deeper sense of knowing we can have the best of both worlds.

If of thy mortal goods thou art bereft, and of thy meager store two loaves alone to thee are left, sell one, and with the dole buy hyacinths to feed thy soul
– Sheikh Muslih-uddin Saadi Shirazi, The Gulistan of Saadi, 1270

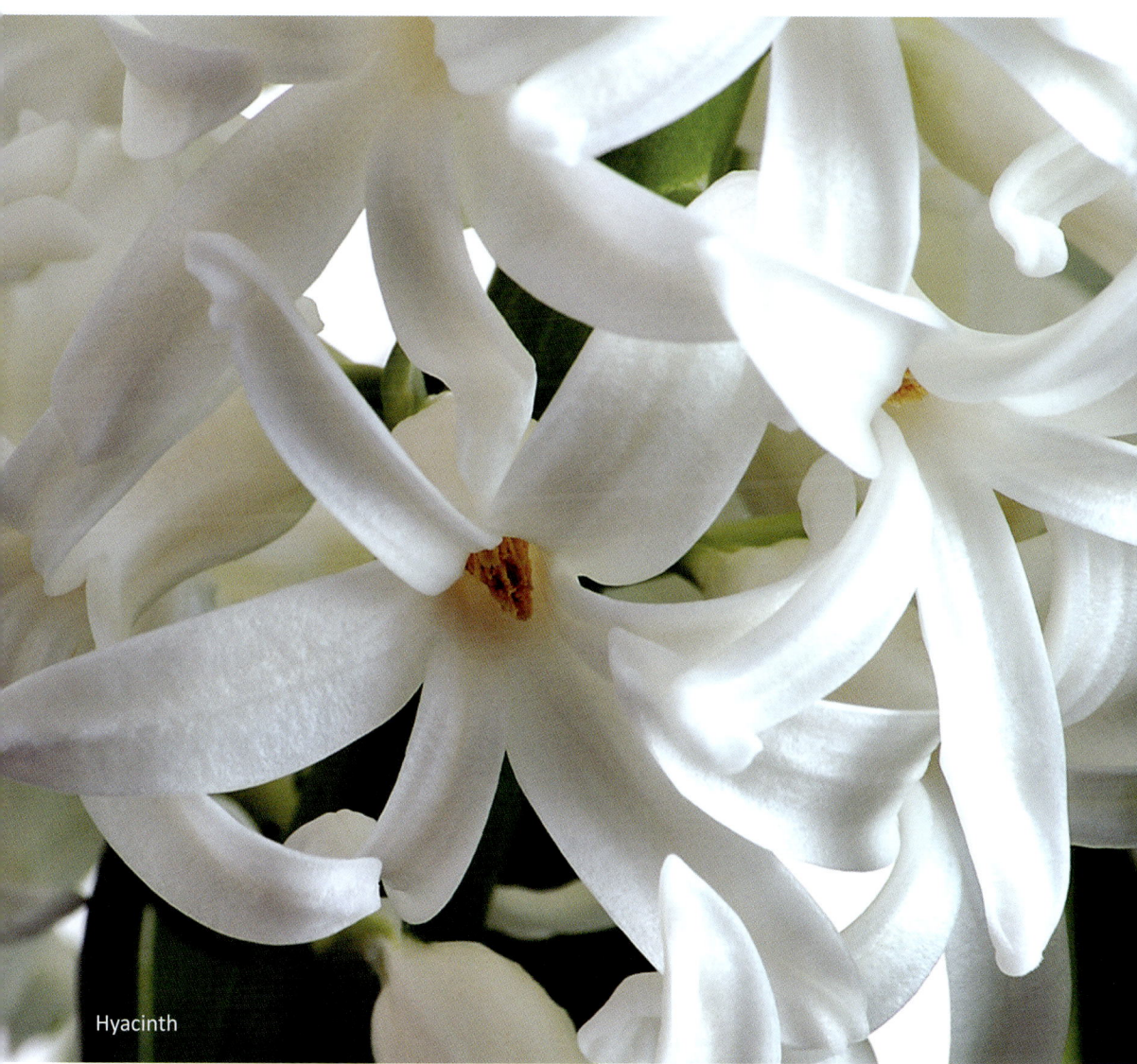

Hyacinth

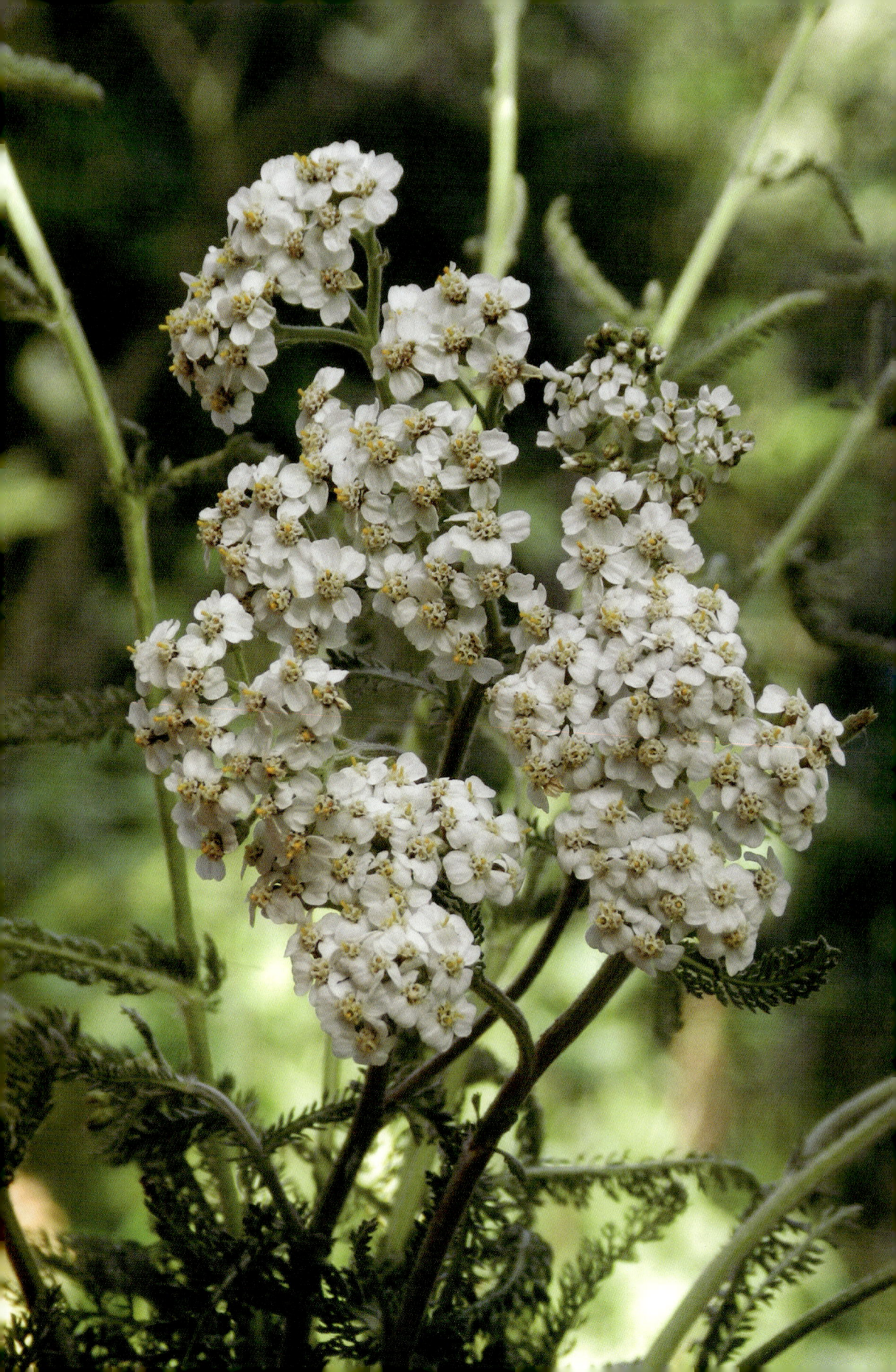

Achillea millifolium: Yarrow

The Flower of Invulnerability

Thou pretty herb of Venus Tree
Thy true name is Yarrow
Now who my bosom friend must be
Pray tell thou me tomorrow
– James Orchard Halliwell (1820–1889)

Other Names: Carpenter's weed, soldier's woundwort, thousand weed, milfoil, herbe militaire, nose bleed, bloodwort, bad man's plaything, staunchweed, noble yarrow, old man's pepper, green arrow

Parts Used: Aerial parts of the flowering plant

Yarrow is an attractive wild flower, found growing all over the globe in hedgerows, lanes and fields. It is a member of the Compositae/Asteraceae family, a cousin of dandelion and daisy. It can be recognised by its numerous feathery aromatic leaves (hence its Latin name *millefolium* meaning a thousand leaves) and flat-topped clusters of small white flowers that bloom from June to October.

One of the most versatile healing plants, yarrow's medicinal properties have been known since at least the time of the ancient Greeks and Egyptians. Dioscorides, a Greek physician in the Roman army writing in the 1st century AD, referred to healing battle wounds with yarrow. Homer described its virtues in the *Iliad*, the famous Greek myths about characters including Helen of Troy, Achilles, Paris, Agamemnon and many a god and goddess besides, each with their own dramas. The plant's name *'Achillea'* commemorates the Greek hero Achilles who was renowned for his invulnerability and apparently used yarrow to heal the wounds of his comrades in battle. Yarrow's first aid use has survived through history; it was used in the First World War for treating wounds, hence its common names 'Soldiers' woundwort' and 'Staunch weed'.

The name 'yarrow' is said to come from 'hieros' which means 'sacred' because of its long association with ceremonial magic. Believed to be richly endowed with spiritual properties, yarrow was preserved in temples and treated with special reverence. Its healing effect on the blood was seen as an ability to influence the 'life-blood', the essence or ego that is carried in it. It was used as an amulet to protect against negative energy and evil, as it was deemed capable of overcoming the forces of darkness and a conductor of benevolent powers.

Yarrow was also used as a love charm and said to be ruled by the planet Venus. In English folklore, a maiden who places yarrow under her pillow and repeats the rhyme above will dream of her future husband. Interestingly far away in China, yarrow stalks have also been used for divination, to reawaken the spiritual forces of the superconscious mind during ritual divination when using the *I Ching*.

Herbal Remedy

The contemporary use of yarrow in healing relates back to its religious, mythological and folkloric history, with its primary effects on the blood and circulation. It is rich in volatile oils (including sesquiterpenes, azulene, borneol, terpineol, cineol, eugenol, thujone, pinene, camphor, achillin and sabinene), tannins and flavonoids (including apigenin, rutin, luteolin, quercetin and kaempferol). It also contains cyanogenic glycosides, aconitic and isovalerianic acid, asparagin, alkaloid (achilleine), cyanidin, silica, sterols, bitters, salicylic acid, amino acids (lysine), coumarins, fatty acids (linoleic, palmitic, oleic), vitamins (B, C, E) and minerals. Its astringent action given by its high tannin content can be felt throughout the body, staunching bleeding internally and externally; from the skin, the nose, the digestive system and the uterus.

Yarrow has a relaxing effect on blood vessels throughout the body, which is attributed to its flavonoids and this can help to lower blood pressure. The flavonoids including apigenin also have antioxidant, anti-inflammatory and anti-platelet effects and with the astringent tannins they tone and stengthen blood vessels protecting them from damage caused by free radicals and inflammation which can predispose to clots and other cardiovascular problems. Another of yarrow's constituents called cyanidin also has an anti-inflammatory effect and can slow the heart rate through its effect on the vagus nerve. A hot infusion of yarrow is a popular remedy for stimulating the circulation and promoting sweating to reduce fevers as well

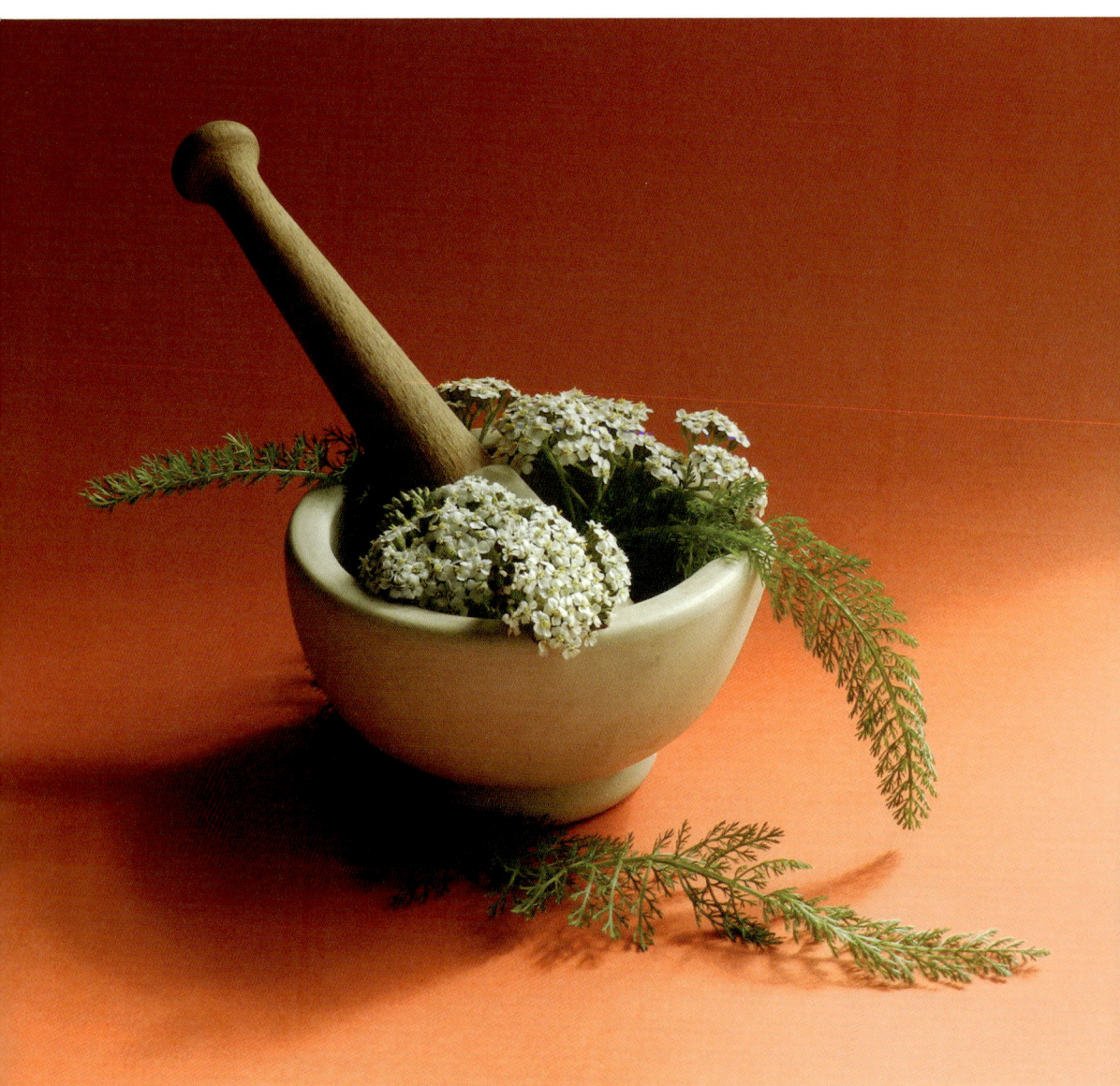

as lower blood pressure. It helps to clear toxins, heat and congestion by aiding elimination via the skin and the kidneys through its diuretic effect. It is used for poor circulation and cold hands and feet, Raynaud's disease and varicose veins. By stimulating blood flow to the skin, yarrow can be used to bring out the rash in eruptive childhood infections such as measles and chicken pox and speed the infections on their way. Its circulatory combined with its antispasmodic effects are helpful in treating leg cramps.

With its aromatic, bitter and astringent tastes and anti-inflammatory flavonoids, sesquiterpenes and salicylic acid, yarrow can cool heat and inflammation in the body including in the digestive tract. It stimulates the appetite and enhances digestion and absorption and makes a good remedy for wind, colic and indigestion, inflammatory bowel problems, IBS and other problems associated with poor digestion. The bitters stimulate the flow of bile from the liver, the great detoxifying organ of the body, and may help prevent the formation of gallstones. With its antioxidant properties given by the flavonoids it has hepato-protective effects, protecting the liver from damage from toxins such as drugs and alcohol.

Its astringent tannins protect the gut from irritation, inflammation and infection, making it useful for diarrhoea, dysentery and inflammatory gut problems such as gastritis, peptic ulcers and colitis. They also help to tighten junctions in the gut wall and remedy leaky gut syndrome and its subsequent health problems. At the same time, yarrow's antispasmodic action can help relieve colic and griping, and its antimicrobial actions given by the sesquiterpene lactones in the volatile oil curb disturbances of the gut flora and help the gut to reestablish a healthy microbiome. It has antibacterial action against several bacteria including *Staphylococcus aureus, Shigella sonnei, Mycobacterium smegmatis, Bacillus subtillus, E. coli,* and *Shigella flexnii.*

Yarrow's astringent effect on the mucous membranes of the respiratory system protect them from invasion by bacteria and viruses, so yarrow can be a good preventative remedy during the cold and 'flu season. Taken as the traditional cold remedy in a hot infusion with mint and elderflower, yarrow make a good antimicrobial decongestant to take at the onset of symptoms, helping to combat infections such as colds and relieve catarrhal congestion. Its antibacterial and antifungal properties help us to throw off infections such as tonsillitis, boils and conjunctivitis. The volatile oils and luteolin in yarrow have anti-inflammatory and antioxidant effects, useful in the treatment of arthritis, gout, allergies and auto-immune problems, and the sesquiterpene lactones help relieve pain as in arthritis and headaches.

Yarrow has a beneficial effect on the nervous system and has a reputation for toughening our boundaries and protecting the more sensitive of us from the harshness of the outside world. It also has a relaxing effect, calming tension and anxiety attributed to the cyanogenic glycosides, isovalerianic acid and the volatile oil. It also has an antihistamine effect which is useful for treating allergies including rhinitis and hay fever. Since immune function and allergic responses are intimately connected to gut function and the microbiome, yarrow's beneficial effect in the digestive system may be related to this. Also, yarrow's astringent effect tightening our boundaries and its subtle effect on the ego, may enhance our immunity by helping us to differentiate between *'me'* and *'not me'* and be instrumental in enhancing our resilience to allergens.

The circulatory and astringent actions of yarrow can help regulate the menstrual cycle and clear stagnation, making it useful for treating painful and heavy periods as well as fibroids. It has oestrogenic properties and can also be useful for tightening muscles in prolapse and urinary incontinence.

Externally yarrow makes an excellent first aid remedy and it has all the components to do this; the volatile oils particularly the blue oil azulene, and salicylic acid are anti-inflammatory and antiseptic, azulene also stimulates the formation of granulation tissue involved in wound healing, the tannins are astringent and stop bleeding, the alkaloid achilleine has a haemostatic effect also stopping bleeding, eugenol in the volatile oil has anaesthetic effects, the resins are astringent and antiseptic, while the silica promotes tissue repair. It is the perfect wound herb as the story of Achilles has told us.

The bruised fresh herb, a strong infusion or a dilute tincture will speed healing of cuts and wounds, ulcers as well as burns. It can be applied similarly to varicose veins, haemorrhoids and skin conditions like eczema. An infusion makes a good vaginal douche, an eye bath for inflamed eyes, a lotion for sore nipples, a gargle for sore throats, a mouthwash for dental plaque and gingivitis and also a rinse after washing hair. A strong decoction of the leaves has been used as an injection into the nostril to stop nose bleeds.

Aromatherapy Oil
The essential oil of yarrow is used in aromatherapy for much the same range of problems, particularly those of the circulation. Its anti-inflammatory and detoxifying properties are useful in arthritis and gout. As an antispasmodic, it can be used to relieve cramps, colic and painful periods. As an astringent, it stimulates the circulation and enhances digestion. It can also be used for heavy periods.

Homeopathic Remedy
Yarrow is used predominantly for bleeding; for bruises, varicose veins, haemorrhoids and bright red bleeding in nosebleeds, blood in the urine, bleeding from haemorrhoids or the stomach, long, heavy periods. This tends to occur in ruddy-complexioned people, after vigorous exercise or exertion, strains or injuries. It includes haemorrhages after childbirth, painful varicose veins in pregnancy and coughing with bloody mucous.

Yarrow is also indicated in red rashes as in chicken pox or measles, hernias from over-lifting with great pain, feeling bruised or shaken after a fall and a continual high fever. There can be vertigo or a feeling that the head is full of blood, piercing pain from the eyes to the root of the nose and palpitations.

The Flower Essence
Yarrow is used to protect against negative outside influences and for psychic shielding, giving us the invulnerability of Achilles. It helps to clarify boundaries between people which is particularly useful for those who are easily influenced and depleted by others and their environment. It is for people who tend to absorb negative influences and are prone to allergies and environmental illness. By 'astringing' the boundaries around us and preventing our energies from 'bleeding' into our environment, yarrow acts to strengthen and solidify our sense of self, our essence, allowing and enhancing our ability to heal, teach, counsel or follow our chosen path.

Edible Uses
When young and tender in spring, the fresh leaves can be finely chopped and added to salads, soups, bean and meat dishes and stir-fries.

Recipe
Mint, elderflower and yarrow tea for colds, catarrh and fevers

1 teaspoon each of mint, elderflowers and yarrow, fresh or dried.

Place in a teapot and pour over 500ml of boiling water. Leave to infuse for 10–15 minutes. Drink hot 3–6 times daily.

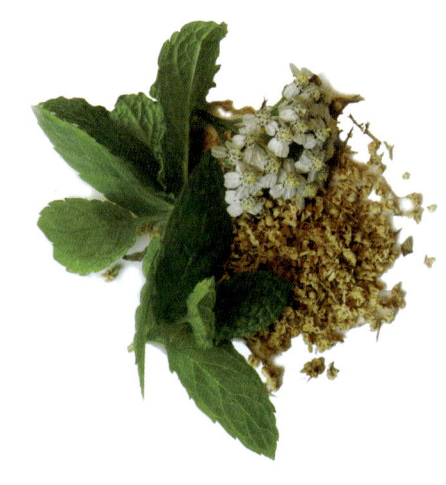

Growing

Yarrow is a hardy perennial and can be found throughout the Northern hemisphere, growing wild in hedgerows, lanes and meadows, on light sandy soils with minute white or pink flowers and is quite drought resistant. Its superficial roots are quite extensive and so help to bind loose soil together to help prevent erosion.

You can propagate by sowing seeds in spring or autumn in well-drained soil and full sun. Alternatively, divide the plant in spring or autumn. Grows 6 – 24" (15 – 60cm) and flowers from July – Sept. Harvest the aerial parts just as it is coming into flower and wear gloves for picking. The stems are very tough and so may require scissors or secateurs.

When put on the compost heap, yarrow has a reputation for speeding up the decomposition of matter by increasing heat and so helps to speed the process of compost making.

Cautions

Avoid the herbal remedy and oil in pregnancy, breastfeeding and a known allergy to the *Asteraceae* family. Yarrow should not be used to treat large, deep or infected wounds, all of which require medical attention. Yarrow may cause allergic skin rashes when harvesting the herb and when applied topically. It may cause photosensitivity. Avoid with anticoagulant drugs.

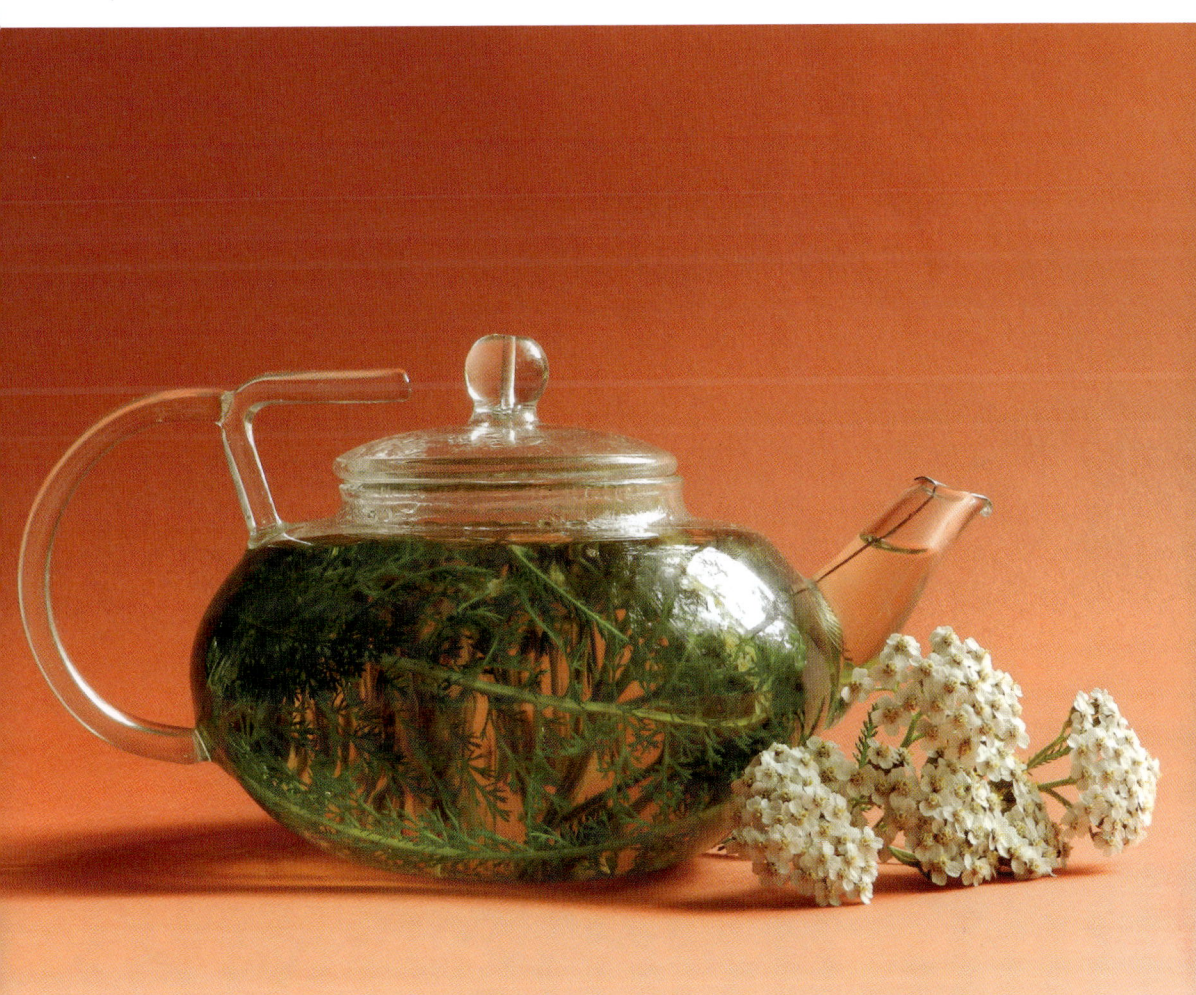

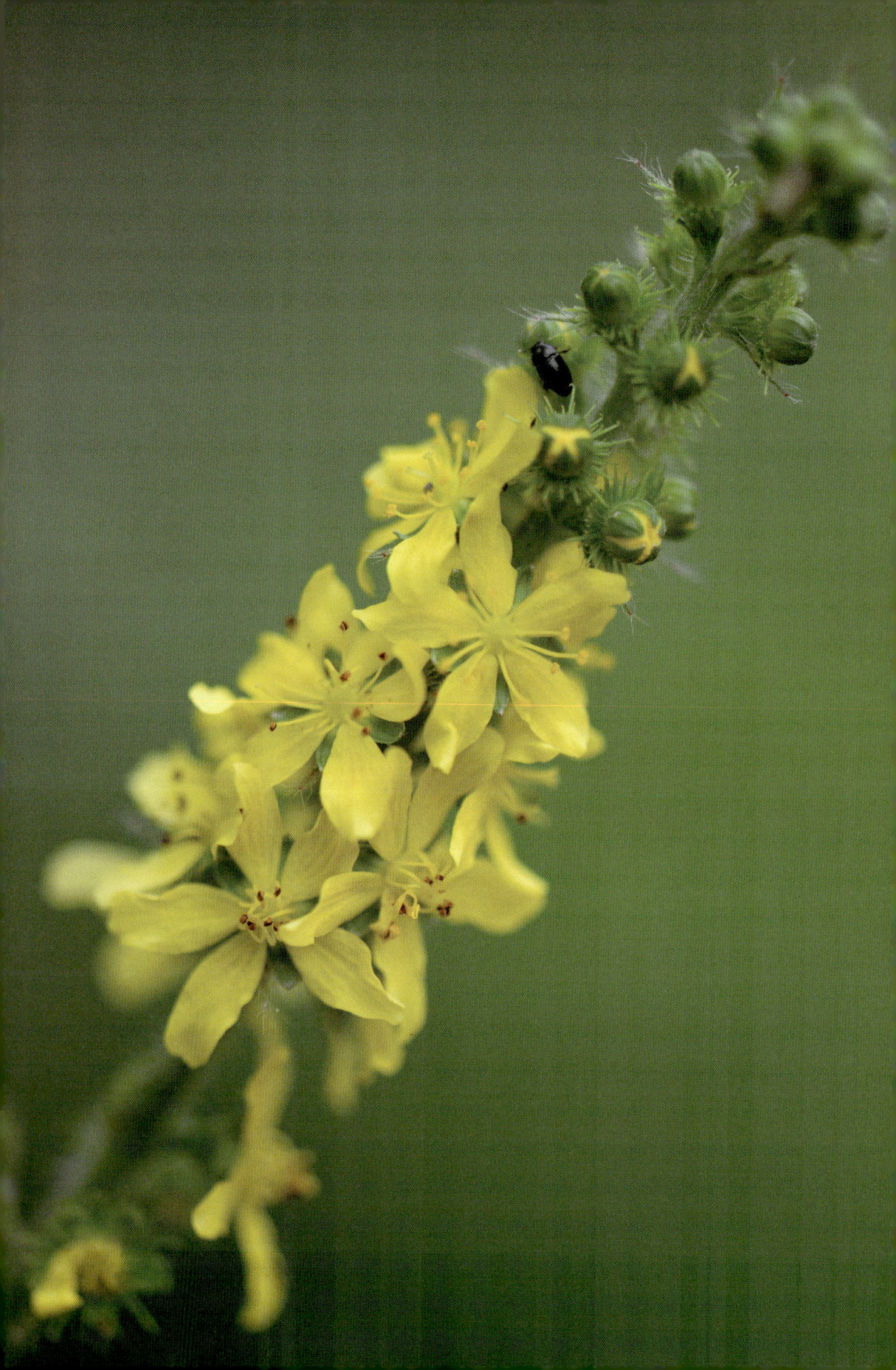

Agrimonia eupatoria: Agrimony

The Flower of Perception

Next these here Egremony is, That helps the serpent's biting
— Michael Drayton (1563–1631)

Other Names: *Agrimonia gryposepela, A. parveflora*, church steeples, cockleburr, sticklewort, liverwort, burr marigold, harvest lice, philanthropos, rat's tail, stickwort, white tansy

Parts Used: Aerial parts, flowers and leaves

Found in summer hedgerows, fields and waste ground, agrimony is easily recognised by its delicate long spike of yellow flowers smelling of apricots, and its beautifully shaped leaves. Its country name 'church steeples' refers to its rising spire of yellow flowers, while names such as 'cockleburr' and 'sticklewort' refer to the seed which attaches itself to passers-by, both animal and human.

Agrimony was praised by the ancient Greeks and Romans for its healing properties. The name 'agrimony' comes from the Greek 'argentone' meaning a white speck in the eye, because of the herb's ability to heal the eyes; the Greeks apparently used it for cataracts. The name 'eupatoria' is after Mithridates IV Eupator, King of Pontus 120–63BC, a skilled herbalist who was apparently the first to use agrimony for liver complaints and to counteract poisons. The Roman physician Dioscorides said that it was *"not only a remedy for them that have bad livers but also for those who are bitten by serpents."*

Agrimony is rich in tannins which stem bleeding and speed healing and on a more psychic level help strengthen our boundaries. This may explain why in common folklore, it has long been held that agrimony could cure musket wounds and ward off witchcraft. It was used since early times in protection spells and to reverse spells and direct them back to the sender. In Anglo Saxon times agrimony was used to heal wounds and treat snake bites and was one of the 57 herbs in the Anglo-Saxon Holy Salve believed to protect from goblins, evil and poison.

Chaucer refers to the use of agrimony for 'alle wounds' and medieval monks grew it in their monastery gardens as a cure for stomach aches and open wounds. Its healing powers, particularly for aiding sleep, were mentioned in an old English medieval manuscript,

If it be leyd under mann's head he shal sleepyn
As he were dead, he shal never drede ne wakyn
Till from under his head it be takyn

Culpeper recommended it to be taken internally and applied externally for gout as well as for bruises, sprains, wounds and snakebites. The Elizabethan herbalist Gerard said it was *"good for naughty livers."* Native Americans in North America and Canada used agrimony as a fever remedy; it has been likened to Peruvian bark for its ability to relieve fever and malaria.

The French drink agrimony 'tisanes' and use it on sprains and bruises in their famous 'eau de arquebusade' made originally for treating battle wounds in the 15th century. The strangest use of agrimony was in an old remedy for internal haemorrhages. It was mixed in with pounded frogs and a little human blood.

In the language of flowers agrimony symbolises gratitude.

Herbal Remedy
Bitter, pungent and astringent, agrimony makes a good cooling and cleansing herb. It contains tannins, flavonoids (glucosides of luteolin,

apigenin and quercetin), coumarins, triterpenic acids, phenolic acids, polysaccharides, glycosidal bitters, mucilage, phytosterols, agrimonin, volatile oil, furanocoumarins, nicotinic acid, vitamins (B1, C, K), silica and iron. With its antioxidant and anti-inflammatory flavonoids and glycosidal bitters, it is generally used for problems associated with heat and inflammation and with its astringent tannins, it has a drying effect which can be useful in reducing catarrh, stemming bleeding and any other excess secretions.

Agrimony acts as a gentle tonic for the digestion. The astringent tannins tone the mucous membranes of the gut, protecting them against irritation, inflammation and infection, which can be very useful in leaky gut syndrome and its subsequent problems. The bitters improve the secretion of digestive enzymes and enhance the absorption of nutrients while the mucilage has a soothing effect.

Agrimony can be used to relieve inflammatory gut problems, to prevent and remedy peptic ulcers and colitis, and makes a good remedy for diarrhoea and the accompanying colicky, cramping stomach pains. It firms up the stools and has analgesic, anti-inflammatory and antimicrobial properties, making it an ideal natural remedy for 'tummy bugs' and for combatting unfriendly bacteria in the gut flora.

With its bitter components, agrimony stimulates the secretion of bile from the liver and gallbladder, enhancing digestion and absorption and improving bowel function. It supports the liver in its cleansing work, clearing toxins from the tissues and can be used for treating liver and gallbladder conditions, including gallstones and cirrhosis of the liver. It also has insulin-like effects and helps to lower blood sugar levels and can lower harmful cholesterol.

Agrimony helps to reduce heat and congestion in the urinary tract. It acts as an astringent diuretic, useful for bedwetting and incontinence, bladder irritation, cystitis and kidney stones. By aiding the elimination of toxins and uric acid, agrimony can be helpful for gout and arthritis as well as skin problems such as eczema and acne. It has an affinity with the reproductive tract and makes an excellent astringent remedy for heavy periods and gynaecological problems such as fibroids and endometriosis.

Its antimicrobial properties are useful against a range of bacterial and viral infections. The polyphenols may be responsible for its antiviral action particularly against *Herpes simplex 1*. It may help inhibit the growth of tumours. Its relaxing action in the chest can be helpful in asthma and irritating coughs, while its antibacterial properties are useful for treating respiratory infections and bronchitis. It can also be given for fevers accompanying infections.

Externally you can also use agrimony for stemming bleeding and speeding healing of cuts and wounds. Its high silica content speeds healing. It reduces the pain and swelling of bruises, sprains and varicose veins, and can be used to relieve aching muscles and inflammatory skin problems such as hives and eczema.

An infusion can be used for nappy rash. As a gargle or mouthwash, you can use it for sore throats, laryngitis and inflamed gums. It makes a good eyewash for inflammatory eye problems and a douche for vaginal discharges and infections such as *Trichomonas*.

Homeopathic Remedy
Agrimonia is used for menstrual and digestive problems. It helps to clear catarrh throughout the digestive, respiratory and genito-urinary systems. It is indicated in painful kidneys, strong smelling urine, deep colicky pain in the lumbar region extending down the abdomen, pain in the uterus and a cough with profuse expectoration accompanied by a need to pass water.

Emotionally an agrimony person may feel as if they have a heavy burden to carry especially if they have to take care of someone else. There is a tendency to avoid problems instead of facing them, to hide their suffering and attempt to be cheerful even when once doesn't feel it, to make light of difficulties in life or find diversions, or block out pain with distractions, alcohol or drugs. They may feel physically weak.

The Flower Essence

Agrimony is particularly for those who appear carefree and cheerful; they are popular and have a good sense of humour. However, their brave face masks inner torture or turbulence which they are careful not to inflict on others. They are concerned to keep peace and harmony, so do not like to upset other people and are distressed by tension and conflict. They will go out of their way to avoid confrontation and to keep other people happy. When ill, they make light of their symptoms. Generally, they hate to sit still or to be alone, for fear their suppressed emotions may come to the fore and they may have to face their darker side or their problems. Agrimony people keep their rose-tinted spectacles firmly on. Such people may indulge in alcohol, drugs or a wide range of exciting activities to distract them from their inner selves.

Agrimony helps such people to acknowledge the real, sometimes darker side of themselves or others. It engenders inner strength to face the problems of everyday life and from the past. In this sense, agrimony is a remedy for perception. The Greeks used it as a remedy to heal the eyes. As a flower remedy it helps one to see things as they truly are.

Growing

Propagate by sowing seeds either from Feb - May or Aug – Nov. It prefers well drained soil and full sun. Alternatively, divide plants in autumn. Grows 6"– 2' (15 – 60 cm) tall and flowers from June – Sept.

Cautions

Avoid in pregnancy, breastfeeding, high blood pressure, constipation or extreme dryness. It may cause sensitivity to sunlight. Those with kidney or liver conditions should avoid it. Avoid with Warfarin and other anticoagulants, insulin and other hypoglycaemic medications (eg. Chlorpropamide). Diabetics should monitor blood glucose levels carefully. Discontinue use 7 days prior to surgery.

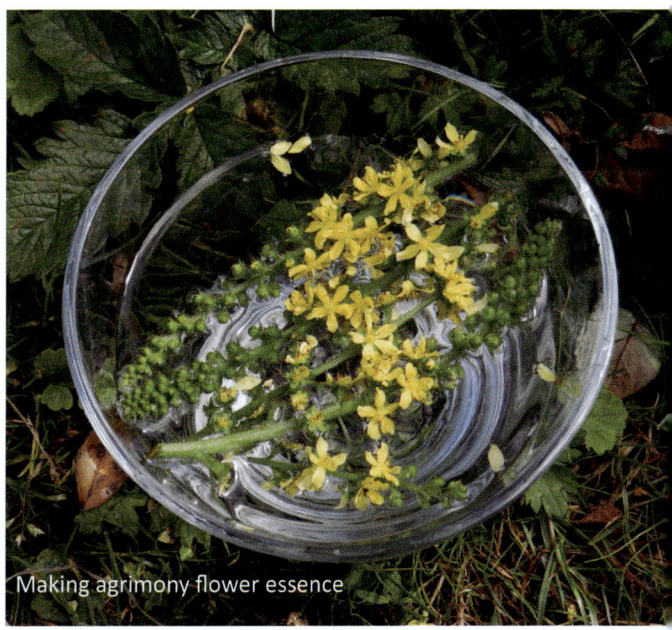

Making agrimony flower essence

Recipe

Toning Liniment/compress
1 part yarrow
1 part calendula petals
1 part St John's Wort flowers and leaves
1 part agrimony

Using equal parts of the herbs, place 250 grams in a glass jar and pour over 500 mls of brandy or vodka to make a tincture. Leave to infuse for at least 2 weeks, shaking daily. Press through muslin or a wine press and store in dark bottles that are clearly labelled.

Use 1-2 tsp in a little cool water, soak a cloth in the liquid, wring out gently and then apply to the area 2-3 times a day. Alternatively pat a little of the liquid with your fingers to the area.

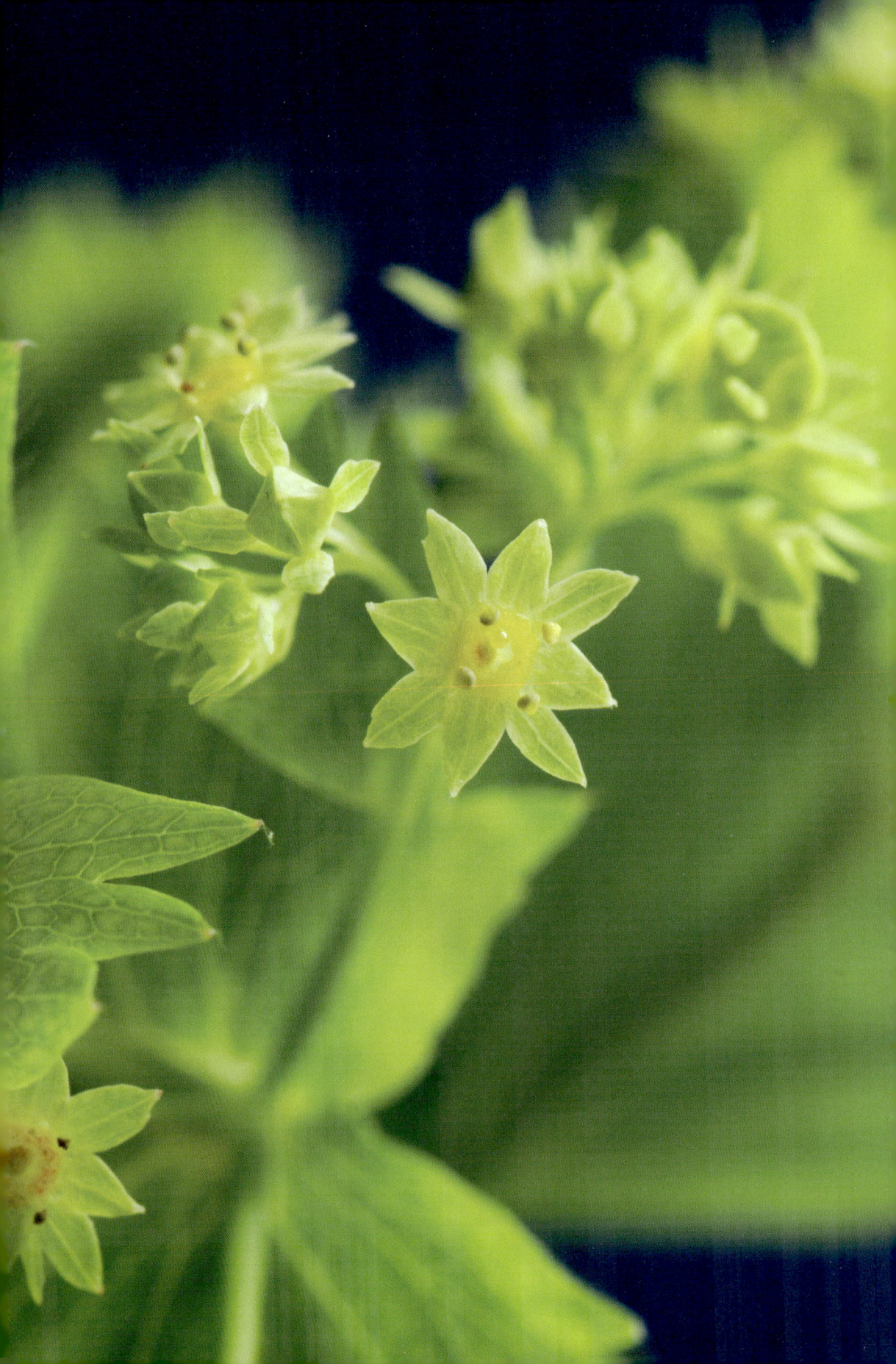

Alchemilla vulgaris/mollis: Lady's Mantle
The Flower of Alchemy

I am forget-me-not
Self-seeding where it will.
I am water hyssop transplanted
From India, Ayurvedic.
I am a hellebore's nectaries
Fleshy with pollen.
I am dewdrops beading
Lady's mantle leaves.
I am dandelion and dock,
Goosegrass and nettle,
Never say weed.
– Virginia Woolf (1882–1941)

Other Names: Lion's foot, bear's foot, dew cup, nine hooks, great sanicle, a woman's best friend, nine monks, breakstone, piercestone, fair with tears, water carrier, water chalice flower, ever-dew, Mary's mantle, Our Lady's mantle

Parts Used: Aerial parts and the root

Lady's mantle is a really attractive member of the Rosaceae family, found in the wild and widely cultivated in gardens. It is a hardy perennial with distinctive pale-green leaves and tiny, lacy green-yellow flowers, which give decorative ground cover in the garden for many weeks over spring and summer. It could be described as an understated or demure plant, but as Mrs Grieve said in her Modern Herbal *"the rich form of its foliage and the beautiful shape of its clustering blossoms make it worthy of notice."*

The name *Alchemilla* comes from the Arabic word 'alkemelych' meaning alchemy, as it was a favourite of the medieval alchemists who considered it magical. In their search for the philosopher's stone, the mystical way of turning baser metals into gold, they collected the pearly drops that form and sparkle on the leaves of lady's mantle, which they called 'water from heaven'. The dew drops, which are actually exuded from the plant itself, were thought to extract the subtle healing and magical virtues from the leaf and were used in many an alchemist's potion.

Lady's mantle was also considered to have magical virtues in other traditions. In Eastern Europe it was thought to protect from or ward off storms if it was burned on the fire and its smoke drifted into the sky. It could also ward off evil spirits and protect farmers from natural disasters if it was hung in windows or doors. According to Scandinavian folklore, a woman would place lady's mantle under her pillow so she could dream of her future children and if she wore it in her hair in bed with her husband, she would definitely conceive.

In the Middle Ages, lady's mantle was dedicated to the Virgin Mary and, as its name suggests, the scalloped-edge leaves were thought to resemble Mary's cloak. In healing, the plant has a strong affinity with women and the female reproductive system. It was highly valued as a wound healer to staunch bleeding and women believed the dew drops would enhance their beauty if they washed their faces in them and that it would be attract love. According to Culpeper, lady's mantle was ruled by Venus and he said,

Lady's Mantle is very proper for inflamed wounds and to stay bleeding, vomitings, fluxes of all sorts, bruises by falls and ruptures. It is one of the most singular wound herbs and therefore prized and praised, used in all wounds inward and outward, to drink a decoction and wash the wounds thereof, or dip a cloth wet with the herb into the wound which wonderfully drieth up all humidity of the sores and abateth all inflammations thereof. It quickly healeth green wounds, not suffering any corruption to remain behind and cureth old sores, though fistulas and hollow.

It must have been highly valued for its ability to reduce bleeding as well as infections, as these would have been dangerous and even life-threatening in those days. It also provided other benefits for women; William Salmon (1644–1713) was an English apothecary and a writer of medical texts who called himself a Professor of Physick. He wrote, "*It is amazing how Lady's Mantle can restore the integrity of torn, ruptured or separated tissue as seen in hernias or perforated membranes.*"

Elizabeth Blackwell (1707–1758) was apparently the first woman to write a herbal. To raise funds to release her husband from debtors' prison, she produced her hand drawn, engraved and coloured 'Curious Herbal' in 1735. She said about lady's mantle, "*The leaves applyed outwardly are accounted good for lank flagging breasts.*"

John Hill, the apothecary and botanist wrote in 1740, "The good women in the North of England apply the leaves to their breasts to make them recover their form after they have been swelled with milk." It was traditionally used to promote fertility. Culpeper recommended drinking distilled lady's mantle water for 20 days to encourage conception.

Andrés Laguna de Segovia (1499–1559), a Spanish physician, pharmacologist and botanist who translated Dioscorides' Materia Medica, recommended two preparations of lady's mantle. Firstly, the root, powdered and mixed with red wine, for internal and external wounds, and secondly an infusion of the aerial parts for greenstick fractures and broken bones in babies and young children. When taken daily for 15 days, lady's mantle was said to reverse sterility due to "slipperiness" of the womb and the astringent and tightening properties of the infusion was so highly thought of that it was "a thousand times sold" to women wanting to appear to be virgins; no wonder lady's mantle was considered a herb of the Virgin Mary!

Herbal Remedy
The whole plant of lady's mantle makes a remedy which lives up to its old name 'woman's best friend'. It contains ellagitannins, salicylic acid, saponins, phenolic compounds, volatile oils, bitters, phytosterols and flavonoids. Its astringent tannins help to dry up excess secretions including catarrh, diarrhoea or bleeding from any cause. It is a highly popular herb for reducing heavy periods, particularly useful for prolonged bleeding due to fibroids and around the menopause. As a uterine stimulant, it can also stimulate menstrual flow and bring on delayed periods. It is thought to have a progesterogenic action and can be used to ease period pains and regulate periods as well as enhance fertility. Taken a few days prior to birth, it can stimulate contractions during the birth as well as help prevent post-partum bleeding.

Lady's mantle has a toning and strengthening effect on pelvic floor muscles and has been used to help prevent miscarriage. It is recommended after trauma such as a termination, miscarriage and after childbirth to aid recovery both emotionally and physically. It promotes normal involution of the uterus after childbirth and reduces risk of prolapse. It also helps the breasts to regain their tone after breast-feeding. It can be thought of for treating fibroids, cysts, pelvic inflammatory disease, polycystic ovaries, infertility, endometriosis, post-partum bleeding, prolapse and genito-urinary infections. It helps to regulate vaginal secretions.

The astringent properties attributed to the tannins, particularly in the fresh root, are excellent for problems in the digestive tract. The

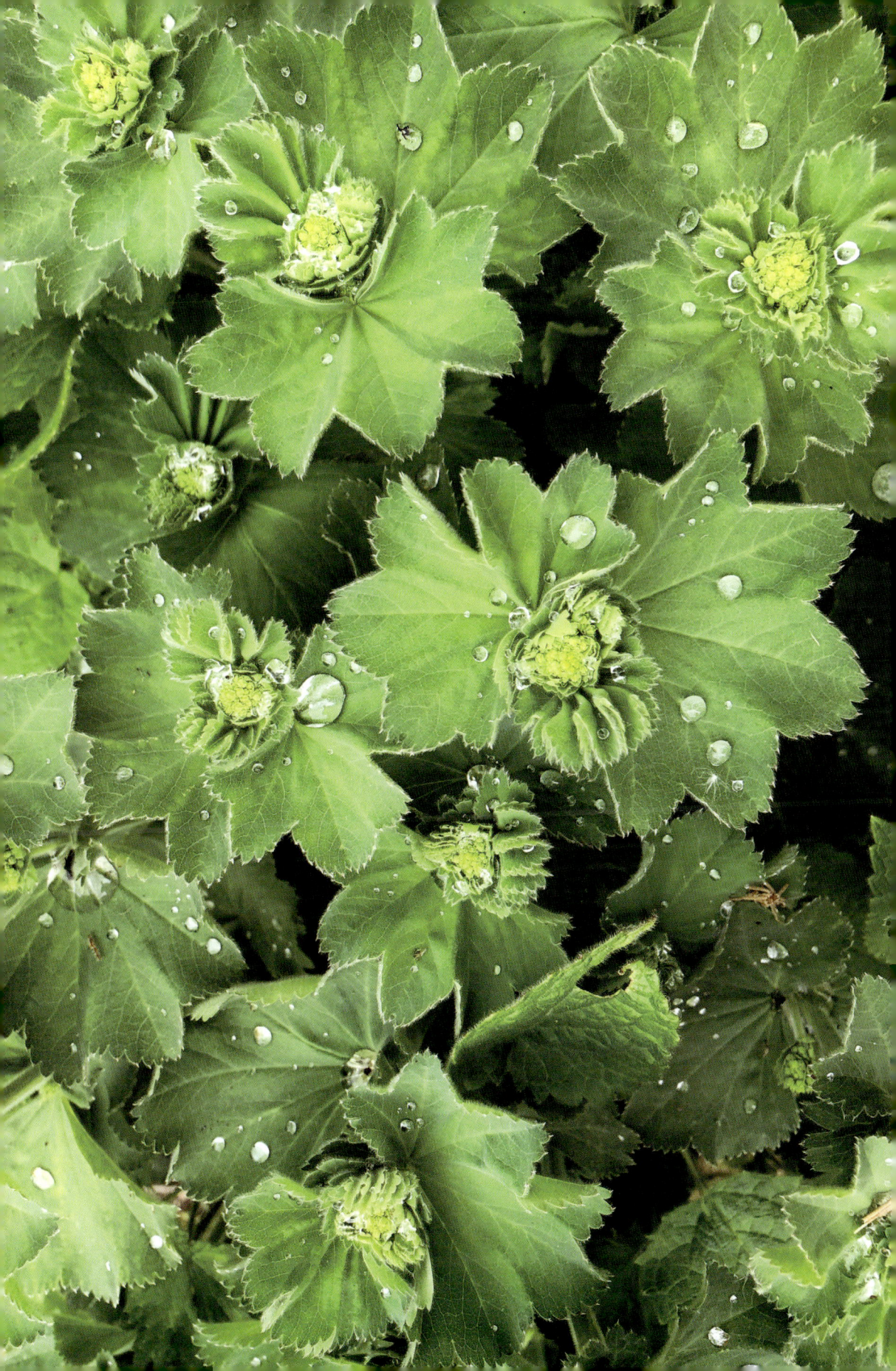

whole plant can be used to tone and strengthen the mucous membranes throughout the gut and is well worth using to treat gastric and duodenal ulcers, diarrhoea, gastro-enteritis and colitis with bleeding. It is often given with good effect for diarrhoea in children. It can be used to tighten junctions in the gut wall and reduce leaky gut syndrome. The salicylic acid helps by reducing pain and inflammation in the digestive and reproductive systems.

There is a lot more to this plant, however. The whole plant contains flavonoids called catechins which have antiviral actions, and the phenolic compounds and flavonoids have antioxidant and possible anticancer properties particularly in relation to oestrogen-dependent tumours such as in the breast, cervix and ovaries. The salicylates have an anti-inflammatory effect and its vasoactive compounds may account for its ability to reduce blood pressure and its cardiotonic effects, possibly aided by its diuretic properties which help relieve fluid retention. It also has thyroid-balancing actions helping to regulate metabolism, and the antioxidant tannins and phenols have a hepato-protective effect, protecting the liver from damage from toxins such as alcohol and drugs.

Externally, the fresh root and leaves make excellent wound healers to stop bleeding and promote healing. This is attributed to their astringent, anti-inflammatory and antimicrobial properties. You can use lady's mantle as a douche or lotion for vaginal discharge, irritation and infections such as *Trichomonas* and *Candida* after antibiotic treatment when the vaginal flora has been disturbed. An infusion makes a good skin lotion for rashes, eczema, pimples, acne, itching, inflamed cuts and wounds, sores and insect bites, an eyewash for inflammatory eye problems such as conjunctivitis and a mouthwash or gargle for bleeding gums, mouth ulcers, sore throats and laryngitis.

In the past lady's mantle, and especially the 'dew' on the leaves, was highly valued as a beauty aid to reduce wrinkles. It is possible that the polyphenols, which include tannins, in lady's mantle help to reduce the impact of aging on the skin. As we age, there is a loss of elastin, a protein in the dermis of the skin. The dermis is the inner layer of the skin which supports and protects the skin and is made of collagen, elastic tissue, blood vessels, nerve endings, hair follicles and sebaceous glands. The tannins in lady's mantle may inhibit elastase, an enzyme that breaks down elastin and causes degeneration of elastic fibres, and in this way it can reduce the effect of aging and the appearance of wrinkles.

The Flower Essence
The uses of lady's mantle as a flower essence continue along the same theme of alchemy and women. The alchemist's 'philosopher's stone' is that which can never be lost or dissolved, something eternal, the mystical experience of the divine within one's own soul. Lady's mantle is a remedy for those women who wish to be more in touch with the divine female power within them, and for those who seek the inspiration or protection of Mary or the goddess within. It is particularly recommended for those who feel alienated from women or from their feminine side, perhaps because of negative experiences during childhood with women who had authority in their lives.

Being an alchemic plant, lady's mantle helps to dissolve away those earthbound or superfluous elements which are concealing the 'stone' within. It aids transitions in life, helping to move away from the past, and release the ties that bind. It is particularly useful during times of change that may bring fear or heartache, such as childbirth, moving home, the break-up of a relationship or a bereavement.

Growing
Lady's mantle can be propagated in spring or autumn by root division. It will grow in poor, slightly acidic soil, and likes full sun or partial shade.

Cautions
Avoid in pregnancy except in last 10 days when it can be used to prevent excessive postpartum bleeding. It may be unsafe in patients using anticoagulants (eg. warfarin) due to its theoretical use as a coagulant and for patients with iron deficiency anaemia as the tannins may reduce absorption of iron supplements.

Allium sativum: Garlic

The Flower of Power

*A feast is not a feast unless to begin
Each guest is given ample Toes of Garlic,
That finest aphrodisiac
To whet his appetite for later revelry*
– Quintus Horace (65–8BC)

Other Names: Bear's garlic, stinking rose, heal all, poor man's treacle

Parts Used: Flowers and bulb

Garlic is a member of the lily family (Liliaceae/Amaryllidaceae) and a wonderfully impressive remedy that has been used in healing for thousands of years, probably by more cultures than any other plant. It originated in central Asia, but it is now found in Europe, North Africa, Asia, and North America. It was first cultivated in English gardens about 1540. An Egyptian medical papyrus dating around 1500 BC included over 200 prescriptions using garlic for problems such as headaches, physical weakness and throat infections. The ancient Greeks apparently ate large amounts of garlic. Galen saw it as a panacea for all ills, while Dioscorides used it as a remedy for asthma, jaundice, toothache, skin problems, worms and as an antidote to poisons. In 1st century India, Ayurvedic physicians used garlic

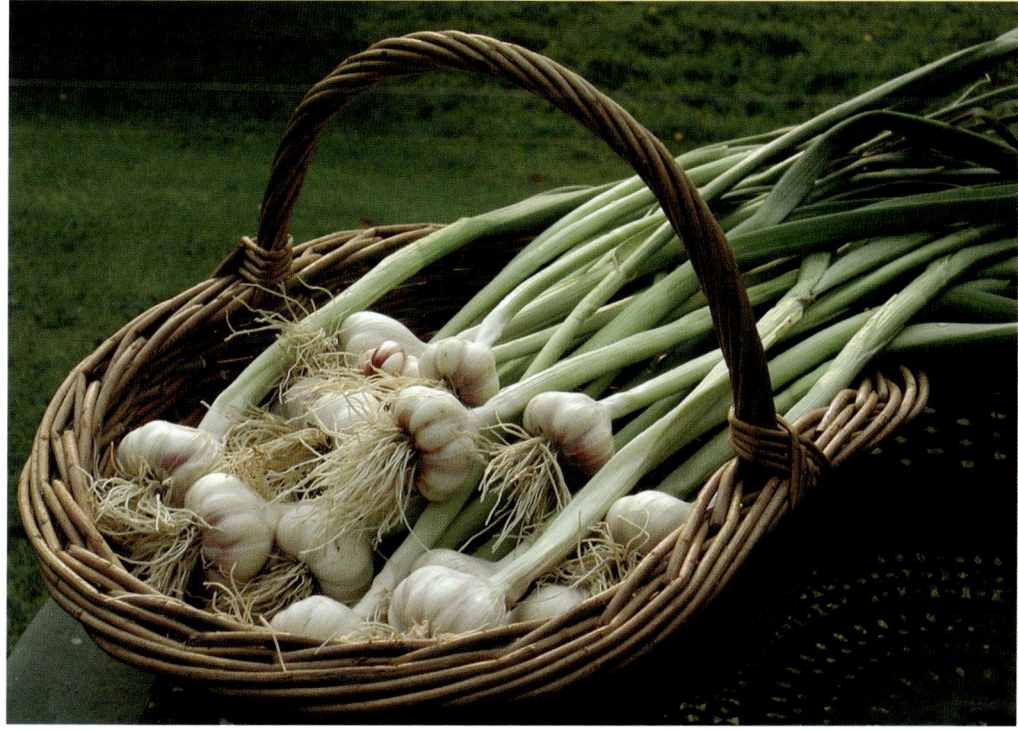

for preventing heart disease and rheumatism, and in China and Japan it has been prized for treating high blood pressure.

Throughout garlic's use in healing there run three main themes – it is strengthening and energy-giving, detoxifying and an antidote to poisoning, and it gives protection against a whole host of evil influences both physical and metaphysical; for centuries it has been used not only for warding off infections but other evils such as vampires, witches, demons and the evil eye.

The ancient Egyptians were well aware of garlic's stimulating and energy-giving properties; the builders of the great pyramid at Giza are said to have eaten garlic to give them strength. The Romans gave it to their workmen and soldiers to give them vigour and courage. The ancient Greeks also saw garlic as a symbol of strength and considered it a panacea and elixir of youth – athletes at the Olympic Games chewed it before taking part to improve their chances of victory. Culpeper said that garlic was ruled by Mars, and its name is said to come from the Anglo Saxon 'gar' meaning spear and 'lac' meaning plant, referring either to the shape of the sharp, tapering leaves, the fact that garlic imparts war-like properties or the fact that its nutritive and stimulating qualities were recommended for those going into battle.

Garlic has also been seen as rejuvenative and aphrodisiac, and when considering the wonderful array of therapeutic actions that garlic possesses, this is hardly surprising. It has been used for centuries as an invigorating tonic and used in many an elixir of youth. The fact that garlic imparts energy and vitality may explain its reputation as an aphrodisiac. It was sold in taverns and on street corners as such, and in Greece during the 5th century BC, street vendors apparently hawked garlic by chanting, *"It is truth, garlic gives men youth."*

Garlic is famous for its powerful defence against infection. Galen described it as 'the rustic's theriac,' meaning 'heal-all' or 'antidote to poison.' It has since become known as 'poor man's treacle.' It has been used for poisoning, diarrhoea, dysentery, cholera and typhoid. It was the principal ingredient in the famous 'Four Thieves' Vinegar' which was used successfully at Marseilles against the plague. Apparently four thieves confessed that while protected by covering themselves with this garlic vinegar, they plundered bodies of the dead in complete safety.

At the turn of this century garlic preparations were still a major remedy for TB. In the First World War, garlic was used to combat dysentery, typhus and to treat suppurating wounds; in the Second World War British doctors successfully warded off septic poisoning and gangrene of battle wounds with garlic.

Perhaps the ability of garlic to drive away infection is linked to its reputation for shielding people from evil and driving away vampires. Like many other strong-smelling herbs, garlic was believed to possess occult magic. In ancient China it was used to ward off the evil eye, and in many traditions garlic was hung in strings from roofs of houses and the sterns of boats to prevent attack by witches, sorcerers, demons and evil spirits. In Homer's Odyssey, it was garlic that Hermes recommended to Ulysses to protect him against the sorceress Circe. Garlic was dedicated to Hecate, the Greek goddess of witchcraft, famous for her knowledge of plants and her magical garden in Colchis on the shore of the Black Sea. Garlic was placed by the ancient Greeks on piles of stones at crossroads as supper for Hecate. There is a Mohammedan legend that tells, *"When Satan stepped out of the Garden of Eden after the fall of man, garlic sprang up from the spot where he placed his left foot and onion from that where his right foot touched."* Greek midwives used to hang garlic cloves around birthing rooms to safeguard the newborn child from disease and witchcraft and all over Europe garlic braids have been hung in doorways of houses and kitchens for centuries to keep away evil spirits and vampires.

Herbal Remedy

The humble garlic bulb, much maligned for its powerful and lingering odour, is a wonderful medicine. It contains sulphur compounds (alliin, alliein), lipids, anthrocyanins, quercetin, kaempferol, glycosides, scordinins, amino acids,

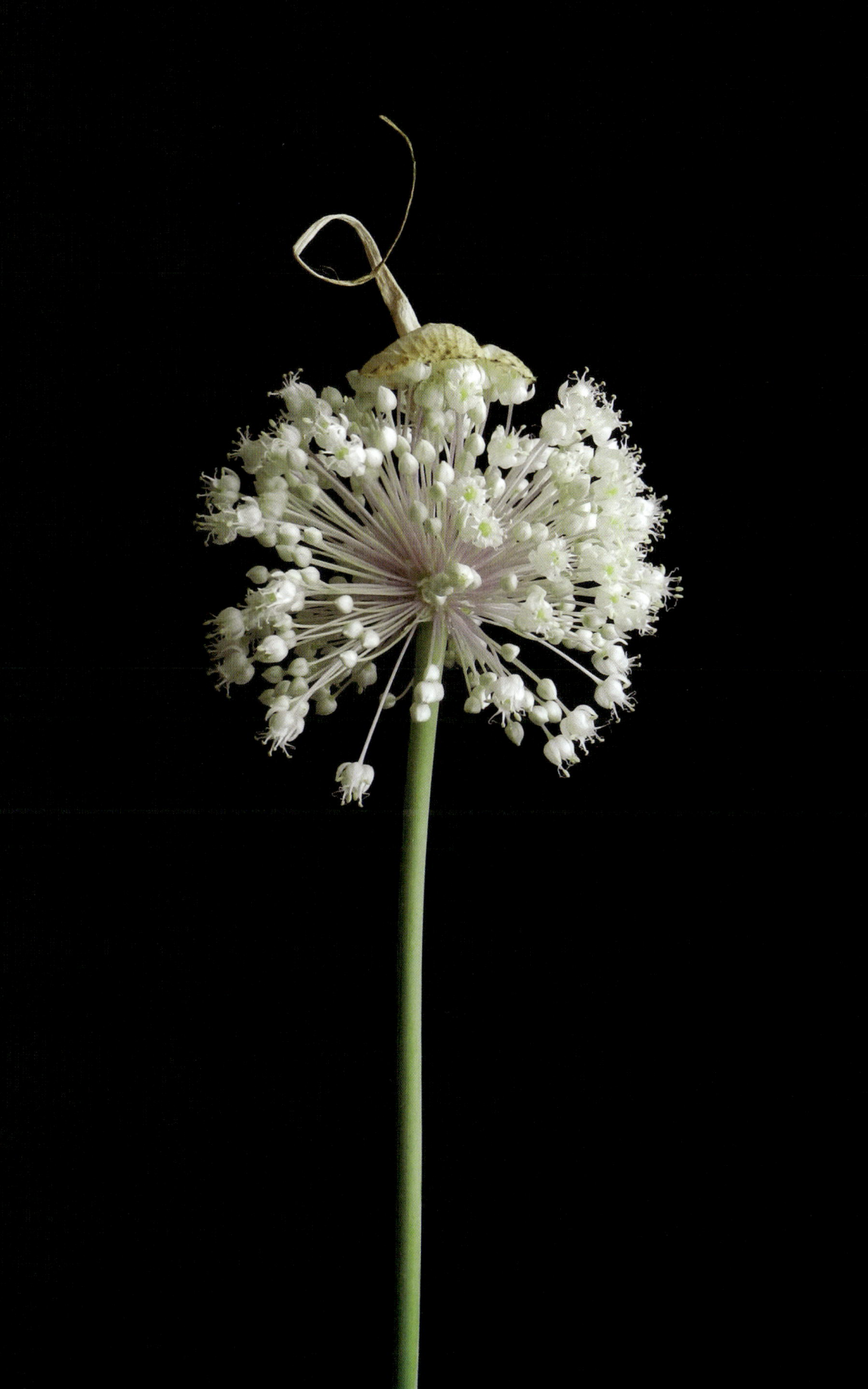

volatile oil, mucilage, germanium, glucokinins, vitamins, selenium and fructo-oligosaccharides. It was used traditionally in many parts of the world as a remedy for digestive problems, intestinal infections, chest infections including pneumonia and tuberculosis, dysentery, ear infections, abnormal growths and circulatory problems. Its ancient use is now explained by the fact that it has powerful antibacterial, antifungal, antiviral and antiparasitic effects which are exerted throughout the body. It is most effective when taken raw and crushed to release allicin, one of its most active constituents.

When absorbed from the digestive tract, garlic circulates in the bloodstream and is excreted via the lungs, bowels, skin and urinary system, all of which are disinfected in the process. Garlic can be used for sore throats, colds, flu, bronchial and lung infections. Like other pungent herbs, garlic acts as a decongestant, helping to clear catarrh, supporting its antimicrobial action in the respiratory tract. Its expectorant properties make it an excellent remedy for acute and chronic bronchitis, whooping cough and bronchial asthma, as well as sinusitis, chronic catarrh, hay fever and rhinitis. By stimulating the circulation and promoting sweating, it helps to bring down fevers.

Garlic has a beneficial effect on the digestion, stimulating the secretion of digestive enzymes and bile, increasing the absorption and assimilation of food and enhancing the movement of food through the gut. Together with its antimicrobial action, this has the effect of eliminating unfriendly gut bacteria and clearing toxins, thereby improving general health. Garlic

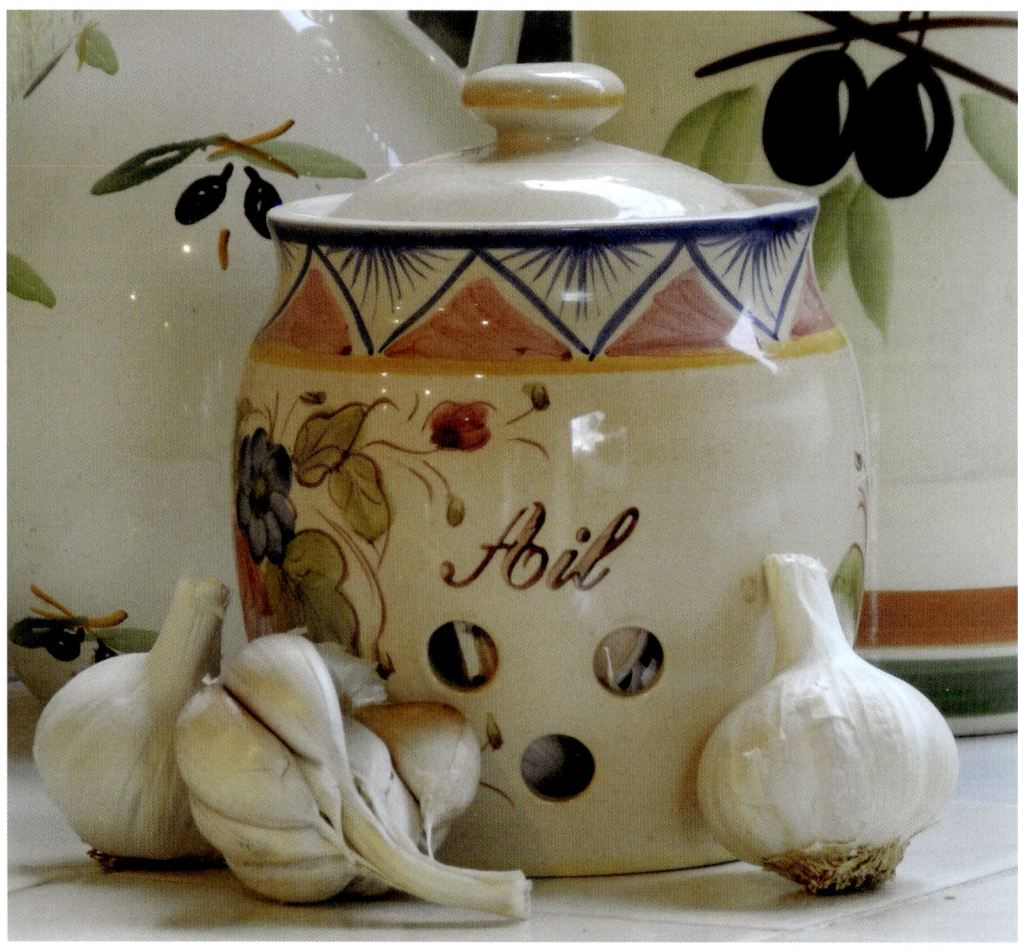

helps to combat infections in the gut and to re-establish the beneficial gut flora after an infection or taking antibiotics. It contains polysaccharides known as fructo-oligosaccharides that have a prebiotic effect, meaning that it supports the beneficial bacteria in the gut while deterring the unfriendly ones. It relieves wind and bloating that can be associated with poor digestion or disturbance of the gut flora. It inhibits *H. pylori* and so is helpful in the treatment of stomach ulcers. It is an effective remedy for worms when taken on an empty stomach, as well as for *Candida* and thrush in the mouth or vagina when used locally. It also supports the pancreas, enhancing the production of insulin and helping to lower blood sugar in type 2 diabetics.

Garlic has antioxidant actions protecting against damage caused by free radicals, and helps to slow the ageing process, verifying our ancestors' use of garlic as a rejuvenative tonic. Its sulphur compounds have anti-tumour activities. Garlic helps to protect the body against the effects of pollution and nicotine. By clearing toxins and warding off infection, it helps us maintain youthful vigour, and with such energy we are hopefully able not only to fend off disease, but also a range of more subtle negative influences.

In confirmation of the ancients' use of garlic for heart disease and high blood pressure, it is clear that garlic can significantly lower homocysteine, cholesterol, triglycerides and low-density lipoproteins in the blood. It can reduce atherosclerosis and the tendency to clotting and lower blood pressure. In this way taking raw garlic regularly can help to prevent cardiovascular disease, including heart attacks and strokes. Its vasodilatory action opens up the coronary arteries as well as blood vessels throughout the body, increasing the flow of blood to the tissues, helping to prevent cramps and circulatory disorders, and promoting a feeling of warmth and wellbeing, especially welcome on cold winter days and nights.

Externally, garlic can be crushed and macerated in oil or made into an ointment to apply to cuts and wounds, painful or inflamed joints, sprains, unbroken chilblains, athlete's foot, ringworm, stings, bites and warts. An oil infusion can be used as eardrops to relieve ear infections and earache and rubbed into the chest or even the soles of the feet for chest infections and coughs. Garlic vinegar can be used for disinfecting and dressing ulcers and septic wounds.

Homeopathic Remedy
Allium sativum suits those who are used to high living, who have voracious appetites and eat more than they drink. Garlic people tend to be anxious and impatient, full of fears, such as fear of not recovering, or fear of being poisoned. They may be sensitive and sad, weep during sleep, and have an impulse to run away.

Allium acts on the intestinal mucosa and can be used for colitis and diarrhoea with disturbance of the gut flora and dull pain in the lower abdomen. It also helps constipation and wind that burns as it is passed, and a sensitive stomach and bowel that is deranged from the least change of diet.

The Flower Essence
Garlic gives us strength and resilience physically, emotionally and psychically. It is particularly recommended for people who are plagued by fears and anxieties and emotionally drained as a result. In a depleted state they can be prone to chronic anxiety and insecurity and are vulnerable to negative influences. This may manifest as a poor immune response with a susceptibility to parasitic or viral infection or a tendency to be prey to emotional or psychic parasites in their lives. This leads inevitably to further draining of vital energy; their face may be pale, and they may feel scattered. Garlic helps to restore wholeness and strength, imparts courage to help overcome fears, and increases resistance to negative energy around us, helping us to maintain our energy and immunity.

Edible uses
Garlic is known to every cook and included in so many dishes that there is not enough space to list them here. However, it is well worth mentioning the delicious wild garlic for its culinary uses. All parts of the plant are edible, the stems, leaves, seeds and flowers, but it is best to use it when young before the flowers are fully out as it can begin to taste slightly bitter the older it becomes. The leaves are some of the earliest wild spring

greens and make wonderful food! They are a tasty addition to salads; they can be made into pesto as an alternative to or with basil, and eaten in sandwiches or with cheese and biscuits. They can be blanched and eaten like spinach, chopped and added to potato and rice dishes, frittatas, omelettes and other egg dishes, used to accompany meat and fish and incorporated into soups, stews and casseroles. The flowers are also edible as well as decorative. They look great sprinkled on a salad, and similarly can be added to salads, egg and pasta dishes, stir-fries and soups. Cooking reduces the flavour of the leaves and flowers, so they are best added towards the end of cooking. The bulbs are a bit like onions or spring onions and can be added to dishes raw or cooked. You can also use them in recipes instead of leeks, scallions or garlic. They can also be fermented or pickled.

Growing
Propagate by planting cloves of garlic in early spring or late autumn in well drained, moderately rich soil and full sun. Harvest late summer when the plant dies down, leave to dry outside for a few days then tie in bunches to hang or store in a cool dry place. Grows 6 – 12" (15 – 30cm) high. Garlic makes an excellent companion plant in fruit and vegetable gardens and under roses to keep aphids away.

Cautions
Avoid excess raw garlic in conditions associated with excess heat; inflammatory skin problems, hyperacidity, peptic ulcers and bleeding. Avoid large doses in pregnancy. Large doses of raw garlic (possibly in excess of 4 cloves a day) may cause allergic reactions, heartburn, flatulence, and gastro-intestinal upset. Raw garlic applied to the skin can cause contact dermatitis. Due to its reduction of platelet aggravation, it may cause post-operative bleeding. Except for small doses of cooked garlic, therapeutic doses of garlic should be discontinued 7–10 days before surgery due to anti-platelet activity.

Care should be taken with patients on anticoagulant/antiplatelet drugs, including Warfarin, Coumadin, Statins and Ticlopine who consume large amounts of garlic. Avoid with antihypertensive medications. Garlic has been found to interfere with the effectiveness of saquinavir, a drug used to treat HIV infection. Diabetics should monitor blood glucose.

Recipes

Wild Garlic Pesto
1 large bunch of wild garlic leaves, washed
1 small bunch of curly parsley, washed
60g pine nuts, toasted
60g parmesan cheese
150ml olive oil
squeeze of lemon juice
salt and pepper

Place all the ingredients into a food processor apart from the olive oil and blitz for a minute or two, then slowly pour in the olive oil until blended. Use for pasta, mash, dipping etc.

Garlic Syrup
4 garlic cloves, peeled and thinly sliced
Honey to cover

Cover the sliced garlic with runny honey and leave for 2 to 3 hours. Crush to extract all the juice.

Take a teaspoonful of the syrup up to 4 times per day during an acute infection

Garlic syrup is a pleasant-tasting way to take garlic and benefit from its antimicrobial and immune-stimulating properties. The honey also has antimicrobial properties and acts as an expectorant and draws out the properties of the garlic.

Probiotic Breakfast
1 large garlic clove
2 dessertspoons of fresh dill leaves
A handful of marigold petals
30 ml Aloe vera juice
2 teaspoon fresh oregano
3 teaspoon fresh basil
1 carton of live yoghurt

Add the fresh herbs to live yoghurt for a gut friendly breakfast or to 30mls of aloe vera juice with a little water or ginger tea for a tasty breakfast smoothie.

Althaea officinalis: Marshmallow

The Flower of Softness

With many a curve my banks I fret
By many a field and fallow,
And many a fairy foreland set
With willow-weed and mallow.

I chatter, chatter, as I flow
To join the brimming river,
For men may come and men may go,
But I go on for ever.
– Alfred Lord Tennyson (1809–1892)

Other Names: Malva, cheeses, schloss tea, meshmellish, drunkards, bullseyes, moorish mallow, white mallow, althea, mortification root, sweet weed, wymote, mallards, schlos

Parts Used: Roots, leaves and flowers

Marshmallow is a handsome and stately perennial with endearingly soft velvety leaves and pink flowers. As its name suggests, it is often found growing wild in damp, salty marshes and by the sea in Europe and Western Asia. In Devon the farmers used to call marshmallow 'meshmellish' and 'drunkards' because it was found growing close to water. Marshmallow is a member of the Malvaceae family, the word 'malva' coming from 'malakos' the Greek word for soft or soothing, referring to the demulcent and emollient properties of these plants. In fact, marshmallow is probably more soothing than any other plant because of its high mucilage content. *Althea* is derived from the Greek 'althane' meaning to cure or to heal as it has been known to ease so many ills.

The use of marshmallow as a nutritious and medicinal herb originated in ancient Greece and later spread to be incorporated into Arabic and Ayurvedic medicine. The Greeks ate the tender leaves and young tops, the Egyptians and Syrians grew it as a food and the Romans enjoyed the

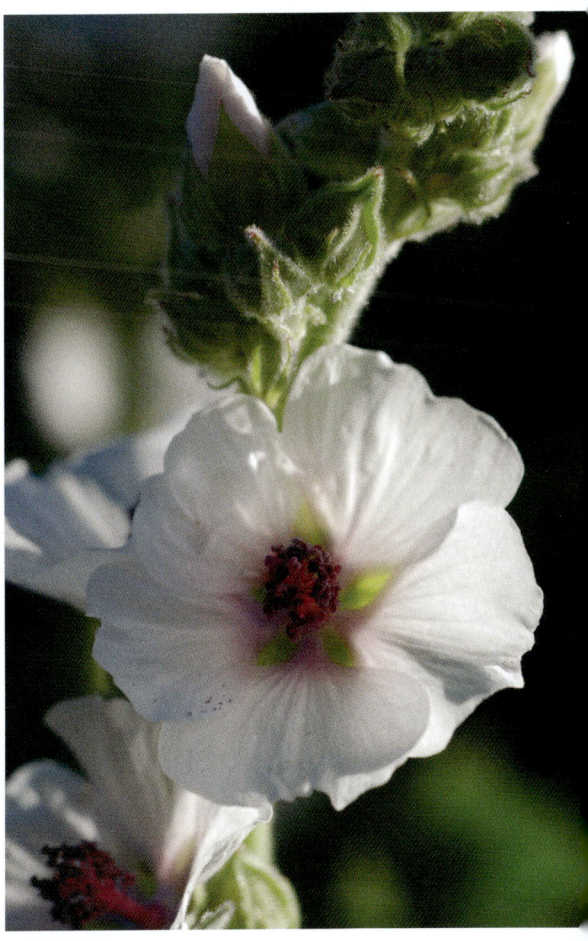

root as a vegetable in barley soup and stuffing for meat dishes. Aristophanes spoke of eating mallow shoots instead of wheat. Followers of Pythagorus considered mallows sacred as their flowers always turned towards the sun. It was for them the symbol of moderation and control of human passions, which they considered necessary for attainment of wisdom and health.

The Romans esteemed the plant 'in deliciis' meaning it afforded great pleasure among their 'dainties' or delicacies and placed it as the first dish on their tables. Pliny said, *"Whosoever shall take a spoonful of the Mallows shall that day be free from all diseases that may come to him."* The laxative properties of the leaves and root were described by Cicero and Horace. In Palestine, according to the Book of Job, the plant was eaten by the poor to eke out their food, *"Who cut up Mallows by the bushes and juniper roots for their meat."*

Marshmallow was also valued for its soothing, pain-relieving properties. In ancient Persia it was given to teething babies to reduce inflammation. Later Gerard said, *"The leaves be with good effect mixed with fomentations and poultices against pains of the sides of the stone and of the bladder; also in a bath they serve to take away any manner of pain."*

Mallow has been a symbol of sweetness and mildness – it certainly has a sweet flavour and smooth texture. Marshmallow is the origin of the soft sweets of the same name. In the nineteenth century, a medicinal sweet was prepared using marshmallow juice, egg white and sugar and used to sooth children's sore throats. Similarly, French pharmacists used to prepare a famous medicinal sweet known as *Pate de guimauve* from the roots to ease teething problems in babies. The modern marshmallow sweets unfortunately do not contain anything of the plant or its constituents.

Herbal Remedy
Marshmallow is a wonderful remedy for any kind of irritation or inflammation, both internally and externally, because of its great soothing and healing properties. It is rich in mucilage and also contains asparagin, tannins, pectin, sterols, coumarins, flavonoids, phenolic acids, amino acids, salicylic acid, minerals including calcium, iron, magnesium, manganese, phosphorus, potassium, selenium, zinc, and vitamins B1, B2, B3, E and C.

The mucilage in the whole plant especially the root is a thick, slimy substance that coats, protects and soothes the mucous membranes throughout the digestive, respiratory and urinary systems, particularly when it is used in a cold infusion. The anti-inflammatory flavonoids and phenolic acids and astringent tannins combine to make marshmallow an excellent remedy to heal inflammation and ulceration of the mucous membranes. With its cooling effect, it can be thought of whenever there is excess heat and inflammation in the body.

When you take marshmallow, the mucilage is not digested and remains unaltered until it reaches the colon, which is why it works well on most inflammatory gut problems. It can be used to regenerate a damaged gut lining and to treat heartburn, indigestion, gastritis, peptic ulcers, IBS, ulcerative colitis and Crohn's disease. It can ease constipation caused by dryness, while it can also reduce excess peristalsis and relieve diarrhoea. It can be a helpful aid to radiologic oesophageal examination, preventing irritation and inflammation and can help blood sugar management in diabetes. Its antimicrobial action has been found to be effective against *E. coli*, so it can be useful in gastro-enteritis and even dysentery.

Marshmallow, particularly the flowers, are rich in antioxidants notably alpha-tocophereol (vitamin E) and these can help to prevent free radical damage that is linked to degenerative disease such as arthritis, cardiovascular problems, cancer, cataracts and other problems related to inflammation and ageing. It can help to reduce cholesterol and blood clotting.

Marshmallow enhances immunity, stimulates production of white blood cells and induces phagocytosis (the process in which white blood cells engulf bacteria and dead cell tissues). It is antimicrobial against bacteria including *Proteus vulgaris, Pseudomonas aeruginos,* and

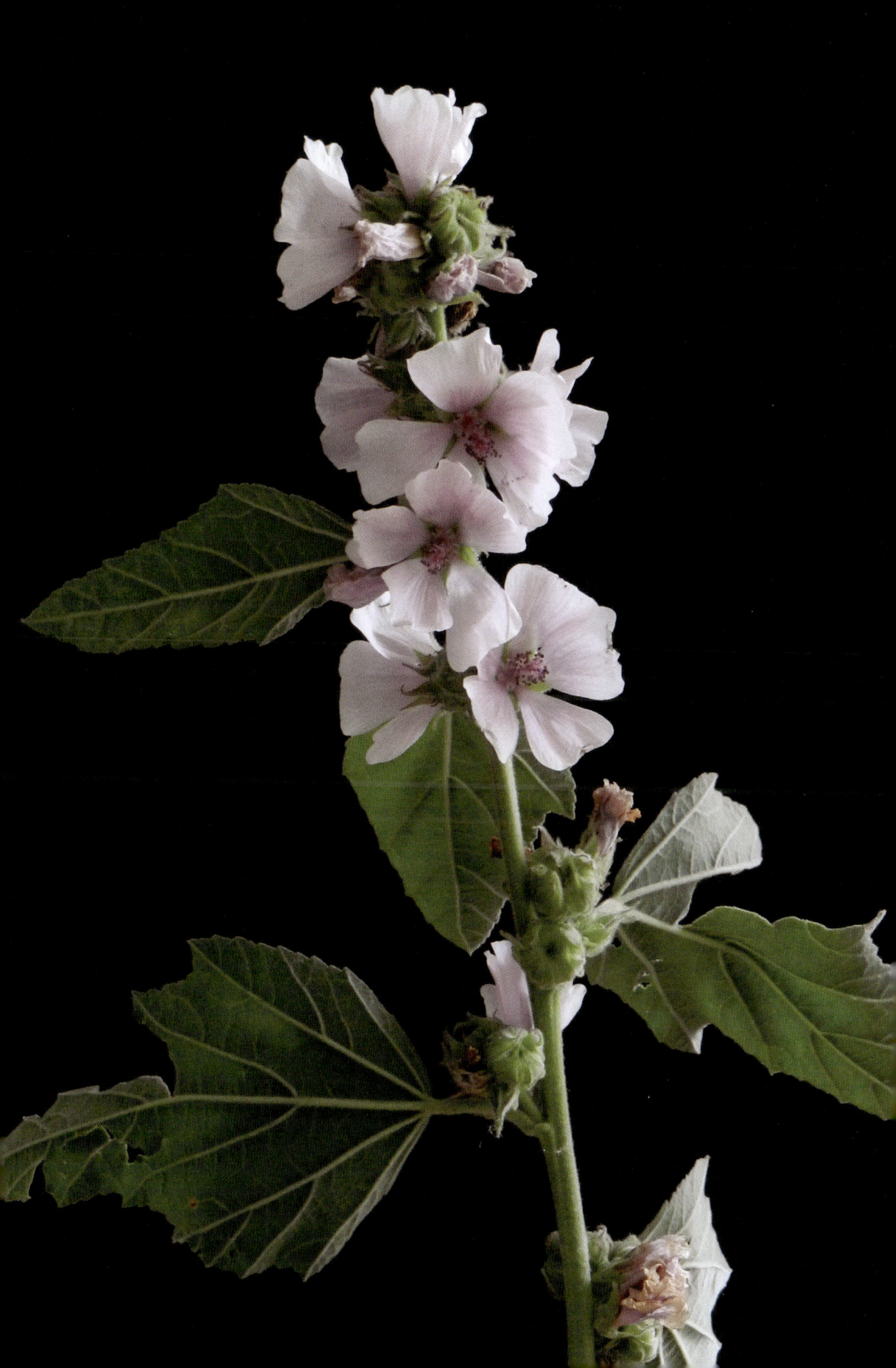

Staphylococcus aureus Its antimicrobial and immune-enhancing actions are helpful in warding off and treating respiratory infections. It acts as a soothing expectorant, easing harsh dry coughs, sore throats, laryngitis, croup and bronchitis. It also helps to clear catarrhal congestion, and may be useful for asthma, especially where there is heat and inflammation in the bronchial tubes.

Marshmallow acts as a soothing diuretic that can relieve burning symptoms of infection and inflammation in cystitis, urethritis and irritable bladder. It was an old remedy for easing the passage of urinary gravel and stones and has traditionally been added to formulae to ease childbirth and to improve the production of breast milk. The scrubbed, chopped roots of marshmallow, as well as the leaves and flowers, can be used as a nutritious and strengthening tonic after surgery, a bout of illness, or when generally run down.

Externally, marshmallow roots and leaves can be used as a soothing, antiseptic gargle for sore throats, tonsillitis, mouth problems and spongy, inflamed gums as it helps combat periodontal bacteria. Teething babies can be given a piece of marshmallow root to gnaw, to cool their inflamed gums. Adults can use the root as a tooth cleaner.

The leaves and flowers can be rubbed onto insect bites, wasp and bee stings, scalds and burns, sunburn and skin rashes, to reduce irritation and inflammation. They help soothe and heal inflammatory skin problems including acne, eczema and sore nipples. They were used in the past for bruises, sprains and strains, as well as joint and muscular aches and pains.

Marshmallow root or leaves can be used with lavender and flax oil and applied to scalds, burns and sunburn. A warm poultice made from

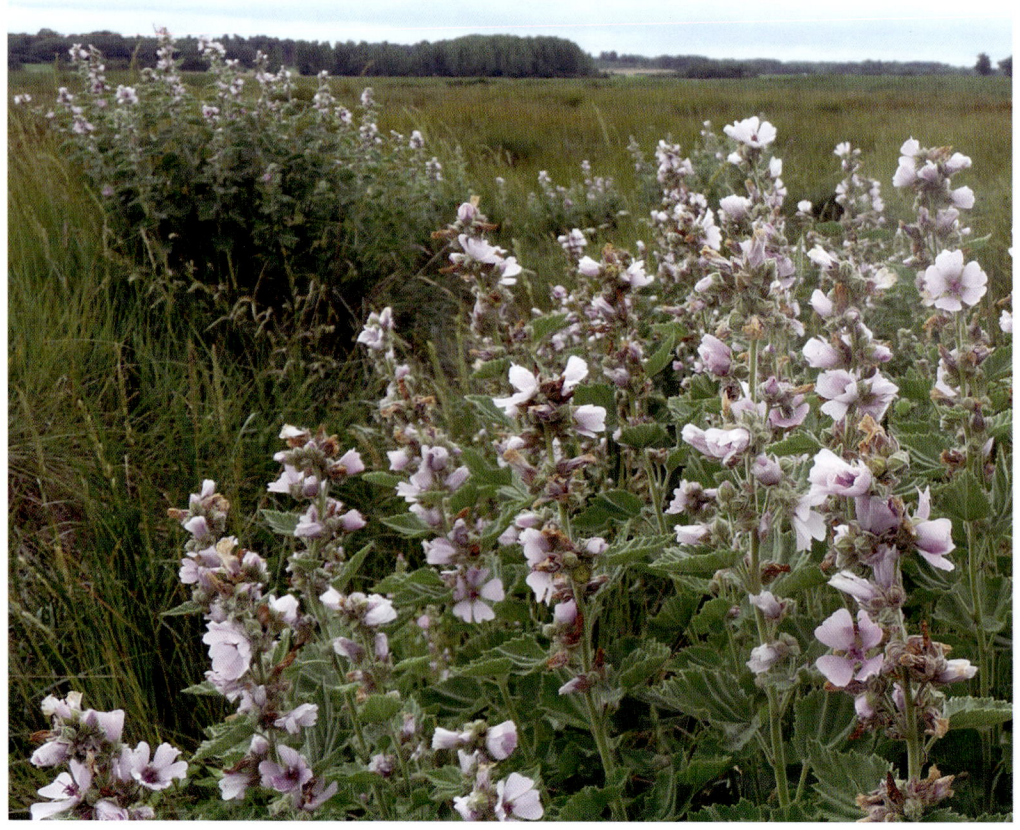

the flowers, leaves or pulverised root will help draw splinters out and can be applied locally for mastitis, breast abscesses, boils and abscesses. A decoction of the root makes a soothing lotion for bathing inflamed eyes.

Flower Essence
Marshmallow flower essence is calming, grounding and softening. It promotes ease in relationships with others and oneself. Just as the sweet, soft marshmallow plant helps soothe irritation and inflammation as well as heal wounds, marshmallow flower essence helps soothe and soften inflamed feelings like impatience, irritability, anger and other emotional hurts and enable us to resolve conflicts and regenerate friendships.

It is particularly good for people who get stuck in a state of tension or anger and have resistance to change or an inability to consider others' feelings. It can ease the situation and allow things to move gently on and soften those who put up protective barriers for fear of getting hurt.

The essence can be taken to ease pressure and tension in the head and neck. It could be helpful in headaches, tension in the jaw and shoulder areas and can be grounding when feeling lightheaded or spacey.

Edible uses
Marshmallow leaves and flowers have a mild taste, so can be added to almost any dish. The young tops and tender leaves and flowers can be added to salads and a handful of chopped leaves can be added to soups in the last 15 minutes of cooking. Let the soup sit for 10 minutes before serving to allow the mucilage to be extracted out of the leaves. Sautéed, chopped mallow leaves or flowers can be added to an omelette or stir fry, or they can be rolled and stuffed as you would cabbage leaves.

The root can be dried and then ground into a powder, made into a paste and roasted to make the sweet *'marshmallow'*. It can also be boiled and fried with onions and eaten as a vegetable. An infusion made with cold water takes up the mucilage and is best for soothing.

Growing
To propagate, sow seeds in late spring in-situ in damp soil or in trays in autumn and leave outside over the winter. Alternatively, divide roots in spring or autumn. Grows 2 – 4 feet (60 – 120cm) high, it likes full sun and flowers from July – Sept from its second year. Marshmallow self-seeds easily. Butterflies love it.

Cautions
Marshmallow is considered a very safe herb and virtually no side effects have been reported. It may cause low blood sugar in some people and reduce absorption of prescription drugs and supplements; take either six hours before or after taking other medication.

Recipes

Cough Syrup
Place 3 tbsp of the fresh crushed leaves and flowers or root and cover with cold water. Let it stand for about 8 hours. Press and strain and add 1 teaspoon honey and juice of ½ lemon.

Take in tablespoon doses 3 times daily in chronic problems and up to every 2 hours in acute problems.

Tea
To one cup of cold water, add three teaspoons of the dried herb or root, or a quarter of a cup of fresh herb, let it stand for eight hours. Press and drain, warm and sweeten to taste.

Strengthening Tonic
The scrubbed, chopped roots of marshmallow, as well as the leaves, could be useful as a nutritious and strengthening tonic after surgery, a bout of illness, or when generally run down.

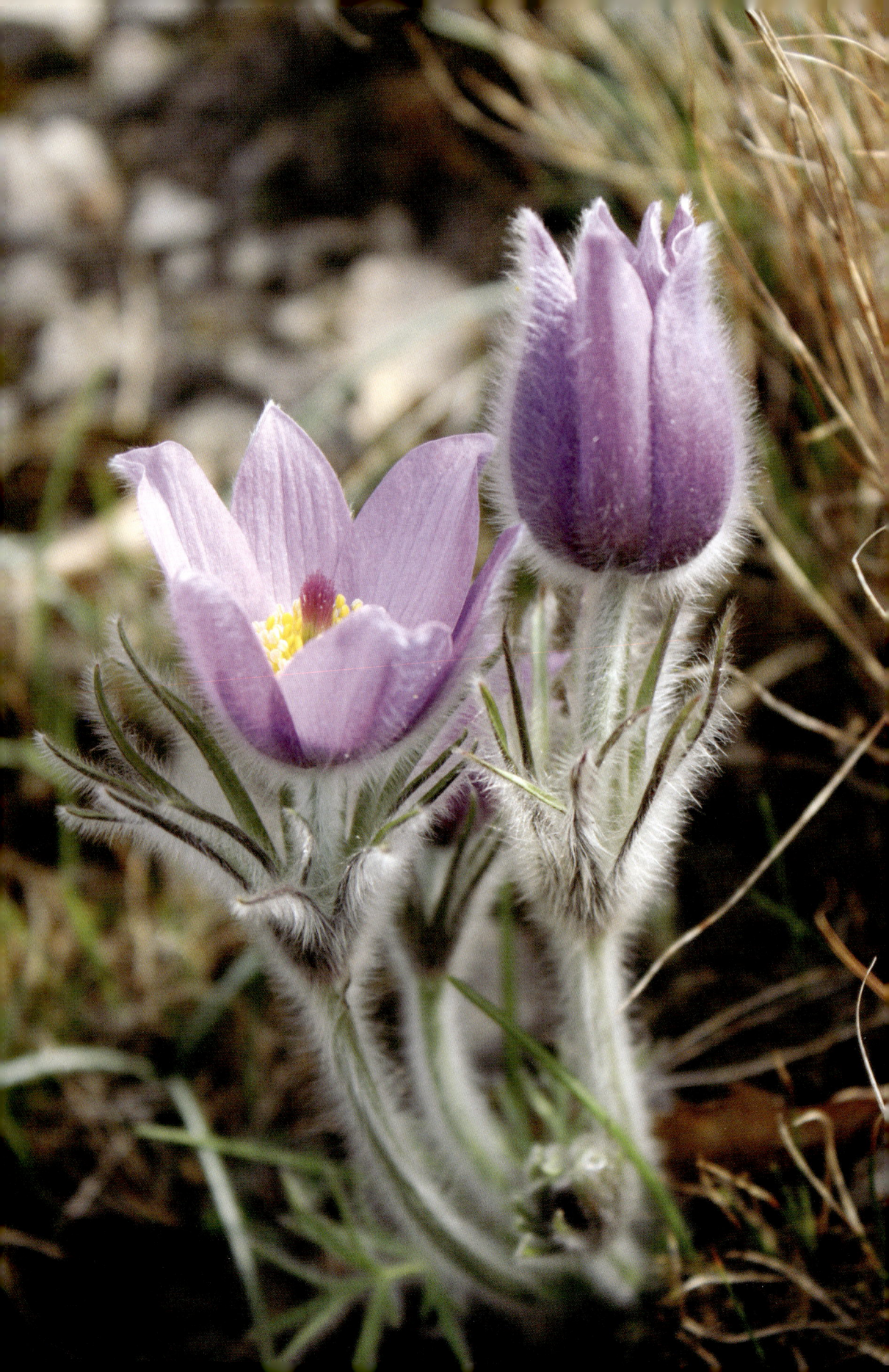

Anenome pulsatilla: Pasque Flower

The Flower of Forsakenness

> *Then came the wind flower*
> *In the valley left behind, pale*
> *As a wounded maiden*
> *with purple streaks of woe*
> – Sydney Dorrell (1824-1874)

Other Names: European pasque flower, pulsatilla, passe fleur, passe flower, easter flower, meadow anemone, flatulence flower

Parts Used: Aerial parts

Pasque flower is often called *pulsatilla* and is a beautiful member of the Ranunculaceae family; in fact, with its silky purple flowers and silvery hairs like a halo followed by feathery seed heads, it is one of the most beautiful wildflowers of Europe. Although delicate looking, it is remarkably resilient, flowering in early spring but often in very wintery weather. It is said that pasque flower was originally called 'passe flower' from the French 'passe-fleur' because it surpassed all other flowers in beauty. In 1597 Gerard renamed it 'pasque flower' as it came into flower in spring and often on Easter day ('*pascha*') in the Northern hemisphere and was popular for dying Easter eggs green.

Pasque flower is also known as the 'wind flower' as the name 'anemone' comes from the Greek 'anemos' meaning wind. In Greek mythology, Anemone was a beautiful nymph beloved of Zephyr, the god of the West wind. The goddess Flora who was his wife, became very jealous and transformed Anemone into the little wind flower and she was abandoned by Zephyr to Boreas, god of the North wind. Boreas wooed her every Spring and she would open only at his bidding. For this reason, in the language of flowers anemone means 'forsaken' and represents all those forsaken in love.

Pasque flower is ruled by the planet Venus and there is another story that tells that the flower sprang from the tears of Venus, the goddess of love, as she wept over the body of Adonis who had been slain, and for this reason also anemone means 'forsaken'. However frail this flower may sound it resiliently withstands the cruel winds of the early spring and it does have remarkable healing powers. The first anemone of the year to be found, it is said, has special healing properties, and it used to be wrapped in red cloth and tied on the arms of the sick.

Herbal Remedy

Dried pasque flower and leaves contain sesquiterpene lactones, glycosides, tannins, saponins, resin, volatile oil, chelidonic acid, flavonoids, glucose, tannins, resins, pectin, calcium and magnesium. It makes a wonderful tonic for the nervous system, soothing and calming anxiety and restoring strength when nervously depleted. By promoting relaxation and sleep, it aids recovery of energy and resilience when feeling run down by helping to conserve nervous energy. It also makes a good remedy for reducing pain. It can be helpful in nervous exhaustion, low mood and depression, insomnia, nightmares, irritability, weepiness, clinginess and fear of being alone.

Pasque flower is particularly good for relieving muscle tension, pain, spasm and inflammation especially in the reproductive system, both male and female. It is one of the best herbs for relieving uterine cramps whether from period pain, during childbirth or after pains. It is also valuable for infections and inflammation in the reproductive system. During childbirth, its relaxant and tonic action in the uterus helps to regulate contractions, and to promote and facilitate the birth. After the birth, pasque flower can be used for any kind of over-excitement, weepiness or depression and can be helpful for afterpains and postnatal depression. It is used for menstrual disorders, including late onset of periods, painful periods and PMS, tiredness or nervous distress related to menstruation. It is also useful during the menopause for weepiness and depression. With its powerful antispasmodic action, pasque flower can also be used for abdominal pain and colic, headaches, asthma and neuralgia.

Pasque flower has a detoxifying action. It has an affinity with mucous membranes, particularly in the respiratory and digestive systems and is excellent for clearing thick, yellow-green catarrh. It also has an affinity with the circulatory system and can be used to improve venous circulation and to treat varicose veins and nosebleeds. It is also helpful to stem bleeding and for anaemia.

With its diaphoretic effect when taken in a hot infusion, it promotes blood flow to the surface of the body and increases sweating. This can help to reduce fevers and bring out the rash in eruptive infections such as measles, which then speeds recovery. Once the rash appears, the fever tends to go down and the patient normally feels a lot better. Its antibacterial action also helps combat infections involved with fever.

With its astringent and antibacterial actions, pasque flower is well worth taking for colds, acute and chronic catarrh, coughs and ear problems including otitis media and earache. Its antispasmodic effect can help relieve tightness in the chest and ease dry paroxysmal coughs and asthma. Its analgesic, antibacterial, astringent and anti-inflammatory actions are helpful in painful inflammatory eye conditions including scleritis, iritis, glaucoma and cataracts.

Externally an infusion of pasque flower can be used as an antibacterial wash for boils and acne and a douche for vaginal thrush. The tincture or an infused oil can be used locally for earache. A lukewarm infusion has been used as a wash to treat eye conditions such as iritis, cataracts and glaucoma.

Homeopathic Remedy
Pulsatilla has similar applications although the pasque flower used is *A. pratensis*. The name wind flower is particularly in keeping with its homeopathic use, for a pulsatilla person is changeable, yielding and gentle, fickle and easily blown around by the wind. Physical symptoms tend to come and go and are all characterised by changeability.

Emotionally, pulsatilla types are like changeable weather – one moment sunshine and showers the next – and they laugh and cry easily. Behind their fickleness is a deep fear of being alone, of being forsaken just like the nymph Anemone.

Pulsatilla has a particular affinity with the female reproductive tract and is used for menstrual disorders, including late onset of periods. It also has applications during pregnancy and in childbirth, and for afterpains and postnatal depression. Like the herbal remedy, homeopathic pulsatilla also has an affinity with mucous membranes and is used for thick, yellow-green catarrh.

Pulsatilla will help where there are varicose veins, sluggish venous circulation, chilliness, anaemia, nosebleeds, fever, measles with catarrh, lethargy and restless sleep with troubled dreams. The patient feels worse in a stuffy atmosphere and better in fresh air.

Flower Essence
Like the windflower blown about by the spring breezes, people needing the flower remedy tend to be changeable, happy then sad, full of vitality one moment then exhausted the next. Like the frail-sounding anemone, they can be tearful, lonely and vulnerable and yet still essentially resilient.

The flower essence allows our gentle, emotional side to flourish while engendering a sense of inner security and groundedness. Pulsatilla enhances our inner strength and stability, allowing us to express ourselves better emotionally and spiritually, while balancing our vital energy.

Growing
Pasque flower is a hardy perennial found wild on limestone or chalk, in dry grassy places. It reaches about 12" (30cm) high. It grows well in well drained alkaline soil and full sun and can be propagated by seed sown in early summer and barely covered with soil. Germination may be slow.

Cautions
Fresh pasque flower should not be used as a herbal remedy as it contains the toxic glycoside ranunculin which breaks down to form protoanemonin and may irritate the skin (gardeners beware!). If ingested protoanemonin may irritate the kidneys or urinary tract. Protoanemonin is unstable and breaks down further to form anemonin when dried which then makes the plant non-toxic.

Avoid use with painkillers, during pregnancy and breastfeeding. Can cause gastroenteritis, vomiting, diarrhoea or convulsions in large doses. Repeated handling may cause skin irritation and hypersensitivity reactions can occur in therapeutic doses. Use under direction of a qualified herbalist.

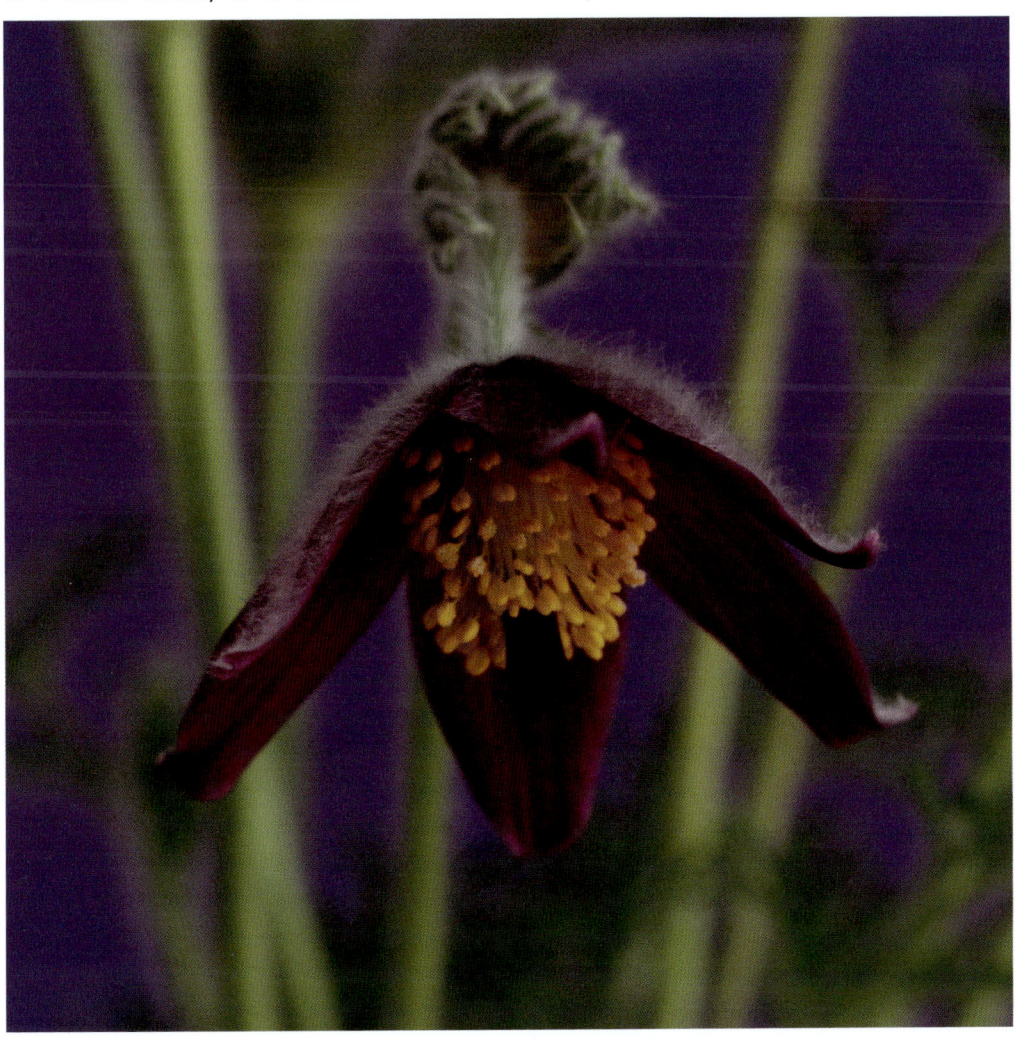

Anethum graveolens: Dill

The Flower of Slumber

Therewith her Vervain and her Dill
That hindreth witches in their will
– Michael Drayton and Thomas Maybank, Nymphidia 1627

Also called: Dill weed, meeting house seed, dillby, dill herb, dilly, European dill

Parts used: Leaves, flowers and seeds

One of the most delightful of all aromas in the garden is that of feathery dill. It is released when we brush against its sweet, aniseed-scented leaves. Dill is a member of the **Apiaceae/ Umbelliferae family and** with its aromatic leaves and umbels of tiny yellow flowers, it can be found growing wild all over its native Mediterranean. The tranquilising effects of dill have been known since the days of the ancient Greek physician Dioscorides and the Roman Pliny in the 1st century AD. Apparently the Greeks used to cover their heads with dill leaves to induce sleep. Its name is said to come from the Saxon word 'dilla' meaning to lull, due to its ability to relax babies and children into a restful sleep. The volatile oil in dill seeds and leaves relaxes smooth muscle throughout the body.

Dill's Latin name *Anethum* comes from the Greek 'aitho' meaning to burn, as dill seeds were popular in the days of ancient Greece to burn as incense. It was known in Medieval England and valued as a vital ingredient of love potions. In these times, it used to be hung in doorways and at windows to keep away witches and the 'evil eye' as Drayton's rhyme above confirms.

Dill has been used in Ayurvedic medicines since ancient times and is still highly popular as a spice in Indian cuisine, for enhancing digestion and combatting worms. It was used by Egyptian physicians 5000 years ago as a digestive aid and a remedy for wind and bloating, and traces have been found in Roman ruins in Great Britain; the Romans chewed the seeds to promote digestion and hung garlands of dill in their dining halls to prevent upset stomachs. The seeds used to be called 'meeting house seeds' as they were chewed during long church services to stop the stomach rumbling. Because of its relaxant and digestive properties, dill seed has long been used in the old-fashioned preparation *Gripe Water*, the mothers' standby that has been given to generations of babies to relieve colic, soothe crying and relax them into sleep.

Culpeper the 17th century herbalist said of dill, *"Mercury has the dominion of this plant and therefore to be sure it strengthens the brain."* Apparently, the leaves have traditionally been eaten with fish to impart a spicy flavour as well as to exhilarate the brain and impart intelligence. Culpeper also recommended a decoction of dill seeds or herb to be drunk with white wine as a *"gallant expeller of wind and provoker of terms"* as it was valued as an emmenagogue to bring on periods and as an aid to childbirth.

Herbal Remedy

As a wonderfully aromatic herb, dill mainly benefits the digestive system. It contains volatile oils which account for its characteristic smell and taste, as well as flavonoids, coumarins, triterpenes, magnesium, iron, calcium, potassium and vitamin C. Any dish or tea with dill would make a good appetiser as dill stimulates the flow of digestive juices and enhances appetite, digestion and absorption of nutrients. The volatile oil in the flowers, leaves and seeds has warming and relaxing effects on the smooth muscle throughout the body and particularly in the digestive tract where they release tension and spasm. Dill is a popular remedy for relieving colic and wind, bloating, indigestion and nausea, constipation as well as diarrhoea. It protects the

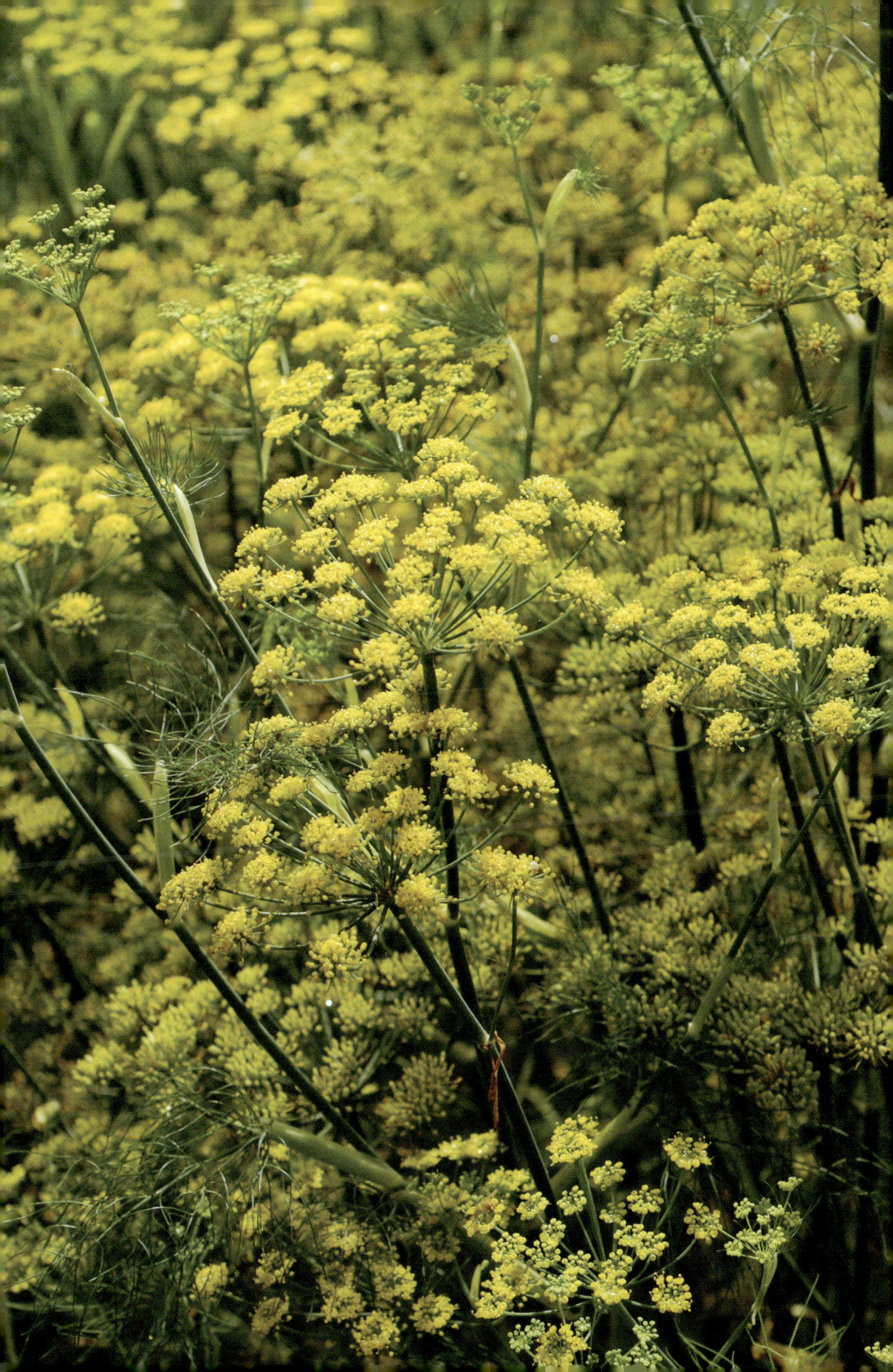

gut lining from irritation and inflammation and helps to prevent peptic ulcers.

The volatile oils in the seeds have antibacterial actions inhibiting the growth of several bacteria including *Staphylococcus*, *Streptococcus*, *Escherichia coli* and *Pseudomonas*. They also have antifungal actions against *Candida* and a vermicidal (combating worms) effect and they may have anti-cancer properties. By improving digestion and absorption and with its antimicrobial actions, dill clears toxins and combats unfriendly bacteria as well as worms in the gut. By helping to reestablish a healthy gut flora, dill can improve brain function as well as immunity. You can chew the seeds to aid digestion and reduce bad breath.

The renowned Ayurvedic text called *Kashyapa samhitaa* says that dill has tonic, rejuvenating and 'medhya' (intellect-promoting) properties. It has been used traditionally to strengthen the mind and to help alleviate tiredness from disturbed nights. It is interesting that while dill enlivens the brain, it also has a wide reputation as tranquilising remedy with a gentle enough action to be useful for babies. Certainly, dill's relaxant properties can be helpful in reducing tension and stress and can be used in recipes for insomnia.

Dill is particularly good for stress-related digestive disorders such as wind, colic and constipation. The relaxant properties of dill can also be felt in the reproductive system and with its emmenagogic actions, it can be helpful for painful or erratic periods. In the East, dill is given to pregnant women prior to childbirth to ease the birth. It increases milk supply in breast feeding mothers. With its antimicrobial, antispasmodic and expectorant effects, dill helps to clear infection and congestion from the respiratory tract; a hot decoction of the seeds can be taken to relieve asthma and harsh, irritating coughs as well as clear mucous and congestion in coughs and chest infections.

As an effective diuretic, dill aids the elimination of toxins from the body via the urinary system and is useful for irritable bladder, cystitis, stones and gravel. Its antioxidant action has a beneficial effect in the cardiovascular system, reducing harmful cholesterol levels.

Externally dill's analgesic and anti-inflammatory properties help relieve pain and swelling. An infused oil can be included in massage oils and liniments for abdominal pain, colic, arthritis and earache.

Aromatherapy Oil
Like the herb, dill seed essential oil has a warm and aniseed-like aroma which is revitalising and restoring. It can have a relaxing and balancing effect on the emotions and can help relieve anxiety and promote sleep. With its relaxant and digestive properties, it can be used for wind, bloating and abdominal pain and was traditionally used in the preparation of gripe water. The oils are ingredients in warming liniments and massage oils to ease tension and spasm in muscles throughout the body, particularly the digestive, reproductive and respiratory systems. It can be helpful for period pain and back pain.

When applied to the skin in a carrier oil, dill oil aids healing in cuts and wounds. When used as a massage oil it enters the general circulation and has a diuretic effect, clearing excess water and toxins from the body. The oil can be added to hair treatments for head lice and works well in spray-on formulations. It can be used as an insect repellent and it is toxic to growing larvae and adults of *Tribolium castaneum*, the wheat flour pest.

The Flower Essence
Dill makes a good remedy for those who feel stressed and nervously overwrought by the hustle and bustle of life. Those who feel over-stimulated or overwhelmed by the world around them, who suffer a kind of 'sensory indigestion', may well have physical signs of stress such as digestive problems and for such people dill can engender a sense of relaxation and inner nourishment. Rather than seeking a remote place cut off from sensory stimulation and living as an ascetic to develop spiritually, dill is used to help us use the world of the senses as a vehicle for understanding our inner selves, rather than a distraction from our higher purpose.

Edible Uses

Dill is a favourite herb in European, Middle Eastern and Eastern cooking; it certainly can transform everyday dishes into culinary delights with a hint of the sunny Aegean. Anything with dill would make a good appetiser as dill has a beneficial effect on the digestion, stimulating the flow of digestive juices and enhancing appetite and digestion.

Recipe

Gripe Water

This can very easily be made by adding ½ ounce (15 gm) of bruised dill seeds to 1 cup (225 mls) of boiling water and allowing it to infuse for 10 to 15 minutes.

Strain and when lukewarm offer a tablespoon (15 mls) to your baby when needed.

With its wonderful taste and aroma, dill leaves add a certain something to *tsadziki* (yoghurt and cucumber) and *spanakorizo* (spinach with rice). It is lovely in salads and as a garnish, particularly with potatoes and fish.

Growing

Propagate by sowing seeds in spring and again in midsummer, in rich, well-drained soil and full sun. It likes a sheltered position. Grow well away from fennel as they cross-pollinate easily. It looks a lot like fennel and both herbs are very easy and rewarding to grow, either in pots on a patio or in the garden. Dill can also be grown or bought in small pots to keep on a kitchen windowsill.

Caution

Caution in oesophageal reflux. Fresh juice may cause dermatitis. Since dill was used traditionally to ease childbirth, the essential oil is best avoided in pregnancy until the last trimester.

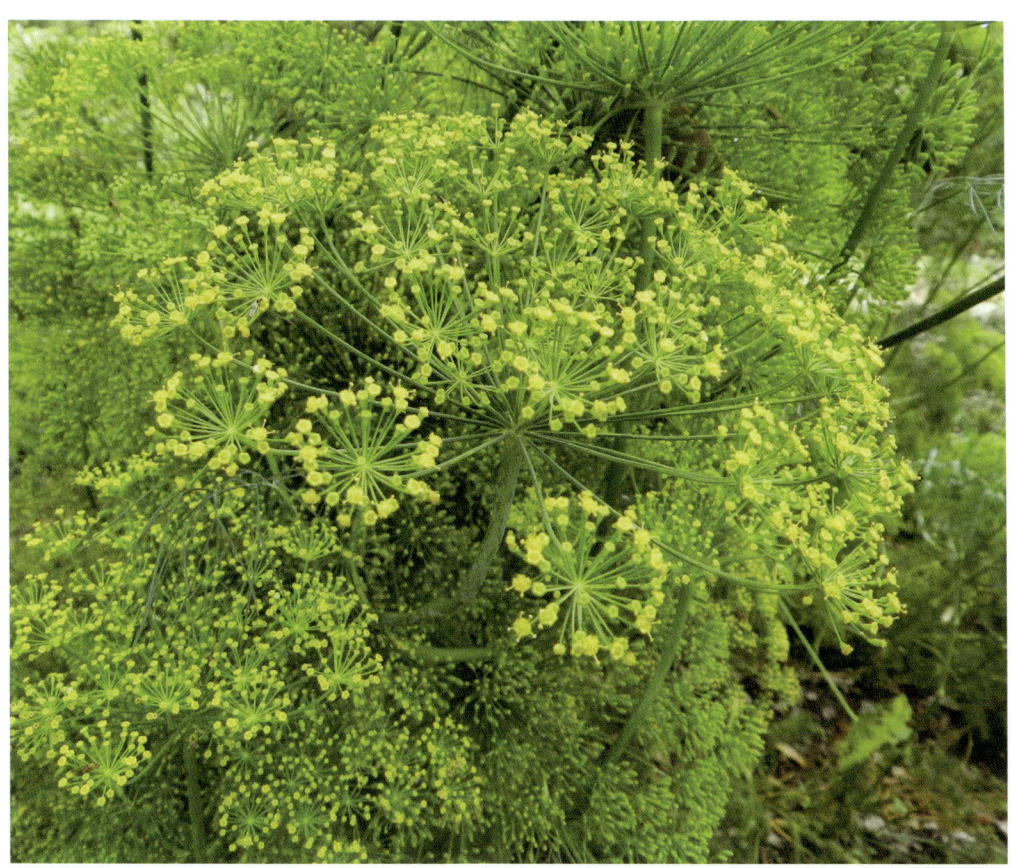

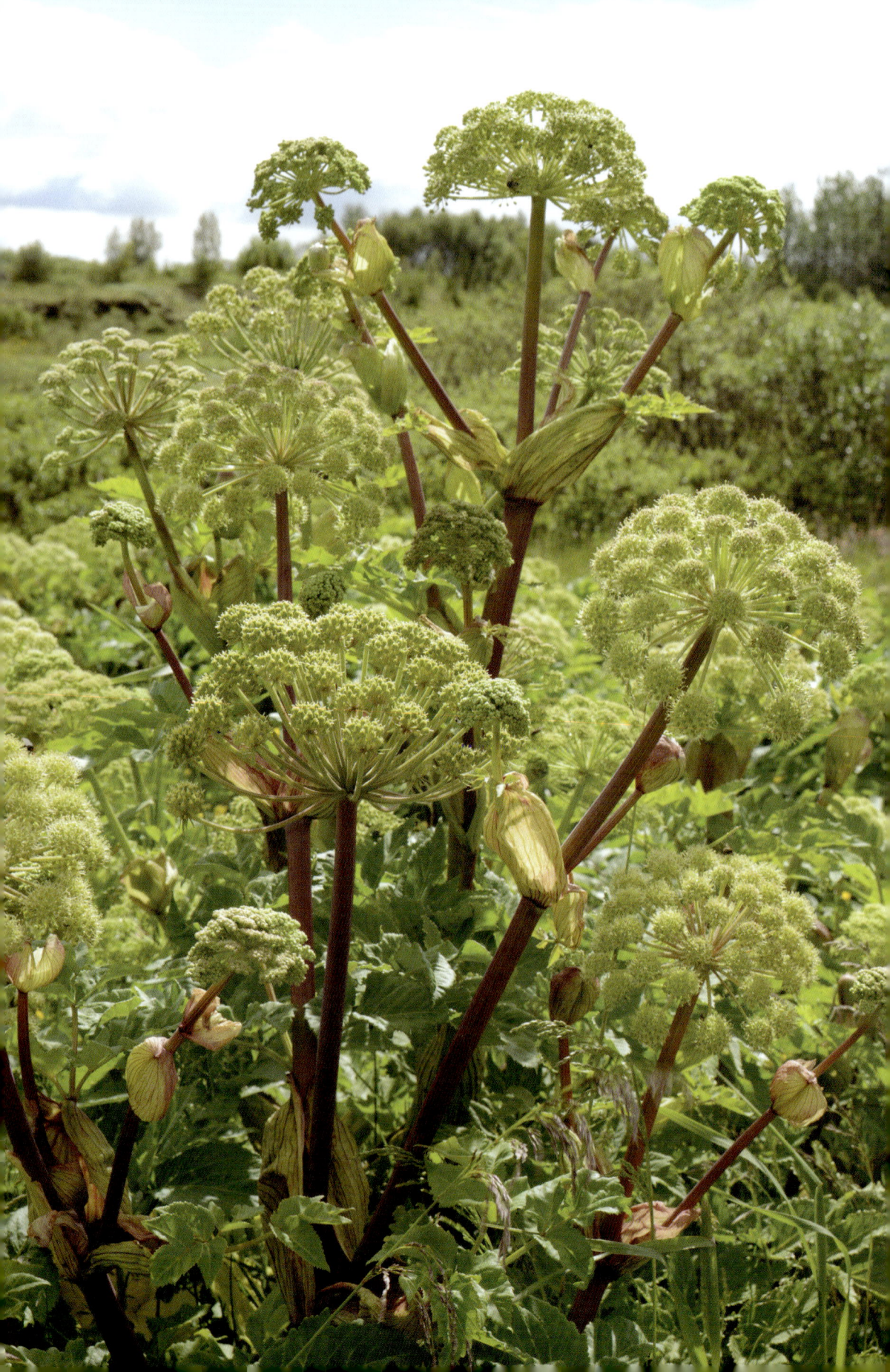

Angelica archangelica: Angelica

The Flower of Inspiration

Contagious aire ingendring pestilence
Infects not those that in their mouth have ta'en,
Angelica, that happy counterbane,
Sent down from heav'n by some Celestial scout,
As well the name and nature both avow't
  – Du Bartas (1544-1590)

Other Names: European angelica, wild celery, archangel, holy ghost, Norwegian angelica.

Parts Used: Root, leaves, stems, flowers and seeds

This tall, statuesque biennial is the largest of the Apiaceae family and can grow up to 8-10 feet (3 metres) tall. The whole plant is aromatic with a wonderfully pungent, sweet taste and smell. It is not to be confused with *Angelica sinensis* also known as Dong Qui, the Chinese species. Historically it was considered a powerfully protective herb. It was held in such high esteem that it was named the 'root of the Holy ghost' some say because it could protect against and remedy almost all ills.

Angelica was used by our ancestors as an antidote to poison and a remedy to combat infectious diseases including the plague. It was considered so powerful that the dried leaves were burned to protect against spells of witches and evil spirits, it was grown in gardens as a protection for garden and home, and pieces of the root were used as an amulet. During the 16th and 17th centuries, angelica was combined with other herbs to make *Carmelite water*, a medieval drink thought to promote longevity and relaxation, to cure headaches and protect against evil forces. The North American Blackfoot tribe used angelica to bring them good luck, for divination, and to bring together group energies for ritual and ceremony.

Angelica is linked in Christian mythology with the springtime festival of the Annunciation. It was thought to be under the protection of Michael the Archangel because it blooms on his feast day, May 8th, in the old Julian Calendar. It was also believed that its potent healing properties were revealed to a monk during an epidemic of the plague, by the Archangel Michael – hence its Latin name. The archangel said the plant could be used to cure the plague and gave instructions that a piece of the root should be held in the mouth to drive away 'pestilential air'. Gerard, author of the Herball or Historie of Plants (1597) recommended, "*If you doe but take a piece of the roote and holde it in your mouth, or chew the same between your teeth, it doth most certainly drive away the pestilentiall aire, yea although the corrupt aire have possesses the hart, yet it driveth it out again.*" It was also taken as an antidote to intoxicating drinks and was considered a symbol of inspiration. In Lapland, garlands of angelica have traditionally been given to poets in the hope that its aroma would promote vision and creativity.

Paracelsus (1493–1541), the alchemist and physician, referred to angelica as a 'marvellous medicine' for treating the plague during the epidemic that he witnessed in Milan in 1510. The herbalist Gerard stated, "*It cureth the bitings of mad dogs and all other venomous beasts.*" Culpeper said it was ruled by the sun in Leo. Norwegians used the roots to make bread and the French used the seeds in a variety of liqueurs, the most well-known of which being Benedictine, gin and Chartreuse. Interestingly, angelica was taken as an antidote to intoxicating drinks.

Herbal Remedy

Angelica has sweet, pungent and bitter tastes and a warming effect. All parts of the plant can be used as medicine, but they are best used dried. They contain volatile oils (including a-pinene, P-phellandrene, carene, limonene and angelica lactones), furanocoumarins (angelicin, umbelliferone, psoralen, bergapten, imperatoren), polysaccharides, phthalates, flavonoids, sterols and resins.

Rich in antioxidants, angelica is an excellent circulatory tonic and has a rejuvenative effect throughout the cardiovascular system. With its warming effect it stimulates blood flow to the periphery of the body and is excellent for people who dislike the cold and damp. It is used for poor circulation, peripheral vascular problems such as Raynaud's disease, intermittent claudication and chilblains. It acts as a calcium-channel blocker in the heart, decreases blood pressure, regulates the heart, reduces the risk of blood clots and the build-up of atherosclerosis, dilates the coronary arteries and enhances the coronary circulation. It can be used to treat high blood pressure, angina and heart arrhythmias as well as to improve lymphatic circulation and reduce lymphatic congestion and swollen lymph nodes.

The pungent components of angelica have a warming and invigorating effect in the digestive system. They stimulate the flow of digestive enzymes, increasing appetite and enhancing digestion, and improving the absorption and metabolism of nutrients. Angelica also has a healing effect on the gut lining which can be applied in the treatment of peptic ulcers as well as indigestion, low stomach acid and nausea. Inhaling the crushed leaves used to be a popular remedy for travel sickness. With its antispasmodic action, which relaxes smooth muscle in the gut, it is a good remedy for easing stomach aches, wind, bloating and colic. In Scandinavia, fresh angelica leaves have been used like chicory, lettuce and dandelion for their bitter properties, to regulate the appetite and digestion, the secretion of hydrochloric acid and other digestive enzymes including bile.

The bitters in angelica have a beneficial effect in the liver; its antioxidant properties have a hepato-protective effect, protecting the liver from damage caused by drugs, toxins and alcohol. Angelica can be used for treating liver problems including cirrhosis and hepatitis. Taken regularly, it is said to reduce the desire for alcohol, which could be invaluable for alcoholics. It clears toxins from the gut and combats unfriendly gut bacteria which can have far-reaching effects including enhancing immunity, aiding the absorption of vitamins and minerals, helping to regulate the production of neurotransmitters such as serotonin and helping to prevent and combat infection. Angelica has antimicrobial action against several unfriendly gut bacteria and fungi including *E. coli, Enterococcus faecalis, Eubacterium limosum, Peptostreptococcus anaerobius* and *Candida*. It can be used to treat auto-immune and inflammatory bowel problem such as Crohn's disease and ulcerative colitis.

Not only can angelica help to build immunity and enhance resistance to infections, it can also be used to treat acute infections when they arise. It was traditionally valued as a remedy for the plague and other epidemics, acute febrile diseases, typhoid fever and malaria. It stimulates the formation of white blood cells, lymphocytes and phagocytes. The volatile oils, particularly in the root, have antibacterial, antiviral and antifungal properties, helping to combat infections including *Herpes, Staphylococcus aureus, Clostridium difficile* and *Clostridium perfringens.* It helps to prevent and treat allergies and has anti-inflammatory properties that can be helpful in arthritis and gout. It may have an anticancer effect by increasing tumour necrosis.

Angelica also has an affinity with the respiratory system and with its warming, antispasmodic and expectorant effects, it is used to treat asthma, colds, catarrh and bronchitis. It can be taken as a hot tea to bring down fevers and for the headaches, chills, aches and pains that herald the onset of acute infections. It is considered one of the best convalescent remedies due to its warming and strengthening properties. It may decrease intraocular pressure and help to prevent glaucoma.

In the reproductive tract, angelica can help to regulate the menstrual cycle, relieve period pain, heavy periods and PMS symptoms including irritability, depression, weepiness and joint pains. It balances hormones, enhances fertility and can be taken to aid contractions during childbirth. It can ease menopausal symptoms including night sweats, hot flushes, depression and mood swings. Angelica has a strengthening effect on the bones and with its hormone-balancing effect, it is useful for the post-menopausal tendency to osteopenia and osteoporosis. It is also a useful diuretic for relieving fluid retention and a urinary antiseptic for cystitis.

Angelica is a strengthening nerve tonic; it enhances mental strength and clarity, promotes inspiration and lifts the spirits. It is particularly useful for stress headaches, nervous exhaustion, mental and emotional fragility, feeling tense, scattered and disorganised, fearful and anxious. It makes a good aid for students before exams. It used to be taken to impart strength to athletes and when recovering from illness, and was considered to have rejuvenative properties. It was chewed by the Laplanders to prolong life.

More recently it has been found to have an antiepileptic effect which could be attributed to the terpenes in the essential oil. It can decrease the behavioural and psychological symptoms of dementia caused by degeneration of the frontotemporal lobe of the brain and it may be helpful in dementia with Lewy bodies associated with Parkinson's disease.

Externally angelica can be used in massage oils or baths to relieve muscle tension and joint stiffness and pain. It can be used topically in pleurisy and bronchitis as an anti-inflammatory compress, as well as in liniments and ointments to ease arthritic pain. It apparently makes an excellent cream to treat chemotherapy-related and radiation damage to the skin.

Homeopathic Remedy
Angelica is indicated in indigestion, nervous headaches and chronic bronchitis. It eases the production of phlegm. If taken regularly, either as a herbal or homeopathic remedy, it is said to cause an aversion to alcohol, helping alcoholics.

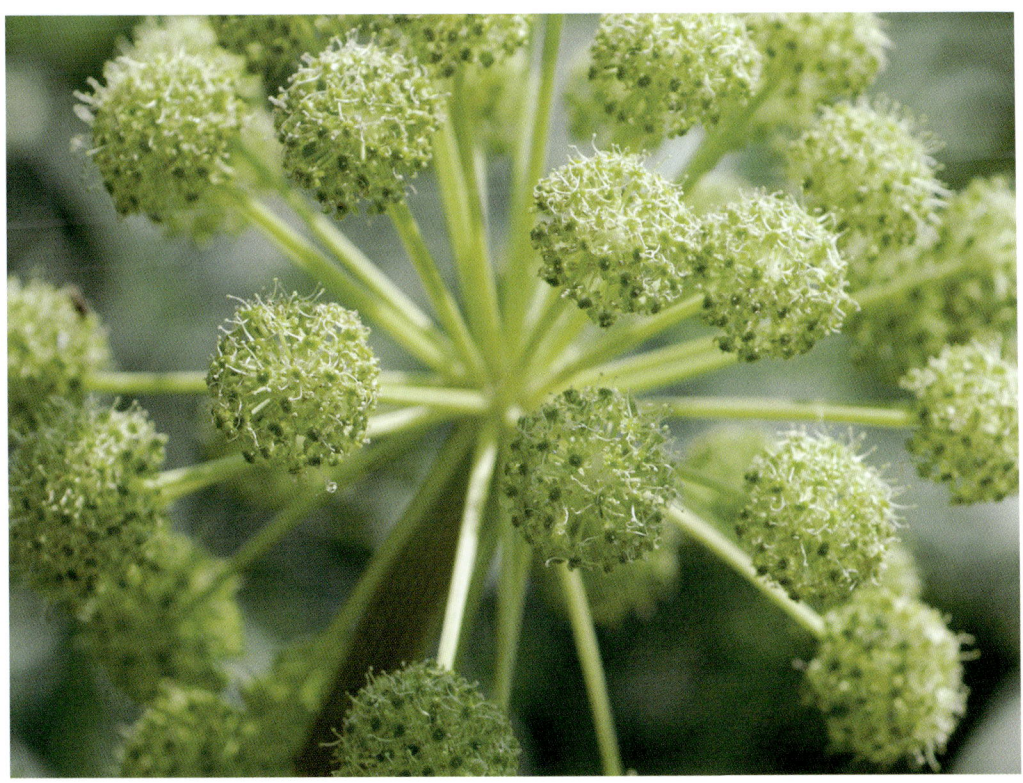

The Flower Essence

For those who feel spiritually lost or isolated, who live predominantly in a materialistic or over-intellectual world, it promotes inspiration and can be used to help people who feel cut off from their inner selves. It is particularly useful during difficult phases in life or when approaching death. It could also be used for those going through the proverbial 'dark night of the soul' to lend strength and courage to endure until life improves.

Edible Uses

Angelica is most well-known for its candied stalks that are used to decorate cakes and puddings, particularly as they not only taste good but have a reputation for expelling wind and strengthening the stomach, rivalled only by candied ginger. The fresh leaves stewed with rhubarb and gooseberries reduce their tart flavour, while the leaves and young stalks can be peeled and eaten sparingly in salads or cooked as a vegetable like celery. The seeds can be used to make liqueurs and as a flavouring in gin.

Growing

Angelica can be grown from seed in late summer or autumn as the seeds benefit from exposure to frosts, or you can pre-chill in the fridge for a few weeks if sowing in spring. It likes damp soil and light shade. If prevented from flowering, it will live for several years, but if it does flower it is biennial. Planted in companionship with angelica, nettles apparently increase angelica oil by 80 per cent.

Cautions

Avoid the use of the fresh root as it may cause photosensitivity; do not handle prior to exposure to strong sunlight and avoid prolonged exposure to sunlight if taking regularly. Care in peptic ulcers, heartburn and acid reflux, bleeding disorders, hypertension and pregnancy. Large doses may affect the heart rate and blood pressure. May increase blood sugar levels and should be avoided in diabetes. Avoid with Warfarin, salicylates and other anticoagulants. Discontinue use 7 days prior to surgery.

Recipes

Angelica, Cardamom, and Cinnamon Elixir for Good Digestion
The combination of warming angelica and the spices makes a great recipe for the digestion especially in the cold.

10 cardamom pods crushed
4 large sticks of cinnamon bark
500 ml glass jar with a screw top lid
Dried angelica root, leaves and seeds
150 ml brandy
120 ml raw sugar

Place the crushed cardamom pods and cinnamon sticks in the jar and fill up with either angelica root, leaves and flowers or seeds once it has been dried.

Mix the brandy and honey in a jug and pour into the jar. Leave it for 2-4 weeks stirring it daily.

After this time, strain the mixture through fine muslin into a clean dark glass bottle, label it clearly and store it in a cool dark place.

You could sip a small amount in some water or neat in a shot glass before a meal as an aperitif or after a meal as a digestif.

Angelica Root Syrup
Place a handful of chopped dried angelica roots in a pan with a litre of water. Bring to the boil and simmer gently for about three hours and then strain through a fine sieve or muslin. Measure the amount of liquid you have left and add an equal amount of runny honey to make a syrup. Stir and then pour into a dark glass bottle, label clearly and then store in a cool dark place.

This makes a delicious remedy for the first signs of a sore throat, runny nose, cold or cough. Take two teaspoonfuls every two to three hours in acute infections and two or three times a day as a preventative.

Artemisia vulgaris: Mugwort

The Flower of Artemis

Remember, Mugwort, what you made known,
What you arranged at the Great proclamation.
You were called Una, the oldest of herbs,
you have power against three and against thirty,
you have power against poison and against infection,
you have power against the loathsome foe roving through the land
– The Nine Herbs Charm from the 10th Century

Other names: Riverside wormwood, felon herb, chrysanthemum weed, wild wormwood, old Uncle Henry, sailor's tobacco, naughty man, old man and St. John's plant

Parts used: Aerial parts, flowers and leaves

Mugwort is a perennial member of the Asteraceae family and can be found growing wild on embankments, roadsides, among rubble and stony ground throughout America, Europe and North Asia. Because it grows so prolifically, many consider it merely a common weed. It has small rather insignificant flowers, but attractive deeply cut aromatic leaves with a silvery underside. The name 'mugwort' may come from the fact that it was used in brewing beer before hops became more popular as a bitter. It may also come from 'moughte' meaning a moth or maggot, because like other members of the Artemisia family, it can keep away moths.

Also in common with the other Artemisias, southernwood (*Artemisia abrotanum*) and wormwood (*Artemisia absinthium*), mugwort is named after Artemis the Greek moon goddess, who is identified with the Roman goddess Diana. Artemis revived the plants each night with her refreshing dew, while her twin brother Apollo, the sun god, sent the sun's rays. Both were essential to the growth and wellbeing of the plant world.

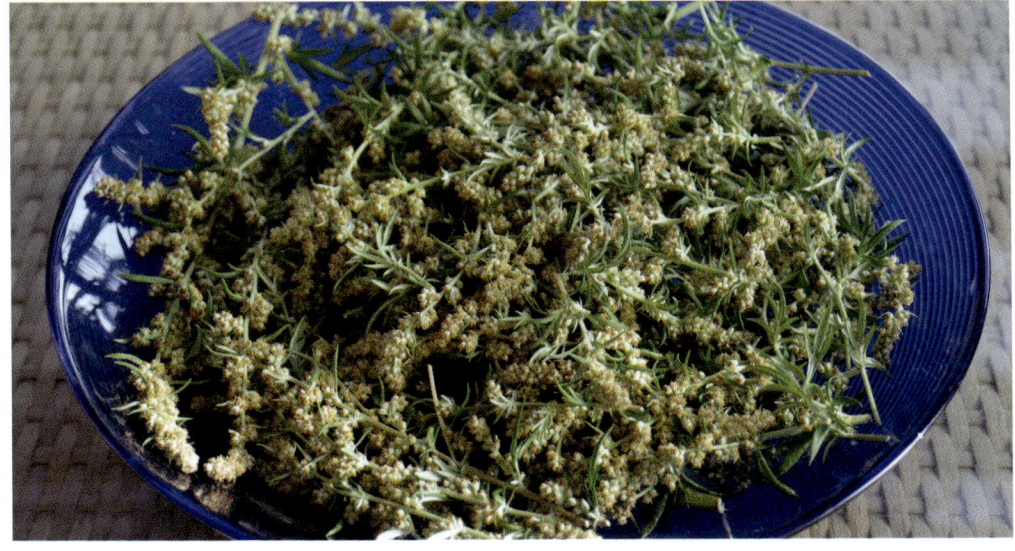

As the moon goddess, Artemis was regarded as the patron and protector of women, to influence their fertility, regulate their menstrual cycles and watch over them in childbirth. For thousands of years women giving birth have evoked her aid and given prayers and offerings to ensure a safe delivery and given thanks to her afterwards.

The healing power of plants named after Artemis reflects her influence in the sphere of women's health and explains why ever since the time of the ancient Greeks and Romans, Hippocrates, Pliny and Dioscorides, mugwort has been valued as an excellent remedy for women and was important in the religious ceremonies devoted to the goddesses Isis, Artemis and Diana. It has been used for balancing menstrual disorders and treating irregular, heavy, painful or suppressed periods, and troubles associated with the menopause. It was used as a traditional remedy for childbirth in Wales; a bunch of the plant would be tied to the left thigh of the woman in labour to ease pain but was thought to be necessary to remove it immediately after delivery to prevent haemorrhage. Mugwort was such an important herb in the Middle Ages it was called 'mater herbarum' meaning the 'mother of herbs.' *The Medieval Womens' Guide to Health: The First English Gynaecological Handbook,* written in the fifteenth century, recommended mugwort for a difficult birth along with the other Artemisias saying,

Make her a bath of mallows, fenugreek, linseed, wormwood, southernwood, pellitory and mugwort, boiled in water and let her bathe in it for a good time.

Culpeper tells us that mugwort is under the dominion of the planet Venus, indicating its close connection to the emotional world of women; it can enhance clarity and inner strength, and is attuned to the receptive quality of women and the world of the psyche and dreams. It was considered to have warming and drying effects and was also recommended for the treatment of urinary problems like cystitis, kidney stones and gravel. Mugwort has been used for centuries for epilepsy, nervousness, fright and convulsions. The 13th century physicians of Myddfai prescribed it for hysteria (it is interesting that this word relates to the womb; for instance, hysterectomy means removal of the womb). In addition, it was a popular remedy for digestive problems related to 'cold' which included stomach pain, wind, diarrhoea and colic. It was also used to treat liver problems and jaundice.

Since early times mugwort was believed to be a magical herb. It has traditionally been used to make dream pillows, to gain visions of the future and important spiritual insights while sleeping on them. One of mugwort's common names is 'poor man's tobacco' perhaps because the dried flowers have been smoked to promote vivid dreams since time immemorial.

Mugwort was also said to be a powerful herb for warding off danger and evil. It was used in spells against a whole range of mortal perils including evil spirits, sunstroke, poison, wild beasts, fire and illness. It was placed in the entrances to houses to keep away infections, and inside the house to stop lightning from striking. In the Middle Ages mugwort was called 'cingulum sancti Johannis,' or 'St John's girdle' as it was said that John the Baptist wore a girdle of mugwort while in the wilderness. It was traditionally worn on St John's (midsummer's) Eve as a garland round the head or waist when dancing round the fire. Afterwards it was thrown on to the fire to protect the person who wore it from danger and sickness in the following year.

Mugwort was used as a talisman against tiredness and valued by the Romans, who apparently planted it by roadsides so that marching soldiers could put it in their shoes. Pliny in his *Naturalis Historia* recommended that travellers should carry mugwort with them. There is an old French saying, *"He who carries artemisia on his travels will never feel weary."* In Nepal, mugwort is called 'titepati' ('tite' meaning bitter, 'pati' meaning leaf). Bundles of the leaves are used for sweeping the floor or hung outside houses and they are also used in offerings to the gods, made into incense and used as a medicine.

Herbal Remedy
The aerial parts of mugwort which include the leaves and the flowers have a bitter and aromatic taste and a warming quality. They contain volatile oils (including thujone, linalool, cineole, borneol

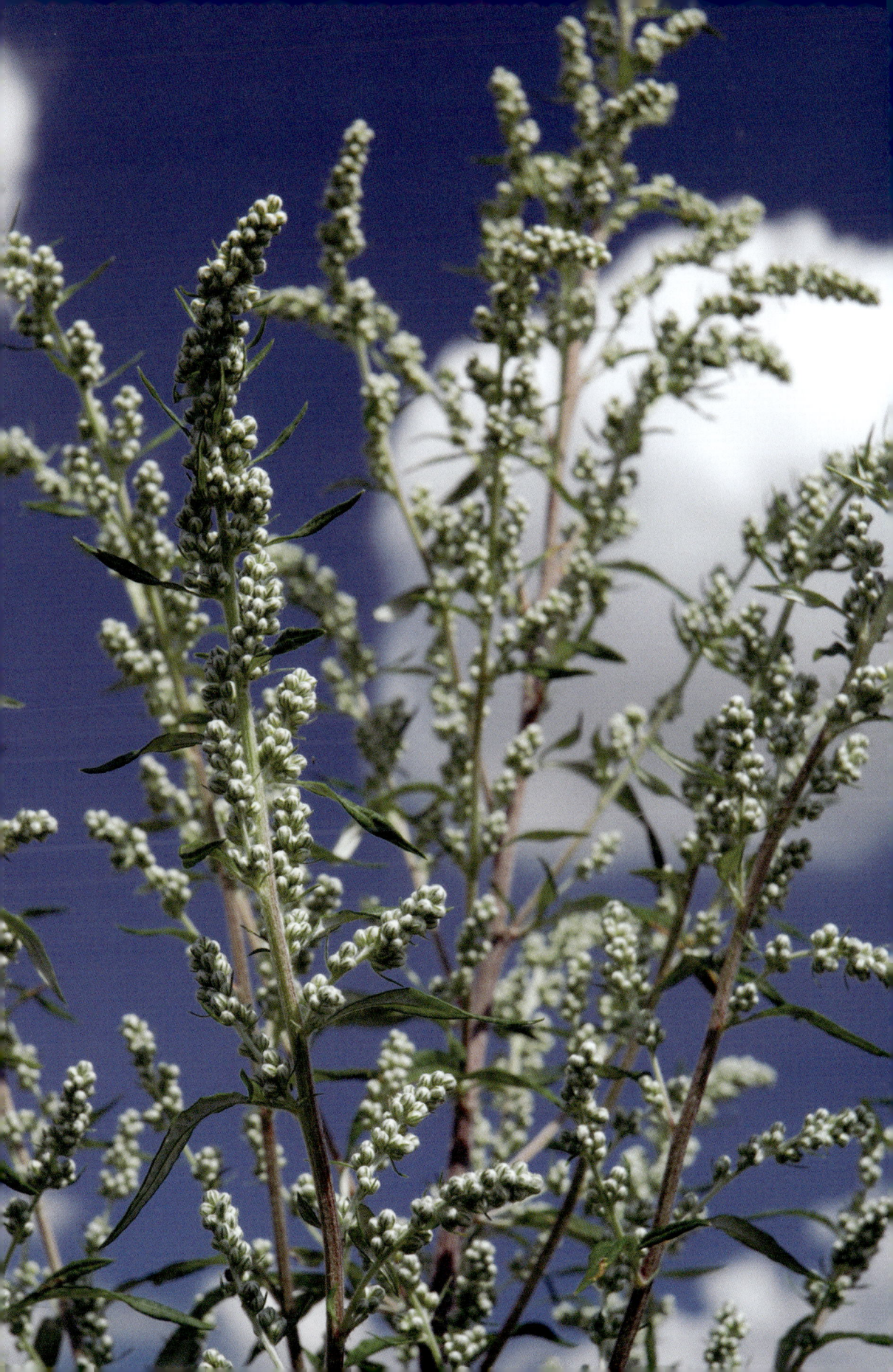

and pinene) phenolic acids, triterpenes (amyrin, sitosterol), coumarins (umbelliferone, esculetin), flavonoids (apigenin, quercetin), polyacetylenes, carotenoids, vitamins, cyanogenic glycosides and sequiterpene lactones (vulgarin). The phenolic acids, volatile oils and flavonoids have antioxidant, antispasmodic, hepatoprotective, antibacterial, antifungal and insect repellent actions which explains much of mugwort's ancient use for dispelling mortal perils, warding off danger and infection. It can inhibit the growth of bacteria including *Staphylococcus aureus, Salmonella enteritidis, Bacillus typhi, B. dysenteriae, Streptococci, E. coli, B. subtilis* and *Pseudomonas aeruginosa, Klebsiella pneumoniae* and fungi including *Candida albicans* and *Aspergillus niger*.

As its history has clearly told us, mugwort is first a woman's herb, recommended for treating menstrual problems including irregular, heavy, painful or suppressed periods, and gynaecological problems such as endometriosis, pelvic inflammatory disease, thrush, fibroids and cysts. It could be included in prescriptions to enhance fertility and facilitate childbirth. Since it acts as an emmenagogue, it may need to be avoided during pregnancy until just before or during the birth. However, in China mugwort is used to stop rather than bring on uterine bleeding and given to women for threatened miscarriage, particularly those deficient in energy and who feel cold. It can also help to relieve menopausal symptoms such as mood changes and hot flushes and may have a phyto-oestrogenic effect.

Like its close relative wormwood (*Artemisia absinthium*), mugwort is an aromatic and warming bitter tonic, excellent for the digestion. It stimulates the appetite and enhances digestion and absorption by increasing the secretion of digestive enzymes and bile from the liver and gallbladder. It makes a good remedy for a weak, sluggish digestion, low stomach acid, poor appetite, acid reflux, indigestion and gastritis, as well as for wind, bloating, accumulation of toxins in the gut and liver problems. It can be good when feeling run down and debilitated from poor digestion or liver function. The phenolic acids, volatile oils and flavonoids have an antioxidant effect, protecting the body against oxidative stress and helping to prevent a range of inflammatory and degenerative problems including cardiovascular disease and diabetes. In the liver they have a hepatoprotective effect, protecting the liver from damage caused by drugs, alcohol and other toxins. In the cardiovascular system they protect the arteries from damage and lower blood pressure and harmful LDL cholesterol and triglycerides, helping to prevent atherosclerosis and heart disease.

With its antispasmodic and antimicrobial actions attributed to the volatile oils, mugwort relaxes tension and spasm in the gut and combats unfriendly gut bacteria, helping to relieve problems such as colic, diarrhoea, constipation and indigestion. It is used for digestive problems related to stress such as nausea, vomiting, colic, indigestion or diarrhoea, and can also be used to expel worms. Its antispasmodic effects can also be seen in the respiratory tract where it can relax the bronchi and help relieve asthma. This has been attributed to many of mugwort's constituents including the alkaloids, coumarins, flavonoids, saponins, sterols, tannins and terpenes.

Mugwort has nervine properties, meaning that it has a beneficial effect in the nervous system. It is relaxing, uplifting and mildly sedative and with its analgesic effect it can ease pain. It is helpful in a range of nervous problems such as insomnia, nerve pain, tremors, headaches and exhaustion and can be thought of in stress-related problems including nervous problems of the gut, muscular aches and pains, headaches and high blood pressure. The flavonoids (jaceosidine, eupafolin, luteolin, quercetin and apigenine) and coumarins (esculetin, esculetin-6-methylether, scopoletin) may have MAO inhibitory effects, meaning that mugwort could be helpful in depression.

As a diuretic, mugwort can ease fluid retention particularly around period time and can be helpful in cystitis. It also enhances the elimination of toxins via the urinary system, which can be beneficial in the treatment of arthritis and gout. Its antioxidant actions are also beneficial here. Taken hot, an infusion of mugwort stimulates the circulation and has a warming effect. It increases blood flow to the skin and promotes perspiration, which helps bring down fevers. Its antimicrobial and detoxifying properties make it a good remedy for treating febrile infections, colds and coughs as well as more chronic problems such as skin problems and arthritis. In addition, mugwort may have anticancer effects particularly in relation to oestrogen-dependent breast cancer and cervical cancer.

The dried leaves of mugwort were used traditionally to make dream pillows for the purpose of gaining visions of the future and important spiritual insights while sleeping on them. Just as ever, they can be made into sleep pillows, smoked or drunk as a tea to promote lucid dreaming and enable you to be more receptive to psychic or prophetic information during your dream states. This oneirogenic effect may be provided by the presence of thujone in the plant. In China mugwort leaves are rubbed together and bound in a cylindrical shape and burnt over certain acupuncture points to stimulate the circulation and warm the point. This is known as 'moxibustion'.

Homeopathic Remedy
The root of Artemisia vulgaris is used mainly for spasms and epilepsy in childhood and in girls at puberty brought on by extremes of emotion such as grief or fright or by excitement. It is indicated when an epileptic fit occurs after a blow on the head, with menstrual disturbances and with teething. It is also prescribed for petit mal attacks (short losses of consciousness), for sleepwalking, catalepsy and dizziness caused by coloured lights when associated with nervousness. Artemisia is also used as a woman's remedy, in particular for irregular, scanty periods, painful periods, threatened miscarriage with violent cramps in the abdomen, and for uterine prolapse. An indication for its use can be profuse sweat with a peculiar fetid or garlic-like odour. It is also used for worms.

Flower Essence
A native of America also called mugwort (*Artemisia douglasiana*), a close relative of *A. vulgaris*, is used as a flower essence. Like the herbal remedy, it enhances the moon-like receptive quality of the psyche, allowing greater clarity and awareness of the dream world. It helps to integrate the insights gained from our dreams and our psychic awareness into our daily lives, and to understand their significance.

Mugwort is used to balance the transition from night to day consciousness, and to help those with a tendency to an overactive psychic life, cutting them off from the physical world of 'reality', remain connected to the practical, earthy aspects of life. It is recommended for people who tend to be irrational, over-emotional and hysterical, prone to disturbed nights because of an overactive dream life.

Mugwort is predominantly a woman's remedy, assisting the 'flowing processes' in the body, such as menstruation and childbirth. It connects menstrual cycles more closely to the lunar cycle. The flower remedy can be added to a herbal oil made from mugwort and used for massage to remedy menstrual problems and aid childbirth. It also stimulates the circulation giving a feeling of warmth.

Edible uses
Mugwort is used to flavour tea and rice dishes in Asia and has been used as a culinary herb for poultry and pork in Western cultures. The young leaves can be used in salads and herb vinegars, dried for teas, and the fresh flowering tops can made into tinctures.

Growing
Artemisia is easy to grow and can be found growing wild in Great Britain, Europe and North America. It can be grown from seed or root division and self seeds easily. It likes full sunlight but can tolerate partial shade and slightly moist, well-drained soil. It does not do well in wet soil.

Cautions
Since it acts as an emmenagogue, mugwort should be avoided during pregnancy and only used just before or during the birth. It is related to ragweed and may cause allergy symptoms that mimic those caused by ragweed allergies. As a bitter, detoxifying herb rather than a nourishing or tonic herb, prolonged use and/or high doses are not recommended.

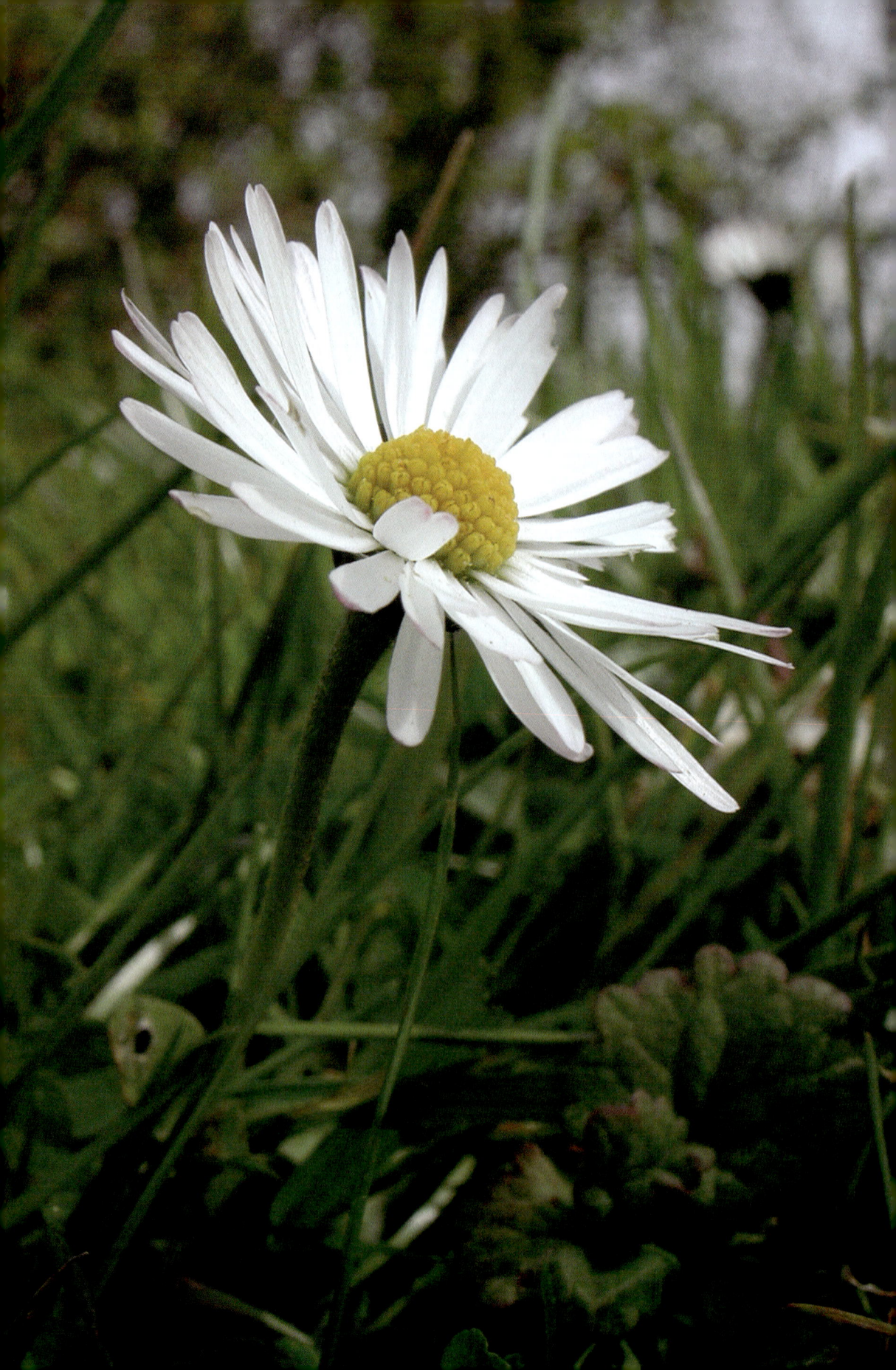

Bellis perennis: Daisy

The Flower of Innocence

Of alle the flowers in the med
Then love I most those flowers, white and rede
such as men callen daysies in our town
– Geoffrey Chaucer (1340–1400)

Other names: Bairnwort, baby's pet, marguerite, bruisewort, day's eye, common daisy, English daisy

Parts used: Leaves and flowers

The cheerful daisy is a sweet little member of the Asteraceae/Compositae family. It has long been a symbol of innocence because of its association with children. Daisy is also a symbol of survival; it can adapt to almost any landscape and type of soil, survive being trodden underfoot and all the indignities of the hoe and the lawnmower and yet continue to bloom for months from early spring to late autumn. Perhaps the resilience of daisies is mirrored by their ability to heal bruises and wounds. They will staunch bleeding from cuts and wounds and taken internally and used locally they can be thought of wherever there is shock or bruising from a knock or a fall. Daisy helps us to survive the knocks of life, like the daisy constantly trodden on yet still comes up smiling.

The botanical name may come from the Latin 'bellis' meaning beautiful, so *'Bellis perennis'* can be translated as 'perennial beauty' perhaps because the daisy flowers for so long. Or 'bellis' may come from 'bellum' the Latin for war, maybe because daisies grew in fields of battle and military doctors of the Roman Empire would soak bandages in their juice to bind the injured soldiers' wounds. Arnica, calendula and witch hazel are all close relatives of daisy, so perhaps it is no surprise that daisy is a wound healer. It was well known by the Crusaders for easing pain and bruising and for healing wounds and broken bones; one of its country names is 'bruisewort.' The name 'daisy' comes from 'day's eye,' a name given because the flower opens in the morning when the sun rises and closes in the evening when the sun sets. Chaucer said: *"well by reason men it call maie, the Daisie, or else the Eye of the Daie."*

Chaucer dedicated many poems to the daisy, as many have done since, as it was his favourite flower. Daisies have always been loved by children too, perhaps because traditionally they were considered a protective herb. The country names 'bairnwort' and 'baby's pet' reflect children's delight in plucking flowers for posies and daisy chains but daisies are equally popular among young girls as a love oracle; pulling flower petals off one by one, they would be told of their fortune, *"The girls who wear a daisy chain, grow up pretty, never plain,"* and whether *"He loves me, he loves me not."* If they slept with daisy roots under their pillow, they would dream of their love. In Medieval times knights would wear the daisy as a symbol of fidelity and a token of their lady's love.

In France the daisy was called 'marguerite' as the flower was said to resemble a pearl or was considered the pearl of flowers. The Greek word for pearl is 'margaritos'. In sixteenth century France, Henry IV's wife Marguerite de Valois revived the daisy's popularity as she bore its name. The daisy was worn in her honour and because it was considered the pearl of flowers.

Daisy was highly valued by our ancestors for its medicinal properties. It was famous among the Romans as a wound herb and Pliny said it would resolve scrofulous tumours. It was used on battlefields to staunch bleeding of wounds and prevent swelling of bruises and sprains. The leaves and flowers were given internally, and the bruised herb applied locally. Culpeper believed that the daisy was ruled by Venus and was "*used in wound-drinks and are accounted good to dissolve congealed and coagulated blood, to help pleurisy and ... pneumonia.*" According to John Gerard, the 16th century herbalist, daisy was used for catarrh, heavy menstrual bleeding, migraine and for bruises and swellings. He said, "*Daisies do mitigate all kinds of pain, especially in the joints, and gout proceeding from a hot humour.*" He also recommended it for curing fevers, inflammation of the liver and "*alle the inwarde parts*".

Daisy was used traditionally as a spring tonic to cleanse the blood, for fevers, coughs and pleurisy, to stimulate digestion, for liver, gallbladder and kidney problems, for swollen breasts and inflammatory conditions of the reproductive tract. Apparently, Henry VIII ate platefuls of daisies to relieve stomach ulcers. According to the doctrine of signatures, the daisy opens and closes like an eye, suggesting that it can ease infections or inflammation of the eye.

Herbal Remedy
The value of this perennial 'weed' as a medicinal plant has largely been overlooked by modern herbalists, even though it is so familiar to us. Lately, as awareness of the advantages of sustainable living and wild food foraging increases, the unassuming daisy is having somewhat of a renaissance. It is quite nutritious as it contains potassium, phosphorus, magnesium, calcium, iron, vitamin A and protein. It also contains phenolic compounds including flavonoids (quercetin, apigenin, kaempferol, isorhamnetin), anthocyanins, phenolic acids (caffeic, ferulic, sinapic, p-coumaric and salicylic acids) and tannins as well as triterpenes, polyacetylenes, saponins, inulin, volatile oils.

Kaemferol has numerous actions including antioxidant, anti-inflammatory, antimicrobial, analgesic, antidiabetic, antiosteoporotic and hormone regulating, and it can reduce the risk of cardiovascular disease and cancer. Other flavonoids including apigenin and quercetin have antihistamine effects which are helpful in reducing allergic reactions such as hay fever, asthma, eczema and urticaria. Flavonoids can strengthen blood vessel walls, helping to reduce cardiovascular problems and they also decrease our susceptibility to viral and upper respiratory infections. Daisy overall has antimicrobial, anti-inflammatory, antioxidant, anticancer and anti-haemorrhagic actions, it has a vasotonic effect which may be helpful in regulating blood pressure and it also reduces cholesterol. It has a beneficial effect in the nervous system, reducing anxiety and helping to dispel tiredness and lethargy.

In the gut, the astringent tannins in daisy help to protect the gut wall from irritation and inflammation, while the soothing mucilage is also protective. Daisy is a good remedy to enhance immunity as it has antibacterial and antifungal activity, particularly when taken as an infusion, effective against *Candida*, *Pseudomonas aeruginosa, Pseudomonas fluorescens* and *Staphylococcus aureus.* Much of this activity is attributed to the polyphenols, flavonoids and triterpenes.

Daisy has mild diuretic properties and will reduce fluid retention and aid elimination of toxins via the urinary system. This can be useful for treating arthritis, gout and skin problems such as acne and boils. The whole plant is rich in tannins that have an astringent effect, useful in catarrh, diarrhoea and bleeding as in heavy periods. Daisy used to be a popular remedy for women's problems, given for swellings in the breasts and heat and inflammation in the reproductive system.

With antimicrobial, expectorant and soothing effects, daisy can be used for coughs, catarrh and sinusitis and is worth combining with other expectorants such as elecampane (*Inula helenium*) and thyme (*Thymus vulgaris*). It has anti-inflammatory, anti-allergenic and analgesic properties attributed to the flavonoids and polyphenols, and can help relieve allergic rhinitis, arthritis and sore muscles. A strong decoction of the roots makes a detoxifying remedy for chronic skin disease such as eczema. It makes an excellent remedy for trauma, bruises, wounds, post-surgery and for injuries to the head when taken internally.

Externally the whole plant makes a great first aid remedy. Its antioxidant, anti-inflammatory, anti-haemorrhagic and antimicrobial actions provide a perfect combination for treating cuts, wounds, sprains, strains, shock or bruising from a knock or a fall. An infused oil of daisy flowers can be applied to painful congested breasts, arthritic joints and gout, varicose veins and haemorrhoids, and to the perineum for bruising and pain after childbirth. The fresh leaves can be chewed to relieve mouth ulcers.

Daisy is a good astringent and anti-inflammatory remedy and an infusion can be used as an eyebath to treat inflamed or irritated eye conditions including black eyes. It could also make a good skin lotion for inflammatory, bacterial or fungal skin conditions including *Staphylococcus epidermidis*. An insect repellent spray can be made from a leaf infusion.

Homeopathic Remedy
Bellis perennis is known as the 'poor man's arnica' as it is given for lumps and bumps from knocks or falls, for bruises, wounds and swellings, and the shock that can cause them. Like the herb, Bellis is prescribed for skin problems such as acne and boils, gout, arthritic pain, varicose veins, women's problems including engorgement of the uterus and breasts. It is prescribed when these complaints follow getting chilled when overheated, or follow injury, accidents or surgery, childbirth or over-exertion.

The Flower Essence
Daisy is a good remedy for both children and adults. It promotes clarity of mind, and the ability to absorb information and organise oneself in relation to it. Daisy enhances concentration and helps to bring together information from different sources into a focused whole. It is particularly useful for those who suffer from the recurrent problems related, for example, to money, relationships, or learning skills, without understanding why. It is also a good remedy for people involved in planning and organisation.

Edible Uses
The fresh green leaves and flowers can be eaten in salads, along with other wild foods such as dandelion and sorrel leaves. They used to be popular cooked as a vegetable and served with meat. The flowers can also be eaten in soups, stews, salads, even sandwiches and make great decorative additions to almost any dish. They have a mild, slightly sour flavour.

Cautions
There are no side effects known although it should be avoided during pregnancy until further research is available. Individuals who are sensitive to other members of the *Asteraceae* family may experience respiratory allergies.

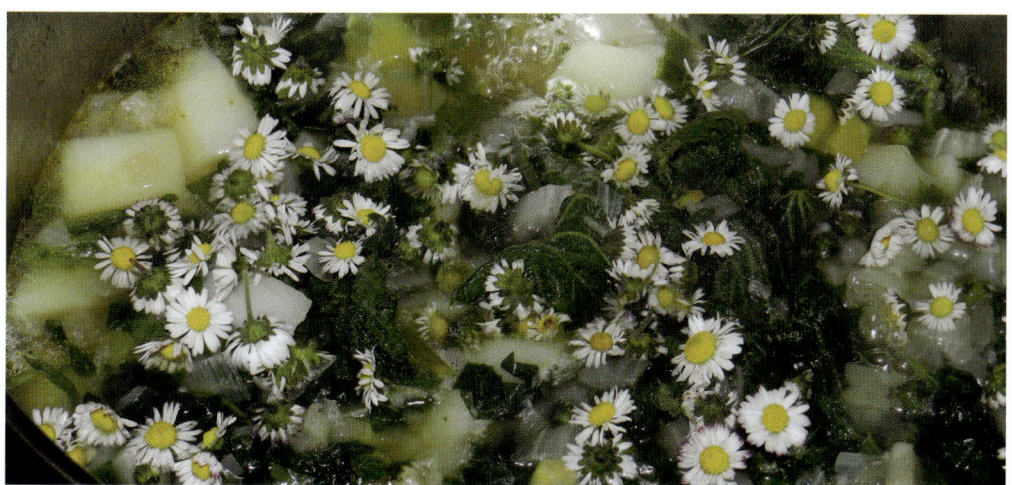

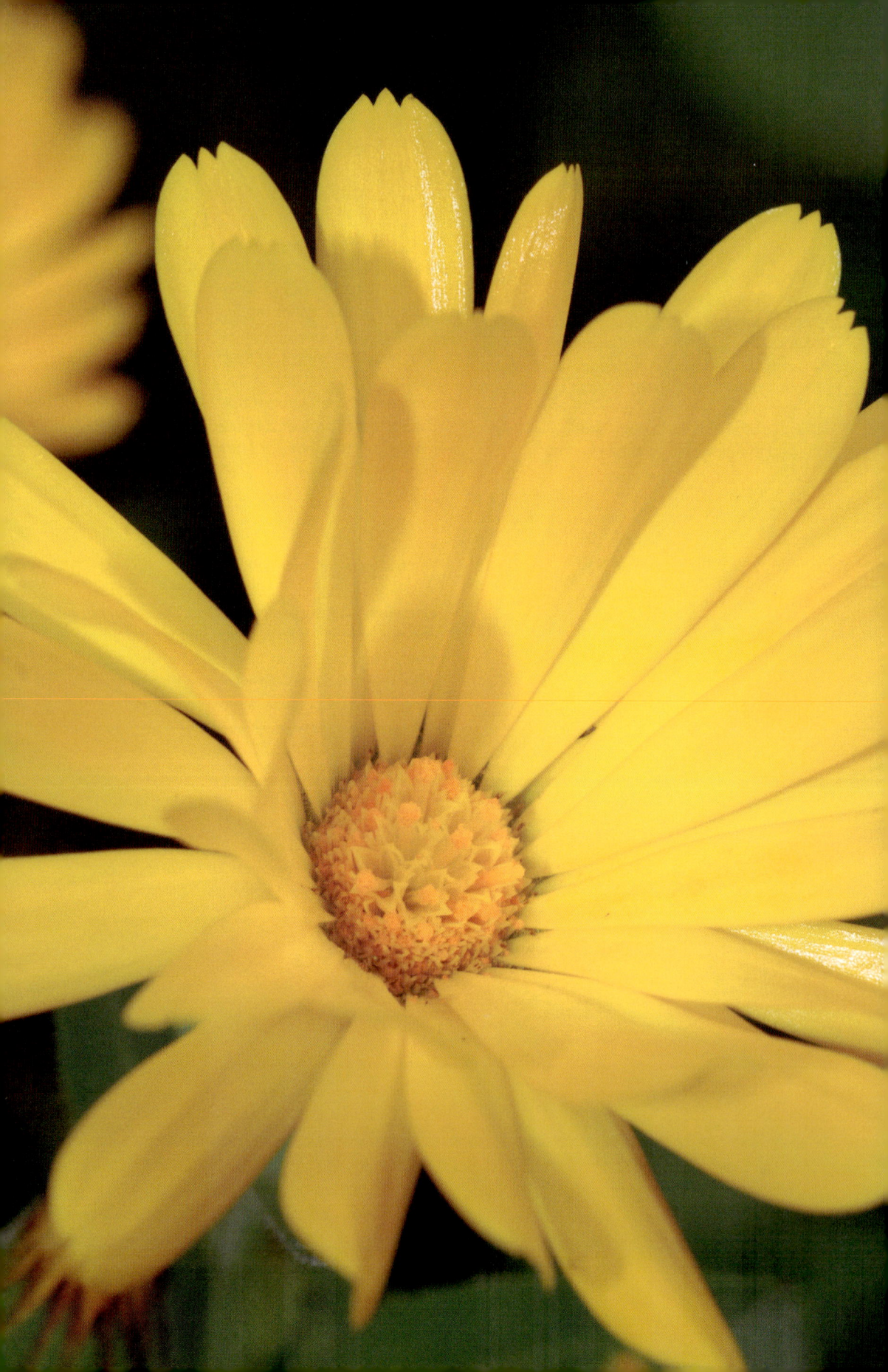

Calendula officinalis: Marigold, Calendula
The Flower of the Sun

The marigold goes to bed with the Sun
And with him rises, weeping
– William Shakespeare (1564–1616)

Other Names: Pot marigold, bull's eye, Mary bud, Mary's gold, poor man's saffron

Parts Used: Flowers

The common marigold, also known as calendula, is a familiar sight in English cottage gardens and much loved for its cheerful orange flowers. It is a member of the Asteraceae/Compositeae family. The English name marigold refers to its use in church festivals in the Middle Ages; the name may come from 'Mary's Gold' as it was dedicated to the Virgin Mary. It was strewn before cottage doors and made into garlands on May day festivals.

The Latin name *Calendula* comes from 'calends' meaning the first day of every month, because in its warm native climate in Egypt and the Mediterranean, marigold is in bloom on the first day of every month throughout the year. In some traditions, marigold is a symbol of endurance. According to Culpeper, marigolds are herbs of the sun and under the influence of Leo. They have always been associated with the sun's journey across the sky because they open when the sun rises and close as it sets.

Shakespeare, as the lines above suggest, was aware of marigold's association with pain and grief. Some say this is because the flower daily mourns the departure of the sun when its petals are forced to close. Others say that it comes from South American and Mexican lore; the Spanish conquistadores murdered many Aztecs in their search for gold, and the little red flecks which appear on some marigolds were said to symbolise their blood. Another story from Greek mythology tells of Caltha, a girl who fell in love with the sun god Apollo but was melted by the power of his rays. In her place grew a solitary marigold.

Open afresh your round of starry folds, ye ardent marigolds!
Dry up the moisture from your golden lids, for great Apollo bids
That in these days your praises should be sung on many harps, which he has lately strung;
And when again your dewiness he kisses, tell him, I have you in my world of blisses:
So haply when I rove in some far vale,
His mighty voice may come upon the gale
– John Keats (1795–1821)

The sad association of marigold with grief and pain is said to be dispelled if marigolds are mixed with roses; the two flowers together symbolise the sweet sorrows of love. Despite it being a symbol of grief, Culpeper and Gerard refer to marigold as a 'comforter of the heart and spirits' and used it for inflammation of the eyes and for 'trembling of the heart'.

Used historically as 'poor man's saffron,' calendula was used as a culinary herb and spice and its remarkable healing properties were well known to herbalists for centuries. It was even considered a magic plant; apparently if you wore marigolds you could see who had robbed you. It was said to protect against all sorts of evil influences and disease, including the plague. The Romans and Greeks used calendula flowers and petals in rituals and ceremonies and made them into crowns or garlands for rituals and ceremonies. Calendula flowers are sacred in

India and have long been used to decorate statues of Hindu deities.

The Romans used the flowers as a tea to relieve fevers, and the juice of the crushed flowers to apply to warts. The flowers were used as a cosmetic and a dye to colour a variety of foods including soups and conserves. In the Middle Ages, St Hildegard and Albert the Great used calendula for intestinal troubles, liver obstructions, insect and snake bites. In the sixteenth and seventeenth centuries, marigold tea was used for eye complaints, headaches, jaundice and toothache. The Shakers apparently used marigold for treating gangrene.

Herbal Remedy
Marigold flowers contain a wealth of beneficial constituents which contribute to it role in healing including flavonoids, volatile oils, sesquiterpene, triterpenoids, polysaccharides, oligoglycosides, saponins, bitters, resin, mucilage, beta-carotene, iodine, manganese and potassium.

The flowers have antioxidant and anti-inflammatory actions which are attributed to the flavonoids and sesquiterpenes, as well as antimicrobial and astringent properties provided by the volatile oils, tannins and a yellow resin called calendulin. They can enhance the function of the immune system, possibly by stimulating white blood cell function and have antibacterial and antiviral activity. They are effective against bacteria including *Staphylococcus aureus, Baccillus cereus* and *E. coli*, fungal infections including *Candida* as well as flu and *Herpes* viruses. The triterpenoids, particularly faradiol, account for much of marigold's anti-inflammatory effects and its ability to reduce swelling and oedema. The mucilaginous polysaccharides, along with the astringent tannins, protect the surfaces they come into contact with including the linings of the mouth, the digestive and genito-urinary tracts, and the skin, protecting delicate tissues of the body from irritation, inflammation and infection.

With its antioxidant and anti-inflammatory flavonoids, marigold is excellent for treating inflammatory conditions of the digestive tract including gastritis and peptic ulcers. The tannins with their astringent effect can relieve diarrhoea, stop bleeding and tighten junctions of the gut wall in leaky gut syndrome. The bitters stimulate the secretion of digestive enzymes and clear heat and congestion from the liver and gallbladder and have a reputation for improving digestion and absorption and preventing gallstones. By supporting the work of the liver, the great detoxifying organ in the body, marigold helps the body to break down toxins.

Marigold is an excellent remedy for treating fungal infections such as thrush in the mouth, the gut and the reproductive system, for combating pelvic and bowel infections including enteritis, parasitic infections and for viral hepatitis. Its antimicrobial and anthelmintic properties inhibit amoebic infections and intestinal worms and clear toxins from the gut. It has a mild laxative effect and has been used for symptoms associated with toxicity or 'liverishness' such as headaches, chronic skin problems, nausea, lethargy and irritability. With its antimicrobial actions and its prebiotic polysaccharides, it makes a good remedy to combat unfriendly micro-organisms in the gut and in this way benefit immunity and the nervous system.

Marigold is used to reduce lymphatic congestion and swollen lymph glands. Taken in hot infusion, marigold promotes sweating and helps to bring down fevers. By bringing blood to the surface of the body, it helps the body throw off toxins and bring out eruptions such as measles and chickenpox to speed them on their way. It is a good remedy for treating fevers and infections in children, such as colds and flu. It also has a diuretic action and increases the elimination of toxins via urine. It can be used to relieve arthritis and gout, aided by its small salicylic content, which adds to its anti-inflammatory action.

Marigold has an affinity with the female reproductive system. It can help to regulate menstruation, reduce tension and spasm in the uterine muscles and relieve menstrual cramps. Its astringent properties provided by the tannins help reduce excessive menstrual bleeding and uterine congestion. It can reduce breast congestion and its associated tenderness and mastitis. Marigold has a reputation for treating tumours and cysts such as fibroids and ovarian cysts, as well as cysts in the breast and digestive tract. During childbirth marigold can promote contractions and delivery of the placenta and for this reason should not be used during early pregnancy. Marigold improves venous return and is used for relief of symptoms related to varicose veins and haemorrhoids. It has a phyto-oestrogenic effect which is helpful during the menopause for easing symptoms such as hot flushes and night sweats as well as mood swings and joint pains.

Externally marigold has pride of place as an antiseptic first aid remedy for cuts and abrasions, sores and ulcers, burns and cold sores, to stop bleeding, reduce infection and speed healing. It is a remarkable wound healer as it brings white blood cells to the affected area and promotes the generation of new tissue for healthy scar formation. The antioxidant action of marigold may be central to its wound healing properties as it prevents the production of free radicals at or around the wound from delaying the healing process, and speeds the healing of the wound.

A marigold infusion makes a really effective mouthwash for inflamed gums and gingivitis, an antimicrobial douche for vaginal infections such as bacterial vaginosis, and an anti-inflammatory eyewash for eye conditions. Used in tincture, infusion or simply by crushing a flower, it rapidly resolves inflammation, reduces swelling from injuries, promotes tissue repair and minimises scar formation. Compresses applied to varicose veins, bruises, sprains and strains will reduce swelling and pain. A crushed flower can be rubbed on to insect bites and wasp or bee stings.

Homeopathic Remedy

Calendula is used for injuries where the pain is out of all proportion to the injury. As a tincture, it is taken internally for its remarkable ability to speed healing. It is particularly useful for wounds which may suppurate, and to prevent cuts, injuries and inflammatory problems becoming infected. It can be used after operations and tooth extractions, for skin conditions, particularly erysipelas, and for catarrhal conditions and deafness.

As in herbal medicine, calendula has an affinity for the female reproductive system. It can be taken for heavy or irregular periods, chronic cervicitis, uterine pain with a feeling of stretching and dragging in the groin, an enlarged uterus and vaginal warts.

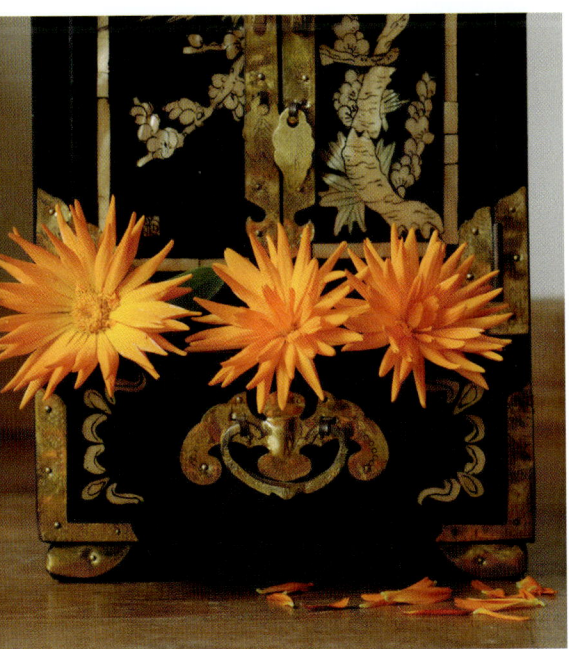

Flower Essence

To the Aztecs, marigold (*Tagetes* sp.) represented the cycles of life. As it followed the sun's journey across the sky, so also it developed from seed to leaves and stem, then it grew buds and flowers that opened with the sun, and once again produced seed, the womb of the flower. Such is the flow of life eternal. As a flower essence marigold is related to the Word, the source of all creation, the womb of all life. As the apostle John wrote, *'In the beginning was the word, and the word was with God ...'* . There is a connection between the Word and marigold's affinity with the womb in both herbal medicine and homeopathy.

Marigold's use extends into the creative force of the written or spoken word and can be used to enhance communication through this medium. It is particularly recommended for people who lack warmth and receptivity in their communication with others, who tend to use sharp and cutting words, where the spoken word may lead to argument or misunderstanding. Calendula helps such people to listen compassionately to others, to understand their message clearly, and to express warmth and caring in return. This can be applied well to those in healing, teaching or counselling professions and to help authors to be aware of the power of the written word. Calendula helps to balance the feminine aspect of receptivity with the masculine aspect of dynamic activity.

Edible Uses

Both the leaves and flowers make an excellent and colourful addition to soups and salads, while in the garden marigold is a good companion plant, deterring infestation of its neighbours. Marigolds have long been popular as a cosmetic herb and a dye to colour a variety of foods including soups and conserves.

Growing

Propagate by sowing seeds in spring or autumn in moist medium rich soil and full sun directly into the ground. Grows 12 – 20" (30 – 50cm) tall and flowers from June to September or first frosts. Deadhead regularly to ensure continued flowering. It self-seeds easily. It is not normally troubled by disease, but is susceptible to mildew in warm, moist weather. Remove affected plants and inspect the plants regularly to nip any further problems in the bud.

Cautions

Avoid during pregnancy or known allergy to Asteraceae family. Caution with sedatives, immuno-suppressive drugs and insulin/hypoglycaemic medications.

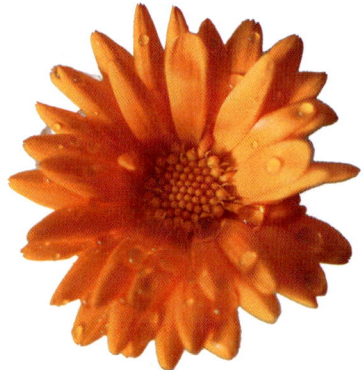

Recipes

Herbal Tincture for Spots and Blemishes
Before resorting to harsh chemicals and antibiotics why not grow your own effective, beautiful and fragrant 'Spot Pot' – containing rose, calendula and basil plants. The rose petals have astringent, antiseptic and calming properties, calendula is an anti-inflammatory – healing and soothing and basil helps to slow the production of oil in the sebum glands.

4 calendula flower heads
4–6 rose petals
4–6 basil leaves

Add all the ingredients to a small pan with a cup of water. Bring to a boil and simmer for about 5 minutes until all the ingredients have softened. Allow it to cool slightly and drain.

Using a cotton wool ball, apply it to affected areas morning and night. Within a couple of days pores will tighten and skin should start to clear.

Calendula Cream
500ml olive oil
50g beeswax
Marigold flowers

Place the oil in a bain marie/double boiler over a low heat and add as many calendula flowers as will submerge under the oil. Leave to heat and infuse for a few hours until the oil turns orange and the flowers look spent. Remove from heat. Press through a fine wire sieve or muslin and then return to the double boiler. Add the beeswax, stirring until it has melted. Pour into ointment jars while still warm. Label clearly and store in the fridge. Should keep for 6 months.

Chamomilla recutita/Matricaria chamomilla/ Anthemis nobilis: Chamomile

The Flower of Equilibrium

*Whilst some still busied are in decking of the bride,
Some others were again as seriously employed
In strewing of those herbs at bridals used that be,
Which everywhere they throw, with bounteous hands and
The healthful balm and mint from their full laps do fly free
The scentful chamomile, the verdrous costmary*
– Michael Drayton (1563–1631)

Other Names: Mayweed, ground apple, the herb of humility, the plants' physician.

Parts Used: Flowers

Two kinds of chamomile are used medicinally: German chamomile (*Chamomilla recutita* or *Matricaria chamomilla*) and Roman chamomile (*Anthemis* or *Chamaemelum nobilis*). They are highly aromatic members of the Asteraceae/Compositae family with very similar properties, but German chamomile is generally preferable as it is less bitter. Roman chamomile is well known for planting lawns, paths and arbours where it releases its pleasing fragrance when trodden on. Shakespeare apparently grew it in his garden

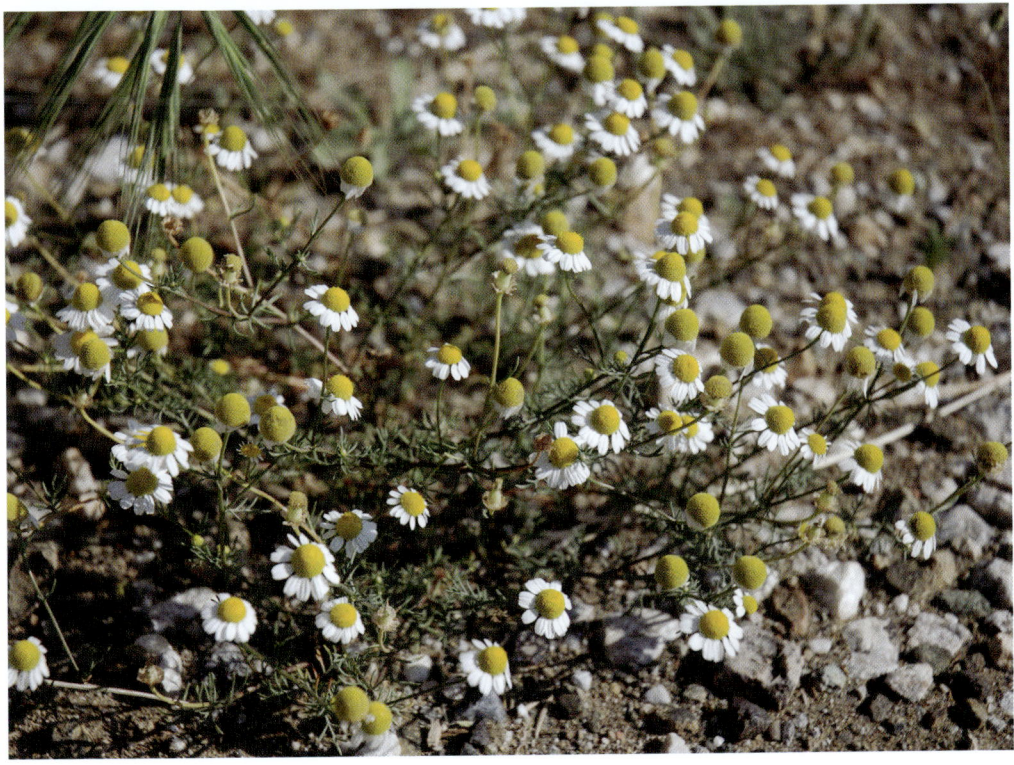

and Sir Francis Drake is said to have played his famous game of bowls on a chamomile lawn. There is a saying, *"Like a chamomile lawn, the more it is trodden, the more it will spread."* It has been called 'the herb of humility' because it grows best when walked on.

Chamomile has been a favourite among garden herbs for over 2000 years. It was well known to the ancient Greeks who thought its scent resembled that of fallen apples and so called it 'khamaimelon' meaning earth apple (from 'kamas' meaning on the ground and 'melon' meaning apple). The Spanish must also have likened it to an apple for they called it 'manzanilla' meaning little apple. The famous Greek physician Dioscorides recommended chamomile as a medicine for fevers in 900 BC and the ancient Egyptians revered it for its medicinal virtues, particularly its power to cure 'ague.' They dedicated it to the sun god Ra as it was considered an effective remedy for heat and fevers and the flower also looked like the sun. When the body of King Ramesses II was displayed in Paris, skin tissue was taken away for analysis and revealed that it had been anointed with chamomile oil; it was probably used in the mummification process of the King for its insect repelling actions.

The ancient Greeks and Romans considered chamomile one of the best remedies for menstrual disorders. The name *Matricaria* comes from 'matrix' meaning mother or womb or it could come from 'mater-cara' meaning beloved mother as it is dedicated to St. Anne, mother of the Virgin Mary, which may indicate its value as a remedy for women's ailments. Chamomile has been used for hundreds of years as a digestive remedy for nausea and sickness in pregnancy, to relax spasm and relieve painful periods, to reduce menopausal symptoms, relieve mastitis,

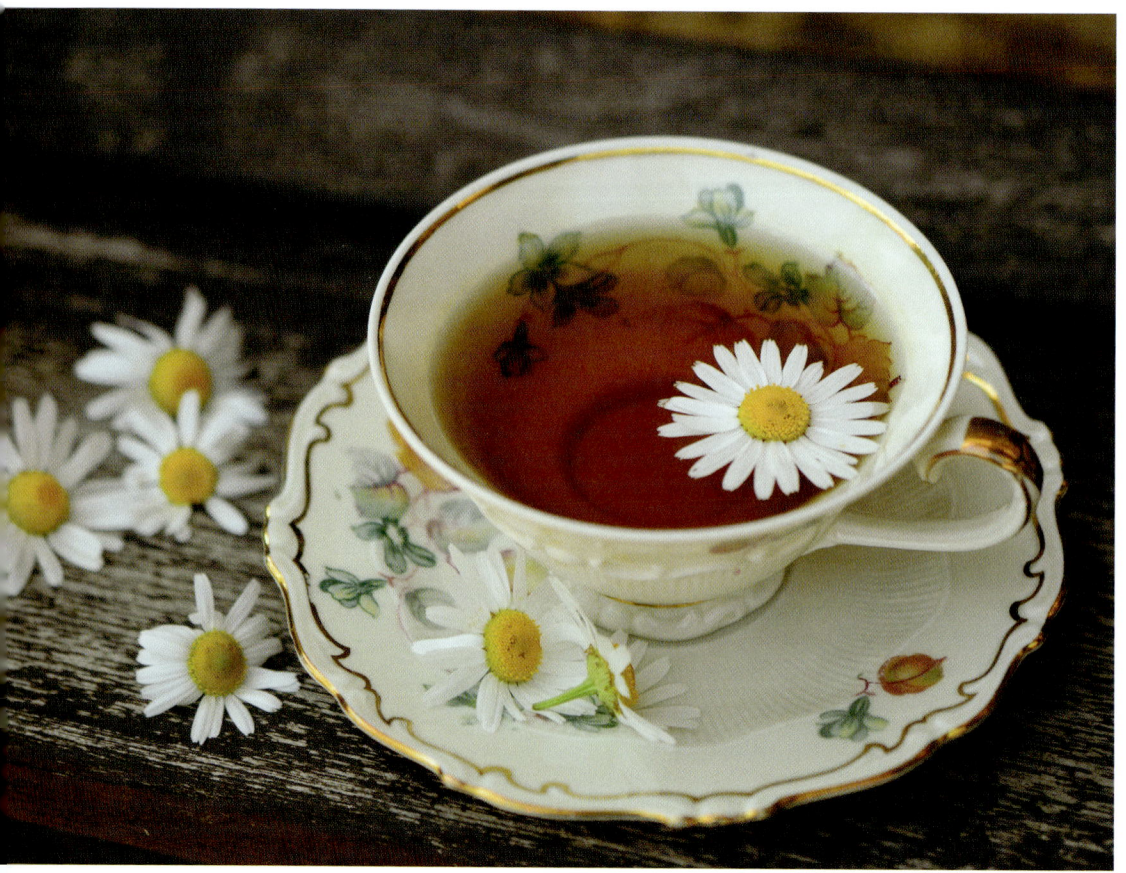

premenstrual headaches and migraines and for absence of periods due to stress or psychological problems such as anorexia nervosa.

Chamomile was used by the Saxons as a calming remedy, and to treat stomach problems. They believed chamomile was one of the nine sacred herbs given to the earth by the god Woden. It was highly valued as a remedy for hysteria, insomnia, nightmares, convulsions, delirium, tremors of alcoholics, melancholy and a whole range of other nervous afflictions, especially of women. In the Middle Ages it was frequently strewn in insanitary halls of castles and great houses to keep infection at bay, and it was burned as incense to mask foul smells and infection. Bunches of chamomile flowers were often hung on babies' cots to protect them from infection and keep them happy and healthy. In 1629 John Parkinson wrote, *"It is a common hearbe, well knowne and is planted of the rootes in alleyes and walkes and on bankes to sit on ... the use thereof is very much both to warm and to comfort and to ease paines"*. Shakespeare apparently grew it in his garden.

In the Victorian language of flowers, chamomile is a symbol of energy and patience in adversity, because of its great ability to restore equilibrium and support the nervous system. The flowers were traditionally used in love potions and at weddings, and to wash the face and hair in order to attract the beloved. It was also respected by our ancestors as a grave plant, to ease the passage of the dead into the world to come.

Not only was chamomile respected as a flower to benefit ailing people, but it was also popular for curing sick plants and was known as 'the plants' physician'. Chamomile tea can be added to a vase of drooping flowers to revive them and chamomile can be planted in the garden to remedy ailing plants or to prevent disease.

Herbal Remedy and Aromatherapy Oil
The main constituent of chamomile is a beautiful blue volatile oil containing azulenes which give it such a distinctive fragrance. The flowers have a combination of bitter, pungent and astringent tastes given to it by its many constituents which include volatile oils (bisabolol oxide A and B, bisbolone oxide A, chamazulene, farnescene), flavonoids (quercetin, apigenin and luteolin), sesquiterpene lactones, coumarins, plant acids, fatty acids, cyanogenic glycosides, salicylate derivatives, choline, tannins, mucilage, calcium, iodine, magnesium, potassium, phosphorus and Vitamin B2.

Chamomile is a wonderful sedative and relaxant with a particular affinity with the digestive system and is a perfect remedy for hot fiery babies, children and adults alike. Its ability to reduce anxiety is attributed to the action of flavonoids including apigenin on the central nervous system. It has mood-enhancing qualities and calms anxiety and nervousness without inducing drowsiness or impairing motor activity. It lifts the spirits and is excellent for tense, stressed people who tend to be hyperactive, irritable, angry and highly sensitive, prone to digestive problems and allergies. It is a great remedy for children's temper tantrums!

Chamomile tea, as we know from Beatrix Potter's Peter Rabbit stories, makes good bedtime drink and an excellent addition to baths for tired, fractious babies and children, soothing irritability or over-excitement and ensuring a restful sleep. It is recommended for restless or hyperactive children, ADHD and other behavioural problems and can be given in a bottle or on a teaspoon to small babies for teething as it helps relieve pain. Its analgesic properties works well in period pain and pre-menstrual headaches and help ease the pain of contractions during childbirth. As a general pain reliever with an antispasmodic action as powerful as papaverine from the opium poppy, chamomile can be taken for headaches and migraine, neuralgia, toothache, earache, aches and pains during flu, cramps, arthritic and gout pains and is especially good for people who are over-sensitive to pain.

Chamomile is famous for soothing all kinds of digestive upsets, especially those related to stress such as nervous indigestion, heartburn and acidity, and for treating digestive infections such as gastro-enteritis. It has the marvellous ability to relax smooth muscle throughout the body and in the digestive tract it can relieve tension and spasm, colic (in babies as well as children and adults), abdominal pain, wind and bloating. By regulating peristalsis, it can be helpful for both diarrhoea and constipation. Chamazulene and bisabolol in the volatile oil have anti-inflammatory effects and are excellent for treating gastritis and peptic ulcers, colitis and irritable bowel syndrome. Chamomile also helps to prevent and speed up the healing of ulcers both internally and externally, contributing to chamomile's value as a remedy for peptic ulcers and varicose ulcers on the legs. The bitters in chamomile stimulate the flow of bile and the secretion of digestive juices, enhancing the appetite, improving a sluggish digestion and supporting the liver. Chamomile can lower blood sugar levels and increase liver glycogen, which is helpful in the prevention and treatment of diabetes.

Chamomile tea is one of the first remedies to consider for children's fevers and respiratory infections such as sore throats, colds and flu. By inducing a restful sleep, it encourages natural recovery, particularly in children for whom rest is probably the best medicine. Chamomile is also an excellent support for the immune system. Its volatile oil is a powerful antimicrobial, active against bacteria, including *Staphylococcus aureus*, and fungal infections including thrush (*Candida albicans*). It may have anticancer effects against various human cancer cell lines.

Chamomile has an antihistamine effect by reducing oversensitivity to allergens such as pollen and house dust and the risk of the severe allergic reaction, anaphylactic shock. It is a really good remedy for all kinds of allergies including eczema, asthma, hayfever and urticaria. Its profoundly relaxing effect helps when dealing with emotional issues underlying such allergies, while the antimicrobial actions help combat unfriendly microorganisms in the gut and promote a healthy gut flora. This has a significant impact on efficient functioning of the nervous and immune systems. The anti-inflammatory properties of chamomile also help resolve problems such as conjunctivitis and tonsillitis, while its relaxant effect on the bronchial tubes helps to reduce broncho-constriction in asthma. Steam inhalations can help relieve asthma, hay fever, catarrh and sinusitis. Its antiseptic oils are excreted via the urinary system where it can soothe an inflamed bladder and relieve cystitis.

As history has shown us, chamomile is wonderful remedy for women's health. It has oestrogenic-agonist activity as well as a progesteronic action and is used to ease menstrual discomfort and cramps, for amenorrhea due to stress or psychological problems such as anorexia nervosa and to reduce nausea and sickness in pregnancy. The tea can be drunk throughout childbirth to relax tension and lessen the pain of contractions. Dilute chamomile oil can be used for massage and for inhalation during childbirth and can be effective at transition stage when pain can seem intolerable. It can also be used for mastitis, premenstrual headaches and migraines and to reduce menopausal symptoms including hot flushes.

Externally, chamomile is an excellent healer. The volatile oils exert a soothing, antiseptic and anti-inflammatory effect on the skin, and stimulate tissue repair. In creams and infusions, dilute oils and compresses, chamomile is really effective for speeding healing of ulcers, sores, burns and scalds, soothing sunburn and a range of inflammatory and allergic skin disorders including eczema, urticaria and infections (eg. impetigo, chicken pox). It is one of the best remedies for treating nappy rash and can be an effective treatment for varicose ulcers. It is not hard to see why chamomile had a long tradition of use as a wound healer. Chamomile can also be used in infusions and creams for soothing sore nipples and as a douche for vaginal infections including thrush. Sitting in a bowl of chamomile tea can be one of the most soothing solutions for cystitis and haemorrhoids.

Chamomile tea makes a good anti-inflammatory and antiseptic mouthwash for mouth ulcers and inflamed gums, a gargle for sore throats, an antiseptic wash for sore inflamed eyes and conjunctivitis. A warm teabag laid over inflamed eyes as a poultice is really effective for all inflammatory eye conditions. An infused oil of chamomile can be massaged into painful, inflamed joints to bring relief and can help to relieve nerve pain such as trigeminal neuralgia or sciatica. Chamomile oil makes a good insect

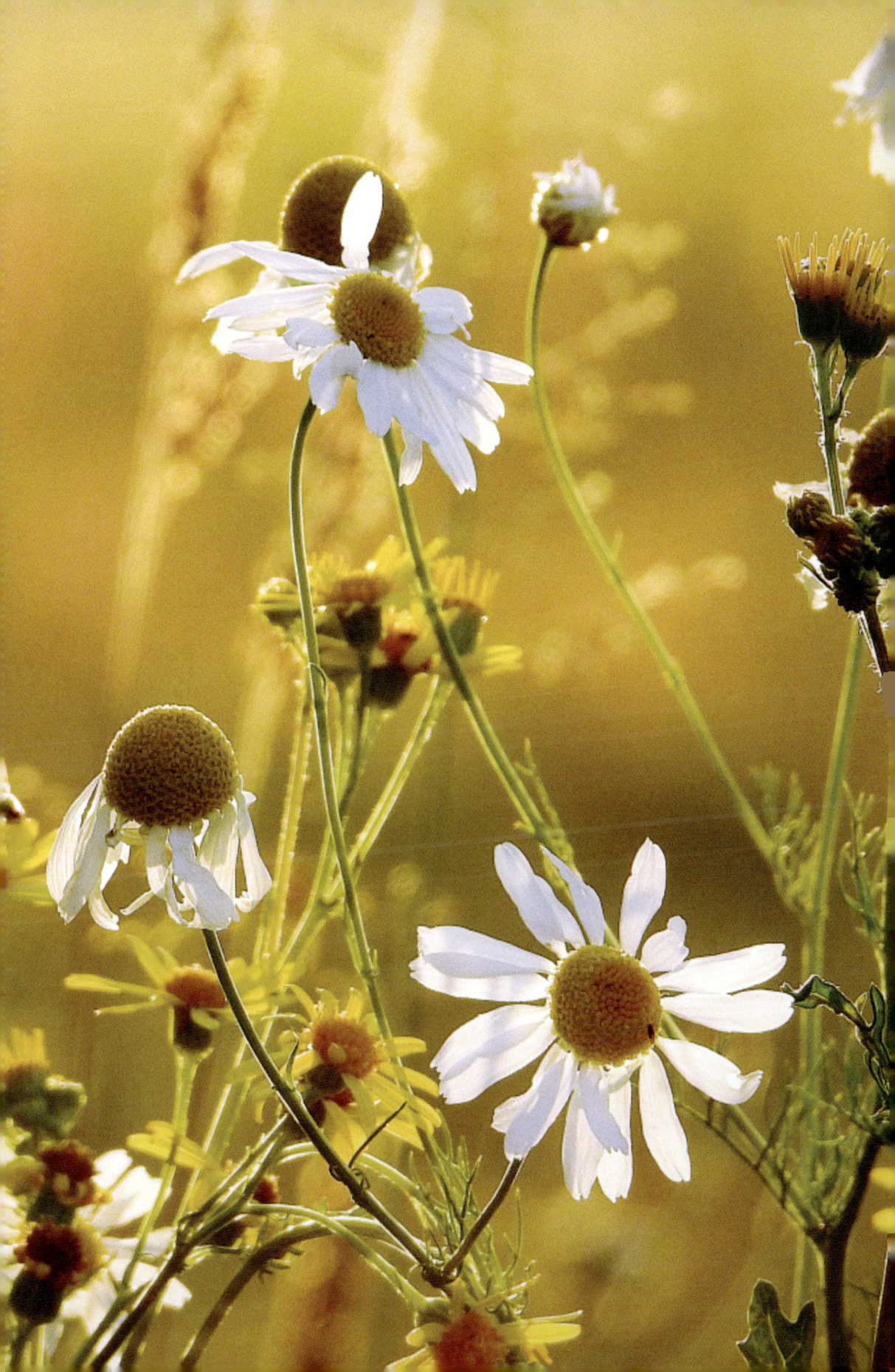

repellent and mixed into a cream can soothe the pain of bites and stings. A wash of chamomile tea used as a hair rinse after shampooing imparts golden highlights.

Homeopathic Remedy
Chamomilla is particularly suitable to people with great sensitivity to pain, which is often bought on or aggravated by emotions such as anger and irritability, as well as by teething in babies and toddlers, and too much tea or coffee. Chamomilla is particularly recommended for a woman in labour when the pain feels unbearable.

Flower Essence
As a remedy of the sun, chamomile helps to ease emotional problems and soothe anger and conflict and to bring out a sunny disposition. It is best for those who are moody, changeable, easily upset, irritable, impatient and angry. It will soothe tension and anxiety and stop it from accumulating through the day to cause restlessness, insomnia or nightmares. Inner tension and disharmony may also cause stomach problems, in both children and adults, as well as depression, hyperactivity, poor concentration and learning problems. Chamomile will help one to stand back from the day-to-day things that irritate and annoy, and upset one's superficial equilibrium, and to find a place of calm and serenity where light, like the sun behind the clouds, is always shining.

Growing
Propagate German chamomile by sowing seeds in spring or autumn in well-drained, preferably chalky soil; do not cover the seeds but water them in. Grows up to 18" (45cm) tall and flowers through the summer. Self-seeds freely. Likes a sunny position.

Propagate Roman chamomile by sowing seeds in spring, taking cuttings in summer or divide the plant in spring or autumn. Do not cover the seeds with soil as they need light to germinate. Prefers light, fertile, well-drained soil and full sun. Flowers through the summer.

Cautions
Some people have allergic reactions, including contact eczema, to members of the *Asteraceae* family. Alweays buy organic chamomile flowers as there may be high levels of pesticides and heavy metals in chamomile coming from Eastern Europe. Avoid with Warfarin and other anticoagulant medications. Caution with CNS depressants, (eg. alcohol, opiates, benzodiazepines, anaesthetics, tricyclic antidepressants, anti- epileptics).

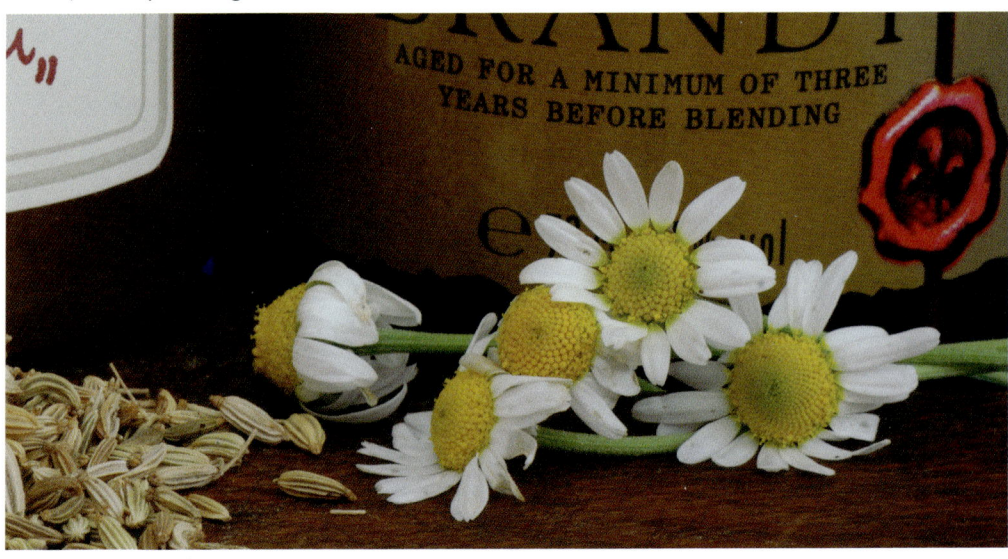

Recipes

Eyewash for Sore Tired Eyes & Conjunctivitis
Equal parts of calendula, chamomile, plantain, coriander and self heal

Place the herbs together in a teapot and pour over boiling water. Leave to infuse until lukewarm to cool. Use sterile eye bath to wash one eye, wash the eye bath thoroughly and then bathe the other eye.

Eye Wrap
Wrap the warmed herbs in a small piece of muslin and place over the eye. Lie quietly for 10–15 minutes 3 times daily.

Rosemary, St John's wort and Chamomile Oil for Muscular Aches and Pains
Place freshly crushed rosemary leaves, chamomile flowers and St John's wort flowers in a clear mason jar and cover them with cold-pressed sesame/sunflower oil or olive oil.
Place the jar, tightly lidded, in a sunny place for 2-3 weeks.
Strain the oil and discard the flowers, pressing them out well.
Use as a liniment or massage oil, applied warm, two or three times daily until pain subsides.
Massage is best followed by a hot bath or shower.

Cooling Stomach tea
1 part Meadowsweet
1 part Marshmallow leaves and flowers
1 part Lemon balm
1 part Chamomile
½ part Vervain

Place herbs together in a teapot and pour over boiling water. Leave to infuse for 20 minutes. Mix 1 dessertspoonful of aloe vera juice per cup of tea and take a cupful 3-4 times daily before meals.

Marshmallow is a wonderfully soothing remedy for irritation and inflammation in the digestive tract. Meadowsweet is the most renowned herbal antacid while vervain and chamomile are cooling and calming, excellent for stress related digestive disorders. The combination also has antimicrobial properties, helping to combat infection such as *Helicobacter pylori* that could be causing the problem.

Healing Salve for Eczema
A fragrant cream made from chamomile, calendula and lavender can soothe and heal at the same time. Chamomile is a wonderful anti-inflammatory herb and acts as an antihistamine. Calendula is one of the best herbs for the skin, cooling inflammation, speeding healing and helping to prevent infection, while delicate lavender has a marvellous ability to heal the skin without scarring and is antiseptic.

Equal parts of:
Calendula petals
Camomile flowers
Lavender flowers

Pour ½ pint /300 mls of warmed coconut oil into a *bain marie* (double saucepan). Chop the herbs roughly and place as much as will fit into the oil and remain submerged. Leave to macerate for a few hours over a low heat after which the oil will have absorbed the constituents and the mixture can be pressed through a muslin bag and the herb discarded.

Whilst the oil is still warm, pour it into sterilised ointment jars where it will quickly solidify. Label it clearly and store in a cool place.

Apply the cream night and morning after gently washing the area with rose water.

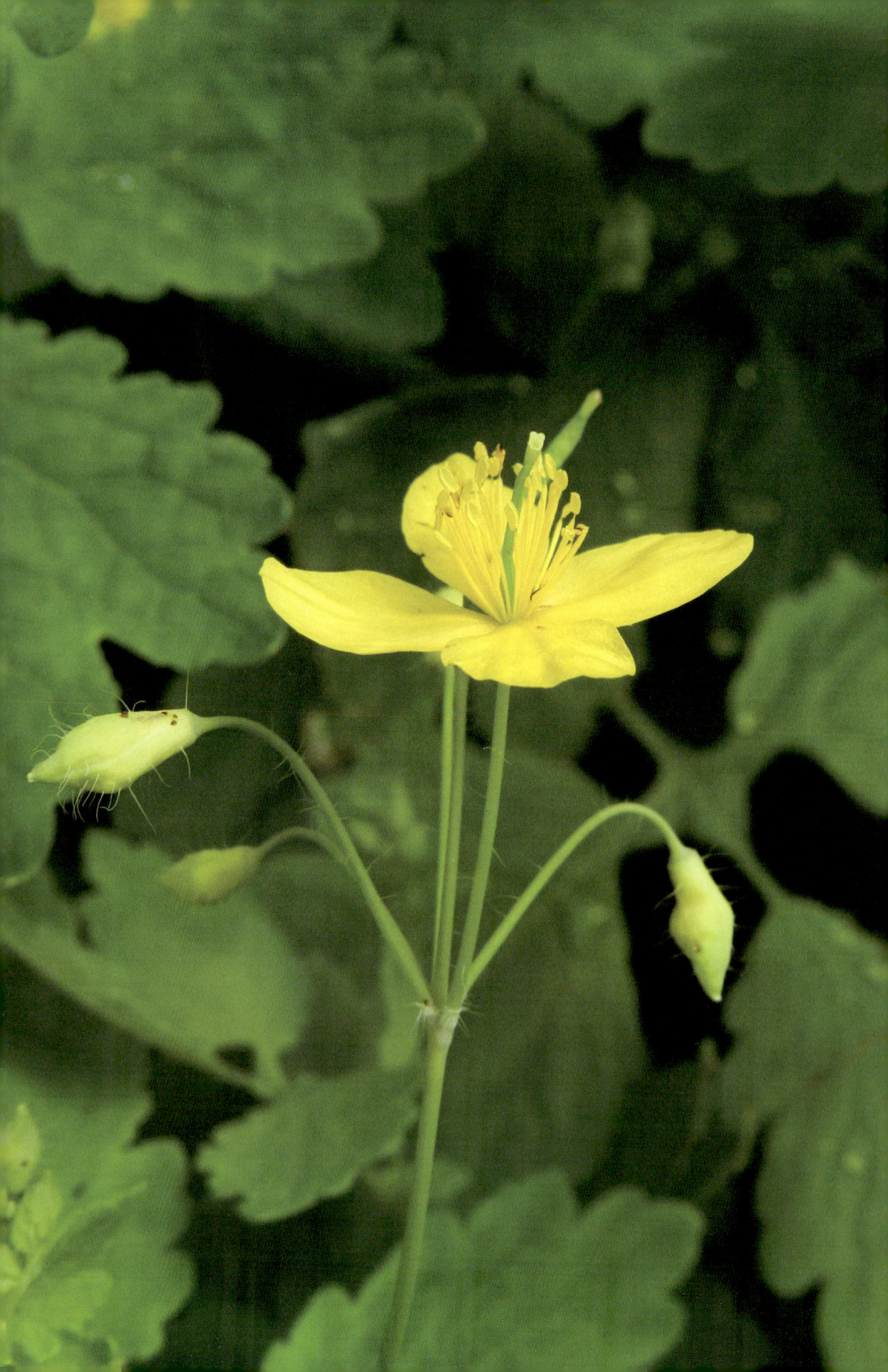

Chelidonium majus: Greater Celandine

The Flower of Vision

It seems to be called Chelidonia because it springs out of the ground together with ye swallows appearing, & doth wither with them departing. Somme have related that if any of the swallowes' young ones be blinde, the dames bringing this herbe, doe heale the blindness of it
Dioscorides (c 40–90AD)

Other Names: Swallow wort, devil's milk, yellow spit, nipplewort, tetterwort, wartwort

Parts Used: Whole herb

Greater celandine is a member of the poppy (Papaveraceae) family and shows many of the poppy's actions in healing; as a herbal remedy it has to be used with great care and is not recommended for home use internally. However, it is safe to use externally and as a homeopathic and flower remedy. It is indigenous to Europe and is remarkably resilient, flourishing where other plants would not survive. It can be found in waste places, growing against walls and fences, and in small cracks in walls and pavements. When cut or bruised it exudes a bright yellow-orange juice that tastes bitter and acrid, much like the juice of a poppy.

The name *Chelidonium* comes from the Greek word 'chelidon' meaning swallow because of an old belief that swallows carried the plant to their nests to open the eyes of their young. It is also thought that the name comes from the simple fact that greater celandine comes into flower when the swallows arrive in spring and fades when they leave at the end of summer. To the alchemists, greater celandine was special, and they used it in their search for the philosopher's stone, calling it 'coelidonum' meaning gift of heaven.

It used to be said that greater celandine symbolised happiness and if put a sprig on your pillow at night it could give you prophetic dreams. Another belief was that if a witch carried a plant in a red bag hung round her neck she would avoid being seen or captured, while other folklore has it that if you scrubbed your floor with an infusion of celandine or burnt the dried herb as incense, it would deter witches.

The leaves and flowers of greater celandine have been used in healing since the days of the ancient Greeks and Romans, as described by Dioscorides and Pliny the elder in the first century AD. As the story of the swallow indicates, the plant has an affinity with the eyes, and its most prevalent use was as a remedy for a range of eye problems that caused visual problems. The Anglo-Saxons used a lukewarm infusion made with honey in a brass or copper pot as an eye salve, which was recorded in 1310. Francis Bacon said, *"Saladyne hath a yellow milk which hathe also much acrimonie for it cleanseth the eyse and is good for cataract"*, while Gerard stated, *"The juice of the herbe is good to sharpen the sight, for it cleanseth and consumeth away slimie things that cleave about the ball of the eye and hinder the sight."* Culpeper also described greater celandine as *"One of the best cures for the eyes — most desperate sore eyes have been cured by this only medicine."* He said it was *"best to allay the sharpness with a little breast milk."* It is still used by medical herbalists for eye infections and inflammatory eye problems.

Apparently, Pliny and Dioscorides recommended greater celandine for toothache, eye problems, gallstones and indigestion. Culpeper recommended that the whole plant should be boiled in white wine and taken with aniseed as it *"opens obstructions of the liver and gall, helps the yellow jaundice… helps the dropsy and the itch, and those that have old sores."* One of its common names 'tetterwort' refers to the fact that greater celandine was used for applying to skin problems such as ringworm and eczema. Greater celandine was much admired during the Middle Ages for its ability to cure eye diseases, throat problems, ulcers and skin problems including eczema, as well as colic and jaundice. Hildegard of Bingen recommended celandine juice to enhance sight and juice mixed with tallow as a cure for skin ulcers in her work *Liber subtilitatum diversarum naturarum creaturarum* written around 1150–1160 AD and published in 1533. Syrenius writing in 1613 said celandine could be used to dye the hair yellow, and to lighten freckles and hyperpigmentation on the face.

According to the doctrine of signatures, the bright orange-yellow juice indicated the plant's use in liver and gall-bladder problems. It was recommended for obstructions of the liver and gallbladder, jaundice, infections, gallstones and pain in the liver area. Paracelsus was aware of the plant's healing properties and classified it as a 'blood' herb for circulatory problems and as a 'yellow' herb for liver ailments and jaundice.

Herbal Remedy
Greater celandine contains isoquinoline alkaloids (berberine, chelerythrine, chelidonine, coptisine and sanguinarine) which are mostly found in the latex in all parts of the plant except the flowers. It also contains organic acids, flavonoids, hydroxycinnamic acids, saponins, carotenoids, phenolic acids, chelidonic acid, latex, vitamin C and proteins. Like the poppy, greater celandine has narcotic properties and is only ever used in small doses by qualified medical herbalists, but it is interesting to note that it has been used for many centuries by physicians and extensively in folk medicine in many different parts of the world especially Central and Eastern Europe without reservations about potential toxicity. It was even given to children.

All over Poland it was common practice to apply the fresh leaves or the juice on wounds, eczema and cuts, and a decoction of the root was used in baths and lotions to treat skin problems. In the Ukraine the root and fresh leaves were rubbed on corns; after a week, they softened and came off. A salve for pustules was made from celandine, olive oil, fir resin and beeswax.

In Russia and Serbia juice of the aerial parts was applied to wounds, skin irritations, allergic rashes such as eczema, psoriasis and boils. In Montenegro the plant has been used on blisters, rashes and scabies.

Greater celandine has also been one of the most popular folk remedies for liver and gallbladder problems, as an analgesic for gallbladder colic, inflammation, gallstones and spasm. In Poland an infusion of the leaves (with half a teaspoonful of the leaves per cup of boiling water) was used for just these problems and to regulate the bowels. Children with jaundice were bathed in celandine and also given it to drink. In the Ukraine, Balkan countries and Serbia, an infusion was used as relaxant in colic attacks, for inflammation of the gallbladder, bile duct, jaundice, and hepatitis.

The plant tastes very bitter and by stimulating the bitter receptors in the mouth, greater celandine stimulates the flow of digestive juices and bile from the liver. It is still used in small doses by some herbalists for inflammation and infection in the liver and gallbladder, for gallstones and also as an anti-inflammatory remedy for arthritis, gout, inflammatory skin and eye problems. Its antioxidant action has a hepato-protective action, protecting the liver from damage caused by toxins, drugs and alcohol. With its antispasmodic and antimicrobial actions, it can ease pain and spasm in the digestive tract, easing wind, bloating, gastro-enteritis, IBS, biliary colic and constipation. It has also been used for stomach cancer and intestinal polyps.

By cleansing the liver and stimulating the kidneys, greater celandine acts as a cleansing remedy, aiding the detoxifying action of the body. As a diuretic, it aids elimination of toxins via the urine, and relieves fluid retention. It can be given for allergies and toxic conditions which give rise to skin problems. As a sedative it can aid sleep, reduce muscle tension and anxiety and relieve pain. It has an antispasmodic effect particularly in the respiratory system, making it potentially useful in asthma.

The main uses of greater celandine have been as an antibacterial, antiviral and antiprotozoal to combat infection, as a spasmolytic to ease pain and spasm, as an anti-inflammatory for stomach and liver problems and as an anticancer remedy. The antibacterial and antifungal activity is attributed to the alkaloids and flavonoids and can successfully treat both Gram-positive and Gram-negative bacteria including *Staphylococcus aureus* and *Bacillus anthracis*. The tincture can combat multidrug resistant Gram-positive bacteria in surgical wounds and infections including *Bacillus cereus, E. coli* and *Pseudomonas aeruginosa*. It is also active against *Staphylococcus epidermidis, Bacillus subtilis, Bacillus anthracis, Klebsiella pneumoniae, Salmonella gallinarum, S. typhi, S. paratyphi, Proteus vulgaris, Shigella flexneri,* and mycobacteria including *Mycobacterium tuberculosis* and *M. smegmatis*.

Its antiviral action is attributed to the glycosaminoglycans and alkaloids present in the latex which may be able to inhibit HIV infections. Extracts of all parts of the plant can combat protozoal infections including *Trichomonas vaginalis*.

The antitumor properties of greater celandine have been known since antiquity and modern research is seeking to verify this. It is thought that some of the alkaloids such as berberine, chelerythrine and sanguinarine stop proliferation of cancer cells. It is also possible that greater celandine might have the potential to slow the progression of Alzheimer's disease. The journey continues into understanding the therapeutic potential of this herb that has been valued for millenia.

Externally, the plant is perfectly safe for home use. With its antimicrobial and antiviral activity, it makes a wonderfully effective remedy for warts and verrucae when the bright orange fresh juice is applied directly. If you do this daily, after three weeks they will have gone. An ointment made from root and leaves can be used for haemorrhoids and an infusion of the flowers and leaves can be used as a skin wash for rashes, eczema and scabies.

Homeopathic Remedy
Chelidonium reflects much of the herbal action. It is predominantly a liver remedy, indicated by a continual bruised pain or ache under the right shoulder blade, with a variety of symptoms indicative of liver or gall-bladder problems.

Like the opium poppy, chelidonium is given for debility and drowsiness, which tends to occur after eating and on waking. It is also a remedy for paralysis. It acts on the respiratory system and is indicated in dry, racking coughs which are worse at night, with little expectoration and no pain. Chelidonium is also given for arthritis, where oedema, heat, tenderness and stiffness are leading indications. The homoepathic remedy can also be given as a heapatoprotective, protecting the liver from damage from toxins such as cadmium.

Flower Essence
The herb was used historically to sharpen the sight, the flower essence is recommended to sharpen the mind and enhance the giving and receiving of information. It is the remedy of communication and has an affinity for the throat area and the thyroid gland. It makes a good remedy for singers, teachers and lecturers as it helps with articulation.

It is useful for people who have difficulty taking in information, such as those who are stubborn and opinionated, or who do not listen, or who cannot concentrate for long. It is said to increase the possibility of telepathic communication and enhance the understanding of information given in dreams. In this way, it affects not only the sight and the mind, but also inner vision.

Growing
Propagate by sowing seeds in autumn or divide roots in spring. It prefers dry chalky soil, full sun or light shade. Self-seeds freely though it is rarely a nuisance. Grows up to 3' (1m) high and flowers in the summer.

Cautions
As a herbal remedy for home use, only use externally. This herb is potentially toxic and has restricted use in UK, available from practitioners only. Avoid in pregnancy, breastfeeding and in children. May cause dermatitis, hepatitis and phototoxicity. It may lower blood sugar so monitor patients on insulin or oral hypoglycaemics.

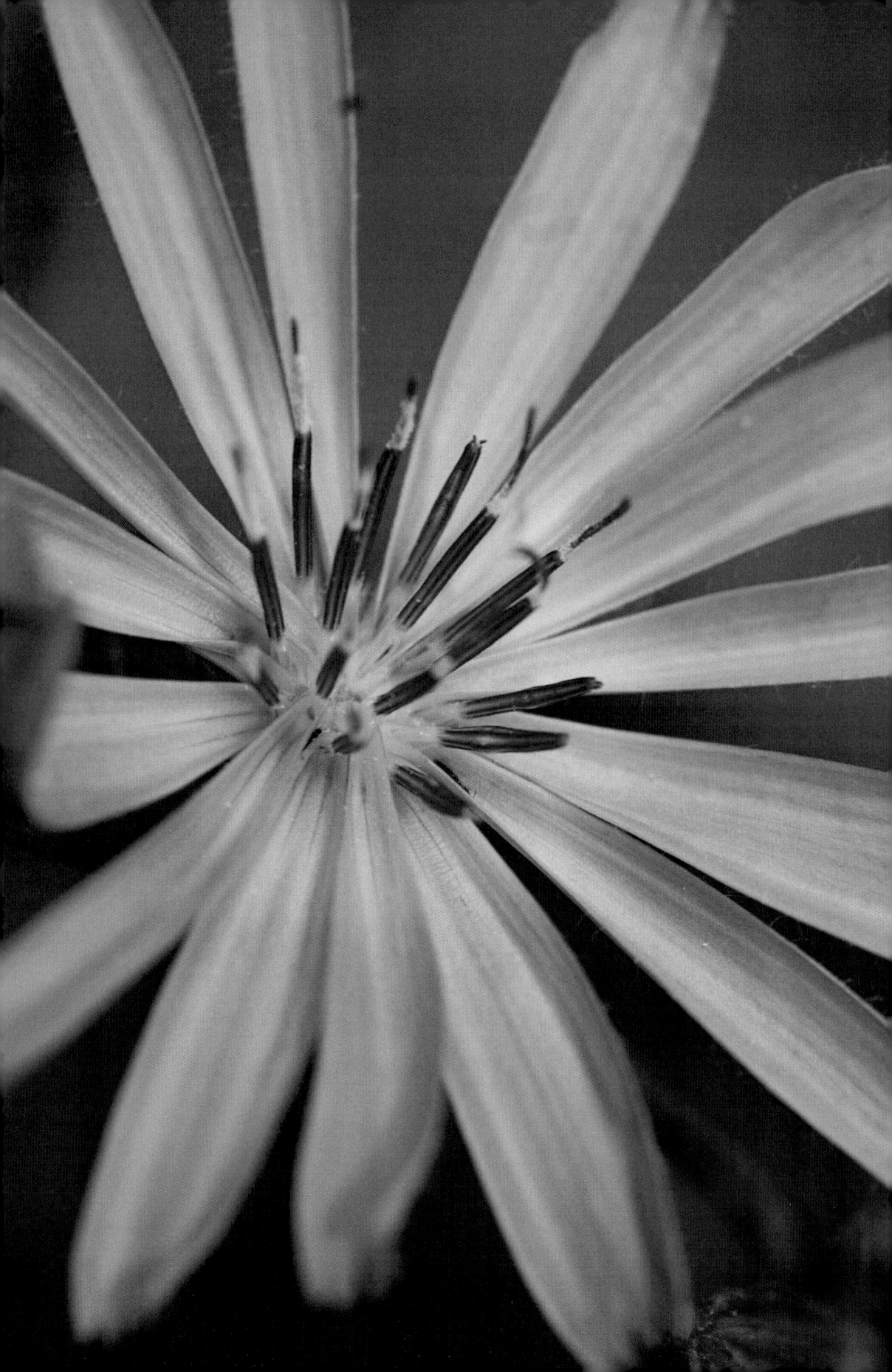

Cichorium intybus: Chicory

The Flower of Assimilation

On upland slopes the shepherds mark
The hour when to the dial true
Cichorium to the towering lark
Lifts her soft eyes serenely blue
– Charlotte Smith (1749–1806)

Other Names: Endive, coffee weed, succory, wild succory, blue sailors, ragged sailors, blue daisy, blue dandelion, blue weed

Parts Used: Root, leaves, flowers and seeds

This resilient wildflower with its beautiful pale blue flowers and tough branching stems can be found in many places in the world in hedgerows, fields and waste land. The flowers apparently open at 7 o'clock in the morning and close precisely at midday and for this reason they were used by shepherds and country folk as a guide to the time and by Linnaeus the botanist in his floral clock. Chicory has long tap roots which have been known since antiquity for flavouring coffee, hence its old name 'coffee weed' and the whole plant has a very bitter taste which has been utilised in many beneficial ways. The flowers are loved by bees.

Cultivated in the Nile area of ancient Egypt for thousands of years, and native to Europe, North Africa and West Asia, this pretty member of the Asteraceae/Compositae family has a long and well-documented history of use since at least the 1st century AD. The ancient Egyptians and Romans were known to eat the root in large amounts to cleanse the liver and the blood. The Egyptians and Greeks drank chicory coffee made from the roasted roots, calling it 'liver's friend'. The young lettuce-like leaves were considered by the Egyptians, Greeks, Arabs and Romans to be a particularly healthy food and were eaten as a cooked vegetable and raw in salads with oil and vinegar. They also used them for blood cleansing and to invigorate the nerves. When bruised, the leaves were used as a poultice for swellings, infections and inflamed eyes.

The name 'succory' may come from the Latin 'succurrere' meaning to run under, as the long tap roots run so far under the ground. Alternatively, it might come from the Arabic name 'chicourey' or the Egyptian word 'ctchorium.' The Germans call chicory 'watcher of the road' since according to an old legend, a beautiful young girl waited every day for her lover to return from sea. When finally, the lover's ship did not return, she died of a broken heart and the blue chicory flower grew in the place where she died. The seeds of chicory have been used traditionally in love potions.

According to the Doctrine of Signatures, the milky juice from the plant meant it was a good remedy for tender breasts in nursing mothers and the delicate blue flowers that opened and closed meant that it would be a good remedy for the eyes. English Tudor poet and farmer Thomas Tusser (1524–1580) said in his long poem *Five Hundred Points of Good Husbandry*, that chicory was a good remedy for ague (malaria), and herbalist John Parkinson (1567–1650) said it was *"a fine, cleansing, jovial plant."* It was used *"when boiled in broth for those that have hot, weak and feeble stomachs doe strengthen the same."*

Herbal Remedy
Chicory has properties similar to those of dandelion. They are both cooling and cleansing,

valuable for treating liver problems, fevers, inflammatory skin problems, anaemia and general debility. The root, flowers and leaves are bitter and stimulate the flow of digestive enzymes and bile from the liver. They increase appetite and digestion, enhance absorption of nutrients and support the work of the liver and gallbladder. The flowers have been used as a tonic and appetite stimulant and to treat gallstones, gastroenteritis and sinus problems. In Italy, a decoction of the flowers is used as a cleansing remedy for clearing toxins from the blood.

The root contains up to 40% inulin, sesquiterpene lactones, chicoric acid, aliphatic compounds, terpenoids, bitter compounds, cichoriin, taraxasterol, tannins, indole alkaloids, pectin, coumarins, vitamins (A, B, C, K) and flavonoids. The aerial parts contain inulin, fructose, resin, flavonoids, sesquiterpene lactones (esculetin), methoxycoumarin cichorine, essential oils and anthocyanins which contribute to the blue colour of the flower. Chicory root has a gentle detoxifying effect; it acts as a mild laxative and diuretic, removing excess water and toxins from the body via the bowels and kidneys. By increasing the excretion of uric acid, and with the anti-inflammatory action provided by the antioxidant phenols and caffeic acid, chicory can be useful in osteoarthritis and gout as well as inflammatory skin problems.

Chicory supports the liver in its metabolic and detoxifying work. By increasing the flow of bile from the liver, chicory root helps break down fats and can be helpful in mild constipation and conditions associated with a sluggish liver such as headaches, skin problems, lethargy and irritability. Its antioxidant action attributed to the phenols and sesquiterpenes, has a hepatoprotective effect, protecting the liver from the adverse effects of stress caused by alcohol, drugs and other toxins it has to break down. It is one of the herbal components of Liv-52, a traditional Indian tonic used widely for protecting the liver and for successfully treating liver problems including cirrhosis. The seeds are one of the main ingredients of *'Jigrine',* a commercial product of India used to treat liver problems. Chicory is also useful for gallstones and can be helpful to diabetics as it reduces blood sugar. It can slow the pace of diabetes progress and delay the development of its complications.

Chicory is an excellent remedy for the gut. It has antibacterial and antifungal properties, which help to curb the growth of unfriendly microorganisms in the gut. The root is an excellent source of inulin, a polysaccharide that feeds the beneficial bacteria in the gut and so supports their habitat and survival in relation to more pathogenic microorganisms. Of apparently more than 30,000 different plant species containing inulin, chicory root contains the highest concentration. The friendly flora help improve the digestive as well as nervous and immune function of the body and are vital for our general health in so many ways. Chicory root enhances digestion and absorption of minerals and synthesis of B vitamins. The inulin is not digestible, so it acts to bulk out the stool and promote regular bowel movements.

With its digestive, laxative, anti-inflammatory, antibacterial, antifungal and antiparasitic properties, the whole plant makes an excellent remedy for a range of digestive problems especially those associated with heat, inflammation, toxicity and disturbance of the gut flora. This includes indigestion, nausea, wind, bloating, gastritis, peptic ulcers, inflammatory gut problems, constipation and IBS.

All parts of chicory can provide good support for the immune system. It has antimicrobial actions; seed extracts are active against bacteria including *Staphylococcus aureus*, *Pseudomonas aeruginosa* and *E. coli*. Root extracts are very effective against *Bacillus subtilis*, *S. aureus*, *Salmonella typhi*, *Micrococcus luteus* and *E. coli*. The leaves and flowers, with their tannins and sesquiterpenes, are good for grazing animals as they have anthelmintic properties and help combat worms and parasites, indicating that it is not only the root and seeds that are of benefit. Constituents in the root, notably magnolialide, may inhibit several tumour cell lines and may be helpful in leukaemia.

Chicory also has antifungal properties active against *Candida albicans* and is a good remedy for allergies such as hay fever and eczema as it can inhibit allergic reactions and lower histamine levels. In parts of the East including Afghanistan, chicory root has been used as a remedy for malaria and we know this use goes back at least to Tudor England. All parts of the plant including the flowers have an antimalarial action, which is attributed to the sesquiterpene lactones, lactucin and lactucopicrin.

Chicory is high in antioxidant polyphenols which have a protective and anti-inflammatory effect on the cardiovascular system. It lowers harmful cholesterol and can be useful for heart problems including arrhythmias, palpitations and fibrillation. A regular cup of chicory coffee can provide preventative care for the heart and circulation.

The seeds have a calming effect on the nervous system and can be used for insomnia. The bitter compounds lactucin and lactucopicrin have an analgesic and sedative action, which can provide help when sleep is disturbed by pain of any sort.

Externally chicory leaves can be made into a paste and applied as a cooling, anti-inflammatory, antifungal and wound-healing poultice to cuts and wounds, as well as infected and inflammatory skin problems such as acne, boils, eczema and prickly heat. In Turkey, an ointment is made from the leaves for wound healing. An infusion of the flowers can be used as a lotion for cuts, bruises and inflammatory skin problems and to bath sore, inflamed eyes. Chicory also makes a good antibacterial mouthwash as it combats several periodontopathic bacteria including *Streptococcus mutans, Actinomyces naeslundii,* and *Prevotella intermedia.*

Homeopathic Remedy
Cichorium is used for sluggish digestion, and heaviness in the stomach with a general disinclination to physical or mental exertion. It is prescribed for over-relaxed bowels, leading to constipation and headaches.

Flower Essence
Chicory flower remedy is for people who are possessive, domineering, excessively interfering and manipulative. Very demanding, they require a lot of support from those around them, needing love, sympathy and a great deal of attention. If this is not available, they can easily lapse into self-pity and use emotional blackmail or illness to get the attention they need. Behind this overbearing personality is an insecure person who fears being alone, or losing friends, family or possessions. They easily feel slighted or hurt and are over-concerned with what other people owe them – their overpowering love and show of affection is very conditional. Chicory helps to create a more secure feeling in oneself, so that one is more able to give love unselfishly – a very useful remedy for mothers and also for children.

Edible Uses
Chicory root is best known as a substitute for or addition to coffee; it helps counteract the stimulating effect of caffeine in the coffee. The root is dried, roasted and granulated and tastes delicious. The sweetness of the inulin once roasted makes a really good blend of sweet with the bitter. As a vegetable, the root can be roasted or boiled. It is also used as a flavouring ingredient for brewing beers instead or in addition to hops.

The young leaves of cultivated forms of chicory are popular in salads, but they are generally blanched to removes the bitterness of the leaves. The wild leaves can be used similarly. For the French, the blanched leaves called *barbe de capuchin* make a favourite winter salad. The young leaves can be cooked and eaten like spinach or other greens, they can be sautéed with garlic and butter or olive oil and added to soups and stews.

Growing
Chicory can be found growing wild, to a height of 3–5' (1–1.5m) and flowering from June to October. Propagate by sowing seeds in late spring in rich soil and full sun.

Cautions
As a herbal remedy, chicory root can reduce absorption of glucose in the gut; caution with insulin and other hypoglycaemic medications. Avoid with Warfarin, salicylates and other anticoagulant medications.

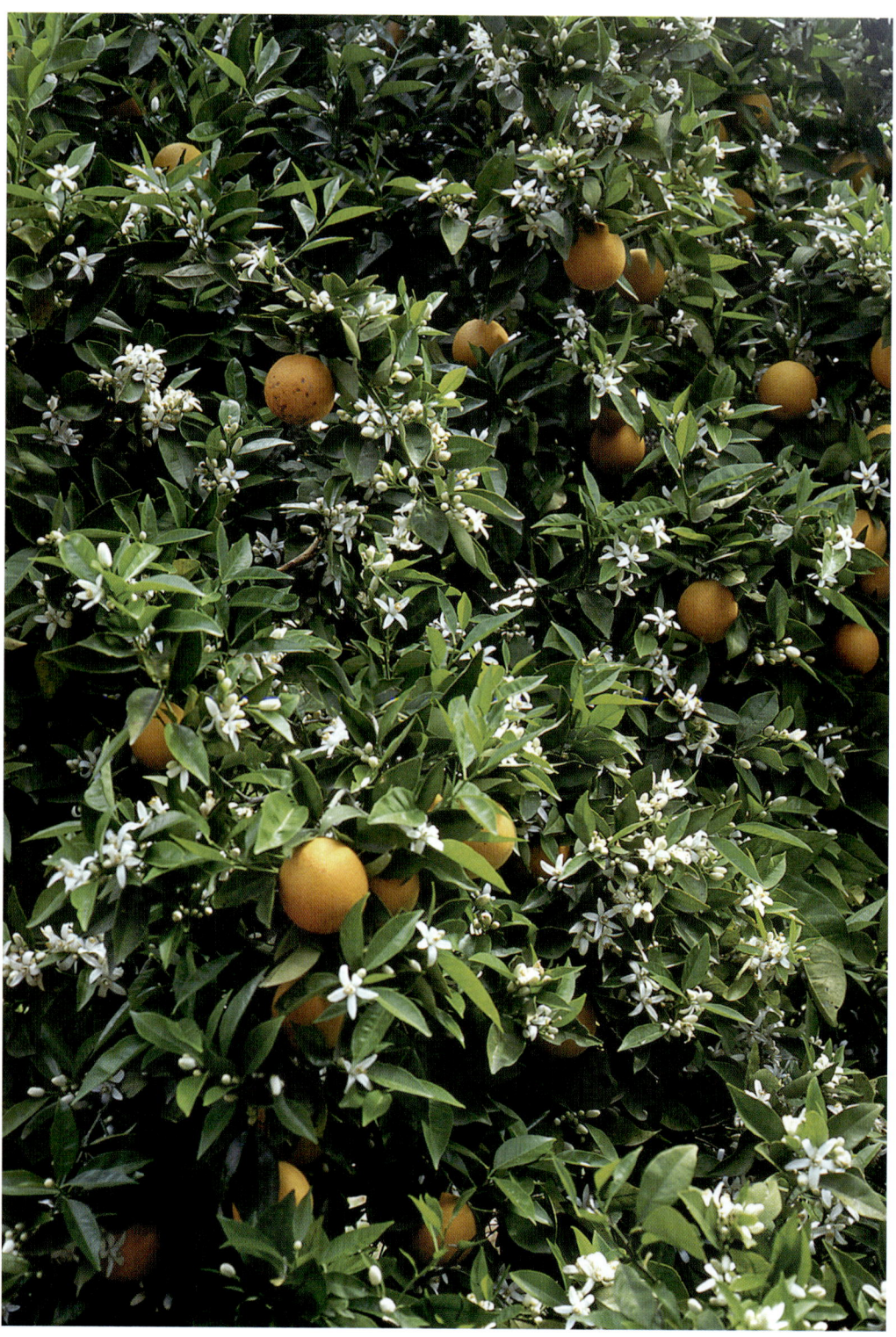

Citrus aurantium: Orange Blossom

The Flower of Morocco

O Love! what hours were thine and mine,
In lands of palm and southern pine;
In lands of palm, of orange-blossom,
Of olive, aloe, and maize and vine!
– Alfred Lord Tennyson 1809–1892

Other names: Essence of neroli, bigarade orange, bitter orange, sour orange, Seville orange, agua de Azahar, boosfeyr, portogalli

Parts used: Flowers

Orange blossom is the delightfully sweet-smelling white flower of the bitter orange or Seville orange tree from the Rutaceae family. The bitter orange is a thorny tree native to China, India and South East Asia and was introduced to Europe by the Arabs and from there spread to America. Its waxy clusters of flowers are loved for their delicious scent that perfumes the air in spring and for their ancient use in perfumery and food. The tree can live up to 600 years! The fruit is important as flavouring. The Seville orange variety is used to make marmalade as the high pectin in the peel helps it to set easily, but it is too bitter to eat as a fruit. The sweet orange *Citrus sinensis* produces the fruit we commonly enjoy. Orange flower water is a by-product of

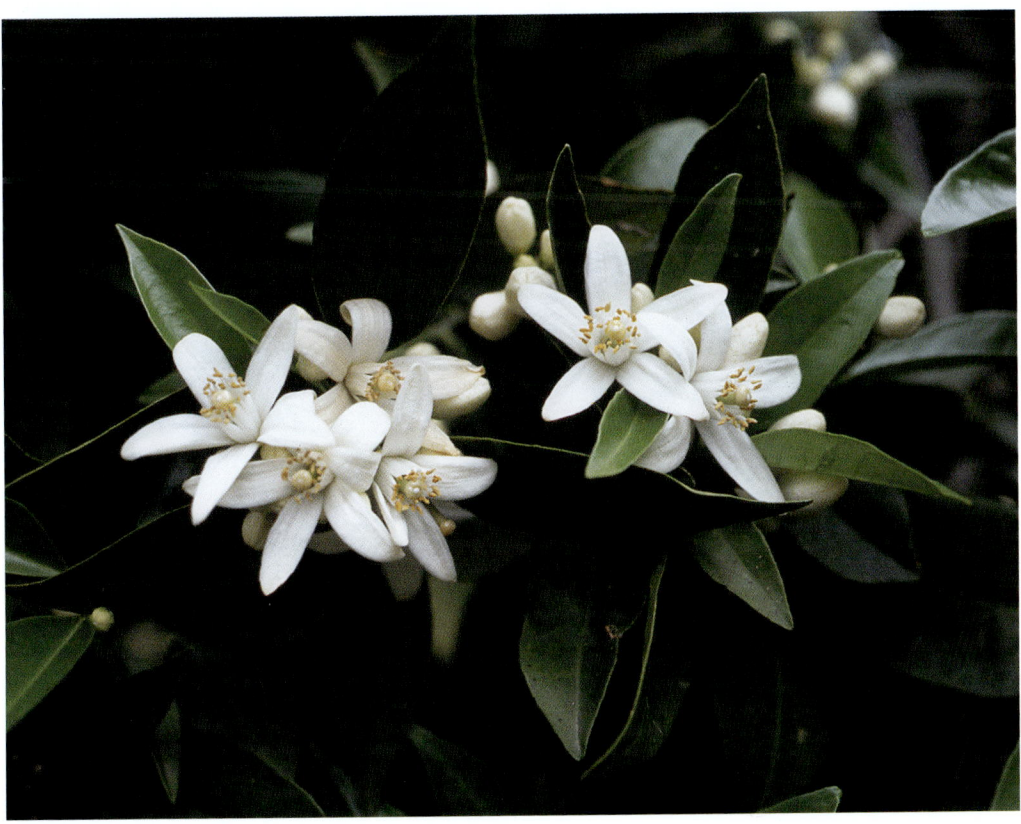

the distillation process to make neroli essential oil from the flowers. It takes 1,000 pounds (454 kilos) of orange blossom to produce just one pint (0.45 litres) of neroli oil, making it one of the most expensive essential oils in the world. It has a wonderfully uplifting sweet, floral and citrus aroma and the floral water has hints of the same.

The bitter orange is mentioned in one of the oldest and the most important writings on Ayurveda, the Charaka Samhita, which dates around 400–200 BC. The word 'orange' comes from Sanskrit 'naranga' or Tamil 'naraththai.' It became 'naranj' in Arabic, 'narantsion' in post-classical Greek and 'aurantium' in late Latin. Unknown to the Romans, the bitter orange was introduced to the Mediterranean by the Arabs, perhaps as early as the ninth century. Highly prized for its medicinal qualities, it was planted in monastery and convent gardens in Italy by the eleventh century and in Spain by the end of the twelfth century. Albertus Magnus was the first medieval writer to describe the bitter orange and he called the fruit 'arangus' from which the Italian 'arancia' and the French and English 'orange' all derive. The beautiful white orange flowers were seen as symbols of purity and innocence as well as good fortune, and until today they have been associated with brides and made into bridal bouquets and floral crowns for weddings.

Distilled waters, also known as hydrosols, have a long history. Orange flower water was first made when the alembic still was invented in 800AD by the Arab alchemist Jabir ibn Hayyan to make essential oils as well as alcohol. The word 'alembic' comes from the metaphoric meaning of 'that which refines; which transmutes' through distillation. The use of the sweetly scented and flavoured orange flower water in cooking dates from then in the Middle East, typically for pastries and other sweet dishes. It gradually spread across the Mediterranean and then into Europe over the course of the following centuries. By the fourteenth century orange flower water was popular in Sicily as a scent for household linen but was not used in cooking. It became known as Essence of Neroli as it was named after Nerola in Italy where an influential French courtier Anna Maria de la Temoiller lived in the 16th Century. She liked the oil and flower water to perfume her gloves and her bath and it became a fashionable fragrance in Italy. From around this time bitter orange was grown in the south of France, particularly to produce orange flower water to use as perfume and for flavouring and it became widely used in European cuisine.

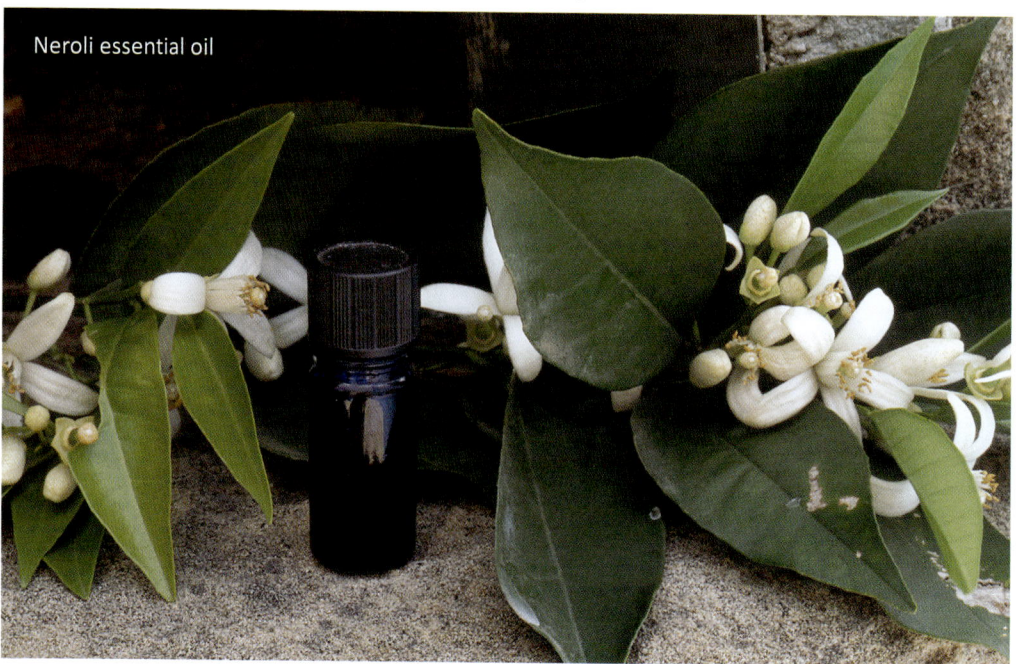

Neroli essential oil

There were several grades of orange flower water based on the percentage of fresh flowers to water used in the distillation process and the price varied accordingly. Double orange flower water was the most commonly produced, using one part of orange flowers to four parts water. Triple orange flower water was made with one part of flowers and three parts of water, while quadruple orange flower water was made by distilling one part of flowers and two parts of water. It became an exotic, costly but popular flavouring in England by the seventeenth century, especially among the upper classes, where serving food and drinks flavoured with orange flower water became almost a status symbol. With its medicinal and cosmetic uses, it was to be found in still rooms, kitchens, dressing rooms and on the apothecary's shelves well into the nineteenth century.

From the seventeenth century, orange flower water became popular for creating special ambiences with its delightful scent. Fountains of flowing orange flower water were set up in the middle of tables, wafting their lovely fragrance around the room or outdoors to accompany alfresco meals in warm weather in Italy and the south of France, but only occasionally in England, probably on account of the unsettled weather! The wafting floral fragrance during the meal was said to refresh tired eyes and revive flagging spirits.

It had many other uses as a medicine in Europe around this time, although orange blossom oil had been used since ancient Egyptian times for medicinal purposes. It was used to promote good digestion and as a tonic to strengthen the stomach. It was also prescribed for those with nervous dispositions as a remedy for 'neuralgic headache' and 'palpitations of the heart' and to prevent convulsions. Orange flower water was often given as a sleeping draught, and yet its scent was considered to have an aphrodisiac effect, especially when made into 'angel water' with one part of orange flower water, one part rose water and a half part of myrtle water, with a dash of musk and ambergris. It was popular for eighteenth century ladies to liberally apply 'angel water' to their bosom exposed by low necklines and pushed up by their corsets, so it was hard to know which played the main part in creating allure!

Orange flower water is still made today in many parts of the world, especially Tunisia, Morocco and Egypt. The trees have become part of the Mediterranean landscape, decorating towns and countryside alike in Spain, Italy, North Africa and the Middle East, filling the air with its enchanting scent in spring. It is still widely used in cooking and as medicines for sleep problems, stomach aches and nervous problems, for children as well as adults. It has also been used in perfumes and colognes as its fragrance is stable and blends well with other aromas.

Herbal Remedy and Essential Oil
The bitter orange flower provides a choice of medicines and aromatic remedies with varying strengths. Firstly, the most expensive absolute, with its viscous oil and heady perfume produced through solvent extraction, called orange blossom oil; next the pale yellow neroli oil, with its sweet, tangy and refreshing scent extracted through distillation; thirdly the cold pressed sweet-bitter orange oil, from the rind of the fruit; fourthly the greener petitgrain from distillation of the twigs and leaves; then the hydrosol called orange flower water, and there is also the tincture of the flowers.

Used either as neroli oil, as a tincture or hydrosol, orange flower is a wonderful medicine. It has antimicrobial, antioxidant and anti-inflammatory actions which help protect against a wide range of infections, inflammatory problems, degenerative diseases as well as cancer. These are attributed to the presence of phenolic compounds, tannins, flavonoids, essential oils, carotene, terpinols, bitter components, terpenes and vitamins C. The essential oil in neroli includes linalool (which is antimicrobial and antiseptic), monoterpenes like limonene and pinene (which act as stimulants, decongestants and anti-cancer agents), linalyl acetate (an anti-inflammatory when combined with linalool) and nerolidol (with antibacterial, antifungal and antioxidant actions).

The way that orange flowers are prepared makes a difference to their medicinal benefits. The hydrosol has much less abundant but still valuable essential oils including linalool, nerolidol, linalyl acetate, d-limonene, α-terpineol and neryl acetate as the major components. The tincture contains tannins, flavonoids, polyphenols, sterols, alkaloids and polyterpenes. The antioxidant phenols and flavonoids are higher in the tincture than the essential oil, which is higher than the hydrosol, as alcohol is a better solvent for these constituents. The essential oil and hydrosol both contain high levels of monoterpenes and sesquiterpenes which have antioxidant activity much like the phenolic compounds, helping to protect the body from damage caused by free radicals.

Orange flowers are a delightful as well as effective remedy for preventing and treating infection. They have antimicrobial effects which are particularly good when the oil is used topically on the skin, but they can also be useful in respiratory infections when the oil is inhaled. The polyphenols, flavonoids, alkaloids and terpenes, particularly in the essential oil and tincture and less in the hydrosol, have significant antimicrobial activity against many different bacteria including Amoxycillin-resistant *Bacillus cereus, Staph. aureus, Listeria monocytogenes, Salmonella Typhimurium* and *E. coli*. They also combat fungal infections.

From its history as well as its wonderful scent, it is hardly surprising that orange flower can be really beneficial for the nerves. Its antispasmodic and sedative effects can help reduce tension and anxiety and lift the spirits. Inhalation of heavenly orange blossom essential oil can quickly reduce stress and cortisol levels and increase serotonin levels. It is excellent for calming fear and well worth using during panic attacks. It could also be helpful when dealing with addiction and addictive behaviour. Orange flower makes a good remedy for sleeping problems and can be helpful for stress-related symptoms including high blood pressure, heart palpitations, headaches and migraine. While being calming it does not cause drowsiness and in fact can be helpful for poor concentration, behavioural problems in children and ADHD.

When the exquisitely scented oil is used in massage oils, in the bath or as inhalations, it helps relax muscle tension, pain and spasms and is useful in cramp, colic, back and shoulder pain and cramping period pains. It has anticonvulsant properties attributed to the linalool, linalyl acetate, nerolidol, farnesol, α-terpineol and limonene in the oil, which help to regulate the brain's activity and to prevent seizures. Its anti-inflammatory and antioxidant actions combined with its sedative effects can be helpful in reducing sensitivity to both chronic and acute pain and inflammation as in gout, arthritis or fibromyalgia.

Orange flower is a delicious but effective remedy for the digestion. It improves digestion and absorption and can be helpful in stress-related gut problems such as stomach aches, wind, bloating, colic, indigestion, constipation and diarrhoea. Its astringent tannins and cooling effect combined with its anti-inflammatory actions can be helpful in inflammatory conditions of the digestive tract such as gastritis, peptic ulcers, Crohn's disease and ulcerative colitis. The antimicrobial properties also help to combat unfriendly gut bacteria, and this can have far reaching effects on immunity and brain function. It also benefits the cardiovascular system by protecting the arteries from free radical damage and can help lower blood pressure by reducing cortisol. Its limonene content may also have a positive effect on the autonomic nervous system, which controls breathing and heartbeat.

Orange flower also has a balancing effect on hormone levels and is a lovely remedy for reducing symptoms of PMS including low mood, pain and bloating. Inhaling neroli oil before and during childbirth can reduce anxiety and ease pain during the first stage of contractions. It can also be helpful during the menopause to reduce symptoms such as mood swings, low libido and hot flushes as it improves oestrogen levels. Its old use as an aphrodisiac seems to hold true.

Externally orange flower is like a gift to the skin and can be used as a hydrosol and as a dilute essential oil. It is generally suitable for all skin types, especially those with delicate or ageing skin. Orange flower has a hydrating and restorative effect on skin and hair, which is good for healing scars, and minimising wrinkles and stretch marks. It contains compounds that can help the skin to heal and regenerate new cells as well as maintain its elasticity.

Orange flower can be used on its own or blended with other ingredients to make a variety of skin lotions or creams. Orange flower milk used to be a popular in skin preparations in the past to soothe and ease the pain of sunburn. Soaps can be scented with orange flower water. Adding a few drops of orange flower water to the final rinse when washing your hair or using it in an atomiser can add softness and shine to hair and a fresh, light scent. You can even add it to your laundry. The oil has antimicrobial and anti-inflammatory actions which can be used in skin treatments for inflammatory skin conditions as well as infections as in pimples, acne, boils and abscesses, ringworm and athlete's foot. It helps prevent infection and speed healing in cuts and wounds.

Flower Essence
As a flower essence the uplifting and calming effects of orange flower are evident. It is used for improving energy, renewing hope and interest in life, banishing melancholy and cultivating joy. It helps us to see the light at the end of the tunnel and the end or resolution of conflict and pressure. It can also give us the strength to endure difficulty and not sink into depression, despair or self pity. It helps us to let go of experiences of abuse both past and present and helps us to manage situations where we might feel we can't go on, as in the death of a loved one, heartbreak, a life-changing accident or illness. Orange flower is the flower of light and hope.

Edible Uses
Along with rose water, orange flower water is the most popular of flower waters for use in cooking and flavouring, especially when it comes to pastries, puddings or cookies, syrups and jams, as its taste is enhanced by sugar. Treats like macaroons, custard puddings, biscuits, jams and jellies were often flavoured with orange flower water in the past and fruit fools made with fresh fruit (especially delicately flavoured ones like apricots and peaches), custard and whipped cream, were often flavoured with orange flower water. In Lebanon it is drunk just as it is with a little water and called '*white coffee.*'

A light and refreshing drink, popular in England for social events in the eighteenth century, was called 'orgeat.' It was made of almond paste, milk, sugar, orange flower water and water. Towards the end of the century, the same ingredients were made into a syrup and served chilled. Today orange flower water can still be used similarly, added to drinks and deserts like cheesecakes, cakes, biscuits, fruit dishes, cereals and milks like almond milk.

Growing
The orange tree likes to be grown in moist but not wet soil and flourishes in subtropical, near-tropical climates, yet it can stand several degrees of frost for short periods. It can be grown from seed as well as from cuttings and is generally self-maintaining, requiring the minimum of attention. Some trees in Spain are said to be over 600 years old and one tree in a tub at Versailles was reportedly planted in the year 1421.

Cautions
Even though neroli oil can be soothing to sunburn, it should not be applied to the skin before lying in the sun or on a sunbed as this may cause an adverse reaction.

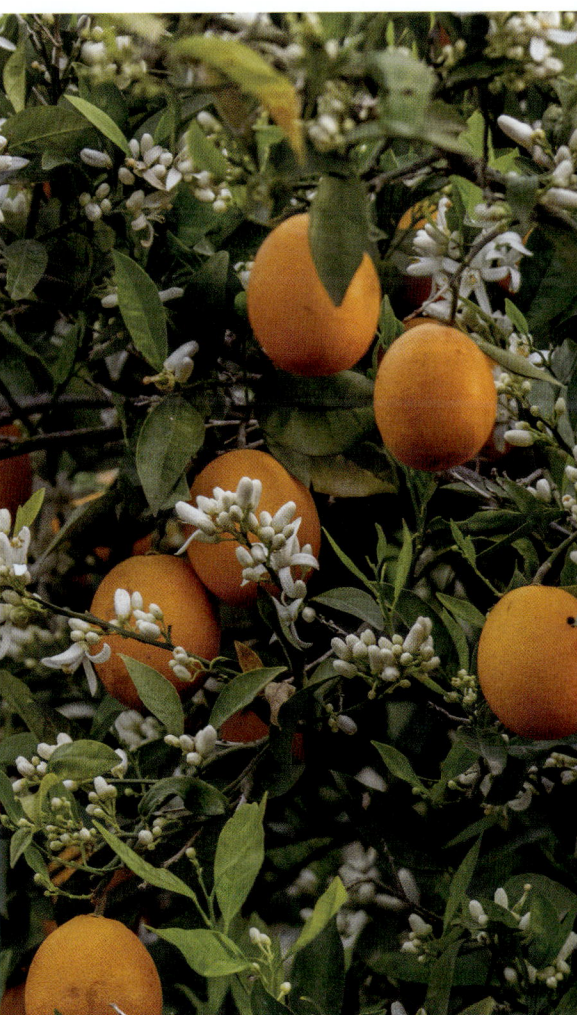

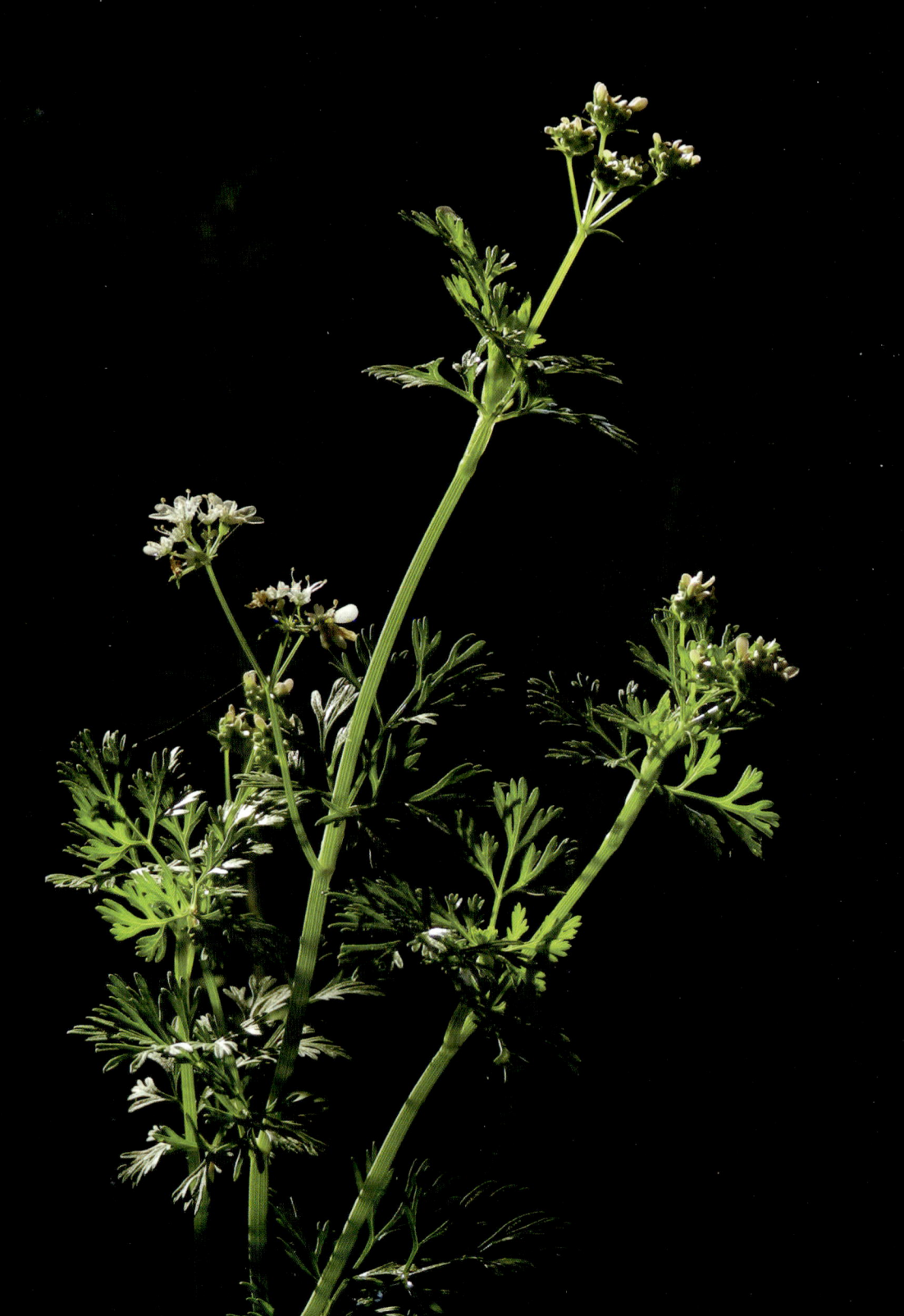

Coriandrum sativumum: Coriander

The Flower of Longevity

*Make yours the seeds of coriander,
For it is a cure for all diseases except swelling,
Which is a fatal disease*
– The Prophet Mohammad (570–632)

Other names: Chinese parsley, cilantro, dizzy corn, Japanese parsley

Parts Used: Leaves, dried seeds and flowers

Coriander is an increasingly popular member of the Umbelliferae/Apiaceae family which includes other fragrant herbs such as dill, caraway and fennel. It is a native of southern Europe around the Mediterranean, and the sweetly aromatic seeds and leaves have been used as a spice and as a medicine for thousands of years in many parts of the world. The unique flavour of coriander leaves can take some getting used to. The name *coriandrum* given to it by Pliny comes from 'koris' the Greek for 'bug' in reference to the foetid smell of its early foliage, which the Greeks thought resembled that of a squashed bed bug! They must have considered its taste and smell quite unpleasant. It was however appreciated by countless others for it was one of the first herbs to be used in cookery and as a medicine, and is still highly fashionable today.

Coriander was mentioned in Sanskrit texts dating back almost 7,000 years and we know that at least 3,000 years ago, it was an important ingredient in cookery and medicines of the ancient Greeks and Egyptians. It has been found stored in remains of palaces in Greece dating to the late Bronze Age around 1,400 BC, and the seeds have been found in early Egyptian tombs. It was also used by a number of Greek physicians, including Hippocrates. The seeds were popular with the Romans, who first introduced coriander into England. From there it was taken to America and was one of the first spices grown in New England. It also travelled further eastwards and was among the few plants from Europe to be popular at an early date in India, both as a medicine and to flavour curries.

In 17th century England the famous herbalist John Gerard wrote, "*Coriander seeds well prepared and covered with sugar as comfits, taken after meat, helpeth digestion.*" Coriander sweets were also common at Victorian and Edwardian dinner tables. The seeds are delicious eaten fresh straight off the plant and apparently the finest ones grow here in England, where they are cultivated mainly for making gin. For centuries they have been used to flavour alcoholic drinks and liqueurs such as Chartreuse and Benedictine. Coriander has been valued domestically not only for its taste, but also for its stimulating and aphrodisiac powers. In Tudor times it was an ingredient of a well known drink called 'Hippocras' which was served at weddings and royal occasions. It was frequently used in love potions including in that prepared by a druggist in the story of Ala-al-Din Abu-al in the Arabian Nights.

According to an ancient Chinese belief, coriander confers longevity, even immortality, on those who eat it. It is mentioned in the Bible as one of the five bitter herbs symbolic of sorrow to be eaten at the Passover. However, in other cultures such as ancient Egypt, it was believed to bring happiness and was among the herbs offered in the temple by the king. A bunch of the leaves and flowers used to be hung in the house to protect from bad influences and illness and to confer peace and security. As a plant of both love and immortality, coriander is said to help unite two people who desire to share their love beyond this life.

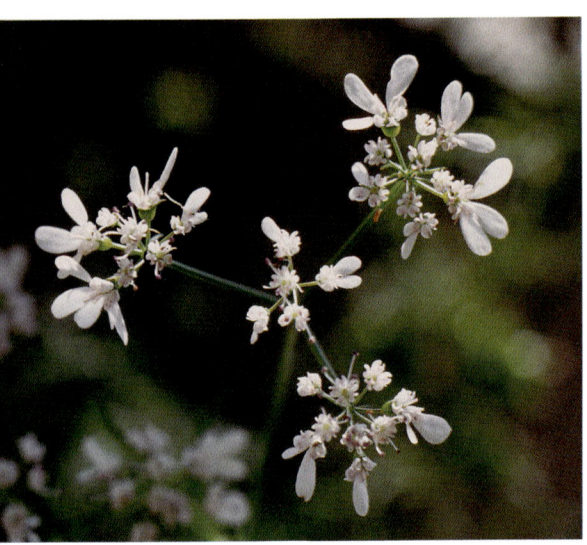

Herbal Remedy

With its sweet, bitter and highly aromatic taste, coriander is a versatile medicine and one that we can benefit from daily through our cuisine. It contains volatile oils mostly in the seeds, as well as resin, malic acid, phthalides, flavonoids, coumarins, tannins and alkaloids. The leaves are rich in antioxidant vitamins A and C, and minerals calcium, potassium and iron.

Coriander is an excellent digestive, enhancing appetite, digestion and absorption of nutrients, in fact it helps to balance the digestion – it stimulates the secretion of digestive enzymes, but cools heat and inflammation. The leaf, often called Chinese parsley, is excellent for balancing the flavour of hot spicy dishes and is used for just this purpose in Thai, Indian, Moroccan, Mexican, Chinese, Indonesian, African and South American cooking.

The volatile oils in the seeds are antibacterial and antifungal and this may also explain its wide use in cooking, particularly useful in the days before fridges when food may have been *'on the turn'*. It is a good herb for prevention and treatment of food poisoning. Relaxant and anti-inflammatory, coriander enhances appetite, digestion and absorption, and is a good remedy for relieving colic, griping, wind and bloating and for treating heartburn, nausea, gastritis, nervous indigestion, halitosis, diarrhoea and dysentery. The seeds can be combined with laxatives to prevent griping. Coriander has long been considered to be a nerve and brain tonic and is a good remedy for stress-related digestive disorders, such as gastritis and peptic ulcers. It can be useful in anorexia nervosa. In India they roast fennel seeds with coriander seeds and a little salt and chew them after eating to combat sleepiness after a large meal. Through their beneficial action on the liver and digestion, coriander seeds can lessen the intoxicating effect of alcohol as well as the soporific effect of large meals. They can help lower blood sugar and could be useful in prevention and management of diabetes.

With its antimicrobial properties, coriander is well worth using for fighting infections and treating fevers, colds, flu, coughs and catarrh. The seeds can be mixed with turmeric and cumin and taken in a hot decoction to make an excellent decongestant for colds and catarrh, asthma and bronchial congestion. This can also promote sweating and break a fever, bring out the rash in eruptive infections such as chicken pox and measles and in this way speed the infection on its way. In other parts of the world, coriander has been used as a cooling remedy for erysipelas (an inflammatory skin condition) and to tone down an over-florid complexion. The leaves taken as a juice or an infusion can be used for treating allergies such as rhinitis and hay fever as well hot, inflammatory skin rashes and asthma.

With its tonic effect on the nervous system, coriander has a reputation for being strengthening and revitalising, and is renowned for clearing the mind and improving memory when taken regularly. It lifts the spirits, relieves lethargy, reduces anxiety and tension, and promotes sleep. It has a mild analgesic action, and can be used to relieve aches and pains, including headaches, migraine and other stress-related problems, muscle and joint pain and neuralgia. The seeds are also used in Ayurvedic medicine for vertigo. The vitamins and flavonoids in the leaves have antioxidant properties, helping to prevent damage caused by free radicals and thereby slowing the ageing process and the onset of degenerative disease. Coriander also helps reduce cholesterol –

Chinese wisdom about longevity certainly does seem to hold true.

Coriander's cooling effects make it an excellent remedy for urinary disorders particularly those with hot burning symptoms such as cystitis and urethritis. Taken in lukewarm decoction, it helps to resolve urinary tract infections swiftly. The diuretic effect of coriander reduces fluid retention and goes some way to explain its cooling and cleansing effect. The leaves, with their high vitamin and mineral content, are excellent for drawing out toxins (particularly useful for those dealing with heavy metal toxicity) and clearing inflammatory skin problems.

The relaxant effects of the volatile oils in coriander seen in the digestive tract are also apparent in the uterus, helping to relieve menstrual problems, particularly period pain. In the Arab world, women have long taken coriander to lessen the pain of uterine contractions during childbirth. Coriander has long been popular as an aphrodisiac. The phytoestrogen content of the seeds may well provide a valid explanation for this. They make a good energising remedy for low libido and are also helpful in amenorrhoea, PMS and a cold infusion of the seeds makes a cooling remedy during the menopause for hot flushes.

Externally the leaf juice or tea can be applied to soothe hot itchy and allergic skin rashes as in eczema and urticaria. A decoction of the crushed seeds can be used as a gargle for sore throats and oral thrush. If the seeds are left overnight in cold water, the water can be used in eye lotions for conjunctivitis.

Aromatherapy Oil
The essential oils play a major role in the use of coriander as a herbal remedy and many of the above uses apply to coriander as an aromatherapy oil. It makes a good aid to digestion; when massaged into the abdomen, it can relieve abdominal discomfort, a feeling of fullness, wind, pain and bloating. Its relaxing and analgesic effect makes it good for easing period pain, tension and pain in muscles and joints and a relaxing soothing remedy for tension and stress. It is a good oil for creating a warm, sensual feeling and helping to relieve stress-related sexual problems.

Coriander is a beneficial oil for the nervous system. Its cooling effects can be calming when feeling overheated, irritable or angry, but coriander can also be stimulating and help to relieve fatigue and low spirits. Its antioxidant components have a neuro-protective effect, protecting the nervous system from the effects of stress, toxins and the ageing process. It can improve memory, concentration and cognitive health, and protect against problems such as dementia and Alzheimer's. Its relaxant effect on blood vessels and the nervous system generally can be helpful in lowering blood pressure.

A few drops in a burner or in hot water for inhalation can help to dispel infection and is useful for colds, catarrh and coughs. When used as a massage oil, once absorbed into the bloodstream, coriander will stimulate the kidneys and reduce fluid retention through its diuretic effect, and in this way has a cleansing action. Diluted in a base oil, coriander can be beneficial for the skin, particularly where there is heat and inflammation. It can be used regularly as a facial cleanser and to help keep a clear complexion.

Flower Essence
As a flower essence coriander helps with emotional maturity. It helps us to blossom in our own time and is good at junctions of life which are particularly transformative such as puberty, menopause and other life changes. It helps to transform challenging personality traits and enhances ease of communication in relationships.

Edible Uses
While the leaves and seeds have traditionally been used in Asian, Indian and Latin cuisines for thousands of years, recently European and American chefs are discovering that the flowers are also tasty, even though they have a more subtle quality. This could be good for some as the unique flavour of coriander leaves can take some getting used to. The small flowers have a lacy decorative appearance, and they taste like a milder version of the leaves, with hints of lemony citrus, spicy and sweet tastes all together.

In India they use coriander seeds in most of their curries, the fresh leaves and flowers can be added to salads, cold soups, bean and potato dishes and vegetable dishes.

Growing
Coriander is easy to grow in the garden or in pots on your patio or windowsill. It grows as an annual, the seeds being planted out in April to May in warm ground. It prefers light, dry soil, and plenty of sun. It is said that when coriander is grown in the garden, it protects the gardener and all who live in the gardener's house.

Cautions
The herbal remedy may rarely cause allergic reactions and contact dermatitis. Care has to be taken when using coriander oil; the scent has an initial stimulating effect but over-exposure to it can have a soporific effect. Caution with insulin and hypoglycaemic medicines, sedatives and other CNS depressants.

Recipe

Cold Coriander Seed Infusion
A wonderfully cooling recipe for the early mornings. If taken on a regular basis, it will cool the body and can help to ease menopausal flushes and night sweats.

3 dessertspoonfuls of coriander seeds
1 cup cold water

Spoon the seeds into a large cup and cover with cold water. Leave it to infuse overnight and strain in the morning.

Drink on an empty stomach and enjoy its velvety smooth texture and cooling qualities.

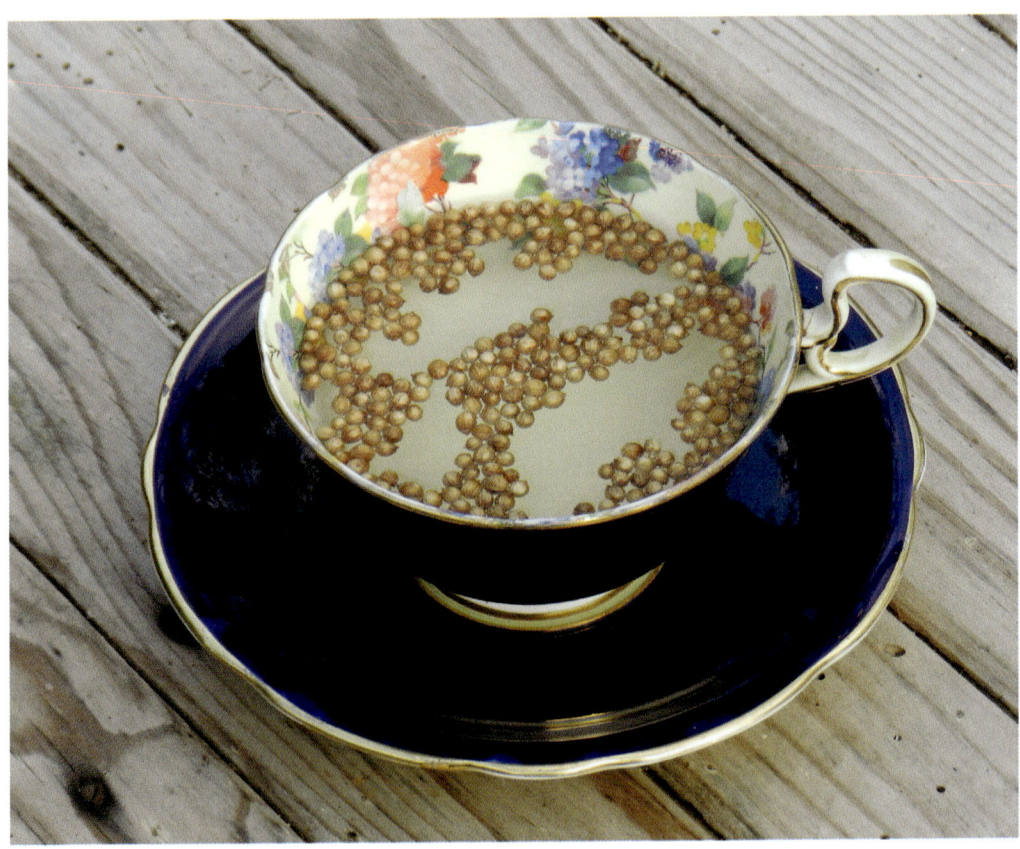

Crataegus monogyna, C. laevigata: Hawthorn
The Flower of the Heart

Shall I compare thee to a summer's day?
Thou art more lovely and more temperate:
Rough winds do shake the darling buds of May,
And summer's lease hath all too short a date
  – William Shakespeare, Sonnet 18

Other names: May tree, bread and cheese tree, moonflower, tramp's supper, whitethorn

Parts used: Leaves, berries, flowers

This delightful member of the rose (Roseaceae) family is a handsome perennial shrub or small deciduous tree, found in the temperate areas of North America and Europe. It is much loved for its wonderful display of fragrant white-pink blossoms that decorate our hedgerows in spring as a herald to summer, and its bright red haws that brighten them in autumn. The smaller branches are thorny, in fact the name hawthorn means 'hedge thorn'. Hawthorn is common throughout the British Isles. Joseph of Arimathea came to Glastonbury in 60AD, and legend has it that he stuck his hawthorn staff into the ground where it grew and flowered.

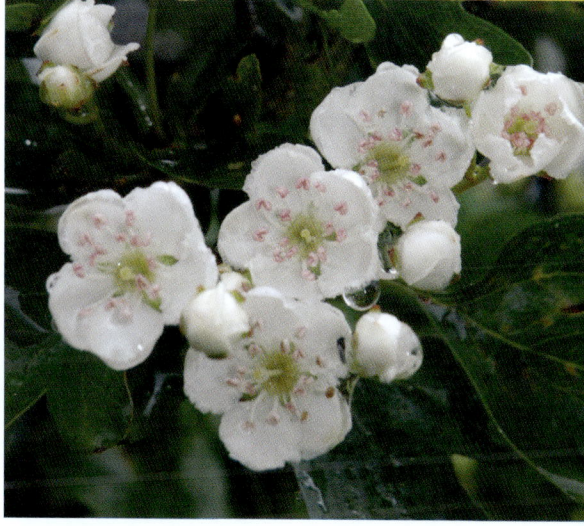

Hawthorn has traditionally been connected with Mayday customs and ancient fertility rites in the Northern hemisphere, where it blooms in May (the 'breeding season'). Mayday began as an ancient spring festival named after the Greek goddess Maia. The girl crowned Queen of the May represented the ancient goddess,

The fair maid who the first of May,
Goes to the fields at break of day,
And walks in dew from the Hawthorn tree,
Will ever handsome be.

The maypole ceremony symbolises fertility and rebirth, as spring is a time of renewed life after the apparent death of winter. The maypole represented an 'axis mundi' around which the universe revolves; the tree stripped of its changing foliage symbolises the changeless centre. The maypole is phallic, the discus at the top from which the ribbons hang represents the feminine principle and the union of the two represents fertility. At this time of year in many places in Europe, hawthorns used to be placed outside the house or the home of a sweetheart and branches decorated the porches.

Hawthorn has been associated with fertility since the days of the ancient Greeks and Romans. At Greek wedding banquets the guests would carry sprigs of hawthorn to symbolise happiness and prosperity for the bride and groom. The bride was sometimes given a sprig of hawthorn to represent her flowery future, intermingled with thorns. In Roman traditions, the bridegroom

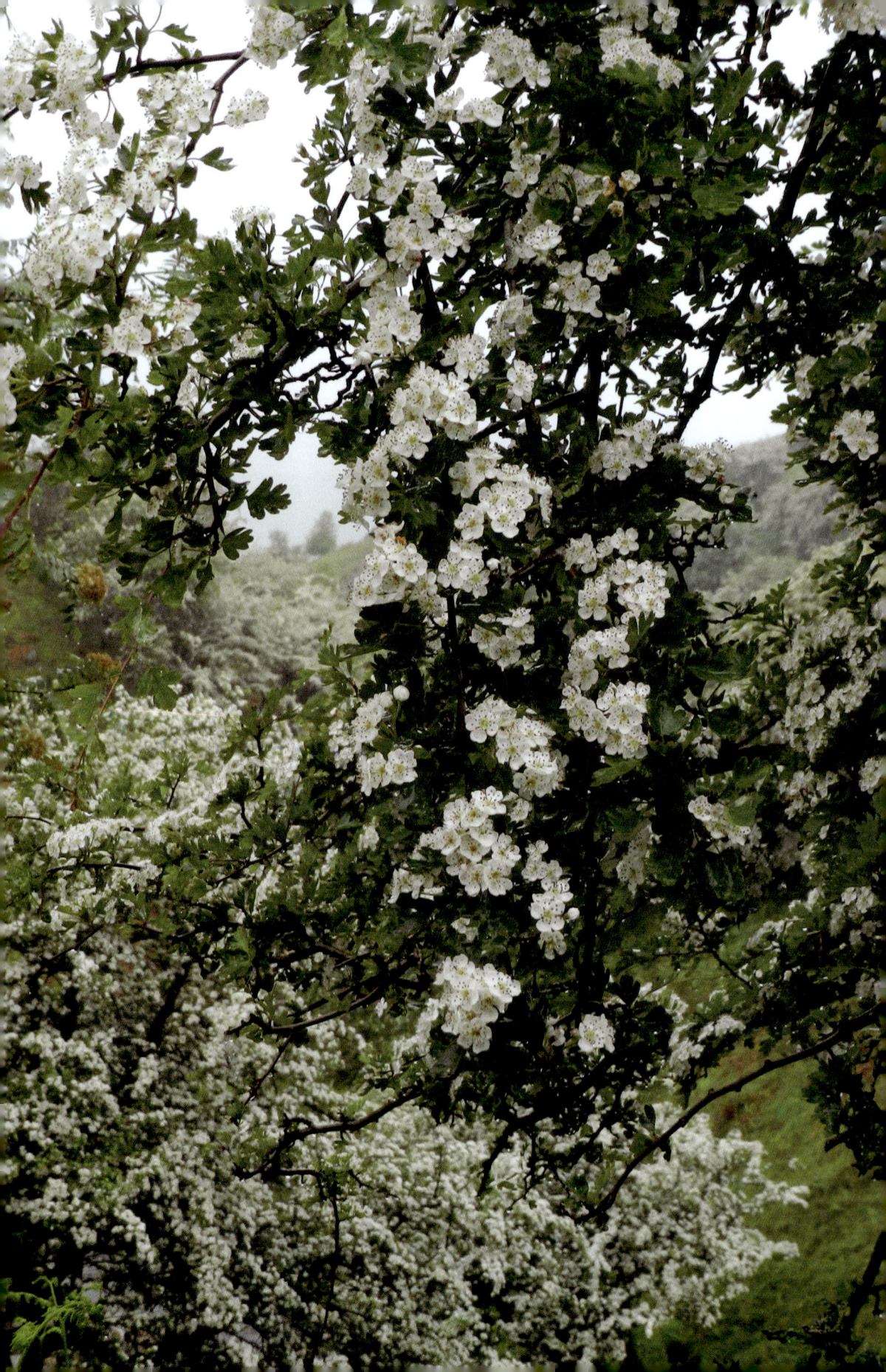

used to wave a sprig as he led his bride to the nuptial chamber, which was lit with torches of hawthorn wood.

Traditionally hawthorn has been held as sacred and as protection against evil. Hawthorn twigs used to be fixed to babies' cradles to protect against harmful influences and illness. When worn or carried, hawthorn blossom was believed to give psychic protection, to lift the spirits and banish melancholy, but was never to be brought indoors. Under the hawthorn tree was believed to be a meeting place of spirits and faeries, and sitting under a tree on Mayday, Midsummer's day or Halloween, one could apparently be enchanted by faery folk.

With the coming of Christianity, the church re-dedicated the hawthorn, like other sacred trees, to the Virgin Mary. It was said that hawthorn was used for Christ's crown of thorns and because of this it was believed for centuries that lightning would never strike a hawthorn tree, as lightening was the work of the devil and could not strike a plant that had touched the brow of Christ. The robin is said to have got his red breast from a thorn in Jesus' crown that pierced his breast and left a little blood stain.

Almost all parts of hawthorn have been used as medicines since at least the Middle Ages. The leaves, flowers and berries were recommended for heart problems, high blood pressure, vertigo, gout, pleurisy, insomnia and to stop haemorrhages. The bark was made into a decoction to bring down fevers and the berries made an excellent remedy for diarrhoea.

Herbal Remedy
Hawthorn is veritably the best rejuvenative remedy for the heart and circulation. It contains saponins, glycosides, polysaccharides, flavonoids, procyanidins, glycosides, saponins, triterpenoids, tannins, pectin, vitamins C, B1, B2, choline, acetylcholine and calcium. The flowers, leaves and berries all provide a wonderful heart tonic and have a vasodilatory effect, opening the arteries and improving blood flow through the coronary arteries of the heart and the general circulation. Hawthorn makes an excellent remedy for high blood pressure and probably by virtue of its antioxidant activity, it reduces inflammation in the blood vessels. It has the remarkable ability to prevent, soften and clear the build-up of deposits in the arteries that cause atherosclerosis, angina and eventually heart attacks and strokes. In this way hawthorn improves the blood supply throughout the body and is ideal for the treatment of high blood pressure associated with hardening of the arteries and for preventing clots and heart attacks. It lowers cholesterol, strengthens heart muscle and regulates heart rhythm. It has further benefit to the heart in its action on the vagus nerve which influences the heart, so that an over-fast heart rate is slowed and heart irregularities settle down.

Hawthorn makes the ideal remedy for all heart conditions, including coronary insufficiency, arrhythmias, palpitations, breathlessness, angina, degenerative heart disease and heart failure. As a peripheral vasodilator, it can be used to improve poor circulation associated with the ageing process such as Raynaud's and Burgher's disease, intermittent claudication and varicose veins. It is recommended for an ageing heart, confusion and poor memory due to reduced blood supply to the brain. It is also used for altitude sickness and anaemia. The antioxidant and rejuvenative effects extend as far as the eyes and hawthorn can be helpful in protecting against eye problems associated with the ageing process including macular degeneration.

As a heart tonic, hawthorn benefits the emotional as well as the physical heart. It is used for heartache, when down-hearted, disheartened and broken-hearted. With its relaxant effect, hawthorn can be used to relieve anxiety and stress, calm agitation, restlessness, nervous palpitations and promote sleep. It is recommended in attention deficit disorder (ADD) and attention deficit hyperactive disorder (ADHD).

Hawthorn has a mild diuretic action, relieving fluid retention and dissolving stones and gravel. It benefits the linings of the joints, the synovial fluid, collagen, ligaments and vertebral discs. Its antioxidant effect helps prevent and remedy inflammatory connective tissue disorders such as arthritis, gout and tendonitis.

The leaves, flowers and berries all have a beneficial and relaxant effect in the digestive tract. They stimulate the appetite, promote digestion, and relieve wind, stagnation of food and accumulation of toxins in the gut which cause indigestion and disturbance of the gut flora. The berries are nutritive, but they also help regulate metabolism and have been used to reduce weight. They have an astringent effect and make a good remedy for diarrhoea. In Russia they are used for amoebic dysentery.

By regulating blood flow throughout the body, hawthorn improves the circulation to the uterus and so can be beneficial for painful and absent periods. It also promotes libido and fertility and is used in threatened miscarriage. It is also beneficial during menopause for reducing night sweats and hot flushes.

Externally a decoction of the flowers and berries can be used as a lotion for skin problems, notably acne rosacea. A decoction of the berries has an astringent action, making a good mouthwash for bleeding gums, a gargle for sore throats and a douche for vaginal discharges.

Homeopathic Remedy
Crataegus is also a wonderful heart tonic. It is used for chronic heart disease with extreme weakness, for heart failure that threatens from the slightest exertion, for pain in the heart area, high blood pressure and arteriosclerosis of the elderly. The berries are used in a mother tincture as a heart remedy.

Flower Essence
On an emotional level, hawthorn works on the heart chakra, opening the heart and working on the expression of love. It can be used when there are any problems either giving or receiving love. It is a remedy recommended to heal broken hearts, and to ease disappointment, anger or bitterness after a failed love affair. It reduces emotional extremes which could contribute to physical illness such as heart disease.

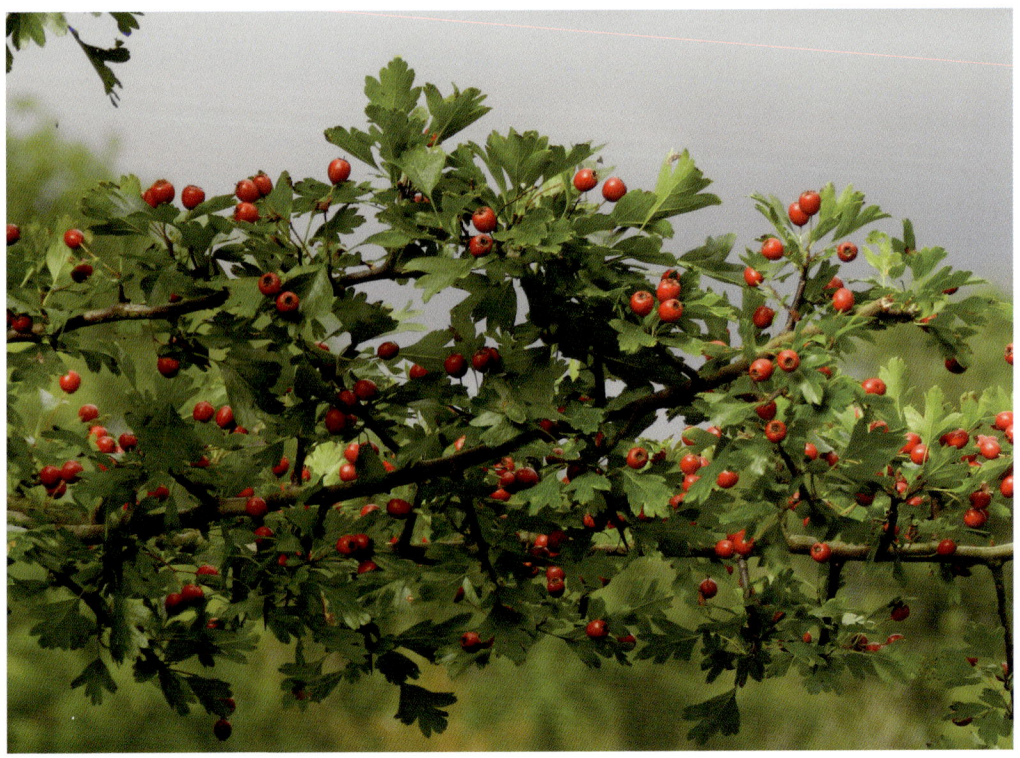

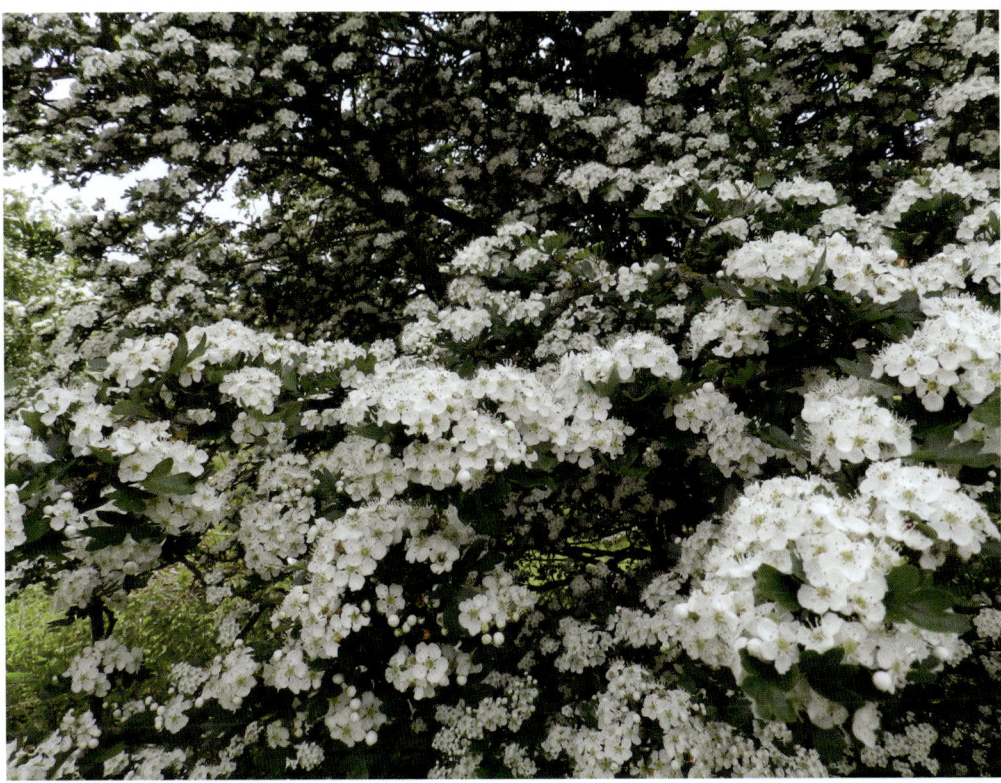

Edible Uses
The leaves and flowers were known as 'bread and cheese' by our parents and grandparents – you can roam the hedgerows and eat the young leaves as you go along. They can be used to decorate salads and desserts. The berries are also tasty – some say they taste of avocado and they certainly have their texture but are fiddly to eat. Being high in pectin, they make a good addition to hedgerow jams and jellies made from autumn fruits.

The fresh pulp can be pressed through a sieve and makes an interesting addition to savoury dishes, and is useful for thickening soups, stews and sauces. Hawthorn ketchup could be made combining the fresh pulp with vinegar, spices and a little sugar and you could add some tomato purèe.

Growing
When buying a hawthorn tree, make sure it has thick roots that are free and not pot bound. Plant out in spring after the last frost. It prefers light, sandy soil. Hawthorn trees can live for over 400 years and can grow 18–25 ft in height and with a 15–29 ft spread. The flowers and leaves are harvested in the spring when the flowers have just bloomed and the berries are harvested in the autumn. Be careful of the thorns!

Cautions
Although hawthorn is considered safe and may be effective in the treatment of angina, congestive heart failure and cardiac arrhythmias, these are serious, potentially life-threatening conditions requiring professional medical care. Avoid hawthorn as a herbal remedy in bleeding disorders. Hawthorn may potentiate the effects of heart drugs including Digoxin and beta blockers. Monitor blood pressure when combined with hypotensives. Caution with anticoagulants, CNS depressants (such as alcohol, opiates, benzodiazepines, anaesthetics, tricyclic anti-depressants, anti-epileptics), insulin, oral hypoglycaemics and vasodilators.

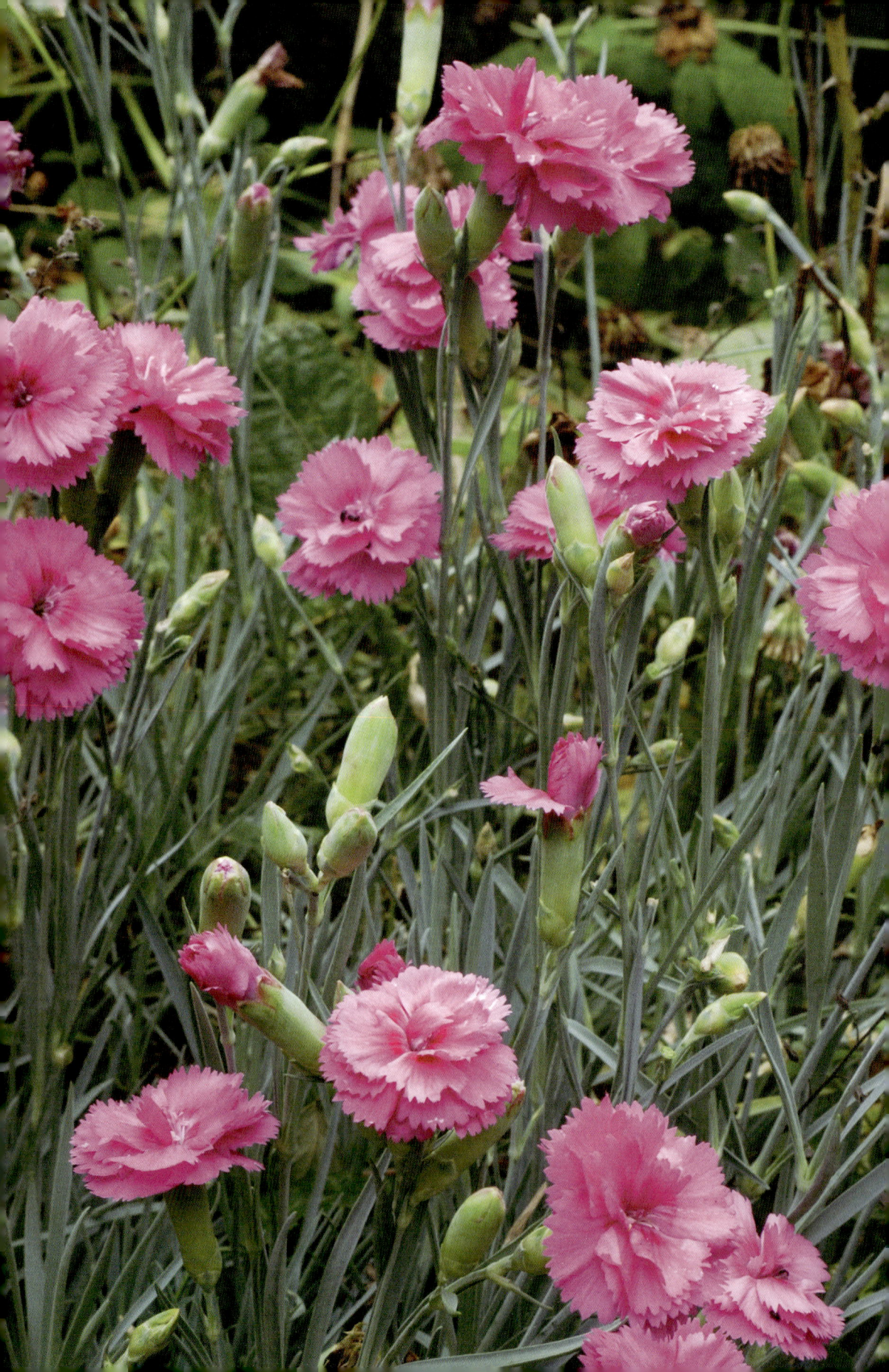

Dianthus: Carnation, Clove Pink and Sweet William
The Flowers of the Gods

One moment Love the rose paused by, but Beauty picked it for her hair.
Love paced the garden with a sigh - He found no fitting emblem there.
Then suddenly he saw a flame; a conflagration turned to bloom.
It even put the rose to shame, both in its beauty and perfume.
He watched it, and it did not fade: He plucked it, and it brighter grew
In cold or heat, all undismayed, it kept its fragrance and its hue.
"Here deathless love and passion sleep," He cried, "embodied in this flower.
This is the emblem I will keep." Love wore carnations from that hour
– Ella Wheeler Wilcox (1850–1919)

Other names: *Dianthus caryophyllus* (carnation), *D. superbus* (fringed pink) and *D. Chinensis* (Chinese pink), *D. plumarius* (pink), *D. barbatus* (sweet William), gillyflower, clove pink, divine flower, bearded pink, China carnation

Parts used: The whole plant

Dianthus are some of the oldest cultivated flowers of the Caryophyllaceae or carnation family and have been treasured for at least 2000 years for their beautiful colours, wonderful scents and their ease of cultivation, all of which have made them highly popular in the cut-flower trade. There are about 300 species found in Asia, Europe and Africa which can be either annual, biennial or perennial. The flowers are hermaphrodite (have both male and female organs) and are pollinated by bees, moths and butterflies. While the original carnation had petals in shades of pink and peach, cultivated flowers now come in all colours of the rainbow, from pure white and shades of pink and red to green, orange, yellow and purple with many striped or variegated varieties too.

The most common varieties are *Dianthus caryophyllus* (carnation), *D. superbus* (fringed pink) and *D. Chinensis* (Chinese pink), *D. plumarius* (pink), *D. barbatus* (sweet William), all perennials. Chinese pink *(Dianthus chinensis)* is the main variety used in Chinese medicine. It is a beautiful and highly scented annual found growing in East Asia and China on dry hillsides, mountain slopes and summits, forests and grasslands, in meadows and by streams and is hardy in temperate climates. It is valuable in the garden for attracting wildlife.

Through their long history, carnations have been associated with many stories and meanings. The name 'dianthus' was apparently given by Theophrastus, the ancient Greek father of botany, and comes from the word 'theos' meaning God and 'anthos' meaning flower, so *dianthus* are the 'flowers of God' or 'flowers of the gods'. This might relate to a story about the moon goddess Artemis, who was hunting when a shepherd playing an instrument frightened her prey. In a fit of anger, Artemis tore out the shepherd's eyes and then felt very sorry. Her remorse resulted in the creation of beautiful flowers that bloomed in the place of the man's lost eyes.

A similar story says Diana, the Roman goddess of hunting, came upon the shepherd boy and took a shine to him. When he rejected her, she ripped out his eyes and threw them to the ground where in their place carnations grew. Another story tells us that the young shepherd was in love with Diana, who seduced and then abandoned him. His tears turned into beautiful carnations as they fell to the ground.

Later with the coming of Christianity, *Dianthus* (as well as many other flowers) came to represent the Virgin Mary, which explains why carnations appear in many paintings of the Virgin from the thirteenth century onwards. According to Christian legend, carnations first formed from Mary's tears when Jesus was crucified and came to symbolise the tears shed by the undying love of a mother in many parts of the world. In a lesser-known painting by Leonardo da Vinci entitled '*A Madonna and Child',* Mary is looking pensive and handing a red carnation to a chubby Jesus, who is reaching to grasp it. A shadow is cast over the carnation intimating the story of the passion of Christ to come. The meaning of the painting, that of motherly and divine love, is encapsulated in a single flower that the contemporary Renaissance and especially Christian viewers would understand.

The name 'carnation' may come from the Latin 'corona' or the Greek 'korone' both meaning a wreath, chaplet, garland or crown, or from 'coronation' as they were often worn as headdresses or crowns on festive occasions, pageants, in religious ceremonies and as a mark of honour in the days of the ancient Greeks and Romans. It may also come from the Latin 'caro' or 'carnis' meaning flesh, which could refer to the natural colour of the flower, or from 'incarnatio' meaning the incarnation of God made flesh in the form of Jesus.

In the fifteenth century their name was 'gillyflower' or 'clove pink' as the scent of the flower was thought to resemble the spice. Also, cloves are shaped like nails which were said to resemble the shape of the nails used to nail Jesus to the cross. The carnation has also been called 'divine flower.'

Historically carnation flowers have been associated with love, weddings and fidelity, and many a carnation is still worn as a buttonhole at weddings all over the world. Red carnations are used at weddings in China and worn or exchanged on a first wedding anniversary in many parts of the world, while in France they are included in bouquets to commemorate loved ones at funerals. In the Victorian language of flowers, carnation is the flower of love and affection, of strong emotions. Carnations were popular for sending secret, coded messages to suitors or secret admirers. Light red flowers mean admiration, deep red mean deep love and affection, white symbolise pure love and fidelity as well as good luck, yellow means disappointment or rejection, variegated means a love not shared, striped means regret, purple flowers represent capriciousness and pink a mother's love and the sufferings of love.

As symbols of both love and distinction, carnations have been used for centuries for many different occasions as they symbolise both. They are often presented in the school colours to graduates or recipients of academic and sports awards. In Japan carnations are the flower of good luck. At Oxford University, students have traditionally worn white carnations for their first exam and red carnations for their final exam. In America they are also worn in corsages (small bouquet of flowers worn on a woman's dress or around her wrist for a formal occasion) and buttonholes for prom and other special or formal events. Pink or red carnations are popular for Mother's Day and green carnation are for St. Patrick's Day. In Korea, carnations are worn on parent's day, May 8th and teachers' day, May 15th.

Sweet William (*Dianthus barbatus*) is much loved for its spicy, clove-like scent and brightly coloured flowers in shades of red, pink, purple and white or combinations of these. The nectar attracts birds, bees, moths, hummingbirds and butterflies into the garden. It is said sweet William was cultivated by monks as early as the 1100s and in the 16th century, it was used in Henry VII's gardens at Hampton Court Palace.

Sweet William is the flower's common name in the United Kingdom. It is not known where it originated from, though it first appeared in a garden catalogue of botanist and apothecary John Gerard in 1596. It could be a corruption of the French word '*oeillet'* which means little eye. It is also called '*bearded pink'* and '*China carnation*.' In Scotland the flower is known as '*stinking Willie'* or '*sour Billy*.' In the Victorian language of flowers, sweet William is a symbol of gallantry. Several members of the carnation family have been used by ethnic communities as traditional medicines throughout the world. Chinese pink has been used for over 2,000 years in Chinese herbal medicine. The whole plant is harvested just before the flowers open and are dried for later use.

The ancient Aztecs used carnation tea as a diuretic and to treat respiratory problems. It has been used in China, Japan and Korea to treat wounds and digestive problems and in China it has been highly valued to relieve tension and anxiety, to restore energy and as a vermifuge to combat worms and parasites. In the *Pharmacopoeia Londinensis*, the landmark publication of the College of Physicians in 1618 as the first standard list of medicines and their ingredients in England, carnation was recommended as an aromatic tonic in cordials and hot drinks to combat fevers, infections and pestilence. In European folk medicine, it was used to relieve nervousness, low spirits, fatigue, stomach aches, liver and heart problems as well as worms, parasites and seasickness. As a mouthwash it has been used traditionally for toothache, throat and gum infections as well as in an eyebath for eye infections. Carnation oil was applied to improve memory and restore energy as well as to heal wounds and remedy skin problems.

Herbal Remedy
Carnation: *Dianthus caryophyllus*
The whole plant with its exquisitely scented flower has medicinal benefits. It contains triterpenes, alkaloids, coumarins, cyanogenic glycosides, cyanidin, pelargonidin and volatile oils.

The antimicrobial volatile oils in the flowers and leaves that lend it that wonderful fragrance help fight off infections, whether viral, bacterial and fungal. The most active compounds of the volatile oil may be thymol and eugenol. They can be used for bacterial infections including *Helicobacter pylori, Bordetella bronchoseptica, Staphylococcus aureus* and *epidermis, Klebsiella pneumonia, Tuberculosis bacteria, Listeria monocytogenes, Pseudomonas spp, E. coli* and *Bacillus spp*. This means that carnation would make a good remedy for gastritis and peptic ulcers and may help to prevent stomach cancer.

It can also be used to ward off and treat chest infections.

The seeds have antiviral actions against *Herpes simplex 1, Hepatitis A* and *HIV* infections and may be helpful in preventing and treating colds and flu. As a hot tea, they promote sweating and helps to bring down fevers. The kaemferide and flavonoid glycosides in the leaves, flowers and stems have antifungal actions which are used for herbaceous plants, as well as food crops such as tomatoes, sweet potatoes and bananas suffering from *Fusarium oxysporum*.

The flowers are considered to be alexiteric (preservative against infectious diseases and the effects of poison) and are used in the food industry to protect against poisoning and food contamination.

Just enjoying the heavenly scent of these flowers, carnations can have a wonderfully relaxing and uplifting effect. In the past they were symbols of both love and distinction and have a connection with the emotional heart and with feelings of self worth. They celebrated our successes and today they can be used similarly to benefit the nervous system, calm the nerves and lift the spirits. With their nervine, antispasmodic and carminative actions, carnations can be taken in teas and tinctures to support us in times of stress. They have a wonderful ability to lift depression, reduce anxiety and ease muscle tension and spasm, particularly in the reproductive system.

Carnations also help balance womens' hormones and make a good remedy for menstrual cramps and relieving PMS. They can be used for endometriosis (in which endometrial tissues normally found lining the uterus, develops in other areas in the pelvis such as the ovaries and fallopian tubes). The analgesic effects of carnation are very helpful when this causes severe pain. With the combination of relaxing and stimulating effects on uterine muscles, carnations could be helpful during the birth to regulate contractions.

With their affinity with matters of the heart, carnations have an action on the physical heart and a cardiotonic effect which supports the

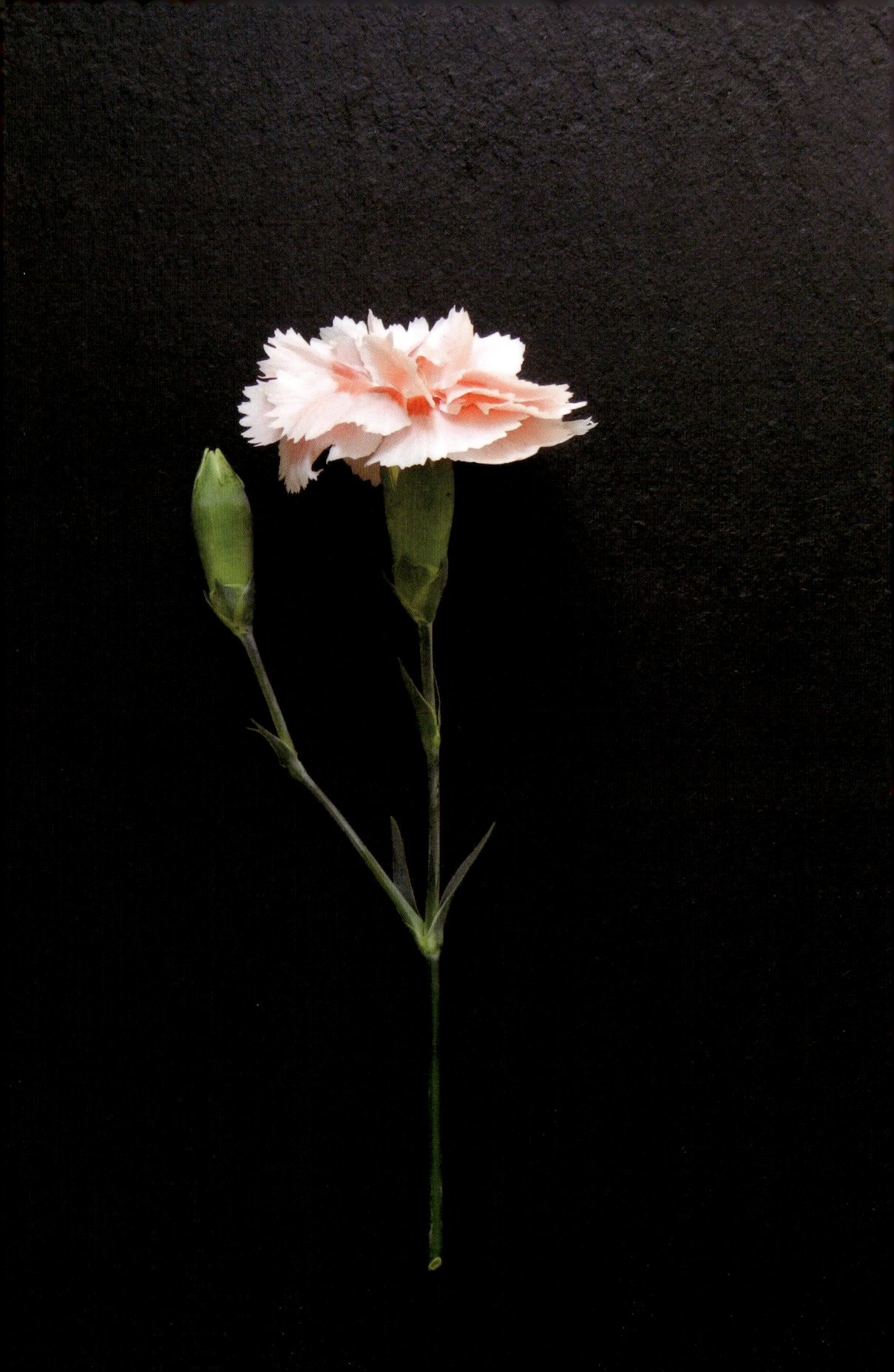

action of the heart and promotes the circulation. With their calming effect, carnations can ease nervous palpitations and lower blood pressure. Their diuretic action can be helpful in this respect. The antioxidant compounds in carnations including anthocyanins, flavonoids, carotenoids and kaemferide triglycoside, help fight free radicals that contribute to the development of cancer, particularly colon cancer and oestrogen-dependent cancers. The antioxidants may also have a protective effect in the brain and the kidneys, helping to prevent free radical damage that accompanies the ageing process.

The lovely relaxing effect of carnations can be felt in the digestive system where it can ease wind, bloating, pain and spasm associated with problems such as IBS. Carnations help to regulate the bowels and can be used for both diarrhoea and constipation. Their antibacterial effect can be helpful in regulating the gut flora and in this way can have a profound effect throughout the body, enhancing immunity and supporting normal function of the nervous system through regulating the production of neurotransmitters.

When used externally, carnation makes a lovely remedy to soothe skin irritations and eczema. It contains saponins with detergent-like properties which form a soapy lather when mixed with water, that can then be used as a soap for cleaning the skin, hair or clothes. The triterpene saponins interfere with the metamorphosis of insects and so make a good insecticidal.

Dianthus chinensis: Chinese Pink
The whole plant is used in Traditional Chinese Medicine where it is known as 'Qu Mai' and its qualities are considered to be bitter and cold. Its constituents include anthocyanins, triterpene saponins, flavonoid glycosides, cyclopeptides, aromatic amide glycosides, pyrane type glycosides and essential oils. It exerts its beneficial effects on the bladder, the heart and small intestine meridians and it promotes urination, drains damp heat from the bladder and dispels blood stasis. **According to Traditional Chinese Medicine (TCM), damp heat in the bladder can cause acute bladder infections, with frequent, burning and urgent urination, blood in the urine, fever, thirst and feelings of heat.** Chinese pink helps to dispel stasis and break up urinary stones and can be used for a range of genito-urinary infections.

Chinese pink is used as a bitter tonic to the digestive system, cooling excess heat and inflammation and stimulating sluggish bowels. It is used for heartburn, acid reflux, gastritis, peptic ulcers, inflammatory gut problems and constipation. Its antibacterial action helps to fight infections and to combat unfriendly organisms including worms and parasites in the gut and to clear toxins.

As a hot tea, it promotes sweating and helps to break a fever. It contains cyclopeptides which may have anticancer and antiviral properties and phenols with antioxidant and anticancer actions, which explains why Chinese pink has been used to treat viruses including HIV and cancers of different types, including oesophageal, colon, liver, cervical and stomach cancer.

Chinese pink has anti-inflammatory, anaesthetic and haemostatic actions and is a good remedy for the female reproductive system. It can reduce bleeding in heavy periods, reduce period pains and since it also has a stimulating effect on uterine muscles, it acts as an emmenagogue and can bring on delayed periods. In Cambodia, Laos, Vietnam and China, Chinese pink is used to cleanse the blood and to check haemorrhages during delivery. It is also used in Korea to treat skin problems including eczema and tumours.

Externally Chinese pink makes a good antiseptic and healing remedy to apply to cuts, grazes, and wounds as well as skin infections such as pimples and acne. Its anti-inflammatory effects can be very helpful for treating skin problems including eczema and to bathe sore or inflamed eyes.

Aromatherapy Oil
Carnation essential oil or carnation absolute is a slightly viscous liquid with a delightfully rich, sweet, spicy and floral aroma, popular in cosmetics, soaps, potpourris, candles and perfumery. It needs to be warmed before using as it becomes solid at room temperature. The main constituents are eugenol, citronellol, coumarins and phenethyl alcohol, benzyl benzoate and

benzyl salicylate. With its invigorating and almost intoxicating scent, carnation is a wonderful oil for the nervous system, easing tension and anxiety, dispelling negativity, apathy and lethargy and lifting the spirits. It boosts confidence, increases energy and motivation and can help us to get things done. It can help you to feel relaxed and yet more alert and may help memory and concentration. At the same time, it has sedative properties and can help us sleep when we are stressed.

It would come as no surprise that carnation oil is highly popular as an aphrodisiac, as it has long been the symbol of love. It is relaxing, enhances confidence and promotes desire. It can even induce feelings of ecstasy and euphoria.

With its antispasmodic effects, carnation oil can be used in massage oils for tense, aching muscles and painful joints. It is good after exercise and sports to prevent stiffness and aching. Massaged into the abdomen, it can ease menstrual cramps, colic, wind and bloating. It can be rubbed into the scalp to stop hair loss and used as an analgesic for toothache.

Carnation oil has anti-inflammatory properties. Diluted in a base massage oil such as coconut oil, it can be used to soothe itchy and inflammatory skin problems such as bites and stings, acne, rosacea and eczema. With its healing and antiseptic properties, it can be applied to sores, cuts, mosquito bites and fungal infections such as athlete's foot. It is a good insect repellent and has larvicidal activity. It can repel the *Culex pipiens* mosquito which can carry Japanese encephalitis, meningitis and West Nile virus. It can also repel *Ixodes ricinus* ticks and yellow fever *Aedes aegypti* mosquitos. With its toning effect, it is great in face creams helping to reduce the appearance of wrinkles and it promotes regeneration of the skin.

Flower Essence
Carnations are the flowers of love, relationships and marriage as well as mothers. They promote long lasting, honest and authentic relationships, strengthening connection and helping them to work out in the best way. White carnation can help you cope with or get over the suffering of love, to let go of resentments caused by betrayal and difficult relationships and ease a broken heart, enabling you to have more happy, healthy relationships now or in the future. It is recommended for nervous exhaustion and burn out and helps prevent and relieve a tendency to mood swings, stubbornness, anger or manic behaviour. It is helps you to find balance, patience and resilience.

Red carnation flower essence is connected to the heart and the heart chakra. It can enhance your belief in yourself and engender feelings of self-worth and self-acceptance and the ability to celebrate being just who you are. It is a good remedy for low self-esteem, feelings of unworthiness and connecting better to yourself as well as to others to find friendship, love, a soul mate and true connection. It is a good remedy for trusting yourself and others, for letting go of issues you have with others such as around fidelity, seeing people clearly, seeing the best in others, releasing fears of commitment and opening your heart to love.

Red carnation flower essence can be used when feeling ungrounded, unable to trust or focus on the present and it helps you to be clear and objective. It is a good remedy for studying, to calm the mind and to bring awareness of the here and now during meditation.

Sweet William flower essence also works on the heart chakra and is a good remedy for relationships. It can help you to find inner clarity and become more aligned with your spiritual purpose and be your best self. It is good if you are struggling to have clarity about your purpose or direction in life and lack interest or inspiration. It helps you to align your will to your spiritual life. It can help to transform a negative view of your life into one of excitement and beauty, to experience a sense of divinity and to grow into the next phase of your life.

It can be helpful if you have fears and reservations about entering fully into relationships, present or future, due to expectations of being let down or hurt based on past relationships. It can enable you to let go of memories of past hurts, to have a more open loving connection,

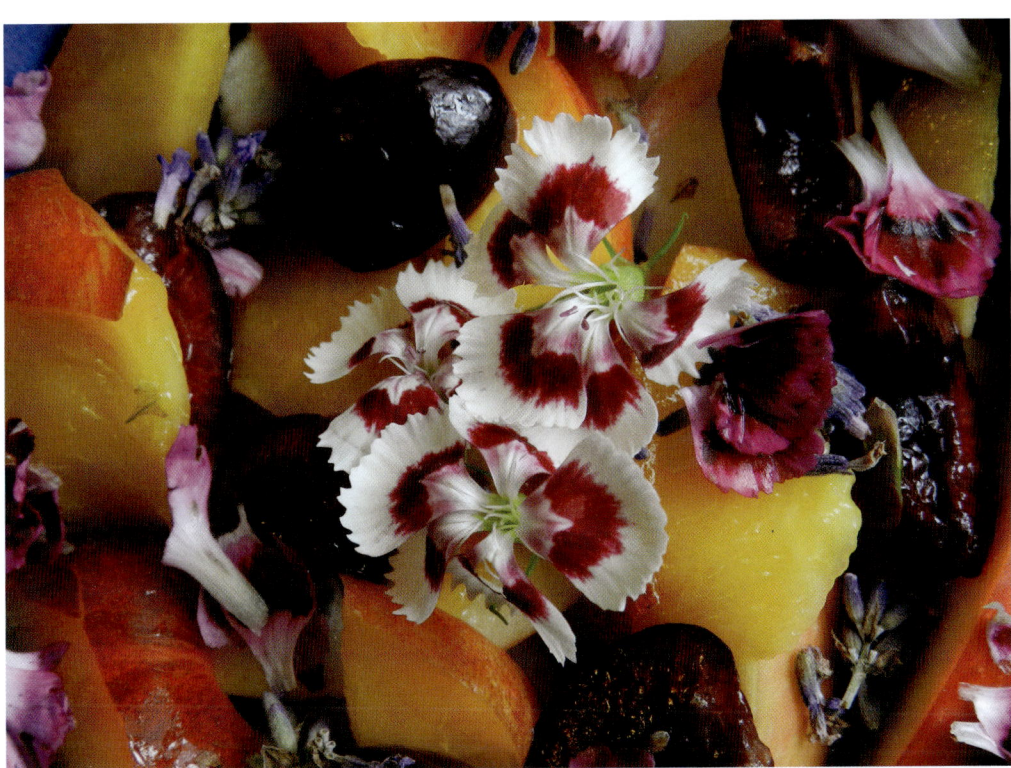

to be clear about what the relationship needs to work well, to have realistic expectations and feel less defended. It can give you a fresh start in relationships and engender honest, open and authentic communication.

Edible Uses
With their delightful cinnamon/clove spicy smell and mild taste, carnation, pink and sweet William petals can be used to beautify salads and any other savoury or sweet dish, for flavouring deserts, decorating cakes and adding to fruit salads. They are delicious made into jams, syrups, ice creams and sorbets. They could be made into cordials, floated in soft drinks or added to home brews such as wine, beer, gin and other alcoholic drinks. You could freeze them in ice cubes to put in teas, lemonades and other drinks. The petals need to be removed from the calyx as the base can taste a bit bitter.

Growing
Carnations and pinks can be sown from seed in the spring in a greenhouse with a little heat. The seed usually germinates in 2 - 3 weeks at 15°c. When they are large enough to handle, prick the seedlings out and plant in individual pots and plant them out in the summer after the last expected frosts. They like well-drained soil, direct sunlight and enough moisture for successful growth. Since some varieties flower freely in their first year and then degenerate, they are usually treated as annuals. They can be propagated easily from cuttings, taken at any time of the year and from root division.

Cautions
Members of the *Dianthus* family might cause allergic symptoms in sensitive people. Avoid the essential oil in pregnancy and breastfeeding and do not use it undiluted for skin application. Large doses of *Dianthus chinensis* can cause contractions of the uterus and should not be taken by women who are pregnant or have recently given birth.

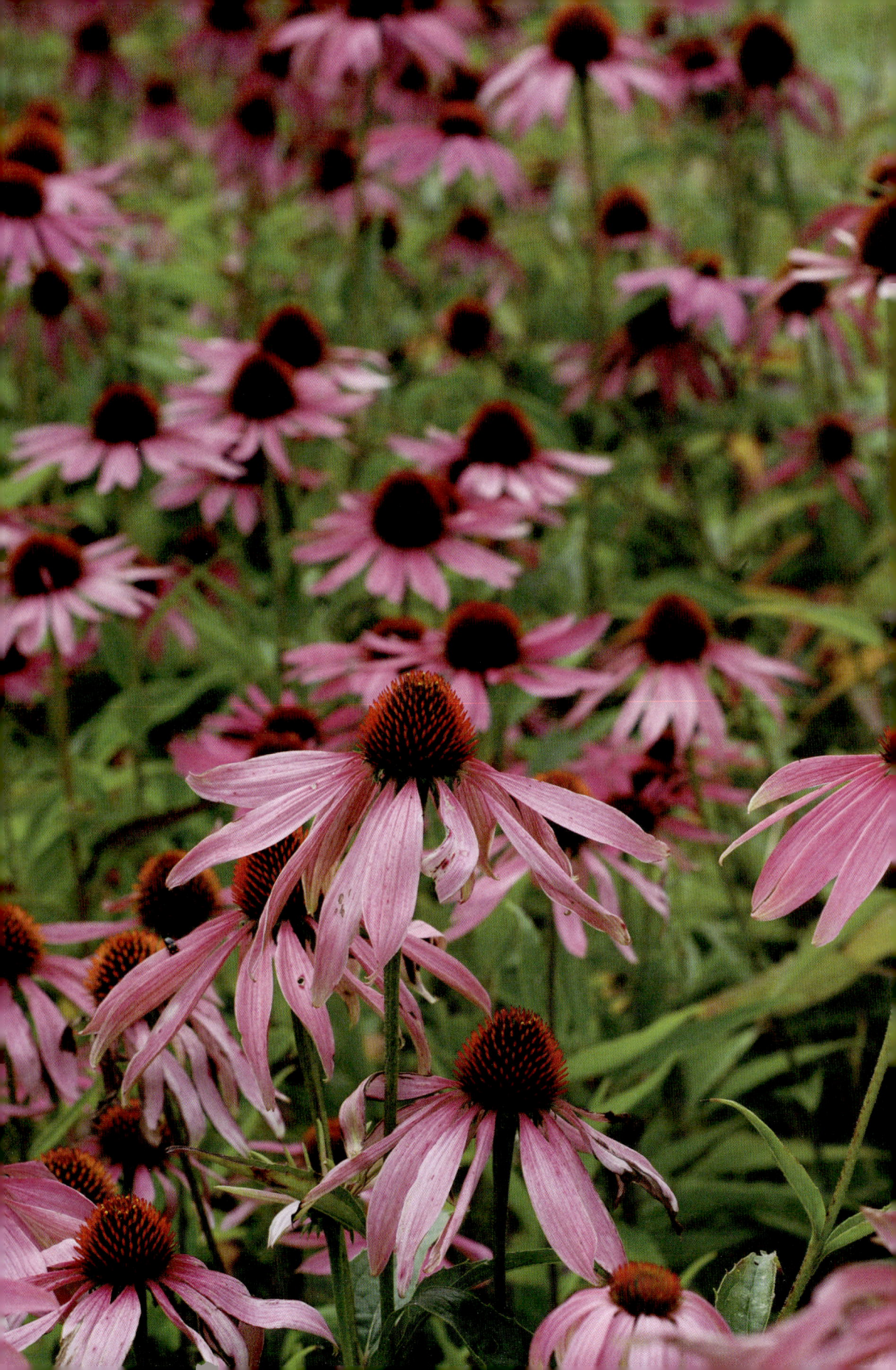

Echinacea angustifolia, pallida and purpurea: Purple Coneflower

The Flower of Immunity

*If we could see the miracle of a single flower clearly
our whole life would change.*
— Gautama Buddha

Other names: Purple cone flower, narrow-leaved purple coneflower, black samson, eastern purple coneflower, snakeroot, scurvy root, Indian head, black Susan, Rudbeckia, hedgehog, comb flower, Kansas snakeroot

Part used: Root and rhizome, leaves and flowers

The Echinaceas are beautiful members of the Asteraceae/Compositae family with pink to purple daisy-like flowers. Their petals fall to reveal black spiny seed heads - the name *Echinacea* comes from the Greek *'echinos'* meaning hedgehog. Three of the nine species of Echinacea that are native to North America have medicinal benefits. These are *E. purpurea*, the common purple coneflower; *E. angustifolia*, the narrow-leafed purple coneflower; and *E. pallida*, the pale purple coneflower. The name *coneflower* comes from its conical flower heads.

Purple coneflower was one of the most important medicinal plants known to the native Americans. They applied extracts to wounds, burns, insect bites and swollen lymph glands and took it internally for headaches, stomach aches, coughs and colds, measles and gonorrhoea. They chewed the root to relieve toothache and neck pain, and commonly used it as an antidote for rattlesnake bites. We now know that Echinacea prevents the formation of an enzyme called hyaluronidase which is secreted by bacteria and also found in snake venom, which destroys the natural barrier between healthy tissues and disease carrying organisms and this way invades the body's tissues.

The root of purple coneflower was the part most commonly used, although tribes such as the Comanche, Cheyenne and the Sioux used the juice and a paste of the macerated fresh leaves and flowers. The root made a good local anaesthetic to deaden sensation and relieve pain. You can feel this on your tongue when taking a few drops of the tincture. The Cheyenne chewed the root to stimulate the flow of saliva, which was particularly useful as a thirst-quencher for those doing the ritual Sun Dance. They also drank the tea to relieve arthritis, measles and mumps.

The white settlers in America soon learned of the amazing immune-enhancing properties of Echinacea and much of its initial popularity was due to the efforts of a patent medicine salesman, H.C.F. Meyer who in 1871 included a tincture of *Echinacea angustifolia* in his 'Meyer's Blood Purifier'. He touted this elixir as a marvellous cure for such diseases as syphilis, malaria and typhoid as well as for gangrene, arthritis, rattlesnake bites and lesser evils such as bee stings, leg ulcers and chronic nasal congestion. By 1920, Echinacea was a popular remedy but with the advent of antibiotic drugs in the 1930s, its popularity began to dwindle in the US. However, its continued recognition as a valuable medicine has largely been due to European interest and research.

Herbal Remedy

Echinacea is one of the most popular herbal medicines today and the first that springs to the minds of many for treating acute infections.

It contains alkylamides, echinacosides, acids, echinacein, polyacetylenes, polysaccharides including inulin, cynarin, flavonoids, essential oil, glycoside, isobutylalklamines, resin, betain and vitamin C. Information on the medicinal benefits of Echinaceas comes from two fronts. From 1895 to 1930 American doctors demonstrated the effects of the roots of *E. angustifolia* on a wide range of complaints including boils and abscesses, blood poisoning, post-partum infection, malaria, typhus and TB.

German studies over the last 50 years using the aerial parts of *E. purpurea* have proved it to be extremely valuable for treating septic conditions, rheumatoid arthritis, antibiotic resistance, whooping cough in children, flu, catarrh, chronic respiratory tract infections, gynaecological infections, pelvic inflammatory disease, urinary infections and a variety of skin problems. You can take it on a daily basis to prevent colds, flu and any other types of infections as Echinacea can enhance immunity. The roots as well as the leaves and flowers have their virtues and it may be best to combine all parts together for the best effects.

Echinacea has an antibacterial and antifungal effect, an interferon-like antiviral action and an anti-allergenic action. Contemporary attention has focused on Echinacea's success in treating the common cold and upper respiratory infections and shortening the duration for improvement. It can be taken at the first sign of symptoms such as sore throats, runny nose and sneezing and needs to be taken every 2 hours in the acute phase for good results. It can also be taken at the onset of coughs, chest infections, tonsillitis and glandular fever as well as for *Candida* and post-viral fatigue syndrome. Echinacea has the ability to inactivate viruses including Human H1N1-type IV, the highly pathogenic avian IV (HPAIV) flu, as well as swine origin IV (S-OIV, H1N1) by interfering with the viral entry into cells. The immune-stimulating effect of Echinacea probably involves many mechanisms, including increased phagocytosis (engulfing and destroying) of pathogens by activating white blood cells called macrophages.

Echinacea is particularly useful for people whose weakened immune systems make them prone to one infection after another. Taken in hot infusion, echinacea stimulates the circulation and enhances sweating, helping to bring down fevers. As a blood cleanser, it helps to clear the skin of infections including boils and abscesses and to relieve allergies such as urticaria and eczema. Its immune-enhancing, antimicrobial and anti-inflammatory effects are helpful in arthritis and gout, skin conditions and pelvic inflammatory disease.

Externally, Echinacea is an excellent anti-inflammatory and antiseptic remedy for treating inflammatory skin problems, infections such as spots, acne, boils and abscesses. It can be used to speed healing and prevent infection in wounds, ulcers, burns, stings and bites. It makes a good antiseptic gargle and mouthwash for sore throats and infected gums and a douche for a wide range of vaginal infections.

Homeopathic Remedy

Echinacea angustifolia is used much like the herbal remedy. It is specific for blood poisoning, poisoned wounds, gangrene, boils and carbuncles, septicaemia, diphtheria and the effects of vaccination. It is prescribed for catarrh, abdominal pain and griping, loose yellow stools, diarrhoea, offensive wind and nausea.

An Echinacea person may feel cross and irritable and does not wish to be contradicted. So nervous they cannot study or concentrate, their head feels dull, and their senses numbed. They may also be depressed and out of sorts, particularly in the afternoon. They generally feel worse after eating, and after physical and mental exertion and better for rest.

Flower Essence

Echinacea is for those who lack a sense of identity because of the anonymity of modern life, or who, because of physical or emotional trauma, feel as if they are *'falling apart'*. They may feel profoundly alienated, unable to contact that inner place of strength and calm. Such threats to the sense of self may underlay many immune-related illnesses. Echinacea strengthens the sense of self and engenders a feeling of wholeness, helping to give greater resilience when under enormous stress.

The Healing Flowers

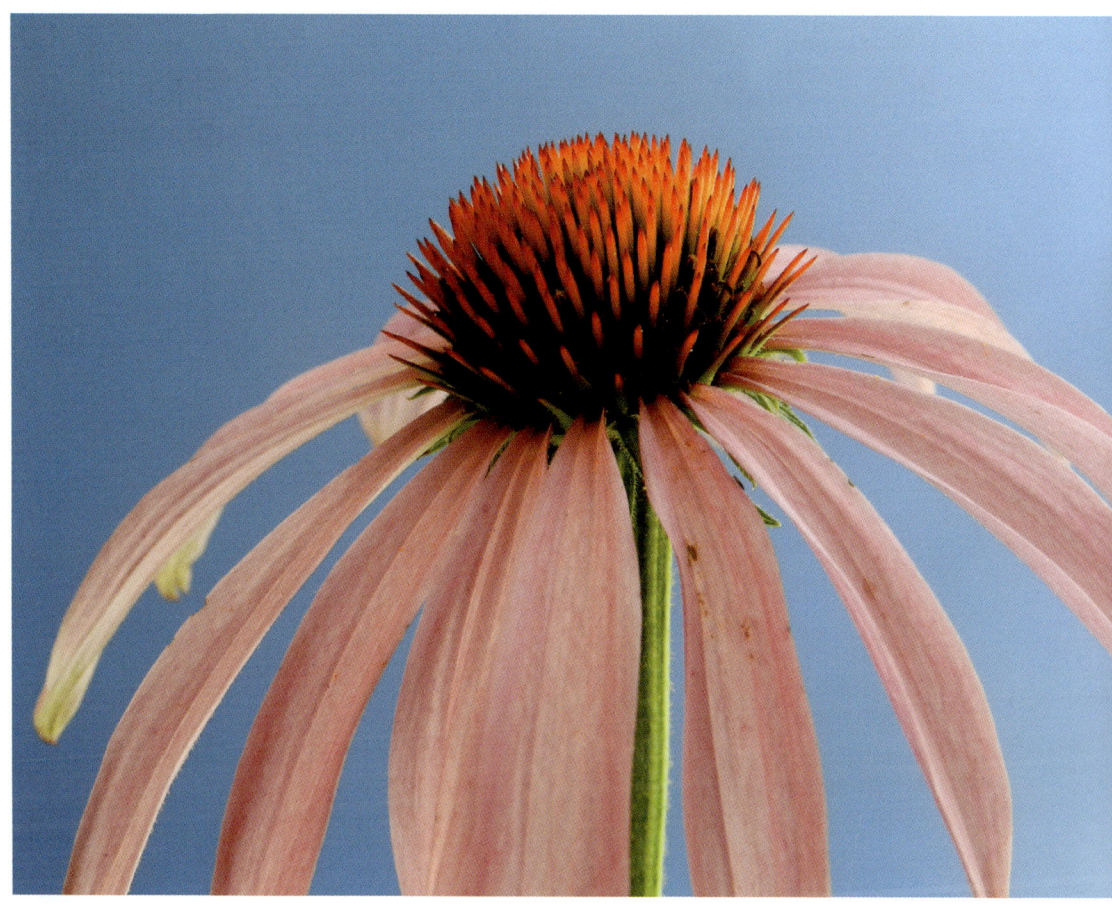

Growing
Echinacea is a beautiful plant with dusky pink/purple, daisy-like flowers and is great value in the garden as it has a long flowering period from July to October. When the petals drop, black spiky seed heads are left. The plant is also called coneflower. *E. purpurea* and *E. angustifolia* are both available at many garden nurseries and specialist herb centres.

Edible Uses
The leaves and the flowers are edible, and the beautiful pink flowers are wonderfully decorative for almost any dish, savoury or sweet. They look good in any vegetable dishes, salads, fruit salads and floated in drinks.

Cautions
In allergies to Asteraceae family pollen (chrysanthemum, chamomile, ragweed, daisy), avoid echinacea flower products (leaf juice or root products should not provoke allergic response). Can cause anaphylaxis, asthma or urticaria. Echinacea may alter metabolism of some drugs. Theoretically it could decrease the effectiveness of immuno-suppressants.

Recipe

Echinacea Tincture
20g fresh Echinacea root
80ml vodka

Wash and chop the Echinacea root, then put in a jar and pour over the vodka to cover completely. Leave for 2-4 weeks. Then press out the liquid, discard the herb, label clearly and store the tincture in a cool dark place.

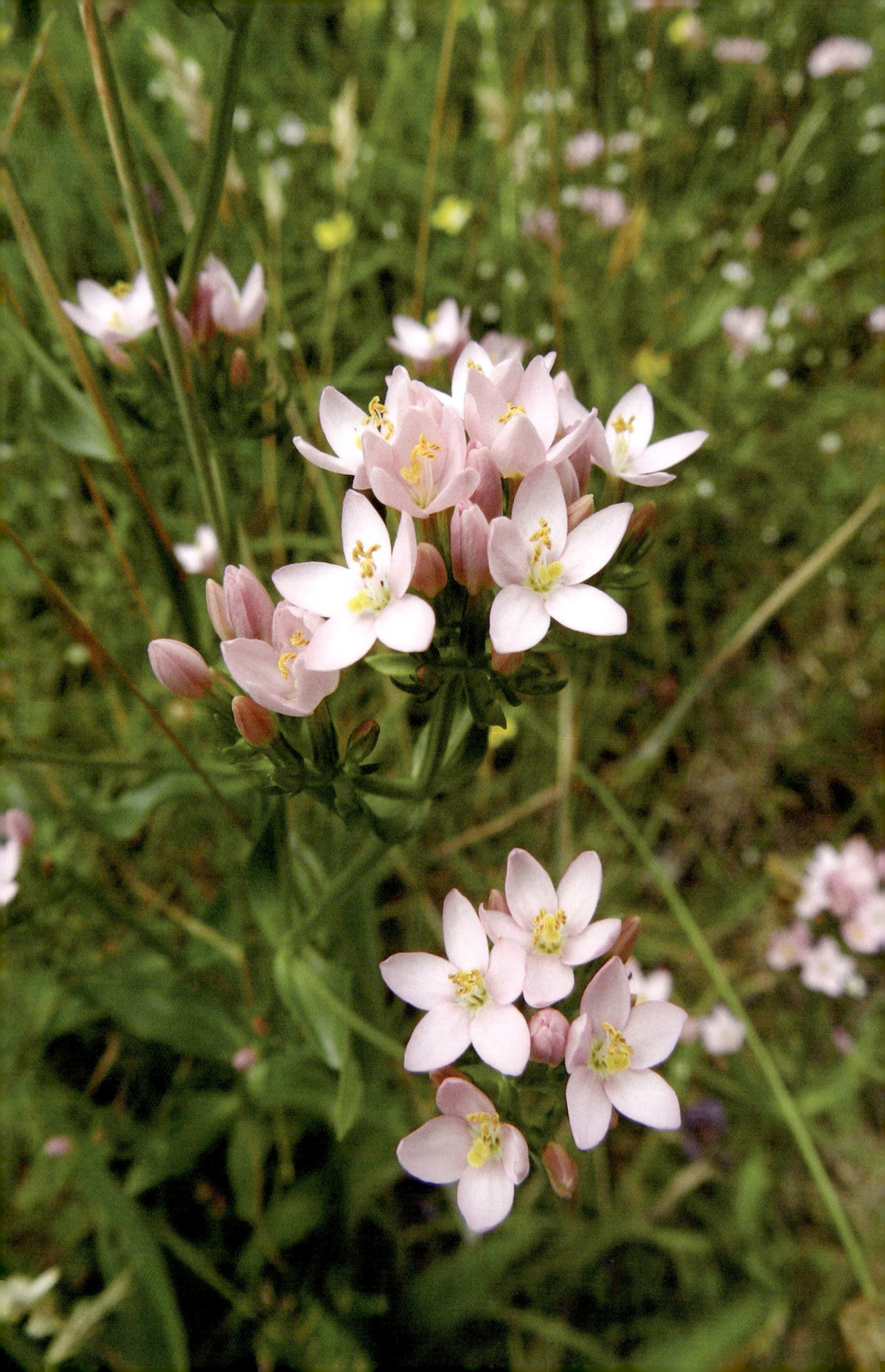

Erythraea centaurium/Centaurium erythraea: Centaury

The Flower of Chiron

*The herbe is so safe that you cannot fail in the using of it,
Only give it inwardly for inward diseases,
Use it outwardly for outward diseases.
'Tis very wholesome,
But not very toothsome*
– Nicolas Culpeper (1616–1654)

Other names: Centaury, red centaury, felwort, centre of the sun, common centaury, feverwort, lesser centaury, Christ's ladder.

Parts Used: Leaves and flowers

This pretty little member of the Gentianaceae family, with its delicate pink or white flowers, grows wild as an annual on chalk downs, sandy pastures and hedgerows throughout Europe. It is said to dislike being cultivated. In the south of England, it has been known as *'herb of the sun'* because the flowers open only in sunshine and close at noon. A single cloud obscuring the sun is enough to keep the flowers tightly closed. Culpeper said, *"They are under the dominion of the sun as appears in that their flowers open and shut as the sun either shews or hides his face."* Century flowers were well known as a floral oracle for testing a lover's affection – if the flowers remained bright pink after they were picked, all augured well.

Centaury derives its name from the centaur physician of Greek mythology, Chiron, from whom humankind is said to have aquired its knowledge of medicinal plants. Chiron taught Asclepius, the renowned god of medicine and the famous warrior, Achilles. Dioscorides, the Greek physician used the 'great Kentaurion' for treating injuries. Its name *Erythraea* comes from the Greek 'erythros' meaning red, alluding to the pinky-red colour of the flower, or maybe the efficacy of the remedy in the treatment of skin rashes.

For 2,000 years, centaury has been revered by many cultures. The Romans believed it had magical powers to drive away snakes, so did the Gauls of the Dark Ages, who used it to antidote snakebites. The Saxons also used it for snakebites and intermittent fevers, hence its common name 'feverwort.' Another name for centaury was the 'universal purifier', since it drove poisons and infections out of the body, as well as negative influences from the psyche. Medieval witches took it to increase their psychic powers and to take them into trance-like states. It was also considered to protect against evil. In Ireland it was known as a herb of good luck. The ancients also called centaury 'fel terrae' meaning gall of the earth, because of its very bitter taste. It has been used in vermouth and other bitter aperitifs and liqueurs.

Herbal Remedy

This delicate and petite plant has a wealth of constituents that contribute to its medicinal use. These include bitter glycosides, iridoids, phenolic acids, alkaloids, sterols, oleanolic acid, resins, flavonoids and xanthones. With its combination of bitter and pungent tastes, centaury makes a good remedy for the digestion, increasing the flow of digestive enzymes, promoting appetite, digestion and absorption of nutrients. It increases gastric motility and its antioxidant action protects the lining of the stomach from free radical damage.

With its effective antimicrobial and vermicidal actions, centaury helps combat unfriendly

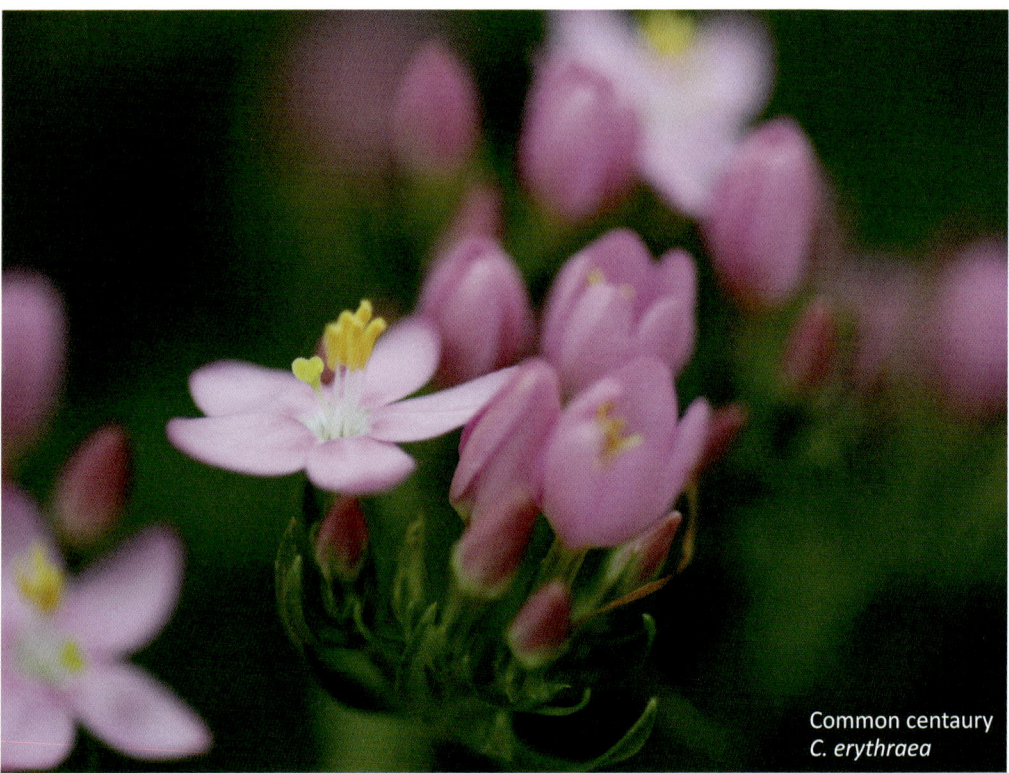

Common centaury
C. erythraea

micro-organisms, worms and parasites in the gut and enhances absorption and synthesis of nutrients, immunity and brain function. It clears toxins from the gut and promotes the flow of bile from the liver. Its bitterness, like that of its relative gentian, accounts for much of its medicinal value. It has an anti-inflammatory action and supports the liver in its cleansing work. The iridoid glycosides in the plant provide hepato-protective actions, protecting the liver from damage from infection, toxins and drugs.

Centaury also relaxes the smooth muscle in the gut and reduces tension and spasm causing colic and eases the passage of stools. It can be used for indigestion, poor appetite, heartburn, gastritis, peptic ulcers, nausea and vomiting, constipation, obesity, gallbladder and liver problems including jaundice and chronic hepatitis.

Centaury has a reputation as a blood purifier, clearing toxins from the system and as a mild laxative, increasing the efficiency of the bowels. With its anti-inflammatory action attributed to the gentiopicroside, it can be taken for arthritis and gout, as well as skin problems including eczema, acne and boils. It will reduce fevers when taken in a hot infusion and has been used as a substitute for quinine. Its inflammatory action can also be helpful in inflammatory eye problems. Generally, it has a strengthening effect, useful when recovering from illness or stress and as a blood tonic in anaemia. Its antioxidant constituents protect the heart and reduce total cholesterol, they protect the blood vessels including the venous system, explaining the use of centaury for varicose veins and haemorrhoids.

Centaury can be considered a good remedy for the immune system and the brain. It helps to combat both bacterial and viral infections and can be used for post-viral syndrome. The xantones in the leaves and flowers are thought to have antitumor and anti-inflammatory activities. One of their bitter glycosides called gentiopicrin, reputedly has antimalarial properties. Centaury also has an affinity for the nervous system and can help to lift the spirits and calm the nerves. Xanthone derivatives in the plant can inhibit acetylcholinesterase (AChE) and this means there is a higher concentration of acetylcholine in the brain, which leads to better communication between nerve cells, which could be helpful in Alzheimer's disease.

Externally centaury makes a good anti-inflammatory and antiseptic wash for cuts and grazes, boils and other skin conditions and to heal ulcers. It makes a good mouthwash for inflamed gums and gingivitis, a cooling eyewash for inflamed eyes and a strengthening, toning lotion for varicose veins.

Flower Essence
Centaury is a wonderful remedy for people who are very sensitive to others and to their environment. They are easily hurt and upset and can become ill as a result of disharmony and negative influences. Centaury people are good-natured and kind, but stronger personalities will readily take advantage of them. As children they are obedient and good, responding well to praise and discipline. They may spend too much of their time helping others, sacrificing their own lives in their service. They can be 'doormats', and martyrs, and neglect their own mission in life in their desire to please.

Centaury helps you to develop your will and recognise your own individuality and personality and to see it as valuable. It turns submissiveness into an ability to relate to others on an equal footing, to say 'No' when necessary and to use service to others as part of your own transformation.

Growing
Propagate by sowing seed in spring or autumn, barely covering the seeds, in full sun or semi-shade. It will adapt to most soils and often thrives in rock gardens and by the sea. Grows 3"– 12" (8–30cm) and flowers from June – September. It will self-seed freely.

Cautions
Avoid in pregnancy.

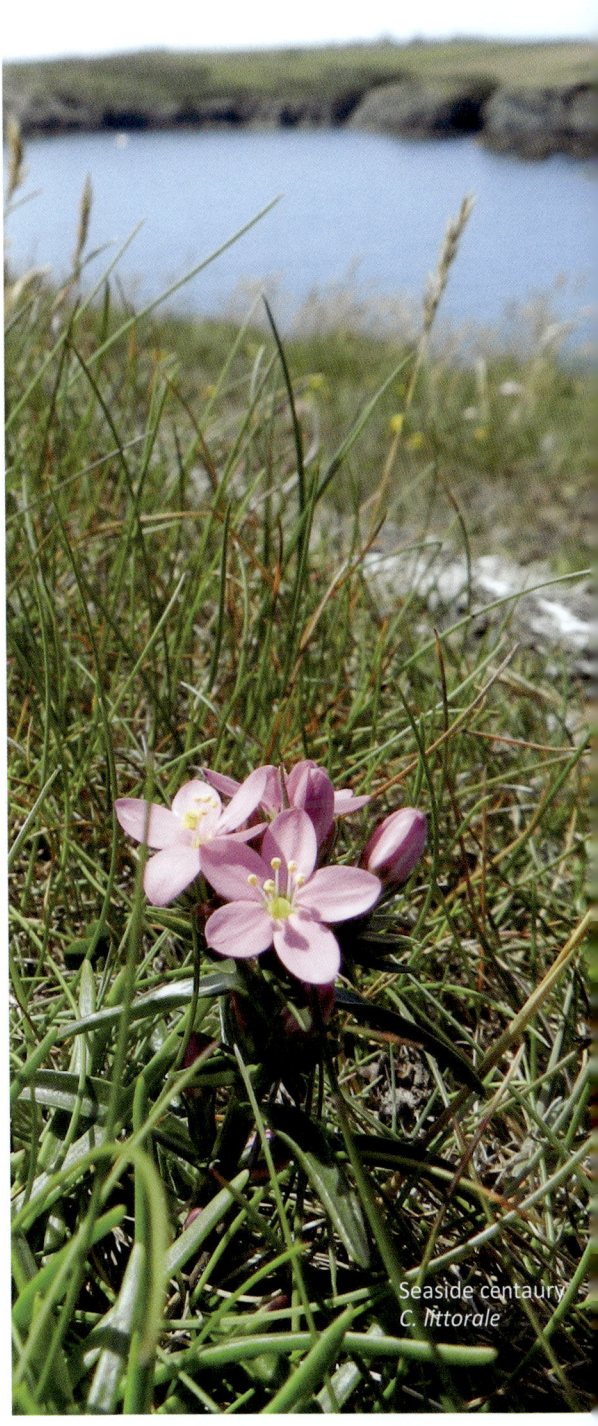

Seaside centaury
C. littorale

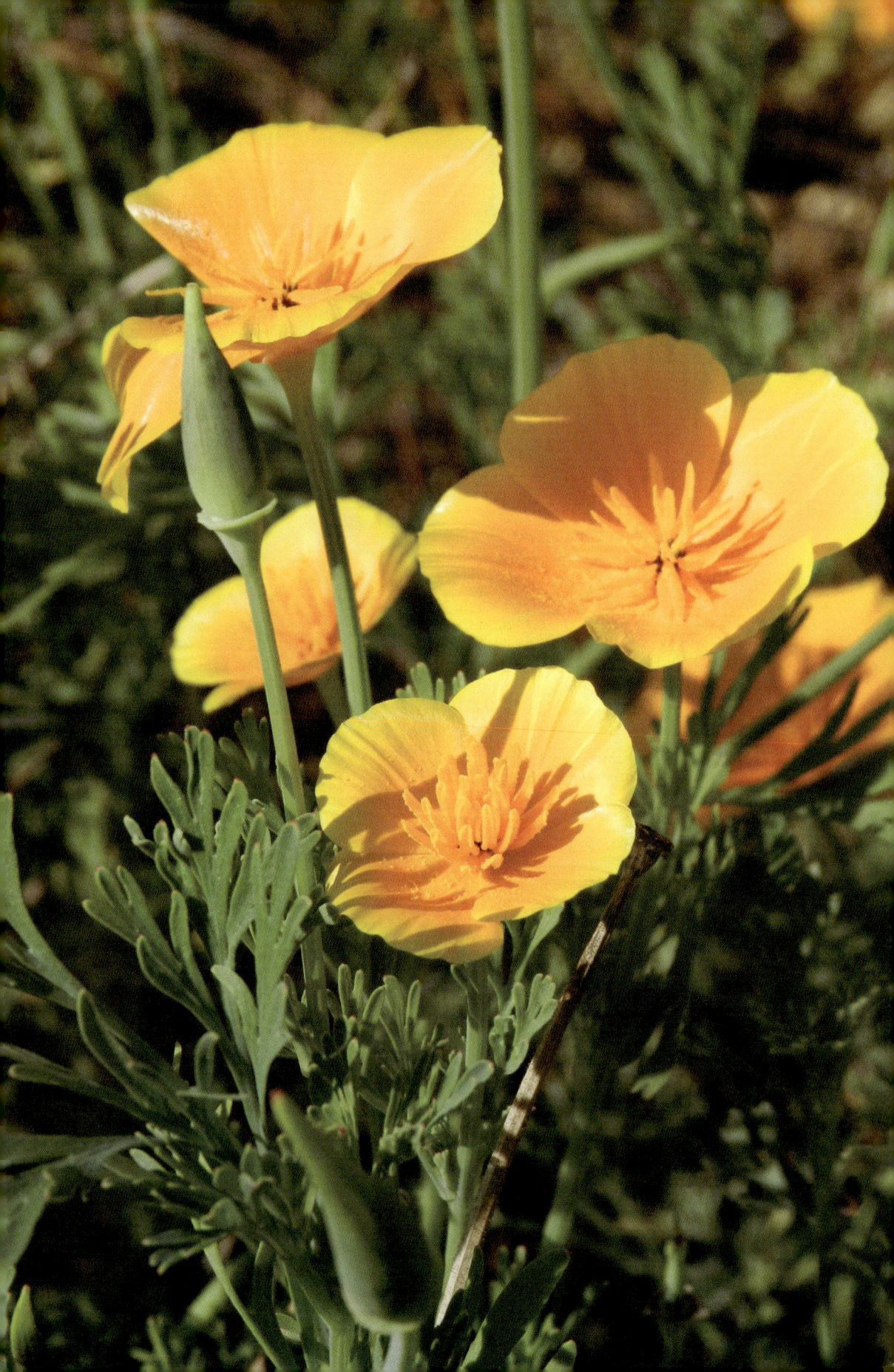

Eschscholzia californica: California poppy

The Flower of Gold

*Pleasures are like poppies spread,
You seize the flower, the bloom is shed*
– Robert Burns (1759–1796)

Other names: Golden poppy, golden cup, California sunlight, cup of gold

Parts Used: Flowers and aerial parts

This vibrantly colourful annual is the state flower of California and native to the west of North America. It has also been found in southern France, Australia and Chile. The flower is usually golden orange in colour, hence its common name 'golden poppy.' California poppy was first introduced to Europe as an ornamental and medicinal plant in the last century and rapidly gained a reputation as a non-addictive alternative to the opium poppy, even though it is a member of the Papaveraceae family. It is a wonderfully relaxing herb, used for colicky pains and toothache by the native Americans and early settlers.

California poppy was first described by Adelbert von Chamisso (c. 1820), a naturalist on a Russian ship called the *Rurik* on a scientific expedition to California in 1810. He named the genus in honour of his close friend Johann Friedrich Eschscholtz, a Baltic German botanist who was also the expedition's physician.

The poppy symbolises the ephemeral pleasures of life – here one minute, gone the next. According to the doctrine of signatures, California poppy resembles a cup of gold, and the saying 'all that glitters is not gold' may be very appropriate to many in the state of California attracted to mind-altering drugs and glamorous spiritual practices.

Herbal remedy
California poppy is a cousin of the opium poppy but far less powerful. It can be thought of as a safe, gentle balancer to the emotions, a calming remedy in times of stress and is a great 'feel good' herb with subtle euphoric properties. When times are hard, the leaves and flowers can be used in remedies to help us to find equilibrium.

California poppy contains isoquinoline alkaloids (including californidine, sanguinarine, escholzine, protopine, crytpopine, chelidonine), flavone glycosides, carotenoids and essential oil. It acts as a gentle sedative and is suitable for calming children and adults alike, helping to reduce stress in the day and induce sleep at night. With its bitter taste and cooling effect, California poppy cools 'heat' in the mind, and makes an excellent remedy for 'chilling you out' – for irritability, anger, frustration, low self-esteem, over-achieving, headaches, being overly critical and analytical and for OCD. It can also be helpful for excitability, restlessness, anxiety, pain and tension.

California poppy can also be thought of whenever physical symptoms are related to stress or upset. Its antispasmodic action relaxes muscles throughout the body, making it useful for treating colic in the gut as well as gallbladder, and for soothing tense, aching muscles and relieving tension headaches. It is recommended in IBS, bedwetting in children, asthma and dry, spasmodic coughs. By calming the nervous system, California poppy influences the heart and circulation. It slows a rapid heart, relieves palpitations and reduces blood pressure.

With its pain-killing action, California poppy can be used to ease pain from inflammation as in arthritis, as well as for nerve pain. It can be

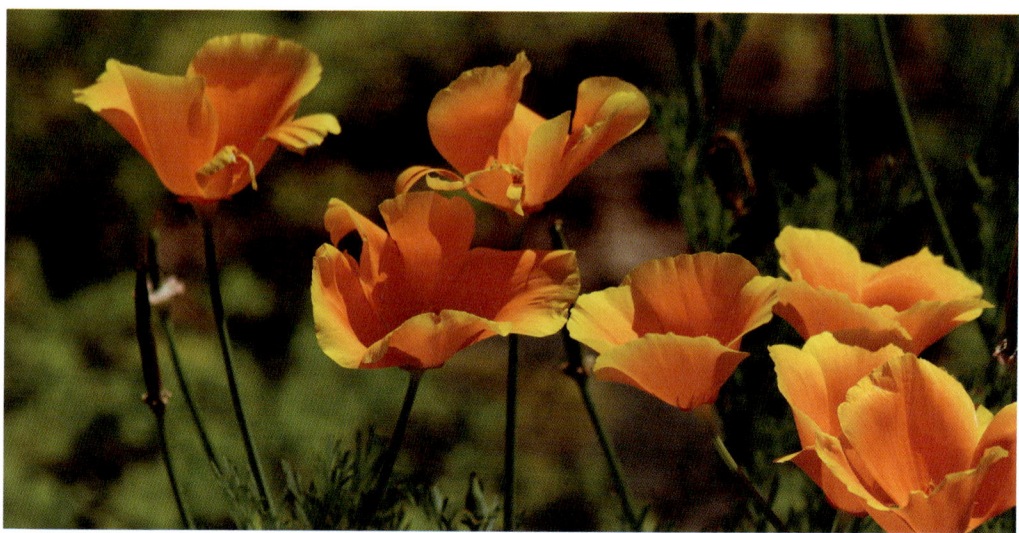

taken to relieve headaches, migraine, toothache, neuralgia, back pain, sciatica and the pain of shingles. It can reduce spasm and pain in lower abdomen and used to ease colic, gallbladder and menstrual pain.

California poppy is worth using when trying to withdraw from addiction, be it to alcohol, drugs, orthodox medicines or tobacco. Its cognitive-enhancing properties can be useful in the treatment of behavioural disorders such as ADD and ADHD in children and young adults. It has also been used to improve intellectual capacity, memory and concentration in the elderly.

Externally California poppy in tincture or tea form can be applied to areas of pain such as headaches and toothache. As an antimicrobial it can be applied to cuts and scrapes. A tincture or paste of the seed pods can be used as a wash for suppressing lactation in breast-feeding women.

Homeopathic Remedy
Eschscholzia is used in tincture form for insomnia, slowness of the circulation and general weakness.

Flower Essence
California poppy is for those who seek spiritual highs from external sources, who are attracted to the glamour and brightness of psychedelic drugs, charismatic teachers or occult rituals. Their spiritual life lacks discipline and solidity and they may be susceptible to techniques or influences which open the psyche too quickly, causing inner disharmony. California poppy helps to develop a more solid inner life, awakening the light within and enhancing self-reliance.

Recipe

Night-time Tisane
Equal parts of:
California poppy
lemon balm
catmint
chamomile

Using 1 teaspoon of herb per cupful of water, place herbs in a teapot, cover with boiling water and leave to infuse for 10–15 mins. Drink a cupful or two before bed.

Growing
Sow seeds in spring in situ in dry, light soil, even gravel. Likes full sun. Grows from 5 to 20 inches tall, with teal-coloured leaves sprouting from its base. The plant is prolific, and self-seeds easily.

Cautions
Avoid the herbal remedy in pregnancy and breastfeeding. Contraindicated in glaucoma. Avoid with MAOIs, tranquilizers, CNS depressants (eg. alcohol, opiates, benzodiazepines, anaesthetics, tricyclic anti-depressants, anti-epileptics) and Pentobarbital.

Euphrasia officinalis: Eyebright
The Flower of Insight

*...To nobler sights
Michael from Adam's eyes the film removed,
Then purged with Euphrasine and Rue
His visual orbs, for he had much to see*
– John Milton (1608–1674)

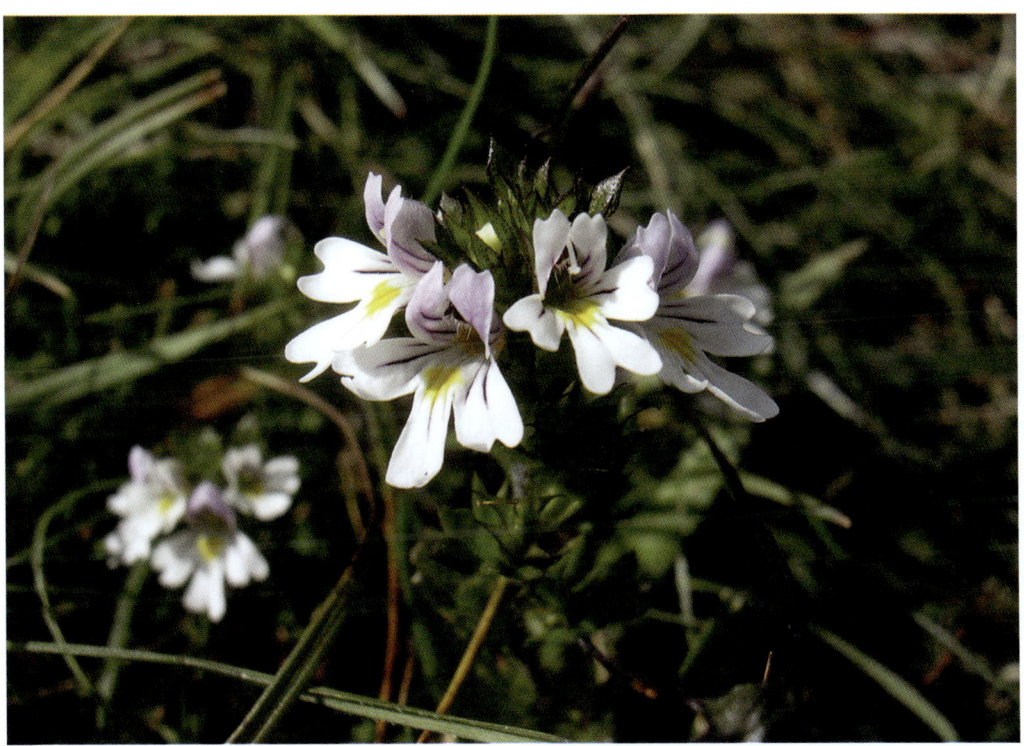

Other names: Bird's eye, fairy flax, peeweets, rock rue

Parts Used: Leaves, flowers

Eyebright is a delicate little plant that grows in dry sunny pastures, commons and hillsides and is loved by bees. It is an annual plant which is partially parasitic, taking nourishment from roots of grasses. It is a member of the foxglove (Scrophulariaceae) family and comes originally from Europe and Asia, although it grows throughout the United States. Eyebright has been famous for centuries for its ability to preserve and restore eyesight.

Its Latin name *Euphrasia* comes originally from the Greek word 'euphrosyne' meaning gladness and also the name of one of the three muses in Greek mythology who represented joy and gladness. This may be because the plant was so highly valued for its ability to improve eyesight and remedy eye problems, that it brought happiness to the life of those suffering from eye problems. 'Euphrosyne' is also the Greek word for the linnet, as the ancient Greeks said that the healing power of eyebright was first discovered by a linnet who used it for her young in the nest. The linnet then gave her knowledge of eyebright to humankind and tells of her gratitude continuously in song.

According to the Medieval doctrine of signatures, the dark spot in the middle of the flower bore a striking resemblance to the human eye and the purple and yellow spots and stripes inside the flower indicated its ability to heal a variety of inflammatory eye problems. Culpeper said, *"If eye-bright were as much used as it is neglected, it would have spoilt the trade of the spectacle makers."*

Eyebright was said to be a visionary herb. It clears the sight and 'gladdens the eye' or lifts the spirits of the one whose sight is improved, and it was also respected for its ability to increase insight and enhance inner vision, the ability to see things as they truly are. It was prescribed for troubles of the mind and according to Culpeper, *"It also helpeth a weak brain or memory."*

In the Middle Ages dried eyebright was often combined with tobacco and smoked to clear congestion in the chest and relieve colds and coughs. In Elizabethan times its bitter taste was valued for flavouring beer and it was made into an ale which was used to clear eyesight.

Herbal Remedy

Although modern herbalists may be more moderate in their claims about the power of eyebright than the ancients, the aerial parts of eyebright still make an excellent remedy for a variety of eye problems. Its antioxidant, anti-inflammatory and regenerative properties are all involved in its beneficial effects and certain of its constituents can be very helpful in reducing eye symptoms and discomfort. It contains iridoid glycosides (aucubin, euphroside), saponins, resin, flavonoids, tannins, phenolic acids, phenylethanoid glycosides, phytosterols, bitters, sterols, vitamin C, lignans and volatile oils. Aucubin has an anti-inflammatory action and can soothe tired and inflamed eyes, the astringent tannins help dry up excess secretions and relieve inflammation of the mucous membranes which can be very helpful in inflammatory problems such as conjunctivitis or blepharitis (inflammation of the eyelids).

Eyebright enhances the circulation to the eyes and can be used to improve eyesight in the elderly. Its antioxidant properties may help the eye absorb more vitamin A and vitamin C. Eyebright also contains minerals including zinc, copper and selenium, which all help to protect against cataracts.

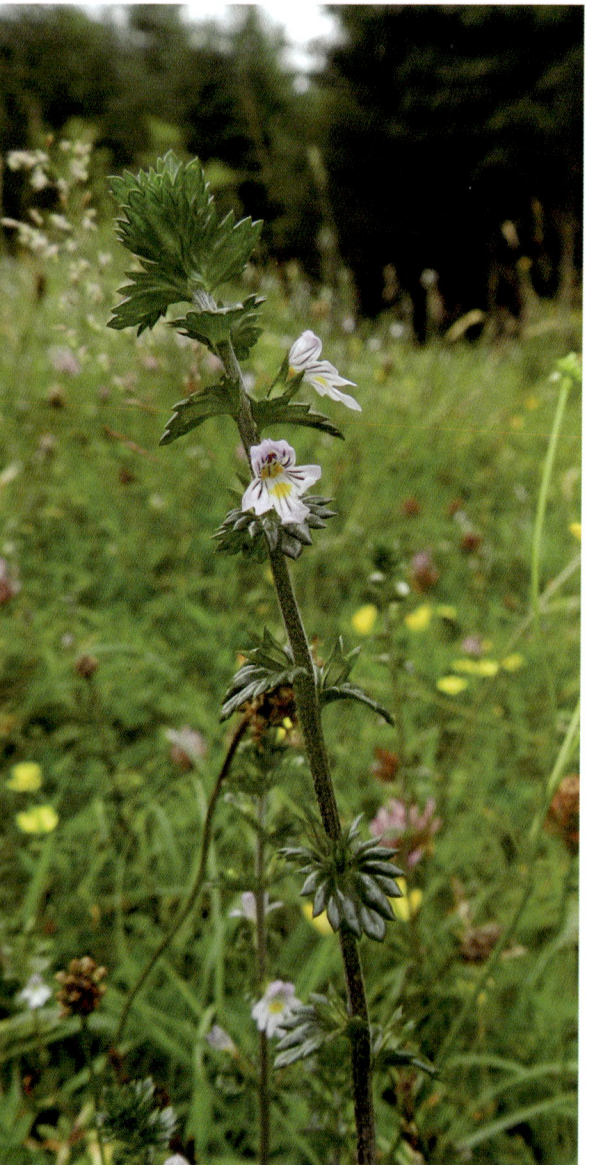

Its antimicrobial and astringent properties are good for relieving inflammatory eye infections such as sties, conjunctivitis, blepharitis and watery eye conditions as well as catarrh. It is particularly good for sore, itchy eyes with a discharge, often seen in hay fever or measles. It can also be helpful for people with oversensitive eyes, which tend to run in the cold and wind, or are irritated by smoky or stuffy atmospheres or by too much light. It can be used either locally in lotions for the eyes or taken internally: 30 drops of the tincture in a glassful of rosewater makes an excellent eyewash.

Eyebright's anti-inflammatory, astringent and decongestant properties are excellent for all conditions involving the lining of the respiratory tract. It can be used in colds, sore throats, post-nasal drip, catarrh, ear infections, sinusitis and sinus headaches. Eyebright contains a flavonoid *quercetin* which can reduce allergic reactions by inhibiting the release of histamine, explaining it use in allergies such as allergic rhinitis/hay fever. It makes a good astringent expectorant remedy for catarrhal coughs. It has antimicrobial action (against *B. subtilis, E. coli, Mycobacterium phlei*) as well as antifungal and antiviral properties.

The bitters in eyebright stimulate the digestion and enhance the flow of bile from the liver, making this tiny plant a good tonic and a cleansing remedy. Several plants that improve the function of the liver are also recommended for the eyes, such as greater celandine, marigold, chamomile and centaury. According to Culpeper, all these herbs, including eyebright, are under the dominion of the sun which governs circulation, vital energy and eyesight. By detoxifying the system via its action on the liver, eyebright helps to clear the eyes and by improving circulation to the eyes, it improves feeble eyesight in the elderly and tired, strained eyes from overwork. By clearing mucus from the system, eyebright will keep the mucosa of the eye clear and healthy.

Eyebright can be used for a range of digestive problems including poor appetite and digestion and poor absorption. As a liver and gallbladder remedy, eyebright can be useful in inflammatory liver and gallbladder problems. The antioxidants in eyebright have a protective effect in the liver, helping to protect it against damage from toxins such as alcohol and drugs.

Eyebright has been used traditionally to lift the spirits, for 'troubles of the mind' and to improve memory and concentration. It can still be used as a visionary herb, enhancing insight and inner vision, helping us to get things in perspective when we lack mental clarity.

Externally the astringent and antimicrobial properties of eyebright can be helpful when used in gargles for sore and catarrhal throats, and in mouthwashes for mouth ulcers. It was used in the past as a snuff for catarrh. A few drops of dilute tincture or an infusion in nostrils can help to clear catarrhal congestion. It can be used in lotions for the eyes – 30 drops of the tincture in a glassful of rosewater makes an excellent eyewash, or the tea can be used on compresses.

Homeopathic Remedy
Euphrasia is an excellent medicine for the eye. Like the herbal remedy, it is prescribed for watery, burning eyes, discharges from the eyes, sensitive eyes aggravated by both light and windy weather, for swollen, inflamed eyelids and eyes as in blepharitis and conjunctivitis. It is good for catarrh, sore throats, colds, catarrhal throats, hay fever and coughs, and for eye and catarrhal problems accompanying measles.

Flower Essence
Eyebright is again the flower of sight, insight, inner vision and perception. It is given to those whose brain feels weak and tired and whose memory is poor. Eyebright increases your sensitivity and perception of others and their conditions, which makes it helpful for those in the caring professions. It helps you to get things in a clearer perspective.

Growing
Because eyebright is partially parasitic, it needs to be cultivated with certain grass species from which it takes nourishment and is best propagated by division of the root in a clump within the grasses. Grows 2–12" high (5–30cm) and flowers from midsummer to autumn.

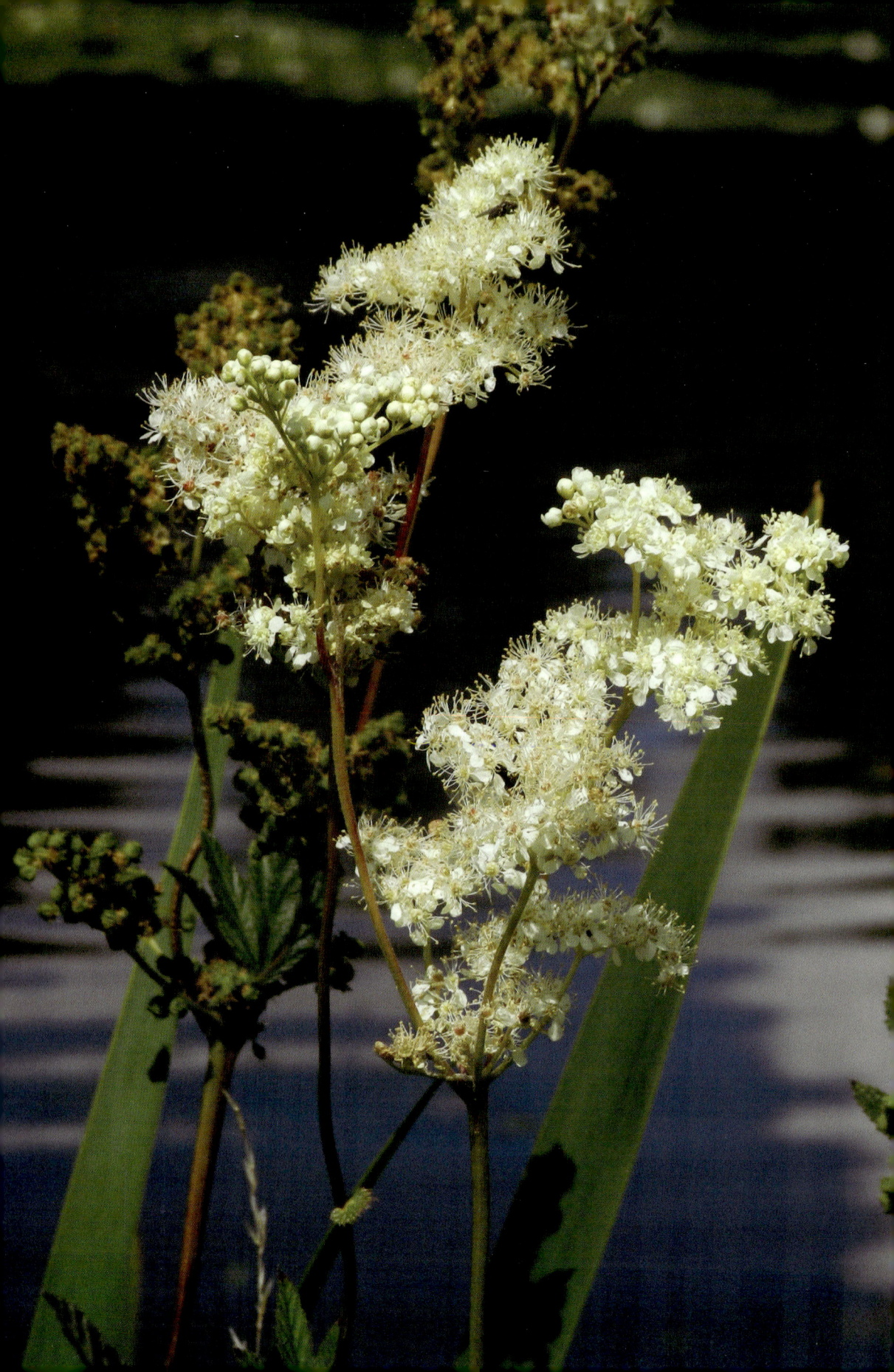

Filipendula ulmaria: Meadowsweet

The Flower of Summer Meadows

*The meadowsweet taunts high its showy wreath
And sweet the quaking grasses hide beneath*
– John Clare (1793–1864)

Other Names: *Spirea ulmaria*, queen of the meadow, lady of the meadow, bridewort, meadwort

Parts Used: Aerial parts of the flowering plant

The elegant meadowsweet flower with its sweet almond scent is a member of the rose (Rosaceae) family that can be found growing in profusion in damp fields and by rivers and streams. The plant well deserves its country name of 'queen' or *lady of the meadow*. It has been used for at least 4,000 years. Traces of it were discovered in the Scottish Hebrides in the remains of a Neolithic drink. It was also found in a Neolithic burial site near Perth. Along with vervain and watermint, it was one of the most sacred herbs of the Druids.

Meadowsweet has been used for centuries in ceremonies to do with growth, transition and change, such as births, funerals, festivals and weddings. In fact, another old name for meadowsweet was 'bridewort' as its feathery white plumes and attractive red stalked leaves were strewn in churches at weddings and made into garlands and posies for brides and bridesmaids.

In Chaucer's England, meadowsweet was made into beer and in the Knight's Tale, the knights about to enter combat were given various magical ointments to apply and a concoction containing meadowsweet called 'Safe' to drink. In Anglo-Saxon times, meadowsweet was called 'meadwort' and used for sweetening mead and in Tudor times, it was a popular strewing herb. It was apparently a favourite chamber herb of Queen Elizabeth I, and loved by Gerard who said that when strewed, the smell of meadowsweet *"makes the heart merrie and joyful and delighteth the senses."*

According to folklore, when gathered on St John's Day, meadowsweet was said to reveal a thief. In Iceland where it also grows, not only is it believed to do this but also to indicate the sex of the robber by sinking in water for a man and floating for a woman!

Medicinally meadowsweet was prescribed for measles, smallpox, dysentery, fevers, diarrhoea, spitting of blood and piles. When crushed, meadowsweet flowers give off the characteristic smell of the salicylic aldehyde and it was this very chemical that led to the discovery of aspirin. In 1838 the Italian chemist Raffaele Piria found that when oxidised it yielded salicylic acid, and in 1853 Strasbourg chemist Charles-Frederic Gerhardt used this to produce acetyl-salicylic acid which became known as aspirin – a corruption of the old Latin name for meadowsweet, *Spirea ulmaria*.

Herbal Remedy
The fragrant meadowsweet contains a veritable treasure trove of medicinal constituents. These include salicylic acid, volatile oils, tannins, flavonoids (rutin, quercetin, kaempferol, hyperoside, avicularin), phenolic glycosides (spiraein, gaultherine), mucilage, coumarins, vitamin C, iron, calcium, magnesium and silica.

As might be expected, the medicinal virtues of meadowsweet are very similar to those of aspirin, but happily without the unfortunate side effects of the latter involving irritation and often bleeding of the stomach lining. The additional tannins and mucilage contained in meadowsweet protect and soothe the gastric lining and its anti-inflammatory action actually enables meadowsweet to be a valuable treatment for a wide range of digestive problems.

Meadowsweet is cooling and drying and one of the best antacid remedies for acid indigestion, heartburn, gastritis, gastro-oesophageal reflux and peptic ulcers. It relieves wind, flatulence and distension and should be thought of in IBS and any inflammatory condition of the stomach or bowels. The tannins have an astringent action in the bowels, protecting and healing the mucous membranes and providing an excellent remedy for enteritis and diarrhoea, especially for children and the elderly; its mild antiseptic action is helpful where there is infection, and its relaxant properties soothe griping and colic.

It seems that reducing acidity in the stomach can help to reduce acid levels in the body as a whole, which is helpful in joint problems associated with excess acidity. For aches and pains, arthritis and gout, meadowsweet offers welcome relief. The salicylates and gaultherine contained in the flowers have a powerfully anti-inflammatory action, well worth using for treating hot swollen joints, and the diuretic properties of the plant help eliminate toxic wastes and uric acid from the system. Meadowsweet also has an analgesic effect, helping to soothe arthritic pain as well as headaches and neuralgia, and relaxant properties which help to relax tense muscles and induce a restful sleep.

Meadowsweet works as a cooling diaphoretic, bringing blood to the surface of the body and causing sweating. Together with its anti-inflammatory and analgesic actions this is helpful during acute infections, colds and flu and to bring down a fever; it also brings out rashes to the skin and can be used in all eruptive infections such as measles, scarlet fever and chicken pox. Once the rash has erupted, full recovery is generally swift. Meadowsweet also helps clear excess heat from the urinary system. With its mild antiseptic action, it makes a good remedy for cystitis and urethritis, fluid retention and kidney problems. The salicylate salts are said to soften deposits in the body such as kidney stones and gravel, as well as atherosclerosis in the arteries.

Externally meadowsweet flowers can be applied to cuts and wounds, ulcers and skin irritations. They are rich in vitamin C, iron, magnesium and silica and speed healing of connective tissue and help to resolve inflammation. The astringent tannins also promote healing and staunch bleeding. A decoction of the flowers can be used as a compress to promote tissue repair and for painful arthritic joints. It can also be used as a mouthwash for mouth ulcers and bleeding gums. Distilled liquid of the flowers was an old remedy to relieve itching and burning eyes. A vaginal douche can be used for cervical dysplasia, vaginal inflammation and infection.

Homeopathic remedy
Spiraea is indicated by symptoms of heat. which can be general as well as local. There may be heat in the cheeks with fever, vertigo, or headache, or a feeling of blood rushing to the face. It is also given for cramp and heaviness in the limbs with sleepiness and a feeling of dullness or heaviness in the head.

Flower Essence
People who feel anxious and tense, and as a result suffer from tightness and tension in the head and neck muscles, benefit from meadowsweet flower essence. It helps you relax and drift peacefully, as on a lazy summer's day on the banks where the plant grows.

Growing
Propagate by sowing seeds in spring or autumn in moist rich soil and sun/light shade, or in trays of compost under glass. Alternatively divide the roots in spring. Grows 3 - 4' (90 - 120cm) and flowers in June – Sept. Keep watered in dry weather. Harvest as the flowers bloom.

Edible Uses
Meadowsweet leaves can be picked when young and used in salads once the stalks have been removed.

Cautions
Avoid the herbal remedy in asthma, bleeding disorders, pregnancy and breastfeeding, people sensitive to salicylates. Possible interaction with anticoagulants such as Warfarin.

Recipes

Tisane for Painful Joints
A mixture of marjoram, nettles, meadowsweet and feverfew can be taken as a tea and also used as a footbath to soothe pain and reduce inflammation of painful joints.

Meadowsweet and feverfew are wonderful anti-inflammatory herbs, nettles are packed full of nutrients including antioxidants and they improve circulation to and from the joints and help clear toxins from the area. Marjoram is warming and relaxing, it improves circulation and is full of antioxidants to help to protect the body from the ageing process, while its diuretic properties help relieve fluid retention, enhancing elimination of toxins.

To Make the Tisane
I part golden marjoram
1 part nettle
1 part meadowsweet
½ part feverfew
Boiling water

Using 2 teaspoonfuls of fresh herb per cup of water, and 1 teaspoon if you are using dried herbs, place the herbs in a teapot. Pour on boiling water and leave to infuse for 10–15 minutes. Drink one cupful three times daily before meals.

A stronger tisane left to infuse for 30 minutes or more can be poured into a bowl and used as a warm foot bath at night.

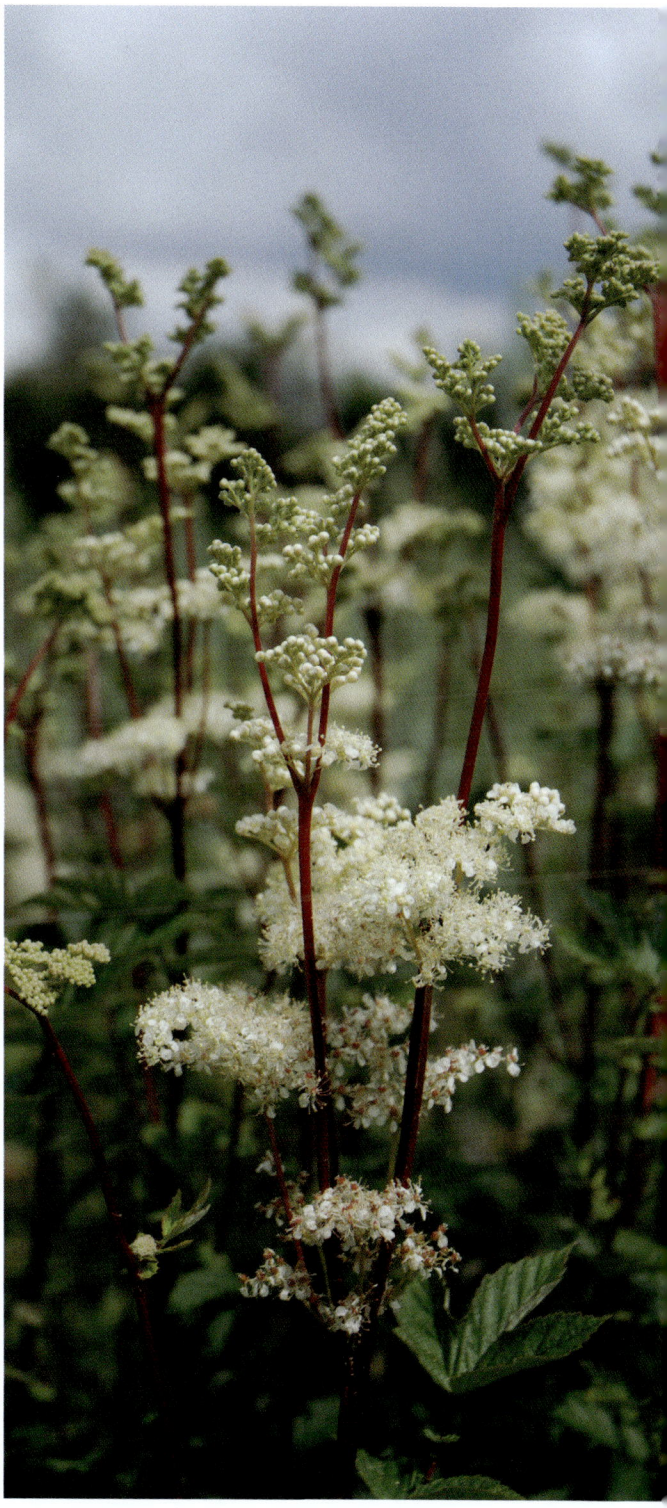

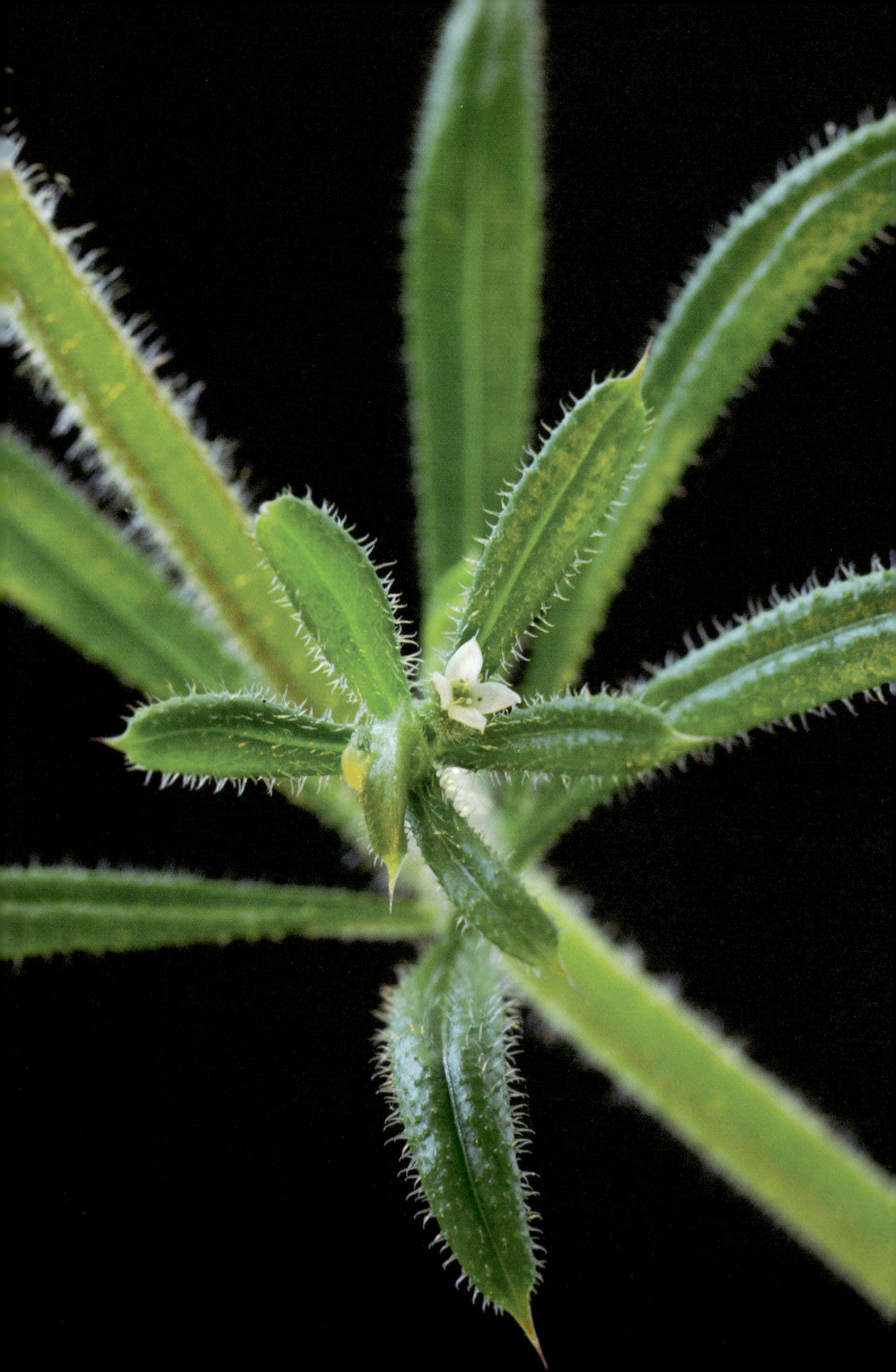

Galium aparine: Cleavers

The Flower of Spring Cleansing

*I am amazed at this spring, this conflagration
Of green fires lit on the soil of the earth, this blaze
Of growing, and sparks that puff in wild gyration*

– DH Lawrence (1885–1930)

Other Names: Goosegrass, clivers, sticky willy, milk sweet, common bedstraw, sticky weed, catchweed, everlasting friendship, grip grass, loveman, sweethearts, bedstraw, stickbud, Robin-run-the-hedge, sticky willow, sticky Jack, grip grass, coachweed

Parts Used: Aerial parts

A familiar hedgerow plant found all over Ukraine, Europe, North America and certain parts of Asia, cleavers is recognised by its long sticky stems (that grow from two to nine feet long) and seeds which stick to anything they touch. It is a crawling or climbing member of the Rubiaceae family and up its stem and along its leaves are tiny curved bristles that cling onto and climb up nearby plants and structures. Its species name *aparine* comes from the Greek word meaning to seize and this is reflected in many of its common names too. Since time immemorial, children have delighted in sticking its stems onto the clothing of unsuspecting friends or family. It is a member of the bedstraw family, so-called for their strewing values in less hygienic times, and many of the plants in this family give off an aroma of new mown hay or honey. Cleavers bears tiny white or greenish-white flowers between May and September.

The genus name *Galium* is derived from 'gala' the Greek word for milk. According to the ancient Greek physician Dioscorides, shepherds used the stems to make a rough sieve to strain milk and apparently this practice still goes on in Sweden. Plants in the *Galium* family also contain enzymes which curdle milk and so they have been used as vegetable rennet; one of cleavers' common names *milk sweet* refers to this. According to Gerard (quoting from Matthiolus),

...the people of Thuscane do use it to turne their milks and the cheese, which they make of sheepes and goates milke, might be the sweeter and more pleasant to taste. The people in Cheshire especially about Nantwich, where the best cheese is made, do use it in their rennet, esteeming greatly of that cheese above other made without it.

Cleavers was an old wives' remedy for losing weight and most commonly taken as a soup. In fact, Culpeper said, "*It is familiarly taken in broth to keep them lean and lank that are apt to grow fat*". Gerard valued it as a cure for bites of spiders and snakes. A cooling drink of cleavers was traditionally taken each spring to '*clear the blood*' and it has been eaten as a spring vegetable for similar cleansing purposes. Culpeper also recommended the herb for earache. According to Thornton's *New Family Herbal* (1810):

Dioscorides mentions an ointment of great efficacy made from the expressed juice of this plant mixed with hog's lard for discussing tumours in the breast; and Gaspian, an Italian, adopted the same with great success. After some eminent surgeons have failed, I have ordered the expressed juice mixed with linseed meal, to be applied to the breast, with a teaspoon of the same to be taken while fasting in the morning; and this plan after a short time has removed very frightful and indolent tumours of the breast.

It is supposed to be useful in scurvy and for haemorrhages of the nose and spitting of blood. Boerhavve says its leaves made into teas are an excellent remedy in epilepsy and gout.

Herbal Remedy
This common weed is a wonderful spring-cleansing remedy. It clears toxins through several pathways at the same time: by supporting the lymphatic system, through its diuretic effect and by its mild laxative action. It contains tannins, citric acid, flavonoids, iridoid glycosides (including asperuloside and aucubin), polyphenolic acids, alkanes, alklaoids, triterpenoids, sesquiterpenes, stigmasterol, sitosterol and carotenoids. It is used to support the work of the immune system, as an anti-inflammatory and detoxifying remedy, as well as for improving the functioning of the lymphatic and blood circulatory systems.

Cleavers has the ability to activate and normalise impaired functioning of the immune system by its impact on lymphocytes and other white blood cells called macrophages. It supports the lymphatic system in its cleansing and immune work and detoxifying the blood and is a popular remedy for treating swollen lymph glands, lymphatic congestion and swollen breasts, glandular fever, post-viral fatigue and tonsillitis. It has antimicrobial, antioxidant and anti-cancer actions and has potential in the treatment of cancers of the skin, the lymphatic system and breasts. The juice of the fresh herb may be the best way to take the remedy in this instance. In tincture form it is active against bacteria including *Staphylococcus aureus, Pseudomonas aeruginosa* and *Bacillus subtilis* and has antifungal activity against *Candida albicans*.

When taken in hot infusion, cleavers has a diaphoretic action, bringing blood to the surface of the body and causing sweating. This is useful in bringing down fevers and clearing toxins via the skin. Its diaphoretic action is also useful to bring out the rash in childhood eruptive infections like measles and chicken pox, speeding the infection on its way.

When taken in a luke warm to cool infusion, cleavers has an affinity with the urinary system. Its diuretic action aids the elimination of excess fluid, toxins and wastes via the kidneys and urinary tract. It can be used for disorders including kidney gravel and stones, urinary infections, cystitis and irritable bladder, prostate problems and fluid retention. It helps to lower blood pressure through diuresis and may be useful for losing weight. Asperuloside, one of the constituents of cleavers, may also have a hypotensive action, helping to lower blood pressure.

Its diuretic properties augment the functioning of the lymphatic system in its detoxifying work and this is helpful in the treatment of chronic and acute inflammatory skin problems like psoriasis, acne, rosacea, eczema, abscesses and boils, as well as gout and arthritis. It is easy to understand why it was used traditionally as a cleansing 'spring tonic' to cool heat and clear toxins.

The slightly bitter taste in cleavers is provided by constituents including the iridoid glycosides and sesquiterpenes which promote liver function, stimulating the flow of bile from the liver and improving digestion, especially of fats. It has a gentle laxative action. The antioxidants including the flavonoids and polyphenols have a hepatoprotective effect, protecting the liver from damage caused by infections, toxins, drugs and alcohol. It may be helpful in hepatitis.

Externally you can use an infusion of cleavers to bathe scalds and burns, cuts and abrasions, as a hair rinse for dandruff or seborrhoea and as an astringent facial wash to tighten the skin and lessen wrinkles. The fresh leaves rubbed together between your fingers can be applied to cuts or wounds, nettle stings, sores and skin inflammations, to check bleeding and speed healing. The juice or an infusion can be used to bathe varicose ulcers, or the fresh leaves can be made into a poultice. It will soothe and cool burns, sunburn, inflammatory skin problems such as eczema, psoriasis and acne and help clear the skin of blemishes.

Homeopathic Remedy
The indications for the use of cleavers as a homeopathic remedy are very similar to those

of the herbal remedy. It is used for problems of the urinary system, as a diuretic for fluid retention, stones and gravel, cystitis and pain on urination. It has been used for cancerous ulcers and tumours of the tongue and for chronic skin problems including ulcers and scurvy.

Flower Essence
Cleavers is a plant that attaches itself to passers-by and as a flower essence, the theme is attachment and bonding. It helps people to form healthy attachments, babies to parents and children to care-givers, and those in other intimate relationships with each other.

When relationships are put under stress by life circumstances and loved ones are separated from each other, it helps to maintain a loving connection, and prevent feelings of alienation or becoming shut down. It helps us to hold on to our relationships in a healthy way and keep ourselves open, so that we can give and recieve the support that relationships provide. We can cleave to each other in our, sometimes rocky, journeys through life.

The flower essence can also be helpful if you feel overwhelmed by attachment and feel the need for more distance from people or circumstances you experience as negative.

Edible Uses
The tops of the young shoots can be added raw to salads or cooked as a vegetable, added to soups, stews, etc. The dried seeds used to be roasted and ground to make a substitute for coffee and the leaves were used to curdle milk as rennet does. Apparently geese also enjoy eating it, hence one of its other common names, 'goosegrass'.

Growing
The wild seed will easily propagate itself in cultivated land and waste places like roadsides.

Recipes

Spring Tonic
Pick equal amounts of cleavers, dandelion leaves, nettle tops and burdock leaves, wash them and pack tightly in a Kilner jar. Pour over enough vodka or brandy to cover. Leave for 4 weeks, shaking occasionally. Squeeze the mixture through muslin, then bottle in dark glass. Label clearly. Take 1 teaspoon 1–3 times a day.

Cleavers Juice
Wash the fresh herb well and put it in a blender or food processor with enough water to make a pulp and then strain it before drinking. Adding fresh mint or lemon balm may make it more palatable.

Otherwise the seed can be sown in autumn or spring directly into most soils in sun or shade, although it prefers damp rich soil and partial shade. It grows vigorously up to 9' (3m) high and flowers through the summer. It is best harvested in late spring just before flowering. It is a food source for several species of butterflies.

Related plants
G. verum: lady's bedstraw, a sweet-scented plant with yellow flowers used to curdle milk and colour cheese.
G. odoratum /Asperula odorata: sweet woodruff, a pretty low-growing plant used to scent linen and keep moths and fleas away, as well as stimulate milk flow in nursing mothers.

Cautions
The hooked bristles of the fresh plant may irritate the skin in susceptible people. Avoid taking with diuretic medicines, including loop diuretics, Spironolactone, Thiazide diuretics, and Triamterene.

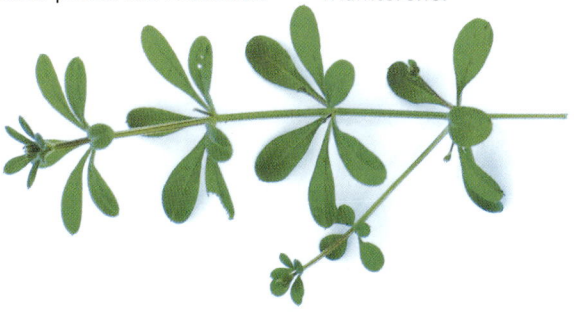

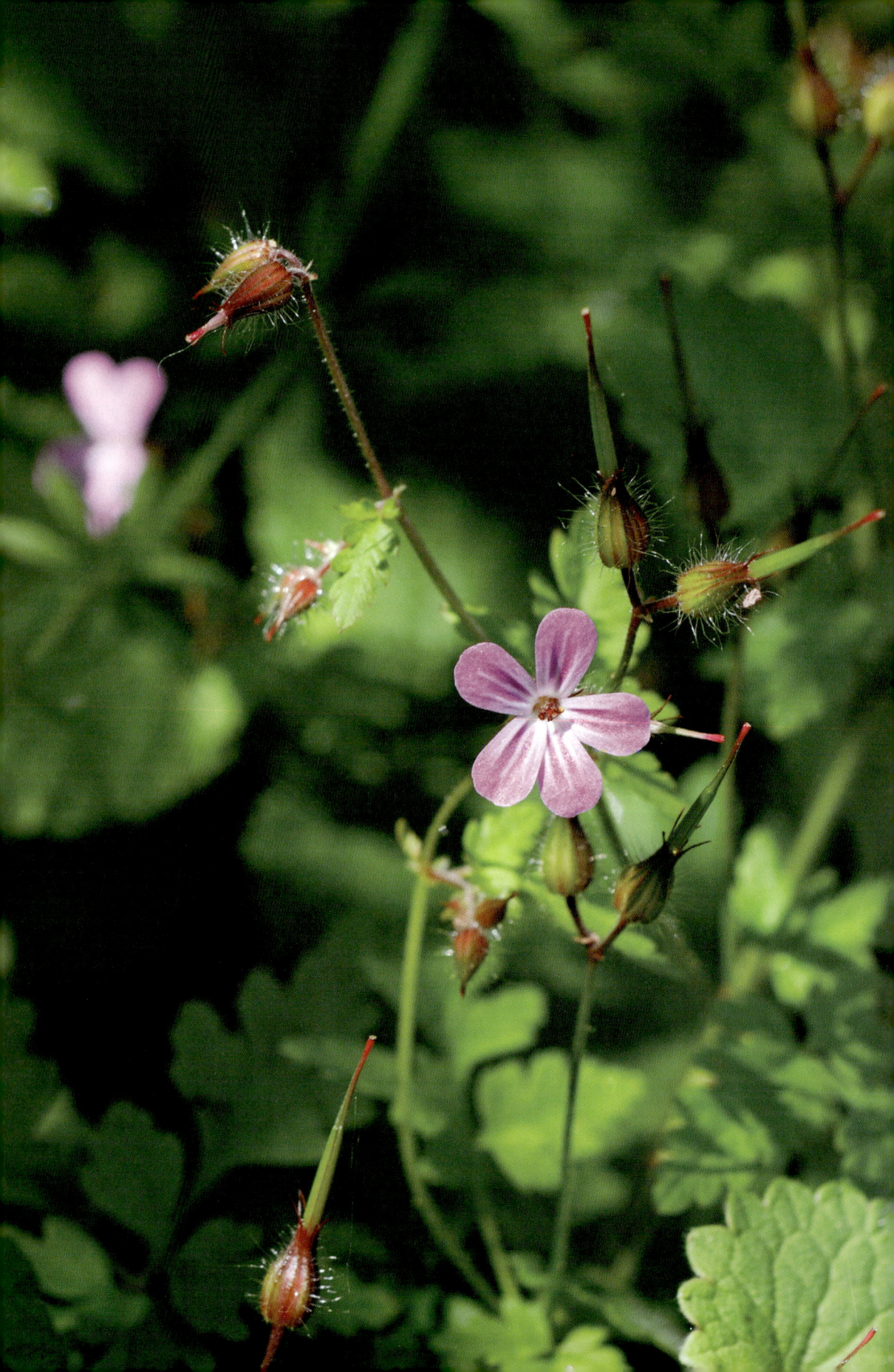

Geranium robertianum: Herb Robert

The Flower of Constancy

...how gay
with his red stalks upon this summer's day!
And, as his tufts of leaves he spreads, content
with a hard bed and scanty nourishment
mixed with the green, some shine not lacking power
To rival summer's brightest scarlet flower
 – William Wordsworth (1770–1850)

Other names: Red robin, cranesbill, death come quickly, storksbill, fox geranium, stinking cranesbill, stinky Bob, squinter pip, crow's foot, Robert's geranium, kiss me love at the garden gate

Parts used: Leaves, stems and flowers

There are many different varieties of wild geranium. In England and Europe, the best-known is the pretty annual or biennial herb Robert, which can be found growing in spring and summer in shaded or partly shaded habitats, such as woodlands, waste lands, woods and even in cracks in walls and steps. A relative of herb Robert called American cranesbill, is an attractive hardy perennial with rose-purple flowers and mottled leaves, found growing wild in woodlands throughout North America. Herb Robert has distinctive red stems, feathery bright green foliage and pretty pink flowers and is also known as 'stinking cranesbill' and 'stinky Bob' because of its strong smell that some say resembles the smell of coriander leaf. The name 'cranesbill' was inspired by the beak-shaped seeds of the plant, which look like the bill of a crane. It also comes from the Greek word 'geranos' meaning crane. It can be gathered between May and October.

Herb Robert could have been named after a Frenchman, the abbot of Molesme in the Burgundian valley of Langres in France, who founded the Cistercian order in the 11th century. Robert had a reputation as a saintly man and a herbalist. Under Robert's instruction, the abbey at Molesme followed the monastic rules of Saint Benedict and became known for its piety and sanctity; perhaps this is why in the language of flowers, geranium means steadfast piety.

It could also have been named after Robin Goodfellow, another name for Puck, the mischievous sprite and jester in Shakespeare's *A Midsummer Night's Dream* as Robin is a shortened version of Robert. Alternatively, it could be named after Robert Goodfellow, an alias used by the legendary bandit Robin Hood. One of its common names 'death come quickly' came from the old belief that if it was picked and taken into the home, a death would soon follow and another name 'crow's foot' is thought to come from the fact that a crow's foot was a symbol of approaching death. If herb Robert was found in the house, it was interpreted as curse from the naughty fairy Puck, Robin Goodfellow. The name 'fox geranium' comes from 'fox' as a corruption of 'folks' referring to 'fairy folk' and specifically to Puck. He needed to be called by the name Robin Goodfellow because in those days you had to be careful about calling a fairy by his or her name, otherwise they could think you are talking badly of them and get angry.

In Medieval times, geranium was used as a protective herb to bring good luck and ward off evil influences and ill-health. According to Culpeper, it was under the dominion of Venus and a symbol of love and the desire to please. The flowers were used in love potions, and also in cordials to lift the spirits and comfort the heart. In the language of love, it means constancy and availability, while to dream of geraniums was taken to mean a change of interests.

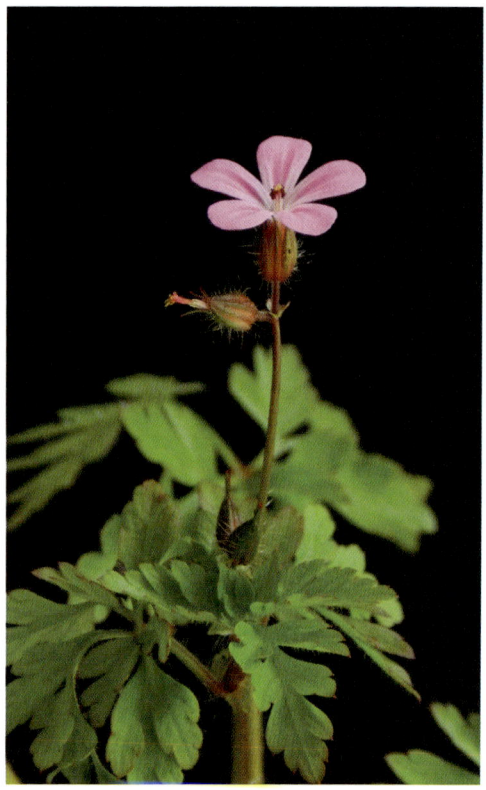

Medicinally, as a herb of Venus, herb Robert was used for promoting fertility, as Venus rules not only love but also the kidneys and the reproductive system. Its names 'cranesbill' and 'storksbill' may come from the fact that the seed heads look like a beak, and this could relate to the myth of babies being delivered by storks. Culpeper recommended it for kidney stones and bleeding. He said, "*It is an esteemed excellent remedy for the stone, and will stay blood, from whatever cause it happens to flow; it speedily heals all green wounds and is effectual in curing old ulcers in the privities and other parts.*" It was also used traditionally in Europe for treating infections, conjunctivitis, jaundice, nosebleeds, gout and dysentery, as a folk remedy for cancer and orally to relieve toothache.

Herbal Remedy

Until recently herb Robert was rarely mentioned in the world of plant medicine. Its North American relative *Geranium maculatum*, with its more powerful astringent action, was popular and herb Robert was largely forgotten. However, it is worth exploring this undervalued plant as it is probably growing right on your doorstep!

The most important constituents of herb Robert are tannins, flavonoids and phenolic acids, giving the whole plant including the root its astringent, antioxidant, antimicrobial, anti-allergic, anti-inflammatory, haemostatic, antidiabetic, diuretic and anti-cancer actions. It also contains carotenoids, vitamins B and C, calcium, potassium, magnesium, iron, germanium and phosphorus. The mineral germanium improves oxygen transport to cells and may support the fight against cancer as a preventative as well as for recovery, supporting its ancient use as a remedy for cancer.

One of the main reasons for herb Robert's health benefits is its antioxidant abilities to scavenge free radicals from the body. The antioxidant properties of plants are closely related to the presence of phenolic compounds and these are better extracted by an alcohol tincture than an infusion. One of the free radicals which can be effectively reduced by extracts is called hydroxyl radical OH, which has been linked to diseases such as cancer, neurological disorders and the build up of cholesterol and plaque in the arteries, atherosclerosis.

The antioxidant actions are linked to herb Robert's ability to reduce inflammation. It can be used in a range of different inflammatory problems including arthritis, inflammation of the liver or gallbladder, headaches, sinusitis, skin problems such as acne and boils, and allergies such as urticaria, eczema and hay fever.

Herb Robert is a good astringent herb due to its high percentage of tannins. This makes it useful for diarrhoea and dysentery, any kind of internal bleeding including heavy periods. It helps to tighten flaccid muscles and makes a good remedy for problems such as stress incontinence and prolapse. Its astringency will also dry up excess secretions, as in catarrh and vaginal discharge.

The essential oils present in the whole plant have antimicrobial properties and are active against a range of bacteria including *Staphylococcus epidermidis* and *Saccharomyces cerevisiae*. The essential oils from the root may well have higher antibacterial and antifungal activity than those from the aerial parts and are effective against *Escherichia coli* and *Aspergillus fumigatus*.

When we take herb Robert, its ellagitannins are metabolisesd by the gut flora into compounds called urolithins, and these have the ability to reduce inflammation. In general, ellagitannins and their metabolites such as urolithins are not absorbed very well, but herb Robert can increase their bioavailability. Urolithins particularly benefit the gallbladder, the urinary and reproductive systems, making herb Robert a useful remedy for liver and gallbladder problems including gallstones. With its affinity with the urinary system and its diuretic action, herb Robert can be helpful for treating urinary problems including fluid retention, kidney stones, gravel and cystitis and aids the elimination of toxins from the body via the urinary system. The aerial parts can also help to lower blood pressure.

Herb Robert is a useful herb for the digestion. It is bitter and cooling and can reduce enzymes such as urease that are involved in *Helicobacter pylori* and the development of gastric ulcers. It may also be of some help in neurological problems such as Alzheimer's disease by inhibiting acetylcholinesterase.

The leaves and flowers of herb Robert are helpful in blood sugar problems and diabetes as they have the ability to lower blood sugar. They can also improve the function of the mitochondria in liver cells, which is particularly useful since mitochondrial impairment is a common feature of several metabolic problems, including diabetes mellitus.

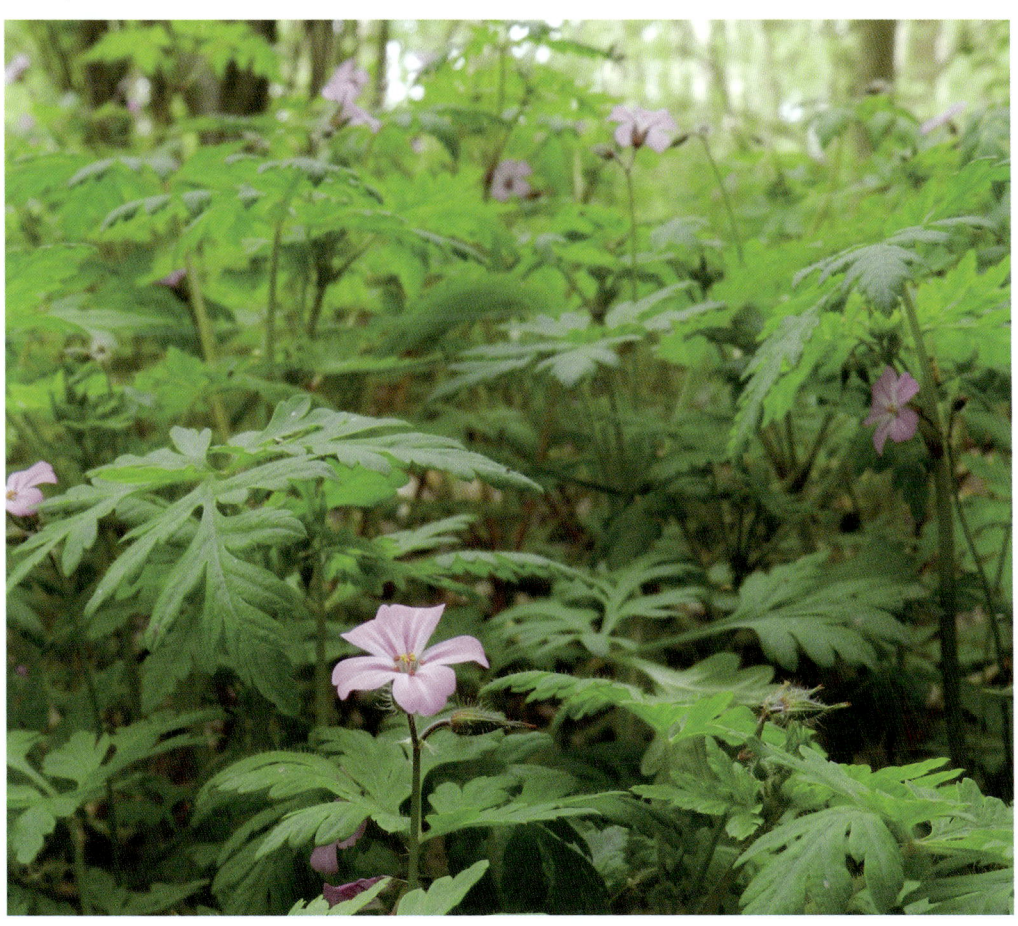

Herb Robert, and specifically its polyphenols, could be helpful in the prevention and treatment of various kinds of cancer. Since the growth of cancer cells increases when blood sugar levels are high, the fact that herb Robert reduces blood sugar is helpful.

The red pigmentation of the stems and then of the leaves as the flowers die down in late summer is attributed to the antioxidant ellagic acid, which can also be found in red fruits such as pomegranates. Ellagic acid may selectively inhibit the growth of breast, prostate, colon and lung cancer cells.

Externally herb Robert makes a good wash for cuts and grazes, sores and ulcers as well as burns, greasy skin and blocked pores that cause pimples. It makes a good mouthwash to combat bacteria associated with the development of tooth decay, *Streptococcus mutans* and *Streptococcus sobrinus*. It can also be used as a wash for the nipples when they are sore and tender (not on the whole breast as this may dry up breast milk). If you rub the leaves on your skin they can act as an insect repellent.

Homeopathic Remedy
Herb Robert is used for anxiety associated with vivid or bad dreams, which is worse after midnight or on waking. Herb Robert types can be self critical, not like company especially of friends, and have repetitive thoughts and difficulty concentrating. They can feel overly busy, restless, stressed, impatient and irritable, sensitive to noise and feel sad and tearful before a period. They can suffer from heat or hot flushes as well as a rapid heart rate, dizziness, head pains that are sharp and pressing, and come on after eating ice cream, washing the hair, or moving the eyes to the left and are better from sleeping.

Herb Robert can also be indicated in nausea, which is worse in the afternoon and evening, after eating or after a bowel movement. It is associated with indigestion, wind, bloating, gurgling, belching, abdominal pain and unquenchable thirst. There can also be constipation or smelly diarrhoea in the morning or that is painful, with burning or stinging and yellow stools.

Herb Robert is useful for people with allergies, with runny nose and eyes, redness and itching, sinus congestion or burning pain inside the nostrils or sinuses. There may be a pressing sensation in both ears, painful breathing that is worse when anxious, or a burning feeling under the sternum and underarm sweat smells of musk. It can also be used for skin problems; greasy skin, acne or pimples on the forehead and nose, or eczema on the cheeks. It can also be indicated for urinary problems, a sore and burning bladder, dryness and itching of the vagina, vaginal discharge, scanty menses or copious menses.

Flower Essence
Herb Robert as a flower remedy is good for people who tend to be hard on themselves and a bit insensitive to others. It can remind us to be kind to ourselves and others, helping us to see things from another's point of view and to be aware that everyone is sensitive even if they don't show it. It is recommended in situations when sensitivity is needed to prevent you from hurting people's feelings with unkind thoughts or words, or being hurt yourself by others. It can also be helpful for shy people who blush easily, those who feel things deeply and get hurt easily. It allows us to accept the fact that we are sensitive and protect ourselves accordingly with firm boundaries, but remain connected to our feelings and aware of those of others.

Edible uses
The fresh and dried leaves and flowers can be eaten in salads and soups or drunk as a tea. The root can be dried and used as a vegetable.

Growing
Sow the seed in a shady area, cover lightly with soil and water regularly. Once established they will reseed themselves easily. Its insect repelling property makes it a good companion plant for vegetables and flowers. Plants seem to grow well next to it. The plant is also said to repel rabbits and deer.

Cautions
It may react with blood thinning medication as it affects blood viscosity.

Glechoma hederacea: Ground Ivy

The Flower of Painters

The smallest flower is a thought, a life answering to some feature of the Great Whole, of whom they have a persistent intuition.
– Honoré Balzac (1799 –1850)

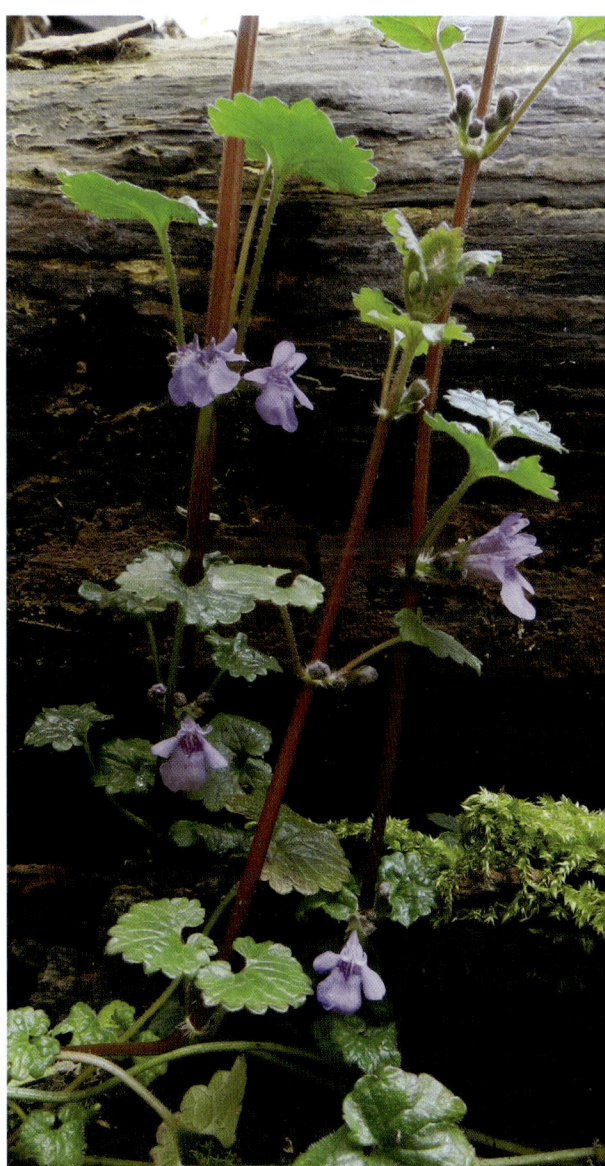

Other names: Gill over the ground, alehoof, creeping Charlie, gillrun, gill go by the hedge, catsfoot, cat's paw, field balm, gill run over, haymaids, hedge maid, wild snakeroot

Parts used: Leaves, stems and flowers

Ground ivy is an appealing little creeping perennial with bright purple-blue flowers. It is a familiar sight in the garden as well as wild damp and shady places, grassland, hedgerows and woods. It is native to Europe and western Asia, and belongs to the Lamiaceae family, which includes mints and herbs such as rosemary, pennyroyal, spearmint, basil, catnip and thyme. It creeps along the ground for 8 to 20 inches (20cm to 50cm) hence its name 'ground ivy' and is a 'plant of the earth' which explains its old Latin name *Hedera terrestris*. It is one of the first wildflowers to appear in spring; it has a tendency to be rather invasive in the garden. The leaves are highly aromatic, with a camphor-like smell with a hint of peppermint and citronella. Its name 'ground ivy' comes from the resemblance of its kidney-shaped leaves to those of the true ivy.

Ground ivy has long been popular as a medicine. During the first century AD Diocorides recommended an infusion for sciatica, and Galen in 2nd century Greece used it for treating inflamed eyes. Later it was used for chronic bronchitis and people sniffed the juice up the nostrils for nervous headaches. It was used for catarrhal deafness and tinnitus, diarrhoea, bile disorders, haemorrhoids and as a general tonic. The 16th century English herbalist Gerard prescribed ground ivy for "*ringing noises of the ears and for those that are hard of hearing*". He also praised it for its ability to cure eye problems, particularly when blended with daisies, greater celandine, sugar and rose water. In fact, he even said, "*It has proved to be the best medicine in the world*".

Ground ivy leaves used to be woven into chaplets for the dead. They were also popular for decorating signs outside taverns, as ground ivy was used in Saxon times for clarifying and flavouring ale, hence its common name 'alehoof'. In 19th century America, physicians used ground ivy for treating coughs, asthma, fever and wind, and it became known among painters that it made a good antidote to lead poisoning or 'painters' colic'.

In the early 20th Century, ground ivy tea was popular in Britain as a cure-all and was used for tuberculosis. Its high vitamin C content made it a popular remedy for scurvy and as a spring tonic.

In British folk medicine, the expressed juice was applied to black eyes and bruises, the dried leaves were used as snuff and the juice sniffed up the nose to relieve headaches. Children were given the tea mixed with nettles for 9 successive days in spring to purify the blood and improve the complexion.

Adding ground ivy to the compost heap is recommended because of its high iron content.

Herbal Remedy

Ground ivy has an affinity with the mucous membranes of the throat, nose, ear, the respiratory and digestive systems, and is excellent for resolving inflammation and congestion, particularly in the upper respiratory system. It contains volatile oils including rosmarinic acid, sesquiterpene lactones, triterpenoids (ursolic acid), polyphenols, sitosterol, saponins, tannins, bitter principle (marrubin), resin, flavonoid glycosides, vitamin C and protein.

With astringent, antiseptic, expectorant and decongestant properties, ground ivy is good for treating respiratory infections and clearing catarrh from the nose, throat, ears and chest. It reduces congestion of the eustachian tubes and ears and may well be helpful in catarrhal deafness and tinnitus as our ancestors recommended. The best way to take ground ivy for throwing off colds, catarrh, congestive headaches, coughs and bronchial congestion is as a hot infusion. It can be given to children to bring down fevers and for respiratory problems including catarrh, glue ear and sinusitis. It can be useful in spasm, congestion and inflammation associated with asthma.

The polyphenols and flavonoids in ground ivy are important because they have an antioxidant action, protecting the body from free radical damage and preventing or remedying inflammation. The anti-inflammatory properties of ground ivy can help to relieve pain and swelling and may prove useful in the treatment of some cancers. Rosmarinic acid is one of the polyphenols found in ground ivy and other members of the *Lamiaceae* family. It has an anti-inflammatory, antioxidant and anticancer actions as well as neuroprotective properties, helping to protect neurons against oxygen-glucose deprivation and prevent degeneration of the brain and memory loss.

Ground ivy can help to regulate NF-κB (Nuclear Factor-KappaB) which is a protein complex involved in inflammatory responses and cellular responses to stimuli such as stress, cytokines, free radicals, ultraviolet irradiation, cholesterol and bacterial or viral antigens. It plays a key role in regulating our immune response to infection and tumour development. Incorrect regulation of NF-κB has been linked to cancer, inflammatory and autoimmune diseases, septic shock, viral infection and improper immune development as well as neuroplasticity and memory.

Sesquiterpene lactones from ground ivy have cytotoxic effects on human cancer cell lines particularly in the breast, colon and the prostate and may be helpful in the prevention and treatment of these cancers. It has a depurative effect, cleansing the blood of toxins. Taken in infusion, (one litre a day for 10 consecutive days) ground ivy is used to cleanse the blood of toxic heavy metals such as cadmium, copper and lead, perhaps due to its diuretic and cleansing properties.

Aromatic, slightly bitter and astringent, ground ivy makes a pleasant tasting digestive remedy. It enhances appetite, digestion and absorption of nutrients. It protects the lining of the gut from irritation and inflammation and can be used for treating acid indigestion, wind, bloating, nausea and diarrhoea as well as gastritis and peptic ulcers. It is particularly useful in prescriptions aiming to both support digestion and heal the lining of the digestive tract. It was traditionally used for expelling worms.

An antiseptic diuretic, ground ivy helps reduce fluid retention and clear toxins from the system. Taken in an infusion, lukewarm to cool, frequently through the day, it makes a good remedy for cystitis, urinary frequency and urinary tract infections. It could be helpful for preventing stones and gravel as it was used for this in the past. It makes a good nerve tonic for easing anxiety and low spirits, and for stress-related conditions.

Externally an infusion or dilute tincture can be used as an antiseptic and anti-inflammatory gargle for sore throats, a mouthwash for inflamed or receding gums, a lotion to bathe inflamed eyes and skin, and a compress to speed healing of bruises, sprains, strain, cuts and abrasions.

Ground ivy has a depigmenting effect which is related to its ability to inhibit the secretion of pro-inflammatory cytokines and melanogenic factors from skin cells. This can be useful in certain skin problems involving pigmentation

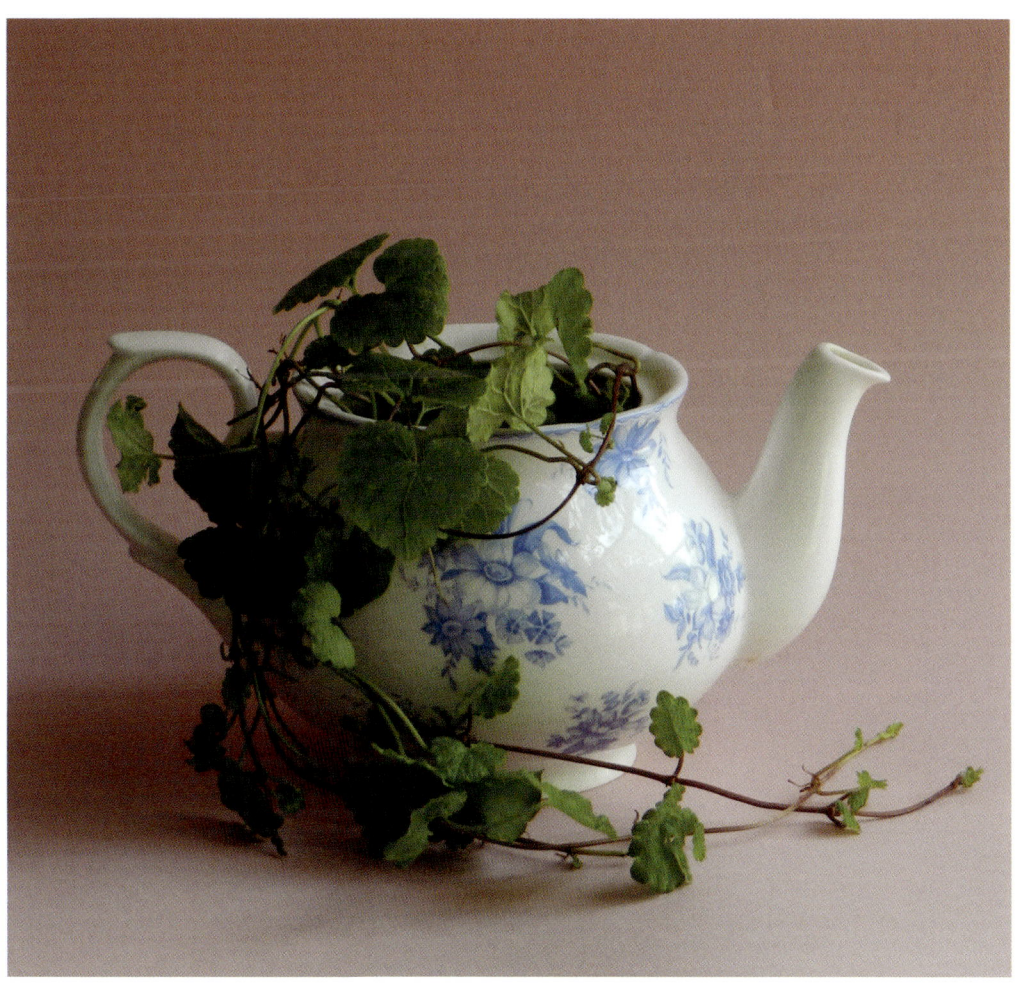

including melasma and excessive pigmentation due to sun damage.

Ground ivy can also be applied to vascular problems such as haemorrhoids, varicose veins and spider veins. Dried and ground it can be used as snuff for headaches and sinusitis. It works well as an infused oil (ear drops) for ear infections.

Homeopathic Remedy
Ground ivy is used for haemorrhoids with rectal irritation and bleeding. It is also used for diarrhoea with rawness and soreness of the anus. It is indicated in coughs with laryngeal and tracheal irritation and inflamed lymph glands. It can improve the perception of our own needs and potential. Frequent symptoms are pains in various parts of the body, tiredness, and protracted itchy skin rashes.

Flower Essence
Ground ivy is used to enhance self-awareness, to help you to be more aware and accepting of your emotional and mental patterns. It helps to clear and transform stuck or outmoded emotional traits and mental attitudes and to bring out the best in you, helping you to be more accepting of who you are.

Edible Uses
The leaves and flowers make a pleasant refreshing tisane. They can be added to salads, soups, omelettes, vegetable dishes and sauces, much like using mint. They can also be cooked like spinach. Some old English jam recipes included ground ivy so that is also worth trying.

Recipe

Ground Ivy Oil
For bruises, wounds and muscular pain.
50 grams freshly dried ground ivy
1 litre olive oil

Place the dried plant and olive oil in a blender and blend. Pour into a dark jar and leave to macerate for about a month and then strain it through muslin. Pour into dark bottles and label clearly. Massage the warmed oil onto the affected part when necessary.

Growing
Ground ivy grows happily in rich, fairly moist/clay soil and sun, semi-shade or shade. It makes good ground cover, with stems reaching 4–12inches (10–30cm) long and can even be rather invasive. It has a long flowering period from March to May. It is an excellent bee plant. Propagate by sowing seed in situ in spring or autumn, covering lightly with soil, or by root division in spring or autumn. It can be harvested during spring and summer especially between April and June.

Cautions
The volatile oil contains pulegone which is known to be toxic to the liver and a gastrointestinal irritant in large amounts. Although present in low concentrations, caution is recommended for use during pregnancy, lactation and in combination with other herbs containing pulegone.

Avoid in epilepsy, liver and kidney disease. Avoid if you have a known allergy or hypersensitivity to ground ivy, or other members of the Lamiaceae family. Patients with compromised liver function should use it with caution. Avoid with drugs that are potentially hepatotoxic (eg Tetracycline, Statins, Acetaminophen, Methotrexate, anti-fungals). Use cautiously in patients with impaired kidney function, as the volatile oil may irritate the kidneys. Ground ivy may contain high amounts of vitamin C, which may decrease the effect of warfarin and anticoagulants.

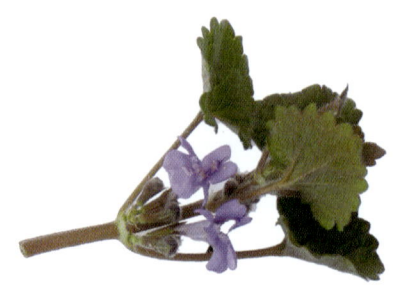

Hibiscus sabdariffa: Hibiscus

The Flower of Fire

Red Hibiscus, I greet your flame,
Hi'iaka, I call your name,
Teach me your sacred song and dance.
My soul full of passion, you enhance
– Hawaiian Poem

Other names: Roselle, omutete, sorrel, saril, flor de Jamaica, Hawaiian hibiscus, rose mallow, Florida cranberry, Guinea sorrel, hibisco, Jamaica sorrel, red sorrel, rosa de Jamaica, rosella, shoeblackplant, tropical hibiscus.

Parts used: Calyces of the flowers

The flamboyant hibiscus flower is widely admired for its extravagantly large and vibrantly coloured flowers that can grow up to 6 inches wide. A beautiful member of the Malvaceae family, hibiscus species are native to tropical and subtropical regions including West and East Africa and South-East Asia and are now found growing in warm places around the world including India, Africa, Sudan, Jamaica, China, Philippines and the United States. The most popular and well-known being *Hibiscus rosa-sinensis* and *Hibiscus sabdariffa*. The latter discussed here is an evergreen shrub which can grow up to eight feet tall and flowers all year round in the tropics, but the blossoms last only a day or two. It is hardy in temperate climates to zone 10, which includes the UK. In temperate zones, the most popular ornamental species is *Hibiscus syriacus*, the common garden hibiscus, also known in some areas as 'the rose of Althea' or 'rose of Sharon'.

With its brightly coloured trumpet shaped flowers, hibiscus is the national flower of Haiti and Hawaii where the flowers are highly revered and associated with Hula, the sacred teaching studied by aspiring sorcerers and healers and the mythological stories of the legendary sisters Pele and Hi'iaka. Hi'iaka was the supreme Goddess of the Hula, daughter of the Earth Mother Goddess Haumea. Hawaiian and Tahitian girls traditionally adorn their hair with hibiscus flowers as the epitome of tropical beauty and these can convey messages; if the flower is worn behind the left ear she is married or has a boyfriend, if worn on the right, she is single and available. The flowers

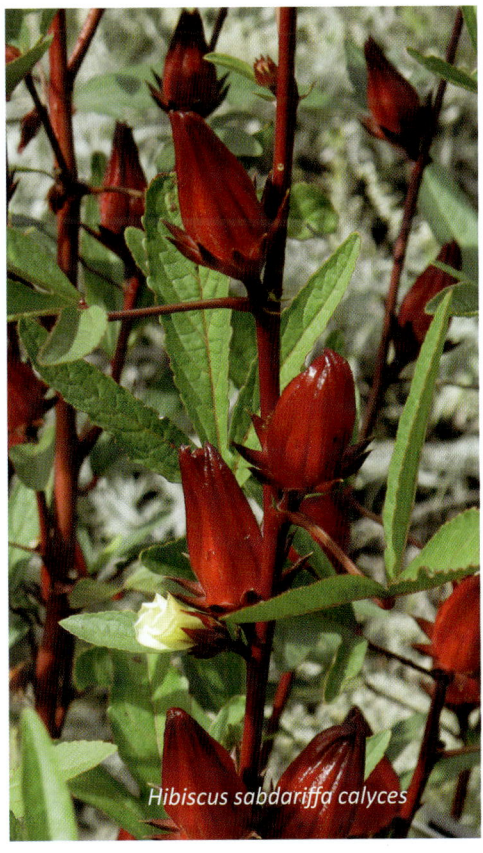
Hibiscus sabdariffa calyces

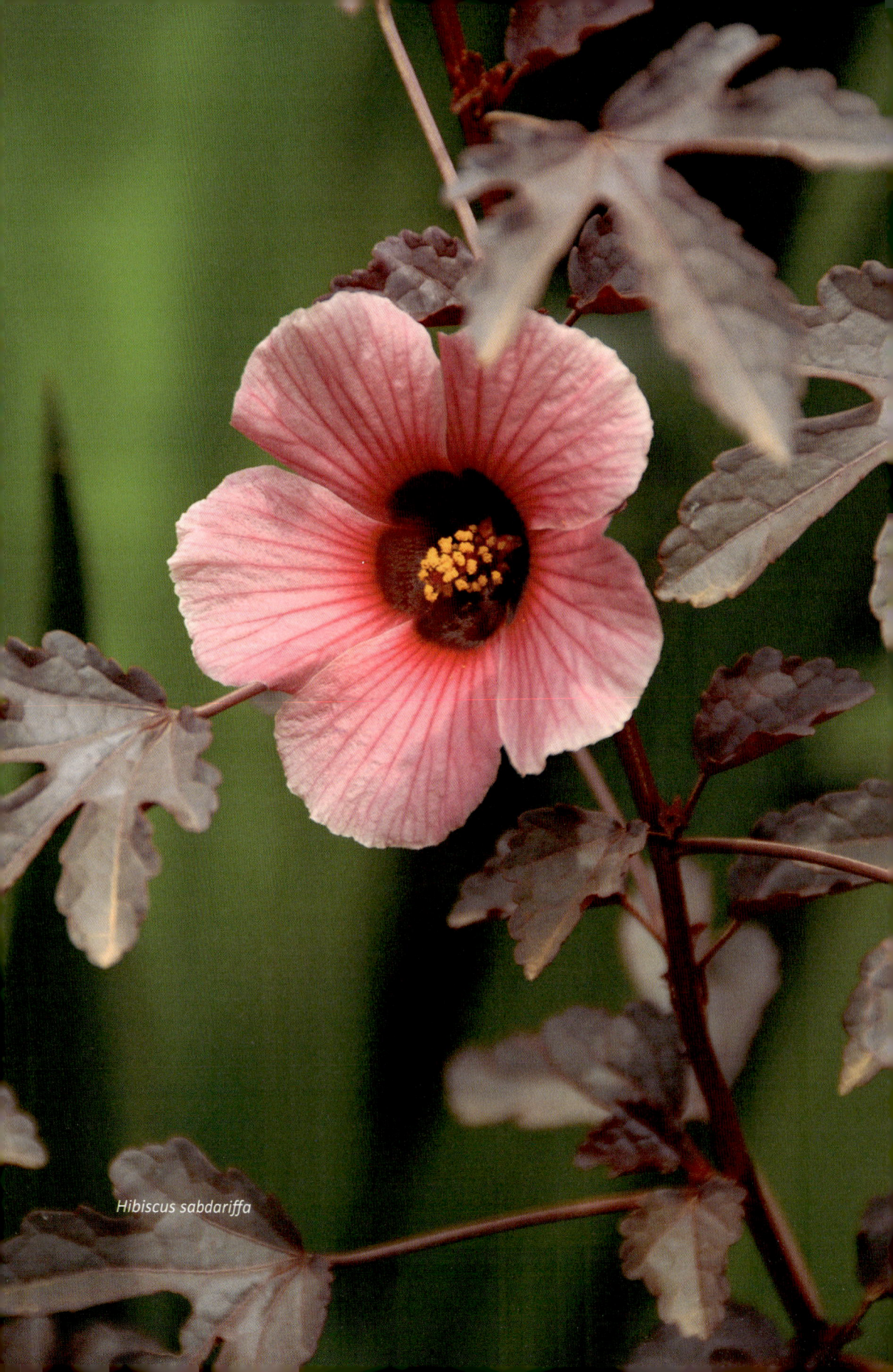
Hibiscus sabdariffa

evoke the exotic and lush vegetation of the tropics and scenes from Gauguin's painting.

Apart from its widely admired showy flowers, hibiscus has large edible calyces. After the petals drop, these deep red calyces (cup-like structures formed by the sepals) remain and grow into seed-containing pods that look like flower buds. Most of the plant's economic value, particularly for making herbal teas, comes from the red calyces, although the leaves, seeds and flowers are also used in traditional medicine in India, Africa, Central America, China and the Caribbean. They are also used as a food, for flavouring and as a source of fibre.

The delicate, short-lived and beautiful hibiscus flowers are considered quintessentially feminine and imbued with symbolic meaning. In North America they are a symbol of the perfect woman and her youth and beauty albeit ephemeral, but the meaning can vary according to the colour. White symbolises beauty, purity and femininity, yellow flowers are associated with good fortune, sunshine and happiness, pink flowers are given in some cultures to young girls to symbolise friendship and platonic love, while red flowers naturally symbolise passion and romantic love. Purple hibiscus flowers are associated with royalty or nobility and also symbolise knowledge and mystery. In China hibiscus symbolises the fleeting nature of fame and personal glory. In South Korea they represent immortality, in Malaysia they are known as the celebration flower and to the Hawaiians the flower symbolises power, respect and hospitality. In the Victorian language of flowers, hibiscus means *delicate beauty* and giving someone a hibiscus flower meant that the giver was expressing appreciation of the delicate beauty of the recipient.

Hibiscus flowers have long been prized for their medicinal and culinary uses. They are believed to have been used for over 6,000 thousand years by various cultures as a cure for a variety of ailments. Ancient Egyptians used hibiscus as a diuretic, as a cooling remedy to help maintain normal body temperature and for treating problems of the heart and nerves. In North Africa hibiscus was applied to the skin to speed healing of wounds and abscesses and used internally to treat coughs, sore throats, respiratory problems, constipation, cancer and liver disease. In Iran hibiscus tea or *sour tea* as it is known there, has long been a popular drink to lower high blood pressure. In other traditions, the tea has been drunk to stimulate the appetite and reduce fevers, to soothe coughs, repair the skin and as a laxative, diuretic, antibacterial remedy. The tea is delicious and refreshing and rich in vitamin C, which explains its sharp tangy flavour and its popular use to fight off cold or flu.

Hibiscus is still widely cultivated for its flowers, fruit and calyces in the tropical and subtropical regions of almost every continent. The tea made from the calyces is known by many names around the world where it can be served both hot and cold. It is known as 'bissap' in West Africa, 'gul e khatmi' in Urdu and Persian and 'orhul' in India. In Jamaica, Trinidad and many other islands in the Caribbean, the drink is known as 'sorrel' and the calyces are used to colour and flavour rum. In Ghana it is known as 'soobolo' in one of the local languages. In Mexico and Jamaica, it is used in a drink called 'Agua de Jamaica' (the flower being 'flor de Jamaica') which is a spicy and sour fruity punch made with hibiscus, ginger, cinnamon or lime. In Cambodia they drink it cold, first steeping petals in hot water until the colours are released from the petals, then adding lime juice (which turns it from dark brown or red to bright red), sweeteners (sugar or honey) and then cold water or ice. In Europe the dried calyces are highly popular as a tasty caffeine-free herbal tea and often used for their calming effects in combination with other herbs such as lemon balm leaf (*Melissa officinalis*) and St. John's wort herb (*Hypericum perforatum*). The stalks are used in making rope in Africa and the seeds are expressed for the oil.

Herbal Remedy
Hibiscus not only looks beautiful but is also a veritable treasure trove of medicinal compounds. All parts of the plant are used. The calyces contain organic acids (mainly citric acid, hibiscus acid, malic acid, tartaric acid and hydroxycitric acid), anthocyanins (also in the leaves, mainly delphinidin-3-*O*-sambubioside and cyanidin-3-*O*-sambubioside), polysaccharides/mucilage, flavonoids and phenolic acids. The seeds contain

high concentrations of ergosterol. Flowers and calyces contain high concentrations of protocatechuic acid, hibiscitrin, caffeic acid and gallocatechin gallate, while the leaves are rich in ellagic acid and catechins. There are also many volatile compounds in the seeds and calyces including aldehydes, alcohols, ketones and terpenes.

Hibiscus has antimicrobial, anti-inflammatory and antioxidant activity, which probably accounts for most of its medicinal actions. Its antioxidant properties have the ability to scavenge free radicals and provide protection against oxidative damage that is implicated in many diseases of modern life including cardiovascular disease, type 2 diabetes, nervous problems, cancer and other degenerative problems associated with the ageing process. It has a protective effect in both the liver and kidneys. It can help prevent fatty degeneration of the liver that can occur with drinking excess alcohol as well as obesity, diabetes and taking certain drugs.

Through its diuretic effect, hibiscus may increase the excretion of uric acid by the kidneys, and help to prevent formation of kidney stones and development of gout. Hibiscus's antioxidant properties may also help to prevent and inhibit the progression of cancer particularly in cancer of the prostate, of the stomach and in leukaemia. It may do this by decreasing cancer cell survival, protecting against potential carcinogens that we encounter and increasing apoptosis, a process by which the body kills off abnormal or unwanted cells.

The traditional uses of hibiscus still persist today and modern herbalists use it successfully to maintain cardiovascular health. The leaves and calyces when taken in teas at least three times a day over a month or more can lower blood pressure and plasma levels of harmful low-density lipoprotein (LDL) cholesterol, triglycerides and total cholesterol. It is thought the antioxidant action of hibiscus, attributed to the anthocyanins, flavonoids and polyphenols, plays a part in this and the fact that hibiscus has the ability to decrease other health problems associated with cardiovascular disease and cerebrovascular disease including type 2 diabetes and metabolic syndrome. Taken regularly hibiscus can help weight loss, which in turn inhibits the development of other diseases related to obesity including diabetes, cancer, hypertension, metabolic syndrome and cardiovascular disease. It can also be given to people with iron deficiency anaemia because the leaves and calyces contain high concentrations of iron and aid absorption of minerals including iron, magnesium and calcium.

Hibiscus is particularly suitable for treating people with metabolic syndrome who have higher than average body fat and abdominal fat, including fatty accumulation in the liver, high levels of triglycerides and low-density lipoproteins (LDLs) and low levels of high-density lipoproteins (HDLs). Hibiscus can not only decrease serum levels of cholesterol, but also reduce body fat including waist circumference and waist-to-hip ratio and decrease fatty degeneration of the liver. The compounds that are thought to affect weight loss and fat metabolism include galloyl ester, chlorogenic acid, caffeic acid, quercetin, tiliroside and anthocyanins.

Hibiscus has been used traditionally as a cooling remedy to assuage the heat of the tropics and to bring down fevers. It also has antimicrobial actions which help to combat infection in the respiratory and digestive systems. It can inhibit the growth of *Salmonella typhimurium* from food poisoning that causes vomiting and diarrhoea and is active against *Staph. aureus*.

Its tannins and flavonoids have an astringent effect in the gut, protecting the gut lining from irritation, infection and inflammation and making hibiscus a useful herb for treating hot inflammatory problems such as acid indigestion, gastritis, colitis and diarrhoea. The leaves, flowers and calyces are rich in mucilage which has a cooling, soothing and protective effect on the linings of the digestive and respiratory tracts. They can be made into soothing remedies for the gut to help regulate peristalsis, reduce spasm, colic, constipation and other stress-related or inflammatory gut problems and can also be helpful in harsh irritating coughs and sore throats. Their beneficial effect on the liver as well as that of the bitter root makes hibiscus helpful for bilious attacks. The seeds also have a laxative effect.

The most common and effective way to use hibiscus medicinally is to drink a tea made from the plant that can include the leaves, flowers and calyces. Infusing it in boiling water for at least ten minutes seems to be the best way to extract its antioxidant phenols and anthocyanins. It can be drunk either hot or cold and is packed full of vitamin C and antioxidants to strengthen the immune system.

Externally both the calyx and seed have antibacterial properties and can be used in mouthwashes to prevent gum infections and cavities. They could also be included in preparations to treat head lice. The leaves and flowers are highly mucilaginous and are used as a soothing emollient for sore, inflamed skin conditions. With their antibacterial action against bacteria including *Staph. aureus* they can be used as infusions or poultices for treating acne, boils, abscesses and other skin conditions.

Aromatherapy Oil
In aromatherapy, hibiscus oil is commonly made into a head massage oil used to support hair growth and repair as it is rich in vitamins and antioxidants. Its antimicrobial actions make it a good addition to skin creams for preventing and treating pimples and acne and it makes an effective and rejuvenating face oil which promotes anti-aging, helps remove scarring from the skin and leaves the skin looking brighter and younger.

Flower Essence
Hibiscus flower essence can provide a spark of passion and creativity within us and help us to feel more inspired. It aids our connection with the heart, helping us to get in touch with our deepest wishes and guiding us on our path in life. It helps us to release pent up tension and suppressed creativity that might be blocking our energy and making us feel stuck or blocked. It gives us the confidence to overcome our inhibitions and fears, to feel rooted and grounded and make positive changes in our lives. It sets us free to dance again as in the Hawaiian tradition of the Hula.

Edible Uses
Hibiscus calyces, leaves and seeds are nutritious, containing vitamins B, C and beta carotene and minerals including calcium and iron. The seeds are rich in fat and protein and also in minerals including potassium, calcium and magnesium. Hibiscus can be used in the traditional way for making herbal teas, fermented drinks and desserts. The bright red calyces are popular for adding colour and flavour to a variety of herbal teas and being rich in citric acid and pectin they are good for making jams, jellies and syrups. They are added to wine and cider and all sorts of cocktails for flavouring and decoration while the tender leaves and stalks are eaten in salads or used as curry seasoning.

The green leaves and shoots can be eaten raw or dried. The calyces can be used to colour and flavour yogurts, ice-creams and syrups and can also be candied and used as a brightly coloured garnish for desserts. A delicious red syrup can be drizzled over fruit or used in a salad vinaigrette, it can be swirled onto ice cream or yogurt and it can be stirred into cocktails on special occasions! The seeds are used to make vegetable oil in China and can be dried and ground into meal or roasted and eaten or used as a coffee substitute. Hibiscus root is edible and used as an aperitif and tonic in the Philippines. The fibrous part of the plant stem is used in the production of twine and cord known as *rosella hemp*.

Growing
Hibiscus will grow happily outside in tropical areas. In temperate climates you need to start the seeds indoors, away from frost and plant outdoors in spring once all danger of frosts has passed. Keep them well watered and once the flowers have bloomed and gone over you will be able to harvest the red calyces. If you pick them regularly, they will keep coming. Keep indoors away from frost in the winter to be safe. The species is hermaphrodite (has both male and female organs) and is pollinated by numerous insects. It will grow in most soil but prefers well drained, moist soils and full sun.

Cautions
Avoid in pregnancy and with diclofenac, chloroquine and acetaminophen.

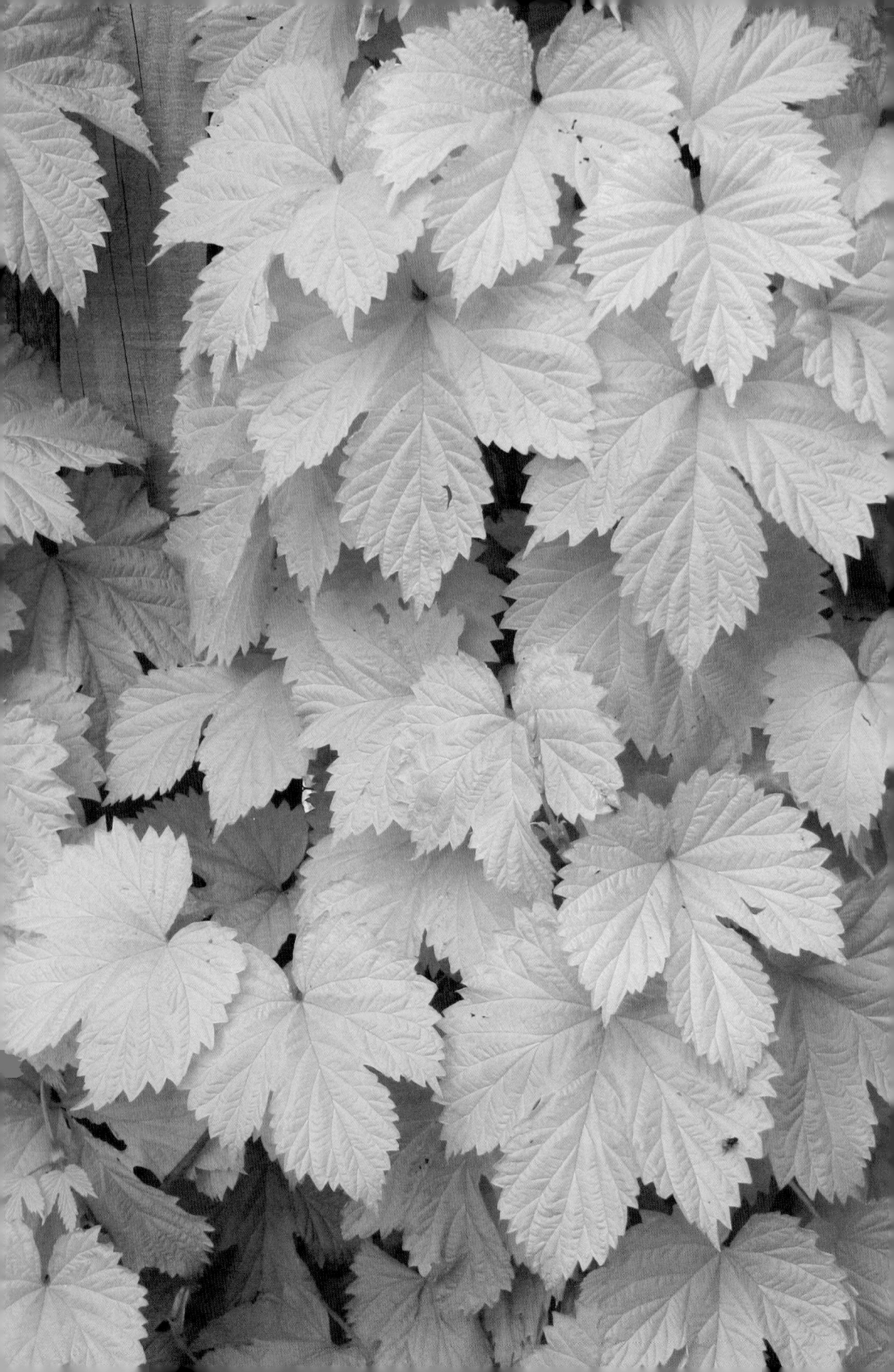

Humulus lupulus: Hops

The Flower of Restful Sleep

I'm getting rather hoarse, I fear,
After so much reciting:
So, if you don't object, my dear,
We'll try a glass of bitter beer –
I think it looks inviting.
– Lewis Carroll (1832–1898)

Other names: Whitebines, bine, bur, seeder, lupulus

Parts Used: Dried strobiles (female flowers)

Hops are trailing plants belonging to the Cannabaceae family that grow wild all over Europe, Central Asia, North America and Australia. They wind clockwise around tree trunks or other supports, clinging to them with tiny barbs. The Romans believed, wrongly, that in this way they sucked life out of the supporting trees, and they called hops '*lupulus*' meaning little wolf. The name *Humulus* probably derives from the fact that hops prefer moist, humus-rich soils. The name hops comes from the Anglo Saxon '*hoppan*' meaning to climb.

Hops are most famous for their relationship to beer. Small yellow glandules on the strobiles of the hops secrete a sticky substance called lupulin which contains several bitter compounds. These help to preserve beer, make it foamy and give it a bitter taste. They were widely used to flavour beer by the 14th century in most parts of Europe, but only used in English breweries since 1524. King Henry VIII of England had forbidden their use as he said they caused melancholy.

The Jewish captives in Babylon drank barley beer with hops to protect them from leprosy. Pliny says that the Romans grew hops in their gardens and ate the young shoots as a vegetable. Hops have been smoked for their narcotic properties and used in sleep pillows to relieve insomnia. They have been a favourite herb of gypsies who use them to relieve uncontrolled sexual desires and quarrelsome natures.

In Medieval monasteries the use of hops to flavour beer was preferred to other traditional beer spices as their calming effects on sexual arousal were an obvious advantage to the monks. Hops were also used medicinally (not by the monks!) to ease the symptoms of sexually transmitted diseases such as gonorrhoea.

For centuries, hops have been valued as a medicine mainly for their sedative effects. *"The manifold virtues of hops do manifest argue the wholesomeness of beere above ale; for the hops rather make it a physicall drinke to keep the body in health, than an ordinary drinke for the quenching of our thirst"* – Gerard's Herball 1636. Culpeper said that hops were ruled by Mars and could be used to cleanse the bloodstream of heat and toxins by stimulating the liver and kidneys.

Herbal Remedy

More than 1,000 constituents have been identified in hops. The dried flowers of hops, called strobiles, from female plants contain volatile oils including sesquiterpenes, flavonoids, asparagin, oleoresins (humulone, lupulene), valerianic acid, phenolic acids, tannins, oestrogenic chalcone xanthohumol, trimethylamine, choline, alkaloids, phyto-oestrogens, gammalinoleic acids, vitamin B6 and C, oils and bitters known as lupulin.

Hops have a sedative action, which explains the use of hops in sleep pillows to this day. A number of constituents in hops such as valerianic acid and humulene in the volatile oil are sedative. Not only do they relieve insomnia, but they also reduce tension, anxiety, irritability, restlessness and agitation and ease pain. Hops reduce the adverse effect of stress on the body particularly the digestive system and at the same time they stimulate digestion. Their antispasmodic action reduces tension in muscles throughout the body including the gut, making them helpful in stress-related stomach and gut problems including wind and bloating, colic, nervous indigestion and irritable bowel syndrome.

Hops have a combination of bitter and pungent tastes, a perfect combination for good digestion. The bitters in hops enhance the secretion of digestive enzymes and of bile from the liver and aid digestion and absorption. The tannins protect the gut wall from irritation, inflammation and infection and aid healing of irritated and inflammatory stomach and gut conditions including gastritis, peptic ulcers, diverticulitis, Crohn's disease and ulcerative colitis. Hops can be used to curb diarrhoea and other signs of gut infections. *Xanthohumol,* a chalcon derived from hops, inhibits inflammation and fibrosis in the liver.

Hops have a beneficial effect on the immune system and have antiviral and antibacterial activity. One of the oleoresins in hops called humulone, that gives beer its characteristic bitter taste, has been found to be effective against the common cold virus and the respiratory syncytial (RS) virus that can cause pneumonia and breathing difficulties in infants and toddlers. The virus tends to spread in winter and can also cause cold-like symptoms in adults. Humulone also has anti-inflammatory properties and reduces inflammation caused by infection from the virus and may also be helpful in other inflammatory problems including arthritis and skin problems. An infusion of hops can be given to bring down a fever and the antispasmodic and relaxant effects of hops can be helpful in tight chesty coughs and asthma.

Humulone also has an antibacterial action, useful against a number of bacteria including *Staphylococcus, Clostridium* and *Salmonella.*

Hops can also inhibit the growth of methicillin-resistant *Staphylococcus aureus* (MRSA), a major cause of both hospital and community acquired infections. The stimulating effect that hops have on the digestion, enhancing gastric secretions and production of other digestive enzymes as well as supporting a healthy gut flora, can help improve immunity. The relaxing effect of hops and their ability to promote good sleep may also be an important aspect of the immune protection gained from hops, since stress can depress the immune response.

Despite the beer-drinking image of tough masculinity, hops are a good remedy for women. The phyto-oestrogens in the plant make hops helpful during the menopause. The phytoestrogen 8-prenylnaringenin (8-PN) found in hops can reverse the rise in skin temperature in menopausal hot flushes. In addition to the oestrogenic activity, hops also have antioxidant and chemopreventive properties which may inhibit oestrogen-induced cancers in the breast and elsewhere. The bitter acids in hops may inhibit the development of leukaemia.

The depressive effect of hops on men's libido means that beer drinking may not be the best thing for enhancing men's sexual energy, but it has the opposite effect on women. Hops have also been used to enhance milk supply in breast-feeding mothers and for suppressed and painful periods. Painful periods are related to the rise of a hormone-like substance called prostaglandin 2 (PG2) which in turn is affected by stress. Hops make a perfect remedy as they decrease PG2 levels, relax muscles in the uterus and reduce stress.

The asparagin in hops acts as a soothing diuretic, reducing fluid retention and hastening the elimination of toxins from the system via the kidneys. This combined with the action on the liver have given hops a reputation as a detoxifying herb, useful for clearing skin problems such as eczema and acne. Its relaxant and antihistamine actions are also useful here.

Externally, hops are used in creams to keep the skin soft and supple and delay wrinkling. Their antiseptic and anti-inflammatory actions are good for wound healing of cuts, sores and ulcers and can be helpful in inflammatory skin problems such as eczema and acne. Hops can be used for their sedative effect and made into herb pillows with lavender to aid sleep. Infused hop oil can be added to a night-time bath to ease aching tense muscles and promote a restful sleep. Inhalations or baths with hops can help relieve pain such as headaches and arthritis and reduce tension, anxiety, irritability and restlessness.

Homeopathic Remedy
Like the herbal remedy, lupulus as a homeopathic remedy has an affinity with the nervous system, the skin, the digestion and the liver. The theme of the effects of drinking alcohol runs through it. It is a good remedy for "unstrung" conditions of the nervous system, accompanied by nausea, dizziness and headaches after a heavy night's drinking.

It is indicated when feeling overexcited, wakeful and delirious when drunk, twitching muscles, nervous tremors, and when felling giddy or stupefied when drunk or otherwise. It can be used in jaundice in children and for burning symptoms of cystitis. A slow pulse, profuse perspiration, drowsiness in the day, scarlatina type skin eruptions, a sensation of something crawling on the skin, peeling chapped skin, painful erections and spermatorrhoea are other indications for this remedy.

Flower Essence
Hops are vigorous climbing plants and they grow several feet quickly in one season and then die right back again. As a flower remedy they promote new growth on physical and spiritual levels. If you feel the need to grow in wisdom or insight, then hops might be your remedy.

Hops can be useful during times of transition in life when you have to grow into a new phase. They are a good remedy for adolescence when the playful energy of childhood transforms into sexual energy and greater bodily strength. Hops also have a relaxing effect and can ease any tension associated with changes in life and help you to feel grounded and in balanced. The flower essence can also help to ease and improve group interaction.

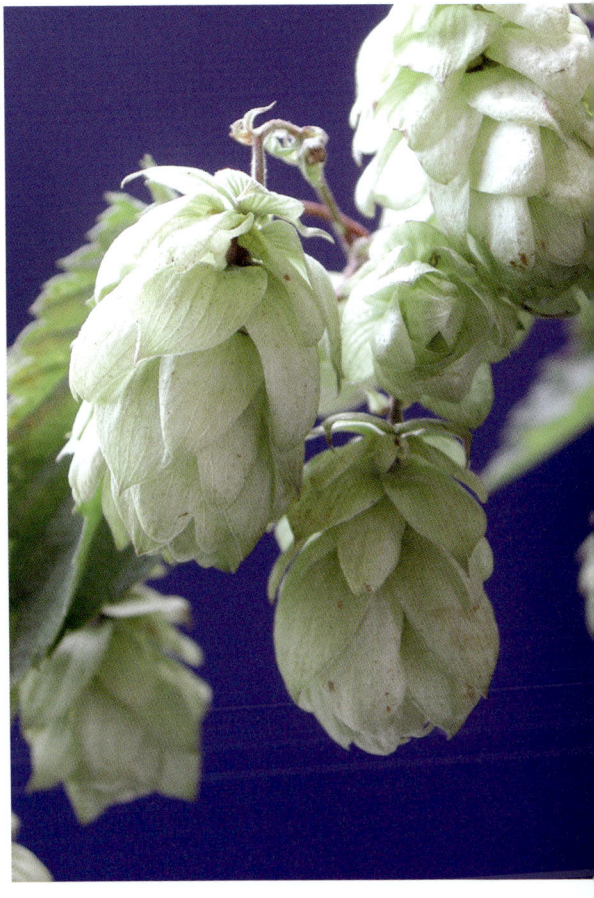

Aromatherapy Oil
Like the herbal remedy hops oil has a rich bitter-sweet aroma and is used to calm the mind and for its relaxing effect on tight or stiff muscles. It helps to calm sexual desire in men, and enhance women's libido, while the oestrogenic effects will be helpful through the menopause. Hops oil can be added to a night-time bath to ease aching tense muscles and promote a restful sleep. Inhalations or baths will help relieve pain and reduce tension, anxiety, irritability and restlessness. Hops oil has antibacterial and antiviral actions and can be used in burners during the cold and flu season to ward off infection. A few drops can be added to bath water, added to massage oils and used for inhalation. It can be thought of in any stress related digestive problem and is good massaged into abdomen for abdominal or period pain. A massage with hops oil should help especially if you are going through the menopause.

Recipes

Hops Tea

A warm cup of hops tea before bed might taste a little bitter but it may save you from counting sheep.

To make a hops tea pour 1 cup (300 mls) of boiling water over 1 teaspoon (5 gm) of dried or fresh hops. Cover and leave to infuse for 10 minutes. Strain and drink.

Hops Sleep Pillow

For a good sleep make a small cotton bag and stuff it full of an equal mixture of freshly dried hops and lavender and put it by your pillow. Change the hops every couple of months as fresh ones work better.

Infused Oil

Make an oil to keep your skin youthful by soaking hops in almond oil for 2 or 3 weeks and then pressing them through a sieve or muslin. Massage the oil into your skin or add some to your bath.

Growing

Propagate by sowing seeds in late summer or autumn in a cold frame to overwinter. Germination can be erratic. Alternatively, grown from summer cuttings or divisions of the plant in spring. Prefers rich moist soil in full sun or light shade. Needs support. Water freely in dry weather. Can reach 6m (20') high and flowers July to August and produces fruit from September to October.

Cautions

Hops are contraindicated in depression and may depress male libido. Fresh hops can cause a skin reaction in some sensitive people. They can cause sedation, bronchial irritation when ground herb dust is inhaled. Caution with CNS depressants (eg. alcohol, opiates, anticholinergics, benzodiazepines, anaesthetics, antihistamines, anxiolytics, tricyclic anti-depressants, anti-epileptics), hormone replacement therapy, oral contraceptives, insulin and oral hypoglycaemics. Avoid in hops allergies or sensitivities. As beer drinkers may know, excessive consumption may cause loss of libido.

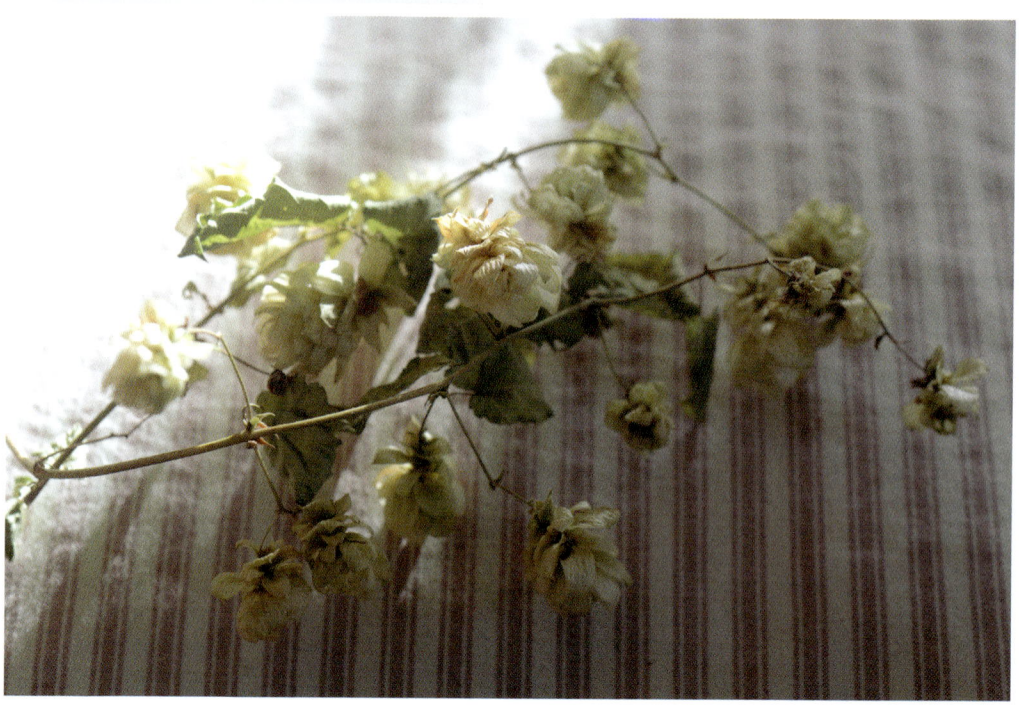

Hypericum perforatum: St John's wort
The Flower of Light

St Johns wort doth charm all the witches away.
If gathered at midnight on the Saints holy day.
And devils and witches have no power to harm
Those that do gather the plant for a charm.
Rub the lintels and post with that red juicy flower
No thunder nor tempest will then have the power.
Old English poem, 14th century

Other Names: Goatweed, klamath weed, tipton's weed, chase devil, sol terrestris, terrestial sun, celestial sun, grace of God, the lord's wonder plant, devil's scourge

Parts Used: Leaves, stems and flowers

St John's wort is a wild plant and a perennial member of the Hypericaceae family found growing in sunny meadows. It has bright yellow flowers that bloom in midsummer on or around St John's day on June 24th and because of this they have long been associated with light, which is reflected in its many ancient names. Culpeper said St John's wort was *"under the celestial sign Leo, and the dominion of the Sun."* Its flowering time made it ideal to celebrate the solstice. It was called 'sol terrestris', 'terrestial sun' and 'celestial sun' as its yellow flowers with golden stamens symbolised the sun, which casts out all evil and dispels the forces of darkness. It is interesting that St John's wort increases sensitivity to sunlight and for that reason makes a good remedy for SAD during the winter.

The name *Hypericum* comes from the Greek words 'huper eikon' meaning 'over an apparition' because of its apparent power to protect against evil spirits. It was also called 'fuga daemoniorum' meaning the devil's scourge, as well as 'grace of God' and 'the lord's wonder plant' and because it was used to keep witches away it was named 'hexenkraut' meaning witches' herb. Mattiolus said, *"certain writers have said that St John's wort is so*

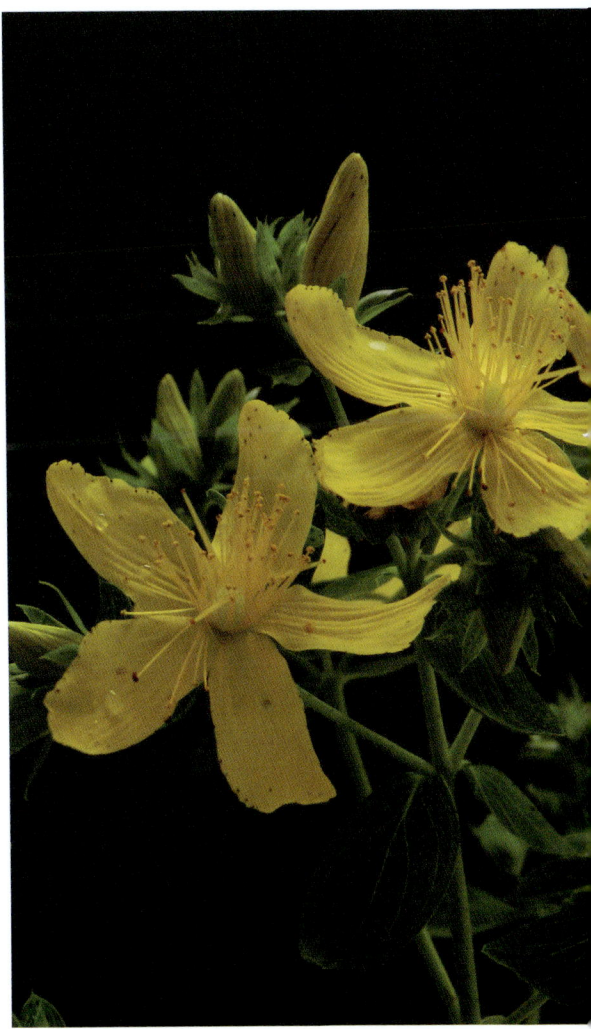

detested by evil spirits that they fly off at a whiff of its odour." In the past it was believed that people who suffered from mental illness, melancholy and epilepsy just had to sniff the juice to drive out their evil spirits. Sprigs of St John's wort were hung at house and church doors on Midsummer's Eve, the pagan summer solstice and the longest day, to protect them from negative influences, thunder, lightning, fire and witches.

It was also believed that if anyone trod on St John's wort flowers after the sun had set, a fairy horse would arise from the earth and carry them around all through the night until the sun rose. St John's Wort had to be collected early while the flowers were still wet with dew, for it was thought to be unsafe to gather them after the sun had risen. In several countries the dew that had fallen on the flowers before daybreak on St John's day was gathered with great care and used to protect the eyes from all harm throughout the coming year. The night of St John was also celebrated by young girls who would hang the plant over their doors or sleep with it under their pillows, to foretell their future husbands as the poem above describes. In the language of flowers, St John's Wort means superstition.

It was also thought in the past that St John's Wort threatened the devil's power so much that he tried to destroy the plant with a needle - hence the tiny perforations in the leaf from which derives the name *perforatum*. With the coming of Christianity, the herb was dedicated to St John the Baptist and Midsummer's Day became St John's day. The red pigment that exudes from the flowers was thought to represent the blood of St John the Baptist. It was also called 'Heart of Jesus oil.'

According to the doctrine of signatures, the red juice from the flowers and the perforations of the leaves indicated that St John's wort was an excellent remedy for healing wounds and stemming bleeding. In fact, the ancient Greeks and Romans, as well as other European warriors including the Crusaders, took St John's Wort to battle with them to staunch bleeding and heal wounds and burns. Apparently, St John's wort was particularly favoured as a wound healing plant by the Knight's Hospitallers who were involved with guarding the Holy Sepulchre at Jerusalem and protecting pilgrims as they travelled to the Holy Land. They also cared for those wounded during the Crusades.

Herbal Remedy
St John's wort contains glycosides (hypericin, pseudohypericin, hyperforin, adhyperforin), flavonoids (hyperosides, quercitrin, isoquercitrin, rutin), catechin tannins, resins and volatile oils. With its bitter taste and cooling effect, St John's wort is a renowned remedy for the nervous system, with a great ability to relax tension, reduce anxiety and lift the spirits. It has been widely acclaimed as an antidepressant and sedative. Its mood-elevating properties take 2–3 months to produce lasting effects and are brought about by enhancing the effect of neurotransmitters in the brain. It is thought it might work by preventing nerve cells in the brain from reabsorbing the chemical messengers including serotonin, dopamine, GABA and norepinephrine. As a result, the neurotransmitters are more effectively used in the brain.

St John's wort is also excellent for treating nervous exhaustion, it increases sensitivity to sunlight and is well worth using in seasonal affective disorder (SAD) during the winter and for jet lag. It improves sleep and concentration and has anticonvulsant actions. It cools hot, fiery emotions like anger, impatience and irritability and is a good remedy for addictive tendencies, nicotine withdrawal as well as feelings of low self-esteem. It has anti-inflammatory and analgesic actions that can be useful in gout and arthritis as well as painful conditions such as frozen shoulder, nerve pain and neuralgia, such as trigeminal neuralgia, sciatica, peripheral neuropathy, back pain, fibrositis, headaches, earache, toothache and shingles. It is useful after surgery and trauma involving laceration of nerve tissue.

The antiviral activity of St John's wort can be helpful in prevention and treatment of viral infections including *Cytomegalovirus, Epstein barr, Hepatitis C, Parainfluenza A* and *B*. It has also shown antibacterial activity against *E. coli, Proteus vulgaris, Pseudomonas aeruginosa, Staphylococcus aureus* and *Streptococcus*

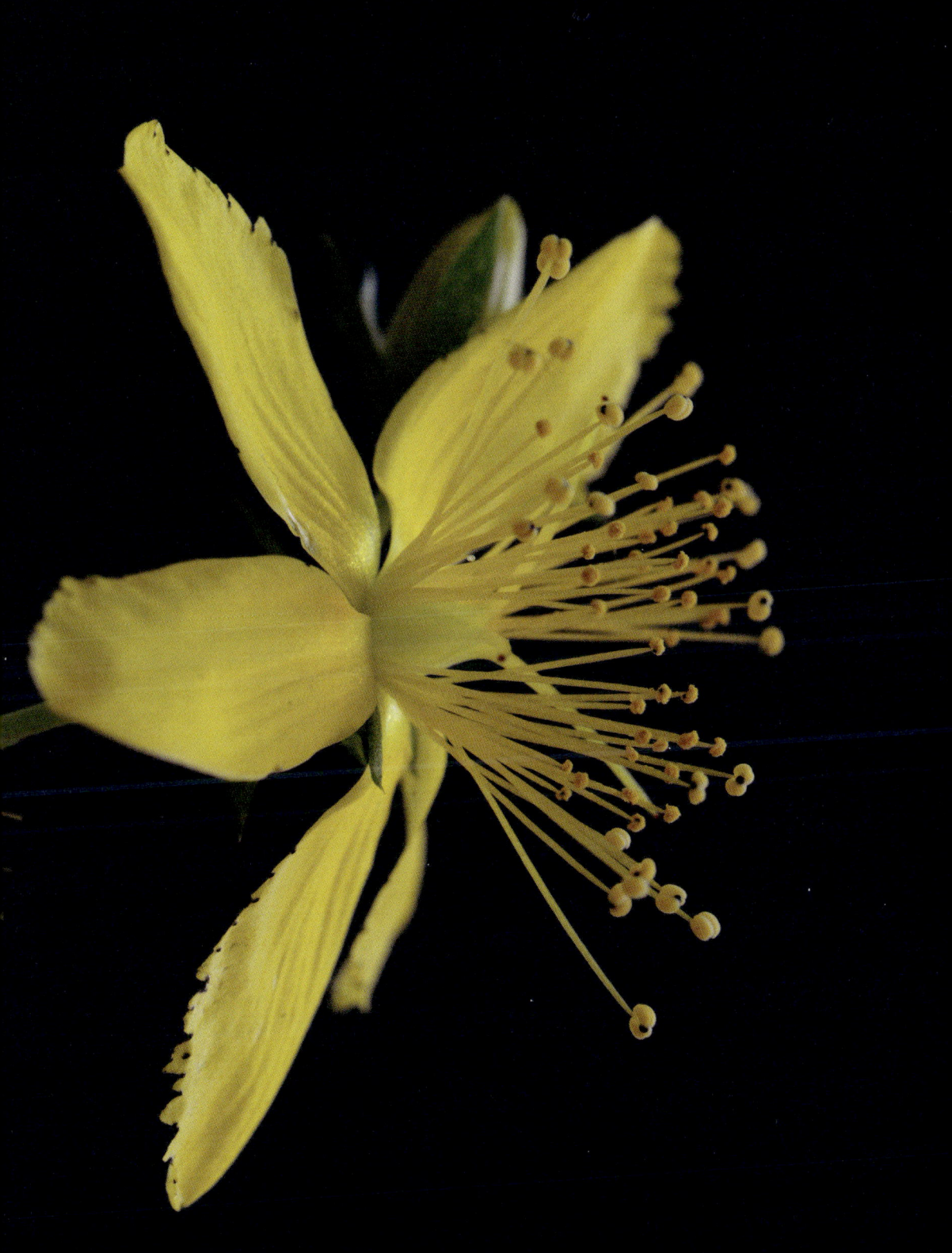

mutans. One of its constituents called hypericin seems to interfere with the reproduction of retroviruses, so it could be helpful for treating HIV and other retroviruses and it has shown potential antitumour activity.

St John's wort can be used to treat ear infections, glandular fever, post viral fatigue and chest infections. Its antibacterial and antiviral action are effective against TB (*Mycobacterium tuberculosis*) and *Influenza A* as well as *Herpes 1* and *2* and *Herpes zoster,* meaning that it is useful for treating cold sores and shingles. Its expectorant action is also helpful in coughs and chest infections. St John's wort may help in the fight against antibiotic resistant superbugs such as MRSA, a type of bacteria that is rapidly becoming resistant to antibiotics.

In the digestive tract St John's wort's anti-inflammatory, astringent and antimicrobial actions contribute to its benefit in treating gastro-enteritis, diarrhoea, dysentery and gut infections, particularly when they are related to stress. It healing properties are helpful in gastritis and peptic ulcers and its hepatoprotective action can help protect the liver from the damaging effect of toxins such as alcohol and drugs.

St John's wort also has a beneficial effect in the urinary system. It has a diuretic action reducing fluid retention and hastening elimination of toxins via the urine. It can be used for soothing burning pain, urinary infections and other urinary problems. It makes a good remedy for bedwetting in children and incontinence through its influence on the nerves and its tonic effect on the urinary system. It is also a useful remedy for gout and arthritis.

St John's wort can be used for a range of menstrual problems, such as painful, heavy and irregular periods, particularly where they are related to stress. It may help the liver to break down hormones. It can be helpful for emotional problems with a hormonal component such as PMS and menopausal mood swings. It is excellent for emotional problems during menopause and reduces blood pressure and capillary fragility causing broken blood vessels.

Externally St John's wort is highly valued for its wonderful healing properties. The infused oil is excellent applied to sites of nerve pain such as sciatica, trigeminal neuralgia, diabetic neuropathy, nerve trauma and damage and shingles to ease pain and speed healing. With its wound healing and antimicrobial effects, it can be used to soothe and heals burns, sunburn, cuts, wounds, sores and to calm inflammatory conditions of the skin. It is also useful for sprains, sprains, joint and muscle pain, arthritis, frozen shoulders, haemorrhoids, varicose veins and ulcers, bruises and sunburn.

Homeopathic Remedy

Hypericum is called the arnica of the nerves; it is used to treat any trauma or injury to areas of the body that are rich in nerve tissue such as the spine, fingers, eyes, lips, mouth and toes. Often arnica should be given first to prevent swelling and bruising, and then hypericum given for pains that are tearing and sensitive to touch or pressure, and for shock.

Flower Essence

St John's wort is again the remedy of light. It is best suited to sensitive people, prone to fears, often of the dark, or of psychic attack, causing restless, disturbed sleep and often nightmares. It is also for those who are oversensitive to sunlight and heat. Such people may be prone to allergies and oversensitive to their environment. St John's wort helps to engender a feeling of being protected from negative influences and to dispel fears by giving a feeling of being strong and full of light. It also allows light to illumine rather than to threaten in one's life.

Growing

St John's Wort is best propagated by root division in spring or autumn. It is happy to grow in most soils but does like good drainage and full sun.

Cautions

The phototoxins in St John's wort may cause photosensitivity in fair-skinned people when taken internally in high doses. Avoid in pregnancy, breastfeeding, bipolar disorders, schizophrenia. May cause CNS disturbances (insomnia, mania, headache, anxiety, neuropathy, tremor, dizziness, palpitations), GI distress (abdominal pain, constipation), hypertension and itching. St. John's wort may interact with some drugs, including those used in HIV infection (such as Indinavir), chemotherapeutic or anticancer, drugs (such as Irinotecan). It may also interact with drugs that help prevent the body from rejecting transplanted organs (such as Cyclosporine). Avoid with anticoagulants, Digoxin, oral contraceptives, antiviral medication, Methadone, SSRIs, MAOIs, tricyclics, Lithium, amphetamines, general anaesthetics. Caution with other medications. Avoid with theophylline and beta-2 agonists, SSRIs, Protease inhibitors.

Recipe

Heart of Jesus Oil

The flowers are covered in little black dots which contain a red pigment. If these are soaked in olive oil in a jar on a sunny windowsill and left for about two weeks, they produce a pinky-red coloured oil, called in the past *Heart of Jesus oil*.

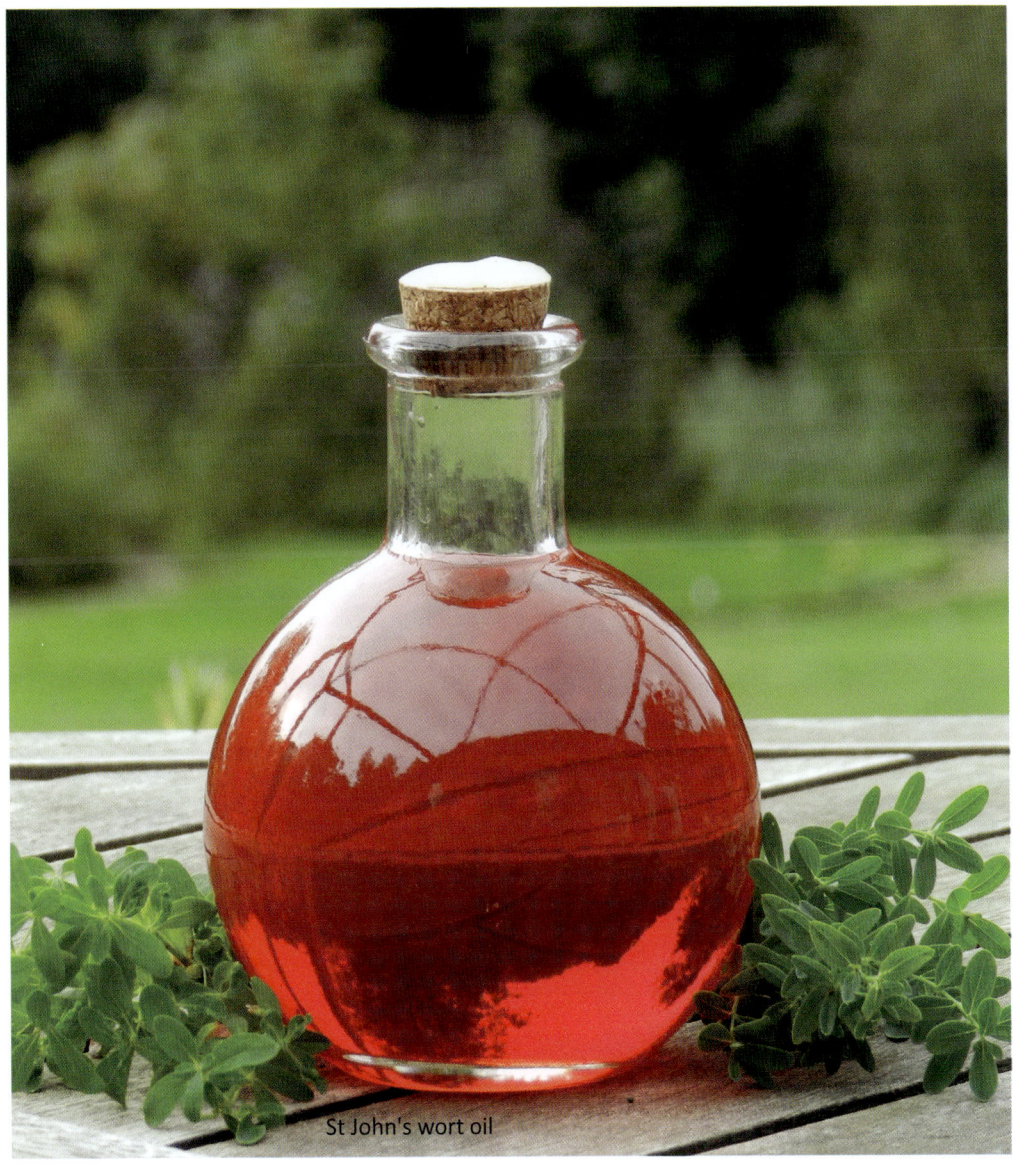

St John's wort oil

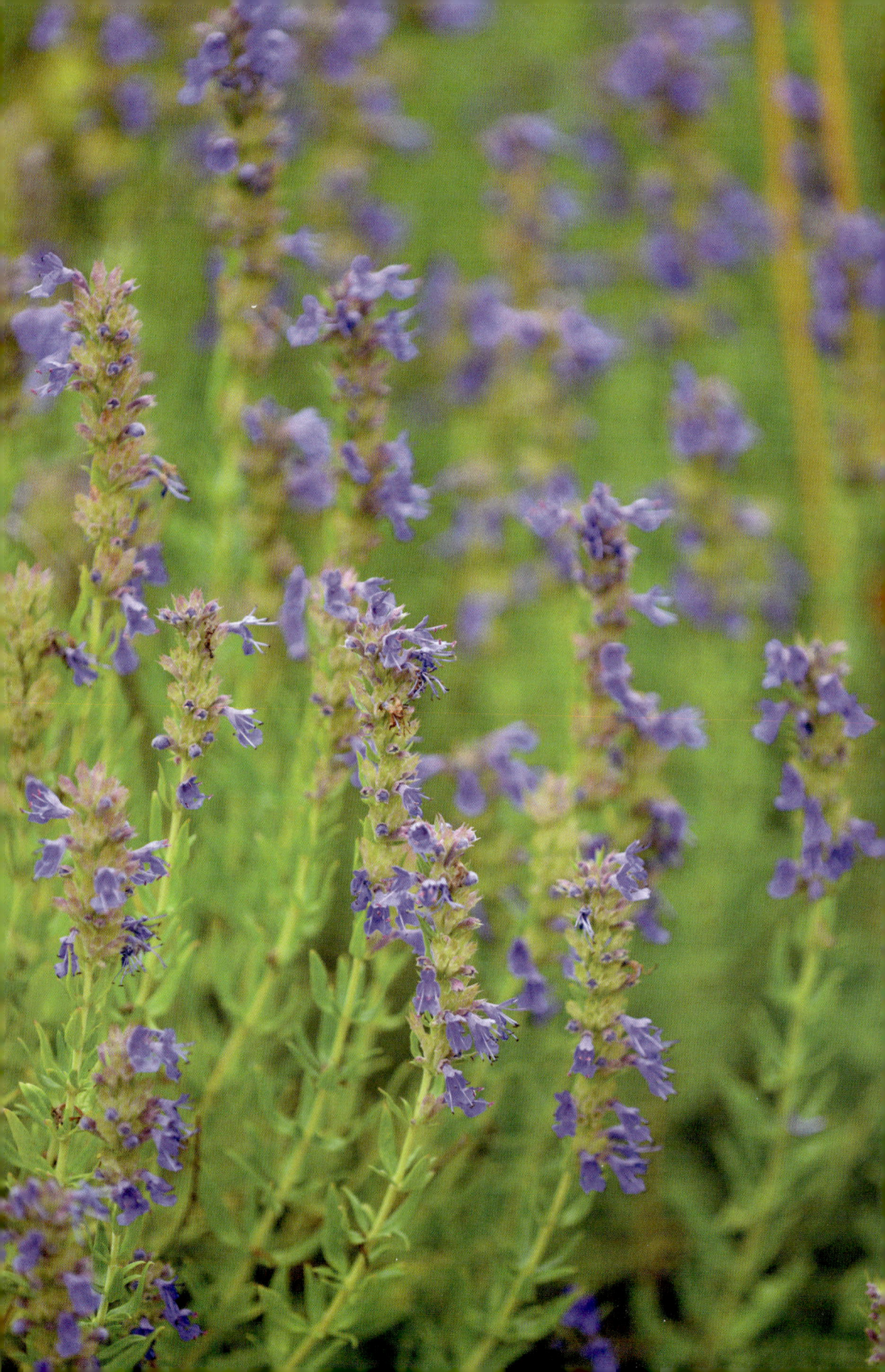

Hyssopus officinalis: Hyssop

The Flower of Forgiveness

*Purge me with Hyssop and I shall be clean,
wash me and I shall be whiter than snow*
– Psalms 51.7

Other Names: *H. decumbens,* common hyssop, garden hyssop

Parts Used: Leaves, stems and flowers

Hyssop is an attractive evergreen member of the mint (Laminaceae/Labiatae) family, with a sweet, powerful and long-lasting scent that has been used often in perfumery, potpourris and herb pillows. Hyssop was planted in medieval monastery gardens and by the 17th century it was often featured as an ornamental flower in English gardens. Its white, pink, blue and purple flowers are loved by bees and butterflies.

The name *hyssop* derives from the Hebrew word 'ezob' meaning a holy herb. To the Hebrews hyssop was a sacred plant, used for cleansing holy places. Since early times hyssop has been a symbol in many cultures of purity, cleanliness, baptism and forgiveness of sins. It is alluded to in the Scriptures: *"Purge me with Hyssop, and I shall be clean"* and was used in the Water of Purification that God commanded Moses to prepare. It was a branch of hyssop to which the soldiers attached the sponge soaked in vinegar that they extended to Jesus when he was dying on the cross. Apparently, it was used in the consecration of Westminster Abbey.

The Greeks valued hyssop in the same way. Dioscorides referred to it as a 'holy herb' since it was an ingredient of incense used in cleansing ceremonies. The Romans valued it to protect them against sickness, including the plague. Pliny said: *"Hyssop mixed with figs, purges; with honey, vomits."* Later it was used to clean churches and houses of the sick including leper houses; it was a strewing herb in the Middle Ages and made into nosegays and bouquets to ward off contagion and bad smells.

Herbal Remedy
With its aromatic, pungent and bitter tastes and warming effects, hyssop is valued for its antimicrobial properties and is an excellent herb for warding off infection and enhancing immunity. It contains terpenes, volatile oils (camphor, thujone, pinocaphone), flavonoids, hysopin, tannins and resins and has an affinity with the respiratory tract making it excellent for people prone to respiratory infections.

Hyssop is a good stimulating decongestant and expectorant for coughs, bronchitis, asthma and pleurisy. The volatile oils in hyssop are mainly responsible for its antimicrobial and expectorant actions; it has been shown to be effective against *Mycobacterium tuberculosis,* the tuberculosis bacillus and the presence of caffeic acid, tannins and other constituents contributes to its antiviral properties – useful in the treatment of colds, flu HIV and *Herpes simplex* which causes cold sores.

When taken in hot infusion, hyssop's decongestant and antimicrobial actions can be used for colds, catarrh, flu and sinus problems. It stimulates the circulation and causes sweating, and this enhances the elimination of toxins through the pores of the skin and help to brings down fever.

Warming and invigorating to the digestive tract, hyssop stimulates the flow of digestive enzymes, increasing appetite and enhancing digestion and absorption of nutrients. The warming volatile oils help to ease tension and spasm in the gut. It can be used for indigestion, wind, bloating, colic,

IBS and to regulate the bowels. With its digestive and antimicrobial properties, it helps to combat unfriendly bacteria in the gut and maintain a healthy gut flora, which in turn has its beneficial effects on the immune system and the function of the nervous system. It can be used wherever there is toxicity in the gut from poor digestion, a bad diet or after antibiotics. It may have the ability to lower blood sugar and could be useful in diabetes.

Hyssop has a traditional use in epilepsy and as a 'cordial' to comfort the heart and lift the spirits. It has been considered a tonic and restorative for the nervous system and recommended in tension, anxiety, exhaustion and depression. It makes a useful supportive herb during times of stress.

Externally, an infusion or diluted tincture of hyssop can be applied as an astringent antiseptic

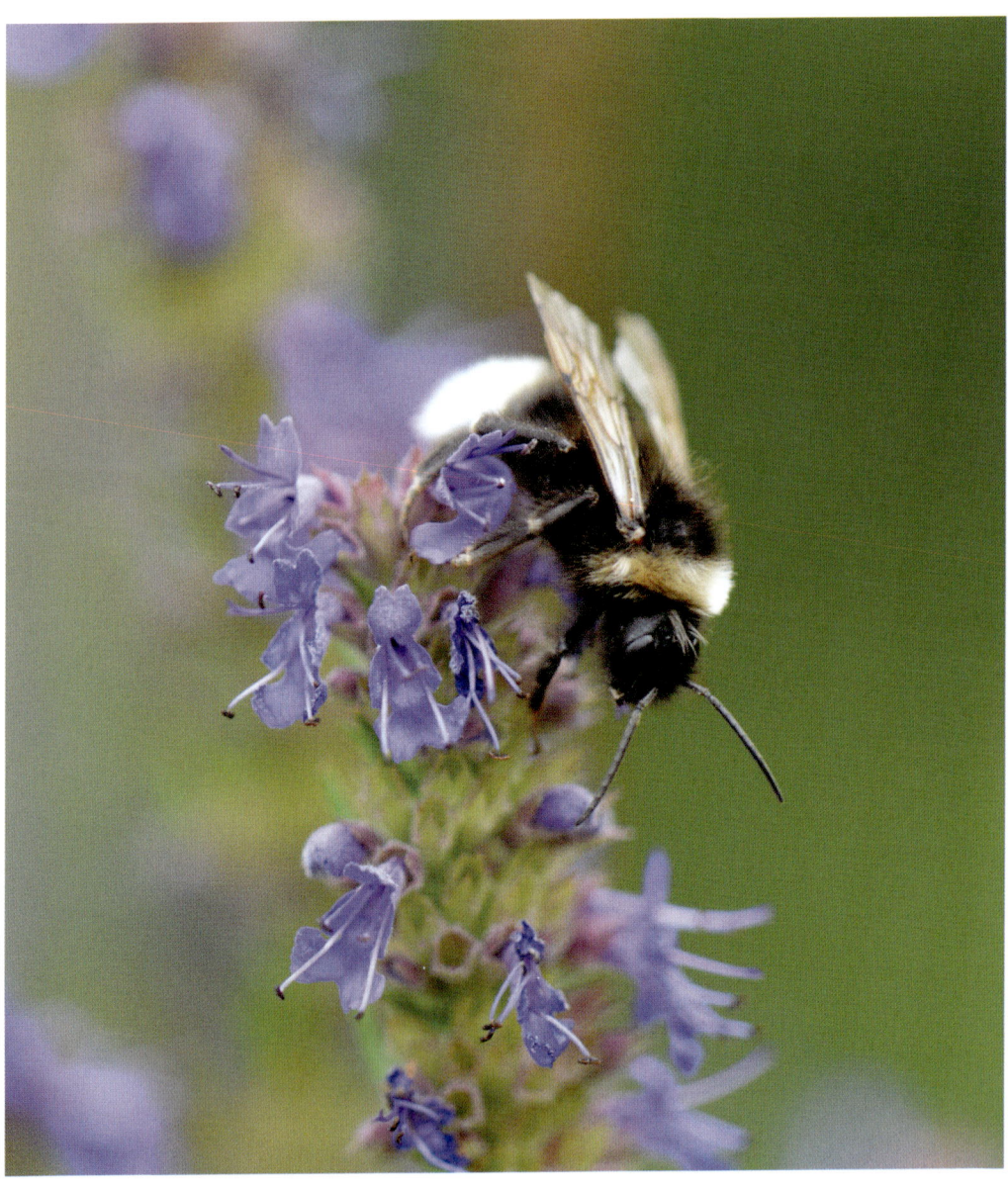

to bruises, sprains, cuts and wounds to relieve swelling, combat infection and speed healing. It can used as a liniment or be added to the bath to relieve aches and pain, muscle tension and arthritis. An infusion or dilute tincture can be used as a gargle for sore throats and tonsillitis and as an inhalation for catarrh and hay fever.

Aromatherapy Oil
Hyssop oil, like the herbal remedy, will also aid digestion and stimulate appetite. Rubbed into painful swollen joints it will help ease the pain. It has also been used for scanty periods, vaginal discharges and as a diuretic for urinary infections and stones.

Hyssop oil makes a nerve tonic to relieve anxiety, tension, exhaustion, depression and to support during times of stress. In a vaporiser it will help to purify the atmosphere, particularly useful where there is infection in the house, and when studying for exams will help clarify the mind and steady the nerves.

As an inhalant it will help to clear respiratory infections and catarrh, and enhance immunity, making it useful in asthma, chest infections, bronchitis, fevers, flu and hay fever.

Flower Essence
Hyssop as a flower essence has similar benefits for purifying and cleansing, emotionally and spiritually, reflecting its use in early times as a symbol of the forgiveness of sins. It will help to release tension throughout the system, when it has its origin in emotional problems and specifically feelings of guilt. In this way hyssop will help one to let go of such feelings and allow self-forgiveness. It is particularly useful for children who may blame themselves for strife between their parents, and for parents who feel guilty because their child-rearing does not mirror their ideals.

Edible Uses
As a kitchen herb, hyssop can add its aromatic and warming qualities to enhance soups and vegetable dishes. It makes lovely tisanes either on its own or with other herbs such as thyme and mint. The flowers can be used for decorative garnishes in salads and fruit salads as well as in desserts.

Growing
Hyssop can be grown from seed in the spring or cuttings taken during the summer. Plants can be divided in spring and autumn. It prefers a sunny position and well-drained soil. Grows up to 2' (60cm) and flowers in late summer. It makes an excellent low hedging plant and a good companion in the vegetable garden as it attracts cabbage white butterflies away from brassicas and other leafy crops.

Cautions
Avoid the herbal remedy in pregnancy and epilepsy. Take away from mineral supplements. Avoid with anticoagulants and Warfarin.

Recipes

Tisane

Mix the herbs together in equal parts and use 2 teaspoons fresh chopped herbs or 1 teaspoon dried to 1 cup boiling water. Place herbs in a teapot and pour on boiling water. Cover and leave to infuse for 10 minutes. Drink hot. Sweeten with honey if desired.

Hyssop Cough Syrup

2 tablespoons dried hyssop or ⅓ cup fresh hyssop chopped,
¼ cup water,
1 cup honey,
1 teaspoon aniseed

Place the honey and water in a saucepan and mix until the mixture is the consistency of syrup. Bring slowly to a boil over a low heat. Skim off any scum that rises to the surface. Crush the aniseed and stir it and the hyssop into the honey. Cover and simmer for 30 minutes. Remove from heat, uncover, and allow to cool. While the mixture is still warm, strain into a jar. When completely cooled, screw on the lid. Store in the fridge.

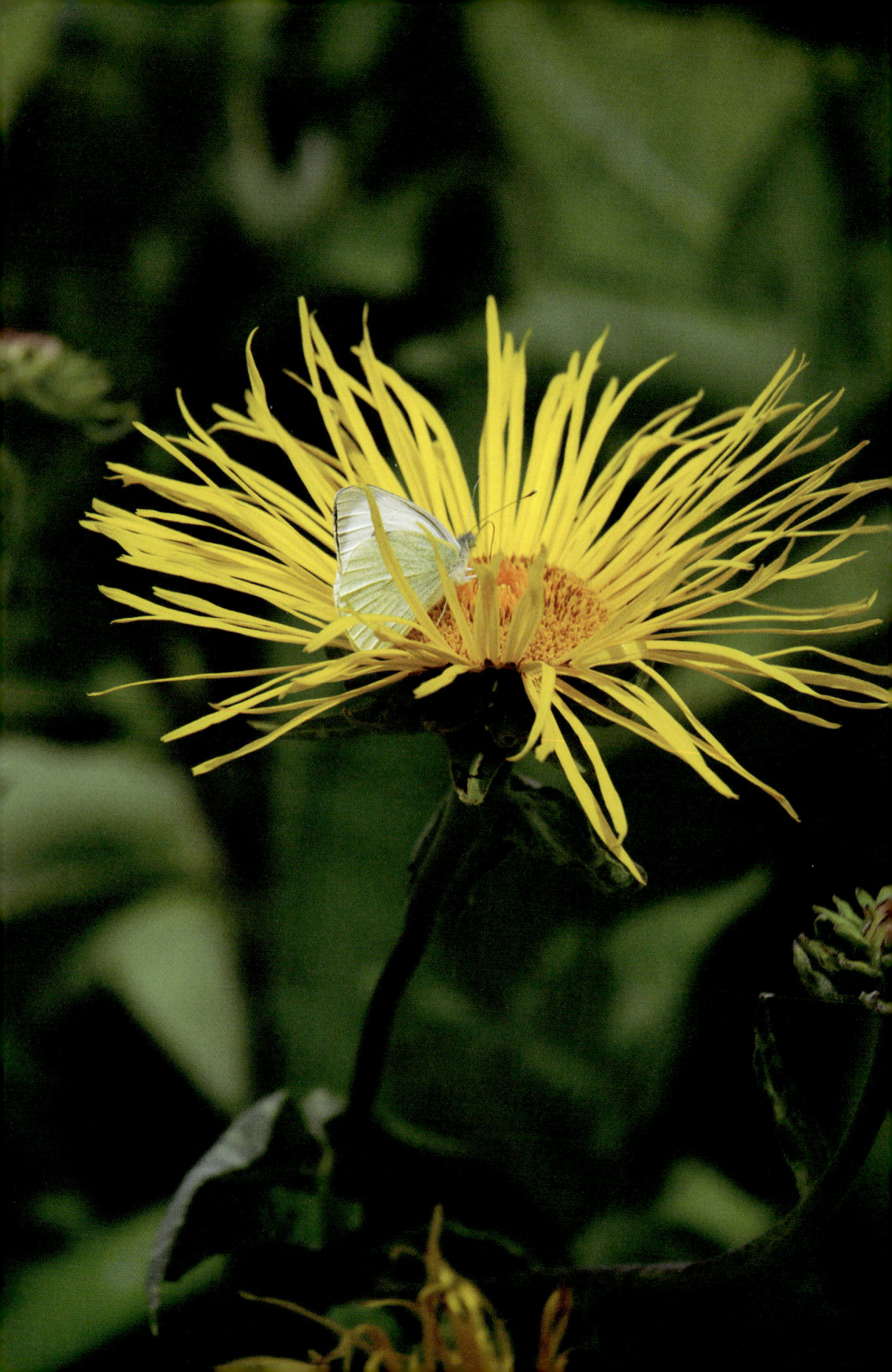

Inula helenium: Elecampane

The Flower of Elves

Julia Augustus let no day pass without eating some of the roots of Enula, considered to help digestion and cause mirth
– Pliny

Other names: Wild sunflower, velvet dock, scabwort, horseheal, allicampane, elf dock, elf wort, else dock, enula campana, horse elder, alant, alant camphor, yellow starwort, marchalan, wild sunflower, horse elder, nurseheal, yellow starwort

Parts Used: Root, rhizome and flowers

Elecampane is a wonderfully stately, statuesque member of the Asteraceae/Compositae family, which can grow up to two metres tall. It has attractive yellow daisy flowers a bit like sunflowers and downy leaves which can grow a metre long. It is native to Europe and northern Asia.

There are different stories about the origin of elecampane's Latin name '*helenium*'. Some say it is named after Helen of Troy whose face was so beautiful it could launch a thousand ships. The plant was said to spring from her tears as they fell to the ground when she was abducted by Paris or that she carried a bouquet of elecampane with her as she went. Gerard tells us: *"It took the name Helenium of Helena, wife of Menelaus, who had her hands full of it when Paris stole her away into Phrygia."*

Others say that it was Helen that first used it to remedy venomous bites and another story says the name comes from the island Helena where the best elecampane plants grew. Before Linnaeus formerly named it, elecampane was known as '*Enula campana*' meaning Helen of the plains.

Elecampane was used both as a food and a medicine in ancient times. Ancient Greeks and Romans regarded elecampane as a panacea for a host of ailments from dropsy, menstrual disorders, digestive upsets to what Galen described as 'passions of the hucklebone' which is probably sciatica. Hippocrates recommended it as a remedy for the kidneys, brain, uterus and stomach. Pliny the Roman diarist said, *"Julia Augustus let no day pass without eating some of the roots of Enula, considered to help digestion and cause mirth"* and also *"being chewed fasting, doth fasten the teeth."*

The root was traditionally infused in port with currants and sugar in medieval Europe and taken as a digestive and to combat worms and parasites. The root was also candied and eaten on special occasions and it was given to children for whooping cough.

In Renaissance times children were given cordials and sweets made from elecampane and liquorice on Easter Monday. It was also popular in France and Switzerland for making absinthe and it has been utilised by the Dutch for making wine and beer.

The medicinal virtues of elecampane were often referred to in Anglo-Saxon writings and it was described by the Welsh physicians of the thirteenth century who called it *marchalan*. It was a common remedy for coughs, bronchitis, asthma and catarrhal congestion. Culpeper said elecampane was **ruled by Mercury and** *"very effectual to warm a cold, windy stomach."* He used it to clear poison, strengthen sight and clear internal blockages while John Gerard recommended it for *"the shortness of breath."* The Native Americans used the root for respiratory problems in humans as well as horses, as did the European settlers in America. They also valued it as an emmenagogue or abortifacient and for treating scabby skin problems in sheep and cattle hence the folk names *horseheal* and *scabwort*.

The root of elecampane was believed to have healing powers beyond the body. It was burned on charcoal to sharpen psychic powers and to create an atmosphere of protection. To the Anglo-Saxons elecampane was the remedy for 'elf-shot' and averting the evil eye, which explains some of the plant's common names such as 'elf wort' and 'elf dock'. It was considered that the work of elves was responsible for the onset of a number of illnesses. When made into incense, elecampane has been used to purify candidates for initiation and is considered to be helpful in times of stress, grief, melancholy or depression. Apparently, the Native Americans used elecampane to help them feel more connected to the earth.

Herbal Remedy
The root of elecampane is thick and mucilaginous and has a unique and deliciously pungent and aromatic taste and smell. It is generally used in Western herbal medicine while the sunflower-like flowers have long been used in Chinese medicine. The roots contain up to 44% polysaccharide inulin, as well as resins, pectin, mucilage, calcium, magnesium, iodine, iron and sodium, vitamins A, C, E, B12, B5, beta-carotene, selenium, bitter principles, sterols (sitosterol, stigmasterol), saponins and essential oils composed of sesquiterpene lactones.

Elecampane is suitable for treating people of all ages and especially beneficial for those feeling run down and debilitated. It cleanses toxins from the body, stimulates the immune and digestive systems and helps combat bacterial and fungal infections. The pungent root makes a warming decongestant and expectorant, and when taken in a hot infusion it is excellent for catarrh, colds, sinus congestion and hay fever. It also stimulates the circulation, promotes sweating and helps to bring down fevers. With its antispasmodic and antimicrobial properties provided by the sesquiterpene lactones, it is one of the best remedies for treating colds, flu, coughs, bronchitis and other chest infections

including pneumonia and pleurisy. One of the sesquiterpene lactones called alantolactone is active against TB. Elecampane is frequently employed as a bronchodilator to prevent and treat asthma, emphysema, whooping cough and croup, and makes an effective remedy for sore throats, tonsillitis and laryngitis. A decoction of the flowers is also considered helpful for coughs or nausea caused by excessive mucous, as well as for treating bronchitis and pharyngitis.

Inulin is a non-digestible polysaccharide in a class of fibres known as fructans and it plays a major role in easing breathing in asthma and bronchitis. During an asthma attack, the lining of the bronchial tubes become swollen and inflamed and restrict the flow of air in and out of the lungs. Inulin coats and soothes the lining of the bronchial tubes thereby reducing inflammation and acts as an expectorant. The saponins also help expulsion of mucus from the lungs. Elecampane may help ease stress on the heart caused by shortness of breath and provide pain relief in patients with cardiovascular disease. It can also lower blood pressure.

Elecampane warms and invigorates the digestion, stimulates the flow of digestive enzymes and enhances appetite, digestion and absorption. Its antispasmodic action relaxes tension and spasm in the gut, its antimicrobial properties help combat infection while the mucilage soothes and cools heat, irritation and inflammation. It is an excellent remedy for clearing toxins from the gut; the inulin acts as a prebiotic and helps promote 'good' intestinal bacteria which ensure regular bowel movements. Its antimicrobial actions help combat unfriendly microorganisms in the gut and remedy disturbance of the gut flora and its antifungal action is useful for treating Candida. It can be used to calm stomach upsets associated with tension and stress, as well as a range of digestive and systemic problems associated with disturbance of the gut flora. The root and the flowers can be used for treating loss of appetite, nausea, vomiting, indigestion, wind, bloating, colic, IBS, irregular bowels, diarrhoea and gastro-enteritis. The root can be chewed to prevent tooth decay and sweeten the breath.

Two active ingredients in elecampane, alantolactone and isoalantolactone, are useful for expelling parasites from the gut including roundworm, hookworm, whipworm and threadworm. Elecampane also has anthelmintic activity against the liver fluke *Fasciola hepatica*. The bitters stimulate the flow of bile from liver and support it in its metabolic and detoxifying work. The antioxidants in the root have a hepatoprotective effect, protecting the liver from damage caused by toxins, drugs and alcohol.

By promoting a healthy gut flora and with its antimicrobial actions, elecampane enhances immunity. It is an effective antibacterial for many types of *Staphyloccal* infections. It also has an anti-inflammatory action probably attributed to the alantolactone, and with its analgesic effects it can be helpful in rheumatoid arthritis and other auto-immune disease. As an antiseptic and soothing diuretic, elecampane root and flowers can be used to relieve fluid retention and resolve urinary tract infections. They make good antispasmodic, anti-inflammatory and analgesic remedies for an irritable bladder and other stress-related or painful problems of the urinary tract.

In Chinese and Ayurvedic medicine two plants with many similar properties, *Inula helenium* and *racemosa*, are used. They have a warm energy, acrid/pungent and bitter flavour and affect the lungs, liver, spleen and stomach. The Chinese use the root prepared by deep frying or baking to strengthen the spleen and stomach, promote energy flow and alleviate pain. It is prescribed for wind, bloating, nausea, vomiting, diarrhoea and painful conditions of the chest and abdomen. In Ayurveda elecampane root reduces *kapha* and *vata* and increases the heat of *pitta*. They use both plants to clear congestion and infection from the respiratory tract and, as a rejuvenative to the lungs, it is considered to promote longevity of lung tissue.

The Chinese also use the flowers and leaves of *Inula japonica* and *I. britannica* which are called 'xuan fu hua'. They are considered to have a slightly warm energy, bitter, acrid/pungent and salty flavour and affect the Liver, Lung, Stomach and Spleen. The flowers were traditionally

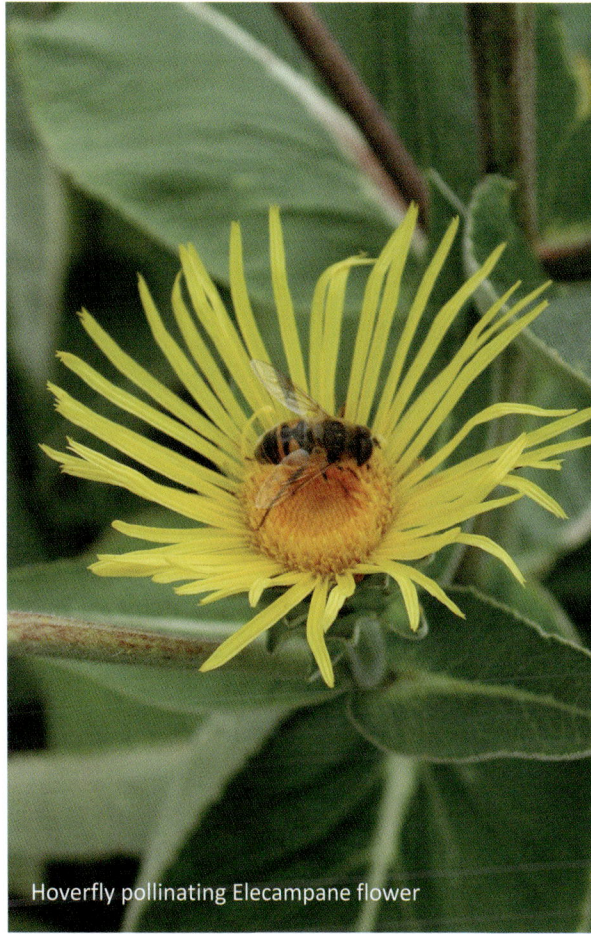
Hoverfly pollinating Elecampane flower

steamed and dried, although today they are fried in honey. They are used to direct energy downward and clear thin or scanty phlegm from blocking the lungs and stomach. They help to relieve coughs, soften hardened phlegm, break up hard accumulations and open areas of stagnation to relieve bronchitis, coughing, asthma, wheezing, shortness of breath, pleurisy, vomiting, hiccough, belching, food stagnation and palpitations with anxiety. The flowers are thought to be particularly good for nausea from chemotherapy and may be useful for upper respiratory allergies. The flowers and leaves are used for their diuretic action.

Antioxidants are very useful for improving the quality of life by preventing or postponing the onset of degenerative diseases. They act as scavengers of free radicals which are responsible for causing a large number of diseases including cancer, diabetes, cardiovascular disease, nervous system disorders, Alzheimer's disease, mild cognitive impairment, Parkinson's disease, alcohol induced liver disease and ageing. The alantolactone and isoalantolactone in the root of *Inula helenium* and *I. racemosa* have antioxidant activity and antifungal actions. Three sesquiterpene lactones isolated from the roots of *Inula helenium* and *racemosa* and the flowers of *Inula japonica* have antitumour activities potentially inhibiting the growth of cancer cells in colon, ovary, breast, prostrate, skin, pancreatic, lung cancers and leukaemia. It also may suppress cell growth and cell apoptosis in oral cancer cells.

The roots and flowers of *Inula racemosa* have a cardioprotective effect attributed to improved antioxidant status and are helpful in allergic conditions because of their ability to stabilise mast cells.

Elecampane has been used traditionally to treat type 2 diabetes. The inulin in the roots may be beneficial as it helps stabilise blood sugar. *Inula britannica* flowers have a preventive effect on autoimmune diabetes by regulating cytokine production and this has been related to the presence of polysaccharides. The phenols and flavonoids, notably rutin and quercetin found in alcoholic extracts of the flowers as well as the leaves and root may be even more effective in managing diabetes. They have a remarkable ability to inhibit the activity of digestive enzymes notably α-glucosidase and α-amylase, which affect carbohydrate digestion and glucose absorption through their antioxidant action. Extracts of the roots of *I. racemosa* and the flowers of *I. japonica* can also significantly reduce blood sugar levels. These species all have antioxidant activity which may be beneficial for the prevention or treatment of oxidative stress-induced complications of diabetes.

Externally a decoction or dilute tincture of the root of elecampane makes a good antiseptic wash for cuts and wounds, for rashes including eczema, for varicose ulcers and skin infections such as acne, ringworm, scabies and *Herpes*.

Its antibacterial and antifungal action is useful for *Staphylococcal* infections including MRSA. Elecampane can be used in massage oils and liniments for easing muscle and joint pain and was traditionally used for relieving facial neuralgia and sciatica.

Homeopathic Remedy
Like the herbal remedy, this is a remedy for the chest and the mucous membranes. It is indicated in bronchial symptoms, a dry cough which is worse at night and lying down, painful larynx, chronic bronchitis with thick phlegm. It is used for period pain, a bearing down sensation and backache, feeling cold during menstruation, as well as cystitis symptoms with frequency of urination. Other indications include pain in the right shoulder, wrist, lower limbs and ankles, as well as heachaches, vertigo when bending down and pressure in the temples and forehead.

Flower Essence
With its affinity with the lungs and the fact that grief is traditionally said to affect the lungs, elecampane makes a good remedy for deep-seated or old grief, helping to open us up and bring it up to the surface so that we can find new strength and wisdom and be transformed in the process.

Edible Uses
The bitter and aromatic root used to be popular for flavouring digestive liqueurs and vermouths, and when fresh and then candied it was used in confectionary. It can be used to flavour puddings, lending a mild camphorous flavour. It can also be macerated with vinegar and used as a condiment. The root is also good in vegetable and meat stews where its pungent and aromatic taste can complement more bland flavours of meat and vegetables.

Growing
Propagate by sowing seeds, barely covering them. Alternatively divide roots in spring or autumn. Elecampane will grow happily in moist soil and sun or semi-shade. It grows 2–5' (60 – 150cm) high and flowers in July and August. It makes a good decorative plant for the herb garden or the back of a flower border. It self-seeds easily if flower heads are left. It is best

harvested in the autumn from plants that are two years old and can be dried for later use.

Cautions
Avoid during pregnancy and breast feeding. Large doses can cause diarrhoea and vomiting. Be aware of possible reactions in people allergic to Asteraceae family pollen (chrysanthemum, chamomile, ragweed, daisy). Caution in inflammation and excess heat. Diabetics should monitor their blood glucose as inulin may inhibit glucose absorption.

Recipes

Four Thieves Vinegar
Apparently, this formula was devised by four corpse-robbers who protected themselves from contagion during the time of the great plague in Toulouse (1628-1631).

The original recipe was as follows:

A handful each of dried wormwood, meadowsweet, juniper berries, wild marjoram and sage
3 pints of strong white wine vinegar
50 cloves
2 ounces of dried elecampane root
2 ounces of dried angelica root
2 ounces of dried rosemary
2 ounces of dried horehound
3g camphor crystals

Other antibacterial herbs can also be used in this formula including sweet flag, cinnamon, mint, lavender, nutmeg and garlic.

Steep the herbs in the vinegar for 10 days then strain through a sieve. Add the camphor and bottle. Rub it on face and hands or inhale the vapours to dispel infection.

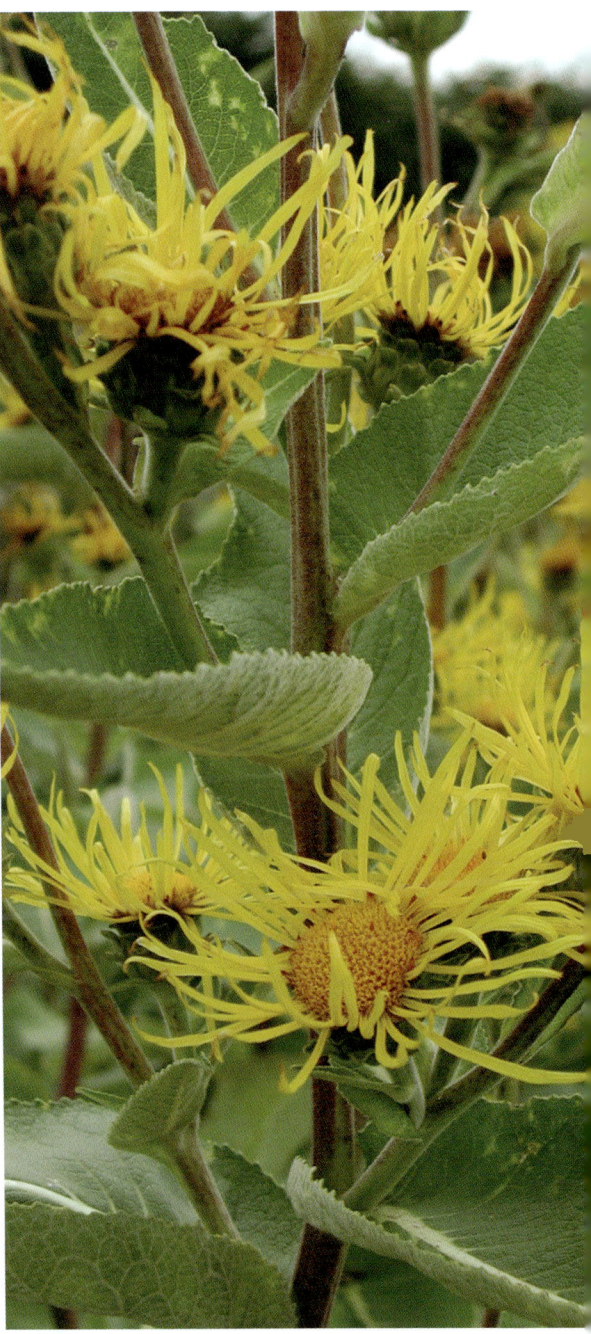

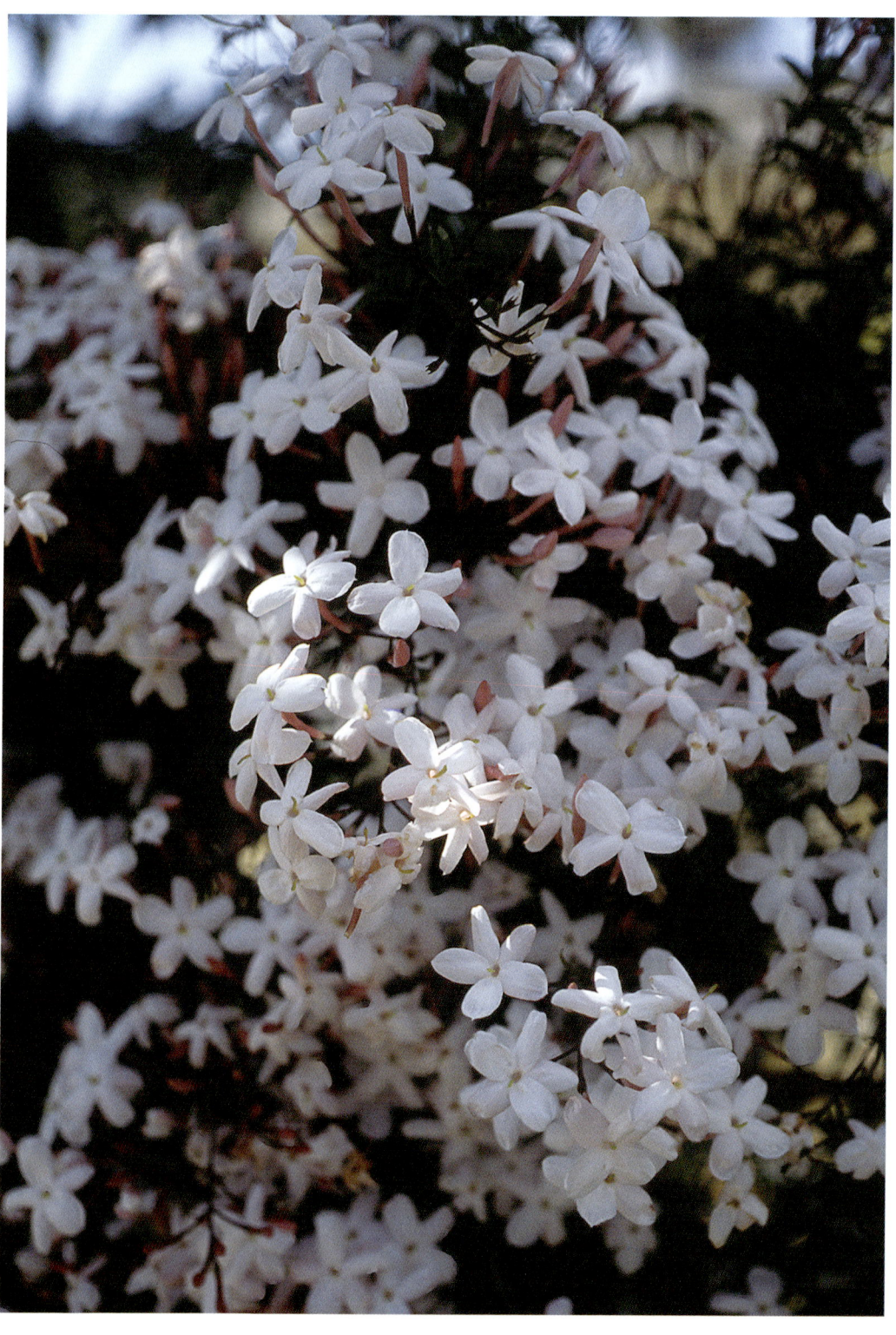

Jasminum officinale, J. grandiflorum: Jasmine
The Flower of Luxury

Twas midnight — through the lattice wreath'd
With woodbine, many a perfume breath'd
From plants that wake while others sleep,
From timid jasmine buds, that keep
Their odour to themselves all day,
But when the sunshine dies away,
Let the delicious secret out
To every breeze that roams about
— Thomas Moore (1779–1852)

Other Names: Star of divine hope, the moonlight of the grove, queen of the night, jessamine

Part used: Flowers

Known in India as 'Queen of the night', the delicate jasmine flower has one of the loveliest and most distinctive perfumes, particularly intoxicating at night. There are between two and three hundred species of jasmine, mostly native to China, India and Iran. They belong to the olive (Oleaceae) family; some are climbers, others are shrubs, some are deciduous, and others are evergreen; some are tender, others are hardy. The common white jasmine (*J. officinale*) is a native of Northern India and Persia, while the Spanish jasmine (*J. grandiflorum*) is a native of the Himalayas and has slightly larger, highly perfumed flowers grown for use in perfumery. The old name 'jessamine' and jasmine come originally from the Persian name 'yasmin' and the Chinese 'yeh-hsi-ming'.

For centuries, the luxurious perfume of jasmine has been associated with feminine sweetness, love and fertility in many ancient traditions including Hindu, Muslim and Chinese culture. In India, jasmine is a sacred flower known as 'moonlight of the grove' and traditionally woven into bridal wreathes and worn by women as scented ornaments. The oil pressed from the flowers has been a favourite scent of Indian women and is used in perfumed hair oils. The Hindus use jasmine flowers to make sweet-smelling garlands for honouring guests. Jasmine is held sacred to Vishnu and to Indra (an ancient Indo-Iranian god) and flowers are used as offerings at religious ceremonies in India in honour of these gods.

The oil and the flowers have long been major ingredients in sensuous perfumes and love potions and valued for their aphrodisiac powers. In the ancient Greek and Roman traditions, they were associated with the moon, the goddesses Artemis and Diana and the maternal, creative aspect of the universe. With the coming of Christianity, jasmine was known as 'the star of divine hope' and dedicated to the Virgin Mary. The star-shaped flowers symbolised 'heavenly felicity' and the purity of the Virgin Mary. According to one legend, on the night Christ was crucified, the world's most beautiful flowers curled up and died. The jasmine flower, then pink, suffered in silence, closing its petals and the next morning it had paled from pink to white. In the language of flowers, white jasmine symbolises deep affection, happiness and elegance. To dream of jasmine was said to mean a romance was on the horizon. In India, jasmine is described as *sattvic*, increasing love and compassion within and enhancing the receptivity of heart and mind.

With its long association with the feminine, it also has an affinity with womens' health and particularly the female reproductive system and has been used in healing for women for many centuries. According to Culpeper, *"Jessamine is a warm cordial plant"* which could be used to facilitate childbirth and remove diseases of the uterus and also to *"dissolve cold swellings and hard tumours."* Culpeper also said that jessamine was *"good for cold and catarrhous conditions but not for hot."*

Herbal Remedy
The heavenly scented jasmine flowers have bitter and astringent tastes and cooling qualities and make an excellent remedy for the nervous system. They contain alkaloids (jasminine), tannins, volatile oils (linalool, benzyl acetate, farnesol), phenolic glycosides, salicylic acid and resin. Jasmine is a lovely remedy for calming the nerves and soothing emotional problems especially when feeling tense, hot and fiery, angry, irritable, frustrated or depressed. It is a good remedy when feeling burned out, overwhelmed or suffering from insomnia. In Ayurvedic medicine, jasmine is considered a *sattvic medhya* herb meaning that is a wonderful herb for the heart and mind to enhance wisdom, compassion, love, joy and contentment, but also that it can enliven the mind and could be helpful in nervous exhaustion.

With its long association with women and the female reproductive system, it is not surprising that jasmine can still make an excellent remedy for a range of menstrual problems. It has a regulating effect on the uterine muscles and helps to prevent stagnation of blood that causes pain and clots. With its antispasmodic and downward moving action, it makes a good remedy for period discomfort and cramps. It can also be used for easing contractions during childbirth and to ease afterpains. Its relaxing effect can be helpful in PMS and menstrual headaches. With its astringent tannins, it can reduce bleeding and is useful for heavy periods, and locally for vaginal discharges and infections. It helps to regulate menstruation and is valued in India for its nourishing effect on the female reproductive system as an aphrodisiac and fertility tonic. In Malaysia, jasmine has been used for puerperal infections (after childbirth), for fevers and as a nerve sedative. Its antimicrobial actions and its ability to clear congestion from the uterine area means that jasmine can be used for cysts, fibroids, salpingitis, cystitis, urinary tract infections and vaginal infections.

The volatile oils that give jasmine its wonderfully evocative aroma make it a very useful remedy for treating infections. They have antibacterial, antiviral and anti-tumour activities, active against bacteria including *Enterococcus faecalis, E. coli, Pseudomonas aeruginosa, Proteus mirabilis, Staphyloccocus albus, Klebsiella pneumoniae* and *Salmonella sp* as well as against the yeast *Candida albicans*. These actions are very helpful in the respiratory system, helping to protect against and resolve infections including sore throats, tonsilitis, laryngitis and chest infections including pneumonia. Its decongestant and anti-inflammatory action can be helpful in catarrh, sinisitus and mucousy coughs as well as sinusitis and rhinitis. Taken in hot infusion, jasmine flowers also help to bring down fevers.

In the gut the antimicrobial actions of jasmine are also beneficial, helping to combat infections causing gastroenteritis and disturbances of the gut flora. The astringent tannins help to protect the gut lining from infection, irritation and inflammation, making it a good remedy for gastritis and diarrhoea as well as leaky gut syndrome. Its antioxidant and anti-inflammatory actions have potential in the prevention of cancer. In Ayurvedic medicine, jasmine is used to cleanse the lymphatic system and can be helpful in swollen glands, as well as different types of cancer, such as breast cancer, bone and lymph cancers including Hodgkin's disease.

The cooling bitter compounds in jasmine flowers have a beneficial effect on the liver and with its antioxidant, anti-inflammatory and hepatoprotective actions, jasmine can be used for healing the liver in hepatitis and cirrhosis. Jasmine also supports the liver in its metabolic and detoxifying work and for this reason can be helpful as a cleansing remedy for hot inflamed skin conditions such as acne and eczema.

Externally the antimicrobial and astringent properties of jasmine can help resolve infections and inflammation. It can be used as a gargle or mouthwash for sore throats, mouth ulcers and gingivitis, and as a lotion or douche for vaginal discharges and infections. It makes a good eyewash when used lukewarm for sore, burning and irritated eyes and a lotion for inflammatory skin problems, infections such as ringworm and scabies, and bites and stings. It is known as a cooling remedy for sunstroke.

Aromatherapy Oil
Jasmine has an uplifting, even euphoric effect on the emotions and has an affinity for women. It is often used to treat emotional problems relating to sexuality, such as impotence and frigidity. Its warming sensual fragrance is relaxing and reassuring, useful in a whole range of stress-related problems, including grief, heartbreak, anger and depression. When combined with clary sage or bergamot, it helps to relieve postnatal depression. Its aphrodisiac effect can be enhanced by combining it with rose, ylang ylang or clary sage.

It is antiseptic, antiviral and antifungal and can be used in treatment of *Herpes* and thrush. It strengthens and relaxes the uterus and is excellent for use for period pain and during childbirth. During the menopause, it reaffirms a woman's confidence in her femininity and sensuality, and brings a feeling of optimism, warmth and wellbeing. The oil can be diluted and used as ear drops for ear infections and as a massage oil for respiratory infections and applied to the skin to treat fungal infections such as athlete's foot.

Homeopathic Remedy
Jasminum officinale is prepared from a tincture of the berries and is prescribed for symptoms of tetanus, including convulsions, vomiting and coma.

Flower Essence
Jasmine is recommended for people with problems of excess mucus clogging the nose, throat and chest and causing a feeling of cloudiness and sluggishness. Jasmine clears the passageways and the head and promotes mental clarity. It stimulates the brain, increases perception and allows the mind to grasp deep questions about the essence of all life and our purpose on this planet. It increases awareness of innate femininity and the wisdom that brings.

Edible Uses
Jasmine flowers are delicious in teas and can also be used to decorate salads, cakes and deserts. They are delicious added to drinks such as elderflower or mint cordial.

Growing
Jasmine is a climbing shrub and can easily be grown from cuttings. It likes moist but well-drained soil. It is happiest in a warm sheltered, sunny site in the garden, where you can sit and enjoy the fragrance of the flowers. It grows quickly, and is ideal for covering a south or west-facing wall.

Cautions
Avoid during pregnancy.

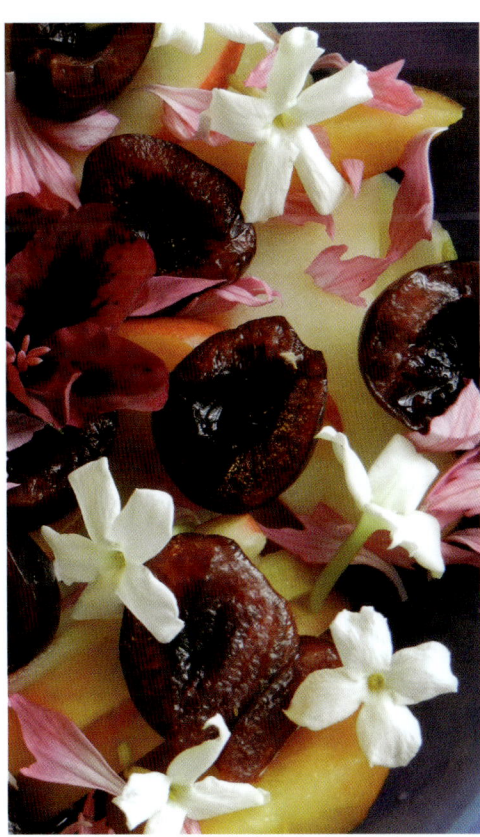

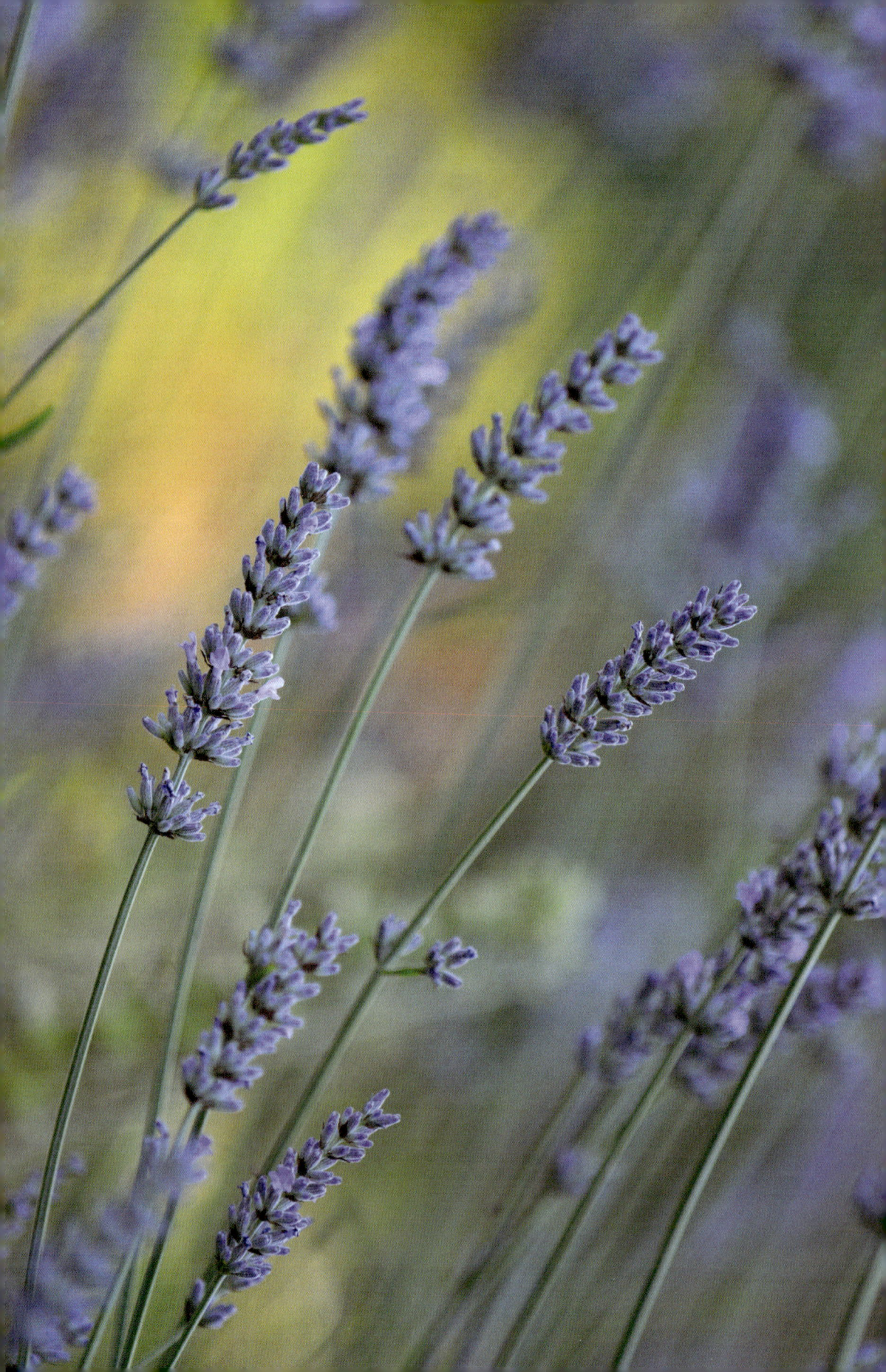

Lavandula angustifolia: Lavender

The Flower of the Virgin Mary

To make a perfume, take some rose water
And wash your hands in it,
Then take a lavender flower
And rub it with your palms,
And you will achieve the desired effect
  – Leonardo da Vinci (1452–1519)

Other names: *Lavendula officinalis*, true lavender, English lavender, garden lavender, common lavender, narrow-leaved lavender

Parts used: Flowers

Fragrant lavender must be one of the best loved traditional cottage garden herbs, with its evergreen grey-green foliage and spikes of highly scented mauve-blue flowers. It is a perennial member of the Lamiaceae/Labiatae family from the Mediterranean coast, now cultivated in many parts of the world for its popular use in perfumery and aromatherapy. Lavender is a joy to every garden. Its fragrance when brushed against not only lifts the spirits, but also dispels insects like mosquitos, while attracting bees. It makes delicious honey.

Lavender water is one of the oldest perfumes; Dioscorides considered its fragrance surpassed all other perfumes, though it was not venerated solely for this but also for its cleansing and purifying qualities. The Virgin Mary is reputed to have been especially fond of lavender because it protected clothes from insects and 'dirty beasts' and also preserved chastity; she is said to have washed the infant Jesus' clothes in lavender water and hung them on a lavender bush to dry.

In ancient Rome, lavender was strewn on floors to sweeten the air, fumigate sick rooms and as incense for religious ceremonies. The Romans used lavender to perfume their baths, explaining the name which comes from 'lavare' meaning to wash. It is mentioned in the 12th century writings of Hildegarde of Bingen. During the Middle Ages and the Renaissance, lavender was very popular as a strewing herb, to perfume and sanitise the floors of houses and churches and to ward off the plague. It was hung in rooms to keep away germ-carrying flies and mosquitos, much as it was hung in linen cupboards by our grandmothers, to scent the clothes and deter moths. According to Mrs Grieves' A Modern Herbal, *"Lavender was hawked around the streets of London with the haunting call, 'Who will buy my sweet lavender?'"* It was dedicated to Hecate, the Goddess of witches and sorcerers and was said to avert the evil eye.

The 16th and 17th century herbalists recognised its medicinal virtues and recommended it for improving eyesight, relieving headaches and faintness and to comfort the heart. It was used to sweeten the breath and for perfumes, in preparation for childbirth and to keep away infection. It was burned in delivery rooms as a disinfectant and used in baths to speed healing and relieve pain after childbirth. It was also used as a traditional remedy for neuralgia, muscle and back pain and to stimulate paralysed limbs.

When inhaled or taken as spirit of lavender made by soaking flowers in brandy or gin, it was an old restorative remedy for faintness, giddiness and debility. Gerard used lavender for treating migraine and *"the panting and passion of the heart"* and Parkinson said lavender is *"of especially good use for all griefes and pains of the head and brain."* Mattiolus the 16th century Italian herbalist said, *"It is much used in maladies and those disorders of the brain due to coldness, such as epilepsy, apoplexy, spasms and paralysis; it comforts the stomach and is a great help in obstructions of the liver and spleen"*. The Arabs used lavender as an expectorant and antispasmodic for the chest, to treat colds, coughs, chest infections and asthma.

Herbal Remedy and Aromatherapy oil
The volatile oils in lavender that create its delightful and penetrating fragrance account for the major part of its medicinal action, so the uses in herbal medicine and aromatherapy are very similar. The scent of the volatile oil can lift the spirits and has a deeply calming effect. The volatile oils include linalool, geraniol, nerol, cineole, borneol and linionene, and they are present mainly in the flowers along with tannins, coumarins (umbelliferone, herniarin, coumarin), flavonoids, antioxidant (rosmarinic acid) and triterpenoids.

As we know from the historical use of lavender, it is a wonderful aromatic remedy for the nervous system, restoring resilience to those feeling stressed, overwhelmed or nervously run down. It calms anxiety and is good for relieving stress-related symptoms such as muscle tension, gut problems, back ache, neck pain, headaches, period pains, palpitations and insomnia. The volatile oils are thought to modulate GABAergic neurotransmission, in this way reducing anxiety and tension. Its pain-relieving actions are helpful here too and can help in the treatment of acute as well as chronic or intractable pain, such as after surgery, childbirth, in back and neck problems and migraines.

In aromatherapy, lavender oil is considered to balance the emotions. It lifts the spirits and stabilises moods. Since it has both a relaxing and a stimulating edge, lavender is used for restoring energy when feeling tired or even suffering from nervous exhaustion, while a few drops of oil in the bath or in a massage oil will help soothe you into restful sleep. Lavender is an excellent remedy for insomnia and to improve the quality of sleep. When lavender is used in massage oils, the constituents and in particular the relaxing linalool are rapidly absorbed through the skin and relax mind and body. It has even been said that tigers and lions in zoological gardens are powerfully affected by the calming effect of lavender's scent and became docile under its influence. Lavender engenders a feeling of ease and contentment and increases mental and emotional resilience so that we can maintain a good mood, even when circumstances could challenge our equilibrium.

With its neuroprotective, anticonvulsant and cognitive effects, lavender holds great promise for the treatment of a whole range of nervous and neurological problems including epilepsy, poor memory and concentration, dementia and Alzheimer's. It has antioxidant and anticholinergic actions and protects the brain from damage from poor circulation to the brain, ageing and injury. When inhaled, lavender oil has an action on the hypothalamus and the limbic system, particularly the amygdala and hippocampus, affecting mood and spirits. It can be helpful in depression and alter EEG brain patterns which are disturbed in epilepsy. It can lower blood pressure, slow heart and respiration rate and has a positive effect on memory, attention span and concentration

Lavender's relaxing qualities can also be felt in the digestive tract, where it can ease spasm and colic related to tension and anxiety. It can be taken in teas and tinctures or massaged as an oil into the abdomen to relieve wind, bloating, nausea, indigestion. It also stimulates the secretion of digestive enzymes, promoting appetite, digestion and absorption of nutrients Its antimicrobial actions help combat unfriendly gut bacteria and make lavender a good remedy for treating gut infections and disturbances of the gut flora and associated toxicity. The tea or tincture can also be taken for stomach and bowel infections causing vomiting and diarrhoea.

Lavender has an affinity with the respiratory tract. Its antimicrobial and anti-inflammatory effects can increase resistance to and help resolve respiratory tract infections. Lavender in teas and inhalations of the oil as well as vapour rubs on the chest can be used for colds, coughs, bronchitis, pneumonia, flu, sore throats, tonsillitis and laryngitis. Lavender has a decongesting and expectorant action, making it easier to clear phlegm from the chest in coughs and chest infections, and its antispasmodic and anti-inflammatory actions reduce swelling and constriction in the bronchi associated with asthma. When taken as hot tea, lavender causes sweating and reduces fevers associated with infections. It has a detoxifying effect in the body by increasing elimination of toxins through the pores of the skin and, because it also has mild diuretic properties, through the urine.

Lavender is a great herb for enhancing immunity. Its antibacterial, antifungal and antiseptic volatile oils account for its ancient use as a purifying and cleansing herb to ward off contagion, the plague as well as the evil eye. They are active against bacteria including *Diptheria, Typhoid, Streptococcus* and *Pneumococcus*. Rosmarinic acid has an antioxidant action, protecting the body against free radicals and exerting an anti-inflammatory effect.

Midwives have valued the pain-killing and antiseptic properties of lavender since medieval times and still do today. Its antispasmodic actions ease contractions and promote downward movement of the baby. Lavender used to be burned in delivery rooms as a disinfectant and used in baths to speed healing and relieve pain after childbirth. Lavender oil can be added to bath water to do just this.

Externally lavender and particularly lavender oil has become a household name for treatment of minor infections and as a first aid remedy. The antiseptic volatile oils make it a useful antiseptic for applying (as a dilute oil, strong infusion or tincture) to cuts and wounds, sores and ulcers. It makes a really good remedy for recurrent mouth ulcers, reducing pain and speeding repair of the lining of the mouth. It stimulates tissue repair and minimises scar formation when the neat oil is applied to burns and when diluted, to skin inflammation and infection as in eczema, acne and varicose ulcers.

The neat oil repels insects and can be used to relieve the pain and irritation of insect bites and stings. Diluted, it soothes pain and swelling of bruises, sprains, gouty and arthritic joints, and when used as a massage oil or added to the bath, it soothes away tension and spasm in the muscles. It can be rubbed onto the chest and used in inhalations for chest infections, coughs, colds and catarrh, flu, tonsillitis and laryngitis. The tea or tincture can be used as a gargle for

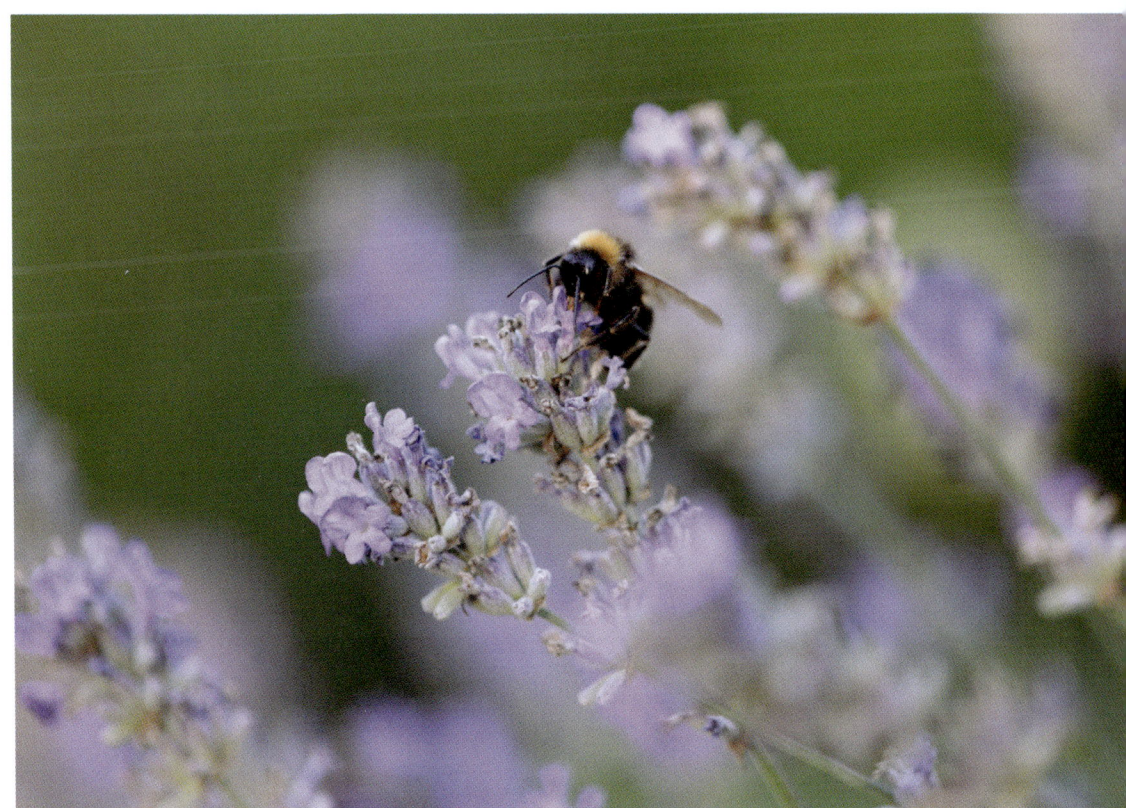

sore throats, tonsillitis and hoarseness, as a mouthwash for mouth ulcers and inflamed gums, and as a douche for leucorrhoea.

The Flower Essence
Lavender can be taken to balance the emotions, to relieve anxiety, depression and reduce stress and conflict. It is particularly recommended to those who have used the herb or the oil over a long period and have become used to it. The flower remedy could be added to enhance their effects.

It is also valuable for people involved in spiritual practices, for it calms the mind and helps to ease emotional conflicts blocking spiritual growth. Lavender is said to activate the crown chakra; it stimulates awareness and alertness and helps to connect people to their higher self.

Growing
Propagate by taking stem cuttings in spring or summer or by dividing the plant in autumn. Alternatively, you can layer older plants by mounding up soil around the stems. Lavender prefers poor light, well-drained soil and full sun. It grows up to 3 feet (90cm) and flowers in midsummer. Lavender makes a good low hedging shrub as well as a lovely border plant. Prune annually in spring or autumn to prevent straggly growth and bare stems.

Cautions
Avoid during pregnancy and breastfeeding. Caution with CNS depressants (including alcohol, opiates, benzodiazepines, anaesthetics, tricyclic anti-depressants, anti-epileptics).

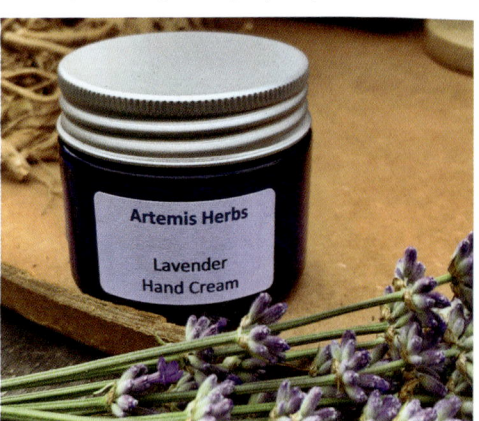

Recipes
Lavender oil or water is lovely for sprinkling on sheets, especially good for people with insomnia, and on clothes when you know you are going to face an especially trying day.

Lavender Water
Combine 4 cups of distilled water and 5 tablespoons vodka in a stainless steel or china bowl. Add 2 teaspoons of essential oil of lavender.

Aromatic Toilet Vinegar
Dry a good quantity of rose leaves, lavender flowers and jasmine flowers. Weigh them, and to every 4 oz of rose leaves allow 1 oz each of lavender and jasmine. Mix them well together, pour over them 2 pints of white vinegar, and shake well, then add ½ pint of rosewater and shake again. Stand aside for 10 days, then strain and bottle. (Mrs Grieves' A Modern Herbal)

Healing Salve for Eczema
A fragrant cream made from chamomile, calendula and lavender can soothe and heal at the same time. Chamomile is a wonderful anti-inflammatory herb and acts as an antihistamine. Calendula is one of the best herbs for the skin, cooling inflammation, speeding healing and helping to prevent infection, while delicate lavender has a marvellous ability to heal the skin without scarring and is antiseptic.

Equal parts of: Calendula petals, chamomile flowers and lavender flowers

Pour ½ pint /300mls of warmed almond oil into a bain marie (double saucepan) and add 30 grams of beeswax. Chop the herbs roughly and place as much as will fit into the oil and remain submerged and leave to macerate for a few hours over a low heat. After this time the oil will have absorbed the constituents and the mixture can be pressed through a muslin bag and the herb discarded. Whilst the oil is still warm, pour it into sterilised ointment jars where it will quickly solidify. Label it clearly and store in a cool place. Apply the cream night and morning after gently washing the area with rose water.

Leonurus cardiaca: Motherwort

The Flower of Mothers

*Venus owns this herb and it is under Leo.
There is no better herb to drive melancholy vapours from the heart,
to strengthen it and make the mind cheerful, blithe and merry*
– Nicolas Culpeper (1616–1654)

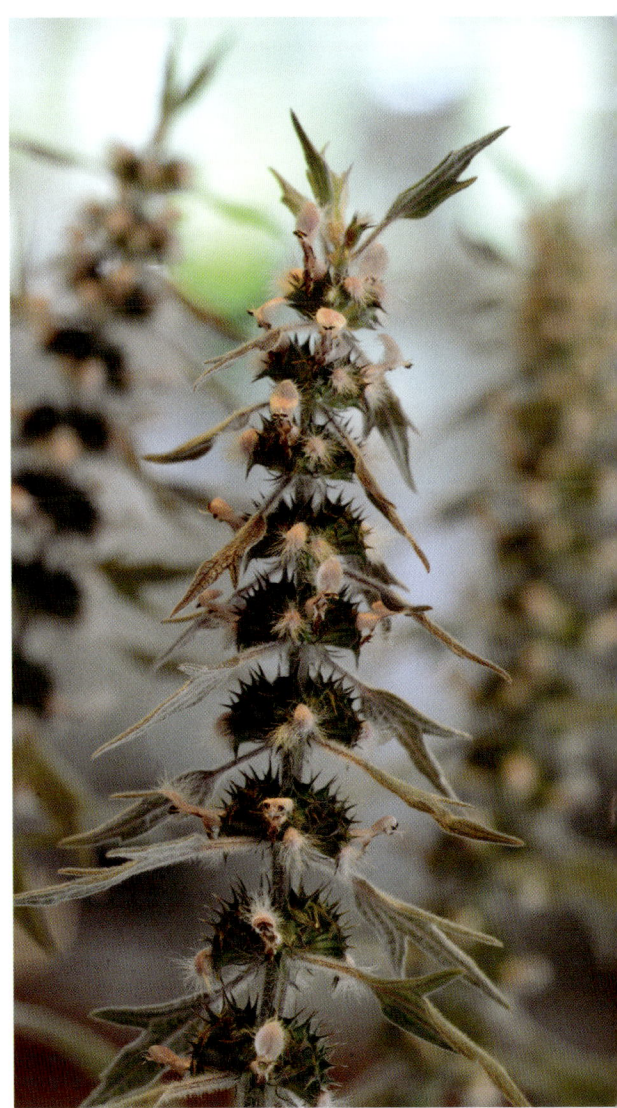

Other Names: Lions tail, lion's ear, throw wort, heart wort

Parts Used: Leaves, stems and flowers

Motherwort is an interesting member of the Lamiaceae/Labiatae family with its five-lobed leaves and whorls of pinkish flowers. A native perennial of central Asia and the United States, it can be found growing wild in many parts of Europe, on banks, paths and in hedgerows in gravelly or calcareous soil. It was named *Leonurus* from the Greek 'leon' meaning lion and 'oura' meaning tail, since it was thought that the leafy stem resembled a 'lion's tail' which is also one of its popular English names. A similar plant, *Leonurus heterophyllus,* is used in China. The Chinese name for motherwort is 'yi mu cao' meaning *benefit mother herb*. The leaves and flowers of motherwort are used in the West, while in Chinese herbal medicine the seeds are also used. Even though the use of motherwort developed separately in Western herbalism and traditional Chinese medicine, many of its uses are the same in both systems.

Motherwort has been praised since the ancient Greeks as a relaxing remedy for women and expectant mothers, which accounts for its name. It has been prescribed for painful or delayed periods and to prepare for childbirth. It has an affinity with the heart, hence its name *cardiaca* and since the Middle Ages, it has been used in Europe for heart palpitations and high blood pressure, and was considered excellent for strengthening and gladdening the heart. The English herbalist John Gerard (c. 1545–1612) said: "*Divers commend it against infirmities of the heart. Moreover, the same* is commended for green wounds." Its ability to lift the spirits, clear congestion from the chest, combat worms, relax tense muscles, relieve cramps and even convulsions was described by Culpeper (1616–1654),

There is no better herb to drive melancholy vapours from the heart, to strengthen it and make the mind cheerful, blithe and merry. May be kept in a syrup, or conserve, therefore the Latins call it cardiaca.... It cleansethe the chest of cold phlegm, oppressing it and killeth worms in the belly. It is of good use to warm and dry up the cold humours, to digest and disperse them that are settled in the veins, joints and sinews of the body and to help cramps and convulsions.

From such early writings, we can surmise that motherwort has been used as a blood thinner, a muscle relaxant, to regulate menstrual cycles, ease childbirth, lift the spirits and relieve low moods and postpartum depression. In China motherwort has also been used to regulate menstruation, and in Europe midwives have long used it for gynaecological problems including uterine infections, as well as to facilitate childbirth. It was called a 'partus praeparator' and was given to women for a few weeks prior to the birth, to prepare the uterus for the contractions of childbirth.

Herbal Remedy
Today, motherwort is still valued as a one of the best tonic herbs for women, valuable in the treatment of a wide range of disorders. The leaves and flowers are intensely bitter and contain triterpenes (including ursolic acid, ilelatifol D, corosolic acid and euscaphic acid), diterpenoids, iridoid glycosides (leonuride), alkaloids (stachydrin, leonurine), flavonoids, tannins, resins and vitamin A. They have relaxing and mildly sedative effects and are used for relieving a wide range of stress-related problems. In Traditional Chinese Medicine, motherwort has been used to promote longevity and strengthen the heart, just as in Western herbal medicine it is considered one of the best heart remedies.

Motherwort is an excellent remedy for the nervous system especially where it affects the reproductive system and the heart. It is good for calming the nerves and reducing tension and generalised anxiety without any clear cause, and can be thought of in any stress-related symptom including insomnia, muscle tension and cramp, heart palpitations, raised blood pressure, menstrual pain, menopausal symptoms, tension headaches, muscular twitches and spasms. One of the alkaloids, *leonurine,* may be responsible for some of these effects on account of its sedative, vasodilatory (opening the blood vessels) and muscle-relaxing properties. The iridoid glycosides, diterpenoids, flavonoids, tannins and essential oils also contribute.

As the name *cardiaca* suggests, its sedative effect is felt in the cardiovascular system and, combined with its hormone balancing effect, means that motherwort makes a good remedy for stress-related circulatory disorders such as nervous palpitations and irregular heart rate. It is particularly useful during menopause for palpitations associated with hot flushes and night sweats. Its vasodilatory action helps to reduce blood pressure and angina symptoms. It also reduces the tendency to blood clotting and atherosclerosis and can lower cholesterol. The ursolic acid has an antioxidant action which may account for much of its effect in the cardiovascular system. Motherwort is often compared to valerian root as far as their hypotensive and sedative properties are concerned. It may be that motherwort's ability to lower blood pressure is as much as three times as powerful as valerian root.

Motherwort has a regulatory effect on the thyroid and can reduce an overactive thyroid. In fact, motherwort has approval status by the German Commission E in cardiac disorders and hyperthyroidism. While most of the effects of motherwort are fairly quick acting, it may need to be taken over many months to help reduce overactivity of the thyroid.

Motherwort also benefits the emotional heart. It was traditionally renowned as a 'cordial' for lifting the spirits and for strengthening and 'gladdening' the heart. It is helpful when feeling downhearted or disheartened and may even help heartbreak. With its bitter taste and cooling effect, motherwort is a wonderfully cooling herb for the heart and mind and is especially recommended for hot, fiery mental and emotional problems, especially those with a hormonal component. It can soothe anxiety, anger and irritability and is a great remedy for PMS and menstrual headaches.

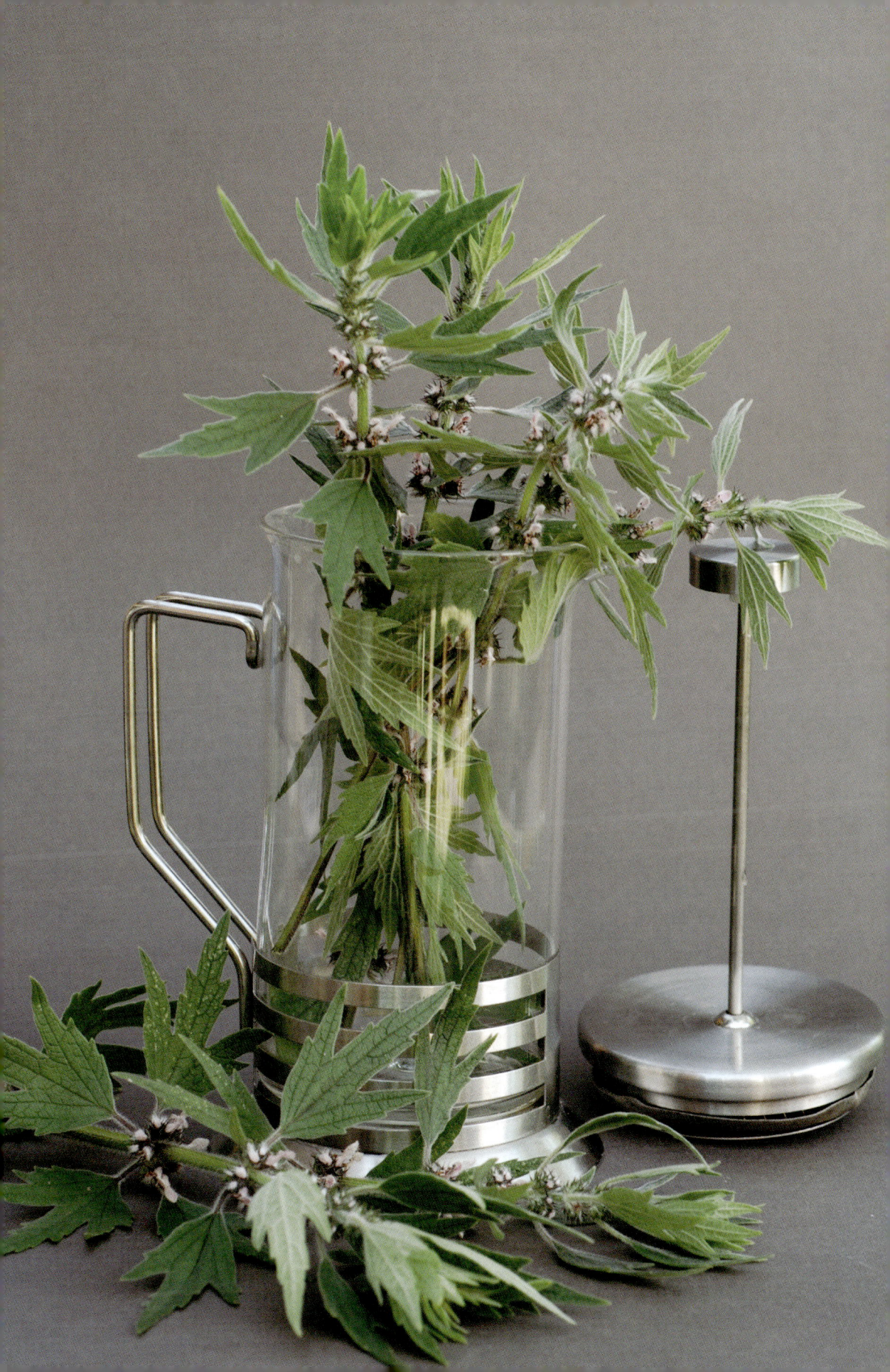

With its particular affinity with the female reproductive system, motherwort is still recommended for its relaxing and tonic effects on the uterus. Its antispasmodic effect on pelvic muscles means it is one of the best herbs for relieving period pain, cramps and vaginismus and it also helps to regulate periods. As an emmenagogue, it stimulates menstruation and may be helpful in amenorrhoea and scanty flow. It is thought to enhance fertility and was traditionally recommended to increase libido.

With its mildly sedative and muscle-relaxing effects, motherwort is recommended in the weeks prior to childbirth for tension or anxiety about the coming birth. It helps to prepare the uterine muscles for childbirth. Taken during the birth, it relaxes the uterus, and combined with other analgesic herbs such as chamomile, skullcap or valerian, it can help to relieve pain and stress. Taken afterwards, it helps prevent post-partum depression and infection, and it can stimulate the flow of breast milk. It can also be used to relieve menopausal symptoms like hot flushes, palpitations, nervous anxiety, sleep disturbances and depression.

The relaxant effects of motherwort may also be felt in the chest and could be useful in tight coughs and asthma. Its anti-inflammatory action can be helpful in sore throats and tonsillitis. In the digestive system, its bitter taste and cooling properties reduce heat and inflammation and make it a good remedy for treating indigestion, acidity, heartburn and gastritis. Its antispasmodic action helps to relieve spasms and cramps and is helpful in stress-related digestive problems. The presence of astringent tannins account for motherwort's ability to protect the gut against irritation and inflammation and curb diarrhoea.

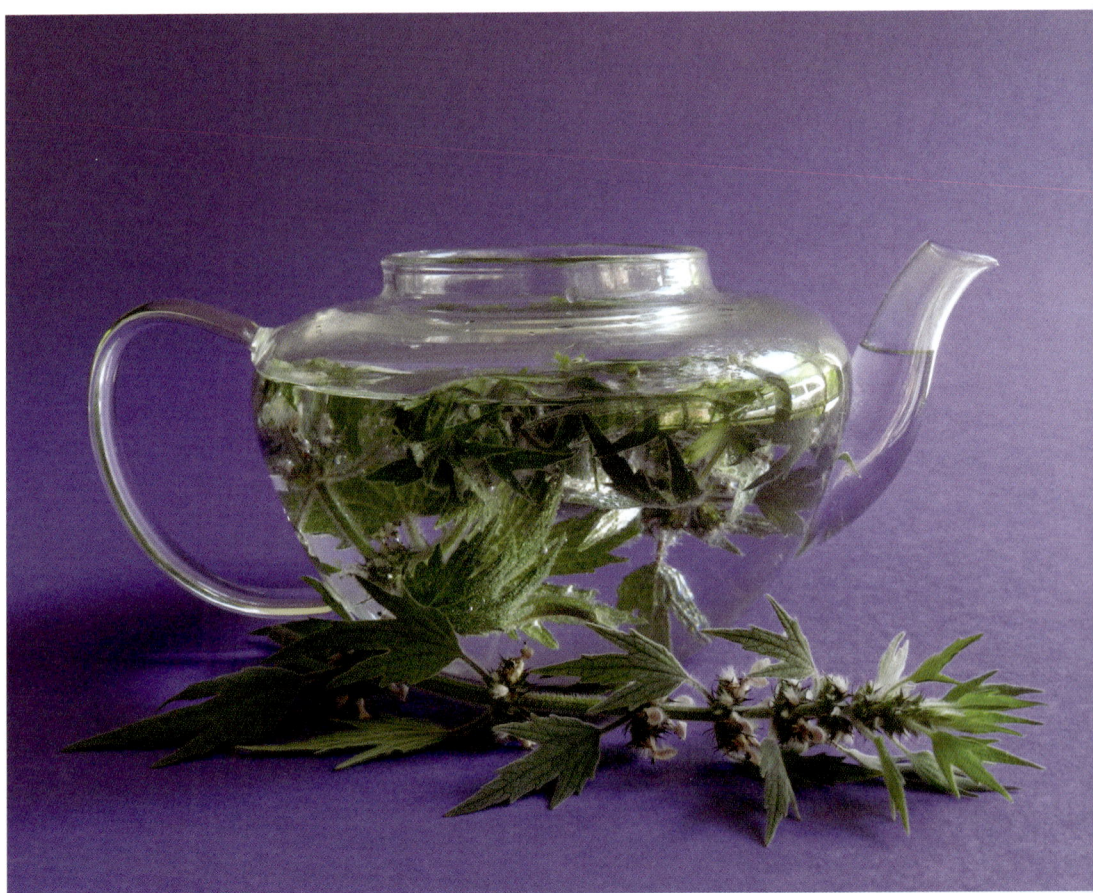

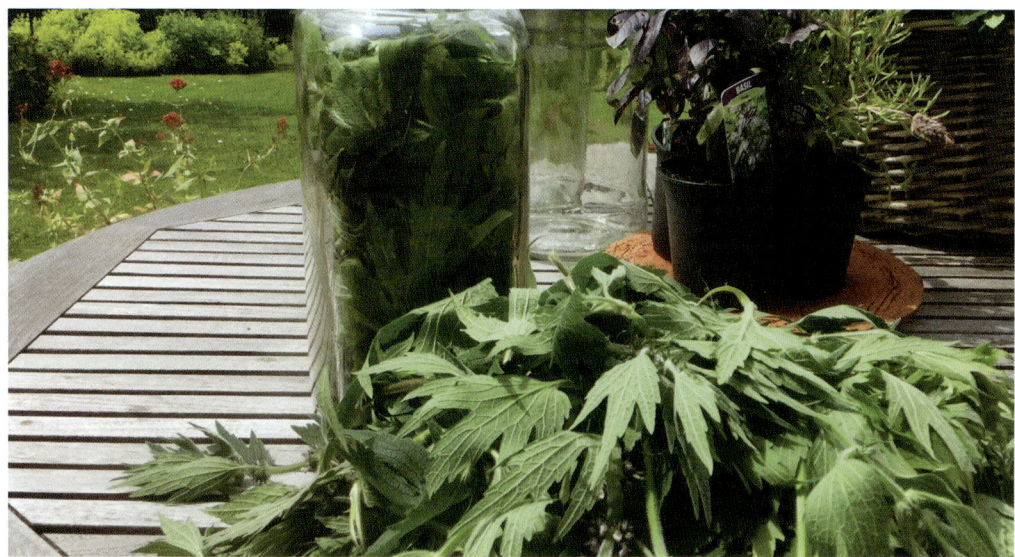

Motherwort enhances immunity and has been found to be active against bacteria and viruses including *Staphylococcus aureus*, *E. coli, Epstein Barr* and *Herpes,* as well as fungal infections. The ursolic acid may inhibit viruses, reduce the risk of cardiovascular problems as well as cancers including leukaemia, lung, breast and colon cancer. Along with other constituents in motherwort including ilelatifol D, corosolic acid and euscaphic acid, it has an anti-inflammatory effect and antioxidant action, reducing damage to the body caused by free radicals, which may contribute to its anticancer action. The anti-inflammatory actions can be helpful in gout and arthritis.

Externally a tea or dilute tincture can be used as a douche or lotion for vaginal infections such as thrush and vaginitis. In Nepal, the leaves are pounded and then applied between the toes to treat fungal infections that are related to walking barefoot in water during the rainy season.

Flower Essence
As a flower remedy, motherwort can be used for pain associated with the emotional heart; for the loss of someone close, the break-up of a relationship, feeling disheartened, downhearted or broken hearted. It could also be helpful to those who find it hard to love themselves and tend to be self-critical. It can be helpful for nervous anxiety and emotional exhaustion especially around the menopause.

Edible Uses
Motherwort leaves and flowers are quite bitter especially as they get older, and once the flowers have begun to go over, they become rather spikey. However, when the leaves are young, motherwort can be used as a vegetable and in soups, and has been eaten in the East with lentil or split peas dishes. Motherwort has also been used for flavouring beer.

Growing
Propagate by sowing seeds in spring or autumn, or by dividing roots. Grows 3 – 5' (90 – 150cm) high and flowers midsummer to mid-autumn. Prefers well-drained, light, calcareous soil and full sun. Self-seeds easily.

Related plant
Leonurus sibiricus: Chinese motherwort – a bitter diuretic, simulates uterus and circulation.

Cautions
Used as a herbal remedy, motherwort might increase menstrual flow. Avoid in early pregnancy. Only use a few weeks prior to the birth. Avoid in bleeding disorders, breast cancer. It can cause allergic reactions. Caution with anticoagulants, Digoxin, CNS depressants (including alcohol, opiates, benzodiazepines, anaesthetics, tricyclic anti-depressants and anti-epileptic drugs). Motherwort may decrease absorption and diuretic response to furosemide.

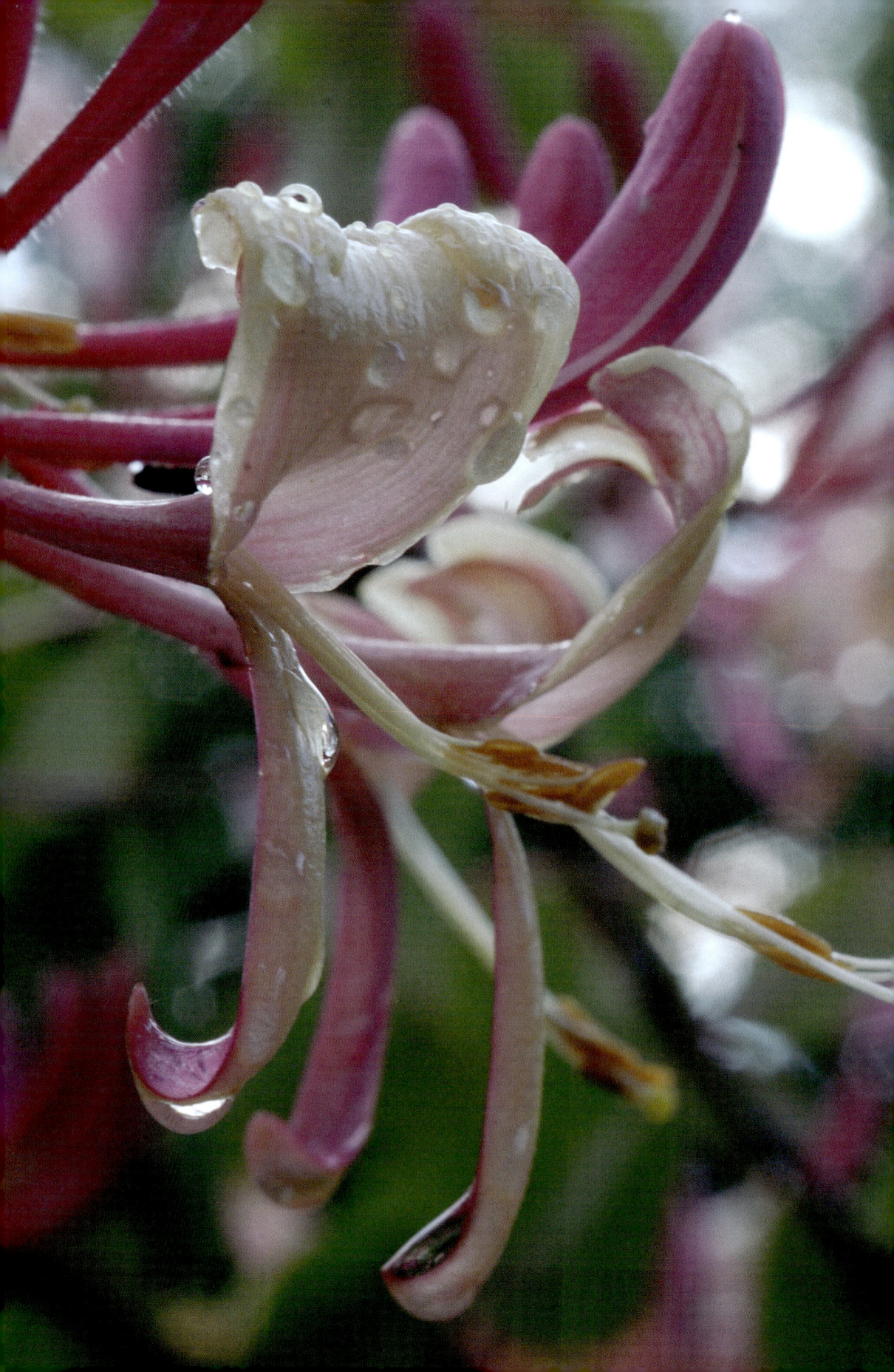

Lonicera japonica, L. periclymenum: Honeysuckle

The Flower of Unity

> *I am drunk with the honey wine*
> *Of the moon-unfolded eglantine*
> *which fairies catch in hyacinth bowls*
> – Percy Bysshe Shelley (1792–1822)

Other names: Woodbine, woodbind, herb of immortality, eglantine, bindweed, Irish vine, trumpet flower, caprifole, honeybind, goat's leaves, Japanese honeysuckle, jin yin hua, honeyberry, blue honeysuckle, sweet berry honeysuckle, edible honeysuckle and haskap

Parts Used: Leaves and flowers

Honeysuckle has been much loved through the centuries for its sweet scent which pervades the warm summer air in gardens, and woods and hedgerows where it can grow wild. It belongs to the Caprifoliaceae family. Its name 'honeysuckle' is one of the oldest English flower names, dating back to at least the early 8th century, and it clearly comes from its honey-sweet fragrance which has inspired many a poet and writer through the ages. Its name also tells us that you can suck the honeyed nectar from the centre of the flower. Its old name 'woodbine' or 'woodbind' describes its twining, climbing nature, scrambling through hedges and woods or winding up garden arches with seemingly inexhaustible energy, for not only does it grow apace, but blooms for a long season. Interestingly, the Chinese believe that honeysuckle increases the span of life. In other cultures, it was known as the 'herb of immortality' because of its ability to flourish even when rigorously cut back.

To our ancestors, honeysuckle's clinging nature represented love and the bonds of devoted affection, and in the language of flowers it means 'we are united in love'. Shakespeare knew all about the symbolism of flowers when he had Titania say in *A Midsummer Nights's Dream*,

Sleep thou, and I will winde thee in my arms,
so doth the woodbine, the sweet honeysuckle
gently entwist; the female ivy so
enrings the barky fingers of the elm.
O, how I love thee! How I dote on thee!

Its sweet fragrance symbolises sweetness of disposition while the heady perfume of wild honeysuckle that might well have turned a maiden's head is a symbol of inconstancy of love. Parents used to forbid their teenage daughters to bring honeysuckle into the house, as it was said to evoke erotic dreams. John Parkinson in his book *Paradisus Terrestris* describes why he, unlike many others since, would not transplant the wild honeysuckle into his garden, *"The honeysuckle that groweth wilde in every hedge, although it be very sweete, ye doe I not bring it into my garden, but let it reste in its owne place, to serve their senses that travell by it or have no garden".*

The name *Lonicera* honours Adam Lonicer, a German botanist of the 16th century. Goats are fond of honeysuckle which itself climbs as nimbly as a goat. The Latin word for goat is 'capra' from which we get the name 'caprifolium'. *Periclymenum* comes from *Periclymenus*, one of the Argonauts in the Greek myths, who had the power to change his shape at will. The honeysuckle flower changes shape and colour daily to attract butterflies and night-flying moths to assist in pollination.

Honeysuckle is one of the oldest medicinal herbs in known history. Of the 100 or so species of honeysuckle, around 12 can be used medicinally

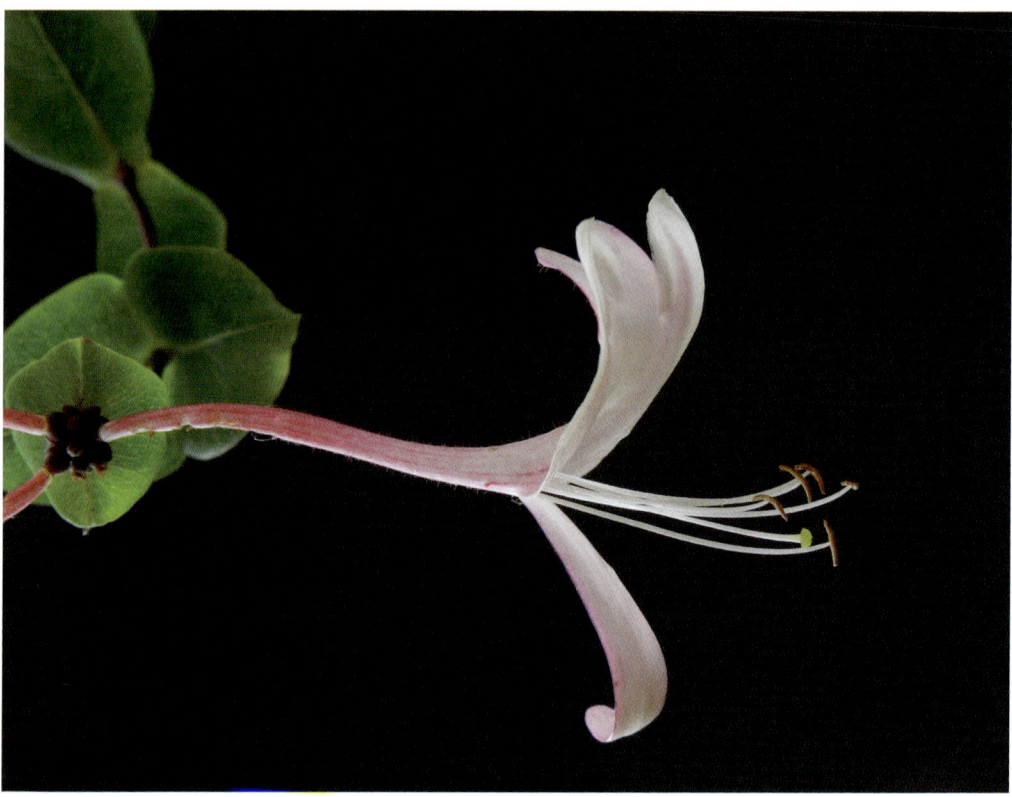

and two have a long history of traditional medicine: European honeysuckle (*Lonicera periclymenum*) and Japanese honeysuckle (*Lonicera japonica*). The use of European honeysuckle has been recorded as early as 659AD for removing heat and fever for reasons ranging from snake bites to childbirth. Japanese honeysuckle, known in China as 'jin yin hua' has been used historically in Traditional Chinese Medicine to treat a range of problems including fevers, diarrhoea and skin infections.

A syrup of the flowers is an old remedy for asthma, croup and irritating coughs. Gerard recommended honeysuckle for hardness of the spleen, shortness of breath, hiccoughs and 'wearisomeness'. Culpeper wrote a long list of ills remedied by honeysuckle, including cramps, convulsions, 'palsies', asthma, 'evil of the spleen' and sunburn and recommended it for speedy delivery in childbirth. He said, *"it is a herb of Mercury and appropriated to the lungs; the celestial Crab claims dominion over it, neither is it a foe to the Lion; if the lungs be afflicted by Jupiter, this is your cure".*

Herbal Remedy

All parts of honeysuckle can be used as medicine and both varieties of honeysuckle described have similar properties. They contain essential oils including borneol, mucilage, glucoside, salicylic acid, flavonoids, alkaloids, phenolic acids, terpenes and steroids. The leaves and flower buds are rich in salicylic acid, meaning that they can be used for symptoms that are relieved by aspirin, such as colds and flu, fevers, headaches, aches and pains including period pains and inflammatory problems including arthritis.

The leaves and flowers not only have anti-inflammatory properties, but also enhance immunity and the fight against infection. They contain antimicrobial compounds active against bacteria including *Staphlococci, Salmonella* and *Coli bacilli*. The high concentration of the terpene called aromadendrene found in honeysuckle contributes to this antibacterial action, as do chlorogenic acid, luteolin and isochlorogenic acid present in the stem. Japanese honeysuckle may have a more significant antimicrobial action. It also has hepatoprotective (protecting the liver), cryoprotective (cold protective), antioxidative and antiviral properties. It is traditionally used in China to clear damp heat and toxins. It enhances immunity and promotes longevity and may protect against breast cancer. Its anti-inflammatory and immune-enhancing actions could be attributed to its antioxidant properties which reduce oxidative stress.

Honeysuckle is an excellent and often forgotten remedy for respiratory and gastro-intestinal infections. Its antimicrobial action is active against cold and flu viruses and several bacteria including TB. It is used with *Forsythia suspensa* in Chinese medicine for infections including tonsillitis, pneumonia, TB and middle ear infection. With added anti-inflammatory, expectorant, decongestant and antispasmodic properties, it is useful for spasm and phlegm and can be helpful in asthma, croup, whooping cough, bronchitis and chest infections. The Japanese use the flowers for sore throats, colds, flu, tonsillitis, bronchitis and pneumonia. A hot infusion of the flowers is decongestant and beneficial for fevers, colds, catarrh, sinusitis, coughs and bronchial congestion.

The plant has a calming effect on the nervous system and is useful where anxiety or tension gives rise to symptoms such as asthma, headaches or stomach cramps. It can also lift mood and boost mental energy and might be helpful in mild depression and for easing feelings such as grief. The Russians apparently prepare an oil from the wood, which they use for tumours and chronic pain. The flowers contain luteolin, a flavonoid with strong antiviral, antioxidant and anti-inflammatory properties that can help protect the brain from neurological impairment and the body generally from oxidative stress. Its antispasmodic effects relax muscle tension, so honeysuckle can be thought of in stress-related problems, particularly those affecting the gut. It has a mild laxative action, but with its anti-inflammatory, astringent and antimicrobial actions, it is also useful for disturbances of the gut flora, diarrhoea, dysentery, food poisoning and inflammatory gut problems including ulcerative colitis and Crohn's disease.

Other constituents, notably chlorogenic and isochlorogenic acids, help reduce blood sugar levels and regulate blood pressure. This means that honeysuckle could be helpful in preventing and treating diabetes. Its antioxidant and anti-inflammatory actions could be helpful in symptoms caused by diabetes, including neuropathy and eye problems. Another compound called inositol plays a role in maintaining the health of the insulin receptors cells, so that insulin can do its job of acting on cell walls to allow the entry of glucose into the cell. If receptors do not work properly, more insulin is released which can lead to insulin resistance and increase the risk of diabetes.

By improving insulin sensitivity, honeysuckle could be helpful in the treatment of polycystic ovaries (PCOS). Inositol also plays an important role in the reproductive system, as it increases levels of SHBG (sex hormone binding globulin) which takes up free testosterone in the bloodstream, and this is also helpful in the treatment of PCOS. With its cooling effect, it is helpful in menopausal hot flushes and prickly heat.

The leaves and flowers have diuretic properties and relieve fluid retention, and with their painkilling and anti-inflammatory effect, they can be helpful in cystitis, irritable bladder, urinary stones and gout. They help to clear toxins from the system via the urinary system and have a cooling action generally, helpful in the treatment of skin problems including spots, boils, acne, psoriasis and eczema.

The fruits in some varieties including *Lonicera caerulea* are edible. They are rich in phenolic compounds and flavonoids called anthocyanins which have an antioxidant action, important for reducing inflammation and preventing problems including atherosclerosis (hardening of the arteries), heart disease, cancer and eye conditions related to ageing. They also relieve inflammation and play a part in regulating metabolism and brain function. Apparently, there are two grams of flavonoids in every hundred grams of the dry fruit, which is similar to blackberries, elderberries, cranberries and blueberries.

Externally honeysuckle leaves and flowers can be used in washes, lotions and creams for the skin. Its antibacterial and anti-inflammatory actions can be helpful in rashes, eczema, psoriasis, pityriasis, rosea, spots and acne. It can improve skin thickness, barrier functions and collagen production and be used for blemishes, areas of hyper-pigmentation and bruises. A cooled infusion or dilute tincture can be made into gargles for sore throats and mouthwashes for mouth ulcers, and an infusion used as eyewashes for sore or inflamed eyes.

Both types of honeysuckle are used as natural preservatives in food and natural or organic skincare, due to their antiviral and antibacterial properties.

Aromatherapy Oil
With its wonderful sweet floral aroma, the essential oil has many of the same properties as the herbal remedy. It can be used for the nerves, to ease stress and anxiety and balance mood. It can be used as an anti-inflammatory in massage oils for pain relief, soothing aching joints and sore muscles and can be helpful in back and neck ache and arthritis. You can add a few drops with Epsom salts to the bath, to relieve muscle stiffness and pain.

Honeysuckle oil can be used in inhalations for colds, catarrh, coughs, bronchial and sinus congestion and headaches. This can also be good for cleaning the pores of the skin and improving the complexion.

Homeopathic Remedy
Lonicera periclymenum (leaves) is used only for irritability and violent outbursts of temper while Lonicera xylosteum (berries) is used for a wider range of symptoms, notably profuse vomiting and diarrhoea, spasms and convulsions. A patient needing Lonicera xylosteum may have a fever with profuse cold sweat and cold extremities, and convulsions – jerking and trembling of the whole body, while apparently unable to see or hear. The eyes are red, the pupil of one eye dilated, the other contracted, the face is red, lips dry and there is great thirst while the tongue is moist, and respiration is rapid and deep. Such symptoms may also accompany kidney problems causing uraemia.

Flower Remedy
Lonicera caprifolium is used as a Bach flower remedy and is particularly suited to those who live in the past and cling to pleasant memories of events gone by, unable to enter fully into the present. Honeysuckle people tend to glorify the past, only remembering the good things and wish that the good old days could return or feel unhappy that they cannot. They may find it very hard to get over the loss of a loved one, particularly if they are elderly, closing themselves to the possibility of new relationships; they may yearn for their old home after a move, or for younger days when they were happy and successful; honeysuckle children may feel very homesick when away at friends' or boarding school or on a school trip. Honeysuckle people may also get stuck in regretful feelings about the past, about missed opportunities or unhappy occurrences or about getting old. The flower remedy helps to bring such people into the present and help them to let go of the past or bring it into perspective so that they can benefit from lessons learnt from experience. Honeysuckle increases the capacity for change and enhances openness to opportunities offered in the present.

Edible Uses
Honeysuckle flowers have a sweet nectar in the centre, which can be sucked directly from them. They can be added to fruit salads, blended into drinks and used as an edible decoration on cakes and desserts. The berries are best avoided as they can be purgative and cathartic and very bitter.

The flower tea has a sweet taste with a hint of vanilla, but if you add more leaves and stem, it can be more astringent and slightly bitter.

Recipes

Honeysuckle Oil Hair Conditioner
Honeysuckle oil in a base of coconut oil can soften the hair and remedy dry ends.

It can protect hair from the effects of harsh chemicals and detergents in commercial shampoos, and from hair dryers and other damaging treatments.

Mix a teaspoon of coconut oil with 5 drops of honeysuckle oil, rub between your hands and then smooth it through the ends of your hair, avoiding the roots. Dry, brittle hair becomes supple, soft and strong.

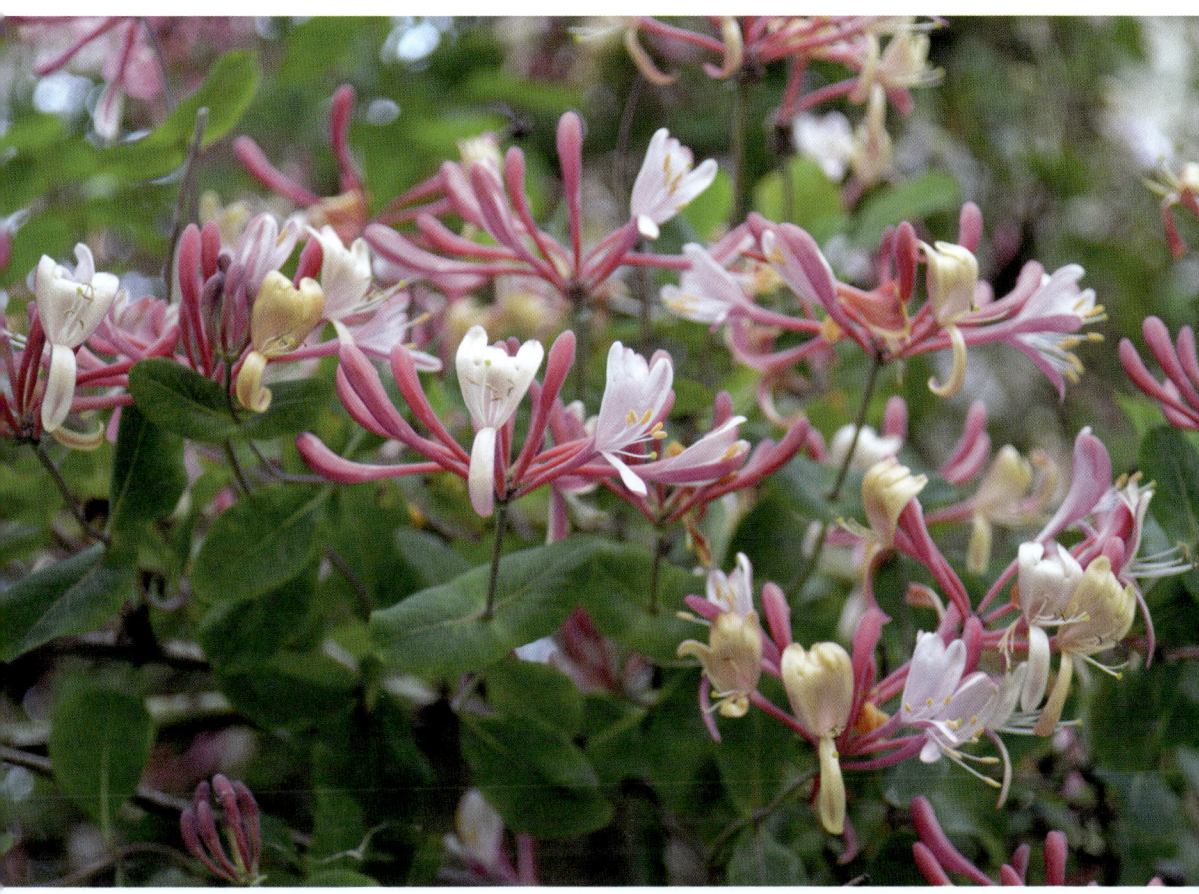

Cleaning Agent
You can use honeysuckle oil as a sweet-smelling antiseptic cleaning agent.

In a spray bottle, mix a few drops of honeysuckle essential oil with 1 cup of white vinegar and 1 cup of water.

Salt Scrub for Vibrant Healthy Skin
10 drops of honeysuckle essential oil
10 drops of grapefruit essential oil
1 cup of pink Himalayan salt
1 tablespoon of hemp oil

Mix together and store in a jar.

Growing
Propagate by sowing seeds in pots in autumn. Germination can be slow. Alternatively, you can take cuttings in summer. Prune and mulch with plenty of compost in springtime. Grows in most good soils, in sun or shade. Needs training up walls, trellis etc. Grows up to 20' (6m) and flowers in summer.

Related Plants
L. caprifolium: yellow flowers and orange berries, similarly antiseptic, diuretic and expectorant.
L. nigra: hardwood shrub, black berries and orange flowers, used in homeopathic medicine.

Honeysuckle branches have been used to make interesting walking sticks. The sticks form naturally as the honeysuckle entwines itself around its branches, causing the branches to become twisted. They used to be popular with Scots music hall performers.

Cautions
Avoid honeysuckle essential oil in pregnancy, breastfeeding and children. Dilute honeysuckle essential oil with a carrier oil to avoid skin sensitivity. Honeysuckle oil may cause photosensitivity. Overconsumption of honeysuckle can cause a laxative effect. Berries produced by some species of honeysuckle are poisonous and should not be eaten. Make sure of the identity of plants used.

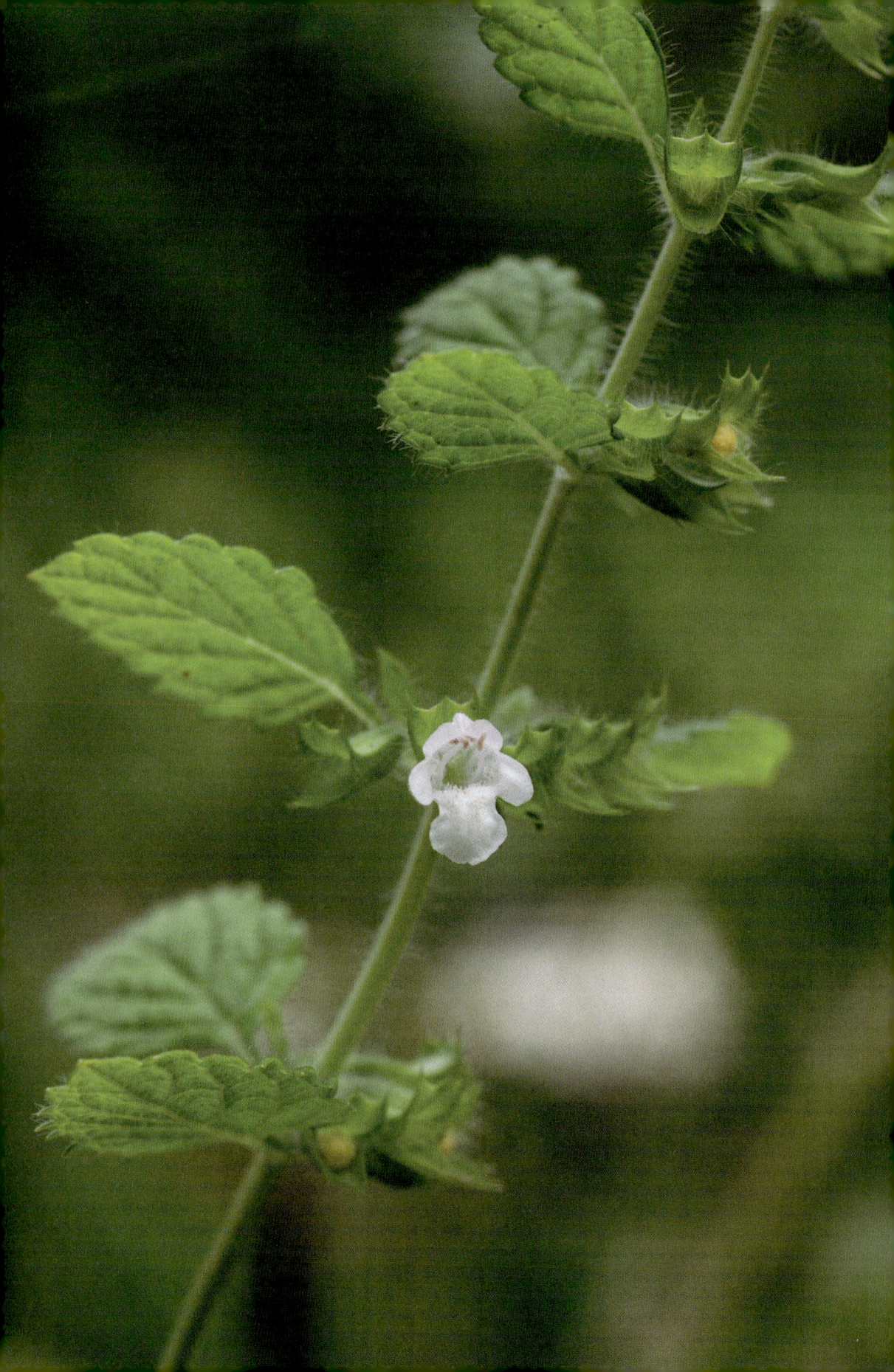

Melissa officinalis: Lemon Balm

The Flower of Bees

Lemon balm causeth the mind and heart to become merry.
– Nicolas Culpeper 1616–1654

Other Names: Melissa, bee balm, sweet balm, cure-all, balm, English balm, garden balm, balm mint, common balm, melissa, heart's delight, honey plant

Parts Used: Leaves, stems and flowers

This delightful lemon-scented plant is a member of the Lamiaceae/Labiatae family, a relative of mint and sage and a favourite in cottage gardens. Lemon balm is an excellent plant for attracting bees into the garden. It was called *Melissa* by the Greeks, as the word means honeybee. Beekeepers still rub their hives with lemon balm to attract bees. Pliny the Elder, the first century Roman naturalist, wrote that lemon balm planted near beehives would encourage bees to return. Later, the English herbalist John Gerard (1545-1612) said rubbing the leaves on a beehive *"causeth the bees to keep together and causeth others to come unto them."*

Lemon balm has long been associated with the feminine, the moon and water and was considered a sacred herb in the temple of the ancient Greek goddess Artemis and Roman goddess Diana at Ephesus in Turkey. In ancient Greek mythology, the 'great goddess' was closely related to the bee. She was said to be the 'the queen bee' and her image in outline was considered to resemble that of the bee. Her priestesses were called 'melissai'. The honeybee was considered to be the form a human soul took when descending from the goddess Artemis herself.

We know that the ancient Greeks and Romans used lemon balm medicinally and knowledge of the herb was recorded as far back as 300 BC in Theophrastus's *Historia Plantarum*. Since lemon balm is native to the eastern Mediterranean, the Arabs were among the first to extol its virtues. The first century Greek physician, Dioscorides, said that lemon balm promoted menstruation and could remedy gout, toothaches, scorpion stings and dog bites.

Lemon balm was probably brought to Spain by the Moors in the 7th century and by the Middle Ages it was cultivated and used throughout Europe. It featured in Middle Eastern remedies for epilepsy and mental illness, apoplexy, lethargy and melancholia. The medieval Arabs used it in their elixirs of life and Carmelite nuns made it into Carmelite tea and water in 17th century Paris, to promote longevity. This can now be explained by the presence of antioxidant substances in the plant, most likely rosmarinic acid. Carmelite water was made from lemon balm with lemon peel, nutmeg and angelica root and was a traditional remedy when nervousness, agitation or depression caused heart pains, palpitations or an irregular heartbeat.

Early herbalists praised lemon balm for its uplifting qualities. The Romans valued it as a medicine to clear the mind, improve memory and lift the spirits. The eleventh century Persian physician and philosopher, Avicenna, recommended it for treating depression or melancholy. According to an old Arabian proverb, *"Balm makes the heart merry and joyful."* Swiss physician and alchemist Paracelsus (1493-1541) said, *"Essence of balm given in Canary wine every morning will renew youth, strengthen the brain, relieve languishing nature and prevent baldness"* while John Evelyn said, *"Balm is sovereign for the brain, strengthening memory and powerfully chasing away melancholy."* Later herbalist John Gerard wrote, *"Bawme drunken in wine is good against the bitings of venomous beasts, comforts the heart, and driveth away all melancholy and sadness."*

Nicholas Culpeper (1616–1654) said the juice of lemon balm *"glueth together green wounds"* and would remedy boils, cure melancholy and was good for the heart, mind, liver, spleen, digestion and fainting. According to the London Dispensatory (1696) lemon balm in wine could prevent baldness. It was recommended to Oxford students in the 16th century to drive away 'heaviness of mind' and to sharpen understanding; in fact, it was known as 'the scholars' herb'.

In Europe, lemon balm was used as a strewing herb and was tossed on floors to freshen rooms. It was strewn amongst church pews until the nineteenth century. In the Victorian language of flowers, lemon balm could be added to a tussie mussie or floral bouquet to signify pleasant company of friends, memories, a cure, and *"don't misuse me."*

Herbal Remedy

Lemon balm is a delightful plant and a wonderfully palatable remedy with its lemon-scented taste and smell. It contains volatile oils (citronellal, citral, geraniol, linalool, pinene, limonene, nerol), flavonoids (isoquercetrin), hydroxycinnamic acids (rosmarinic, courmaric, caffeic, chlorogenic acids), polyphenols, tannins, bitters and minerals. Its flavour and aroma are due largely to the volatile oils citral and citronellal, although other phytochemicals, including rose scented geraniol and lavender scented linalool, also contribute to its scent.

Refreshing lemon balm, once a main ingredient in elixirs of life, is a wonderful herb for the heart and mind and a lovely cooling remedy for all conditions of excess heat. It influences the limbic system in the brain, which is concerned with mood and temperament. It is excellent to take when stress causes anxiety, fear of failure, low self-esteem, insomnia and depression. Its relaxing and sedative actions ease tension and

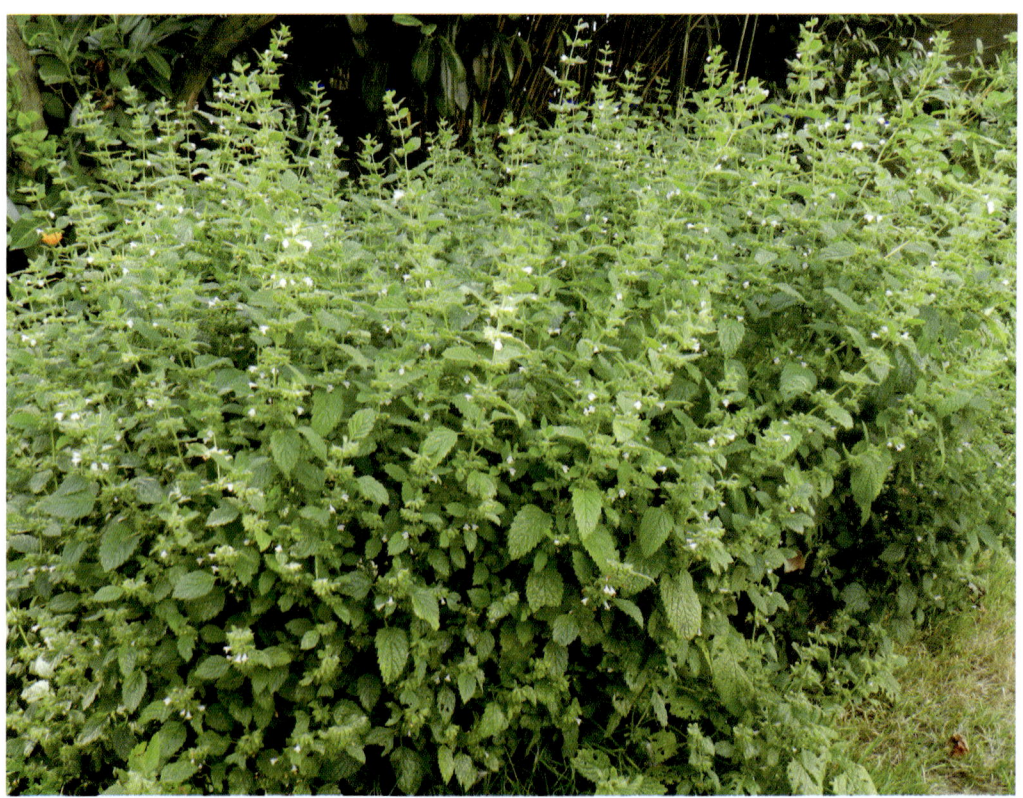

anxiety, even mania and hysteria, enhance relaxation and induce natural sleep. Part of the calming effect of lemon balm may be attributed to the constituent apigenin. Lemon balm can be taken as tea frequently through the day and also at night for insomnia. The dried leaves are a frequent component in sleep pillows. A strong infusion in a warm bath at night will help calm excitable children.

Lemon balm is also restoring. It lifts the spirits, improves memory and helps tired brains to concentrate. It is excellent when studying or working, it soothes stress and exam nerves and can relieve nervous headaches, migraine, vertigo, tinnitus, insomnia and neuralgia. Lemon balm also influences the heart and can be used to calm nervous palpitations and hypertension.

Lemon balm is an excellent remedy for a whole range of infections, bacterial and viral, including colds and flu, *Herpes simplex,* mumps and possibly HIV. It has anti-inflammatory, antifungal and antihistamine action and is a good herb for treating allergies such as hay fever and eczema. Lemon balm contains tannins, which are astringent and contribute to lemon balm's antiviral effects, and eugenol acetate, which is probably responsible for lemon balm's antispasmodic effect. Its relaxant effects and mucus-reducing properties are helpful in the treatment of catarrhal congestion, chest infections, harsh, dry irritating coughs and asthma. Taken in hot infusion, its diaphoretic action promotes sweating and helps to reduce fevers and clear catarrhal congestion.

Lemon balm has an anti-inflammatory action and a thyroid inhibitory effect, useful in the management of hyperthyroidism. Several of the constituents in lemon balm may contribute to its antioxidant action and anti-inflammatory effects. These include phenolic acids, terpenes, rosmarinic acid and caffeic acids. Together they help to protect the body against damage caused by free radicals and oxidative stress, and in this way help to prevent a wide range of problems associated with the ageing process including cardiovascular disease, diabetes, degenerative disease including arthritis, cancer, and loss of memory and brain function. Lemon balm has particular affinity with the digestive system and is excellent for remedying stress-related digestive problems. It cools inflammation and soothes nervous indigestion, gastritis and peptic ulcers, colic, wind, IBS, nausea, diarrhoea and constipation. It also benefits the liver and gallbladder. A mild infusion is excellent for children's nervous tummy upsets.

In the reproductive system, lemon balm's antispasmodic action helps relax tense muscles and relieve painful periods and with its sedative and mood elevating effect, it can be used for irritability associated with premenstrual tension. It also helps to regulate periods. During the weeks prior to childbirth, it can be taken to help prepare for the birth, to ease and speed the process and reduce pain. With its cooling and uplifting properties, it can also help relieve menopausal flushes and depression. Its antiviral action is applicable to genital *Herpes* which responds well to internal and topical application. A relaxing, antimicrobial diuretic, lemon balm can be taken in luke-warm to cool infusions to treat urinary tract infections, irritation, pain and burning in the bladder.

It has long been said that lemon balm was called *Melissa* by the Greeks as the word means *honeybee*, because it would attract bees to the hive. Interestingly, lemon balm contains several compounds found in the worker honeybee's nasonov gland, which helps bees communicate about food sources and hive location. Both contain citral and geraniol, and honeybee pheromone contains nerolic acid, which is similar to the nerol found in *Melissa officinalis*.

Externally a strong infusion in a warm bath or inhalation of the essential oil at night will help calm excitable children and can be used as a wash for cuts and wounds. Its ability to combat bacterial infections makes it useful for surgical dressings. When diluted, the essential oil can be massaged into the lower abdomen to relieve period pains, and into muscles elsewhere to ease tension and pain. It can also help joint pain and neuralgia.

As an antiviral remedy the dilute oil is effective when used topically for mumps and *Herpes* (cold sores and shingles blisters). It also relieves wasp and bee stings. Its antihistamine action is helpful for allergy sufferers and it can be used in creams for allergic skin conditions such as eczema, and urticaria. The dried leaves are a frequent

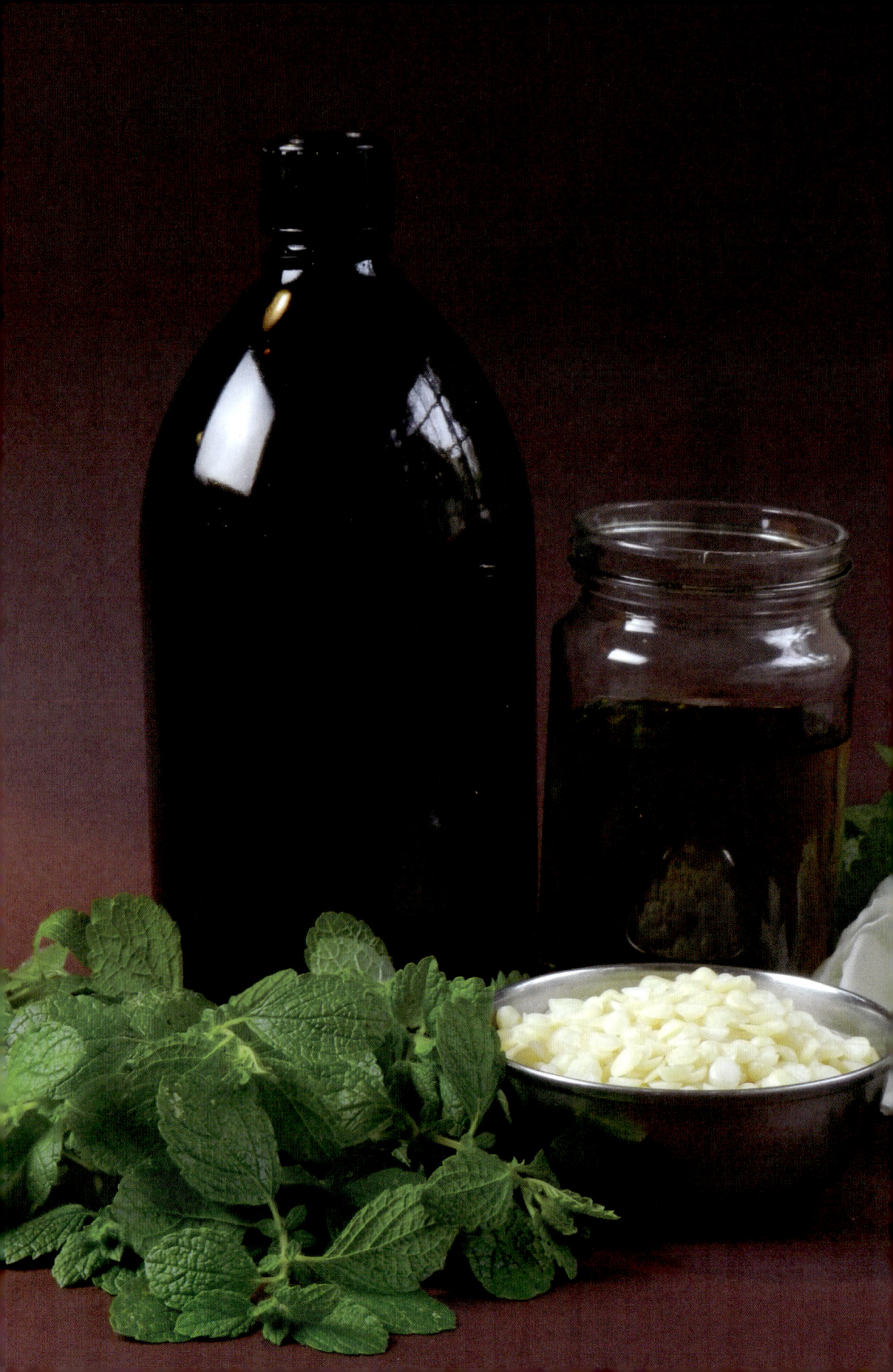

component in sleep pillows. The diluted essential oil can be used in ear drops for infections and in mouthwashes for gum infections and toothache.

Aromatherapy Oil
Like the herbal remedy, Melissa oil calms and slows the heart, relieving palpitations and reducing high blood pressure. While it has relaxant properties, it also acts as a tonic and rejuvenative. It can be used to calm nervousness and anxiety, release tension and tension headaches, and relieve insomnia. It makes a good digestive particularly in stress-related problems such as colic and indigestion. Its antihistamine action is helpful for allergy sufferers and it can be used in creams for allergic skin conditions, and relieves wasp and bee stings.

As an antiviral remedy, the dilute oil can be massaged into the skin in mumps and cold sores. It is cooling for fevers, and makes an antimicrobial inhalant for colds, catarrh, coughs and chest infections. Its antispasmodic action relieves harsh irritating coughs and asthma. Massaged into the lower abdomen it relieves period pains, and generally relaxes muscles and eases tension pain. It will help joint pain and neuralgia. The oil can be used in eardrops for infections and in mouthwashes for gum infections and toothache.

Flower Essence
Just as Paracelsus recommended lemon balm to renew youth, strengthen the brain and relieve a languishing nature, so too the flower essence can help to renew health and vigour, lift the spirits and balance the emotions. It is excellent for those whose health and strength have been depleted by stress or overconcern for other people, restricting their lives and inhibiting their spiritual growth. Restoring and relaxing, it gives support during emotional difficulties and increases inner strength and courage.

Edible Uses
The leaves and flowers can be added to flavour summer drinks and fruit cups, soups, stews, casseroles, meat and vegetable dishes, and make a delicious tea. They can be added to salads, butters, cheeses, fish, egg dishes, vegetables, jams and jellies, sauces and marinades, dressings

Recipes

Lemon Balm Infused Oil
Fill a jar with dried lemon balm. Cover the herb with olive oil or almond oil and use a tightly fitting lid. Shake it daily for 2 weeks then strain the oil through a piece of muslin or a fine sieve.

Add a few drops of vitamin E and refrigerate to extend its shelf life.

Lip Balm
Melt 1 ounce of beeswax in a pot.
Add 1 cup of lemon balm infused oil

Stir and heat on low until melted and mixed well. Pour the balm into tins or small jars.

and herb vinegars, cakes and tarts, sorbets and ice cream, fruit dishes and summer drinks.

Growing
Propagate by sowing seeds in moist fertile soil and full sun or light shade or divide the plant in the autumn. Cut back in the summer to encourage a fresh supply of leaves. Grows in clumps up to 3' (90cm) high and flowers in midsummer. Self-seeds easily. The variegated plant is delightful.

Cautions
Caution during pregnancy and breastfeeding. Avoid with thyroid drugs, sedatives, barbiturates, CNS depressants (eg. alcohol, opiates, benzodiazepines, tricyclic anti-depressants, antiepileptics).

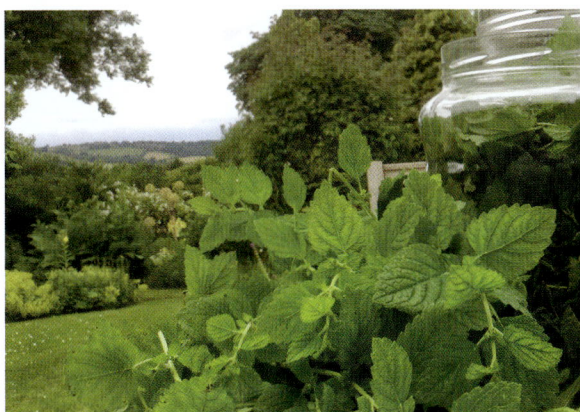

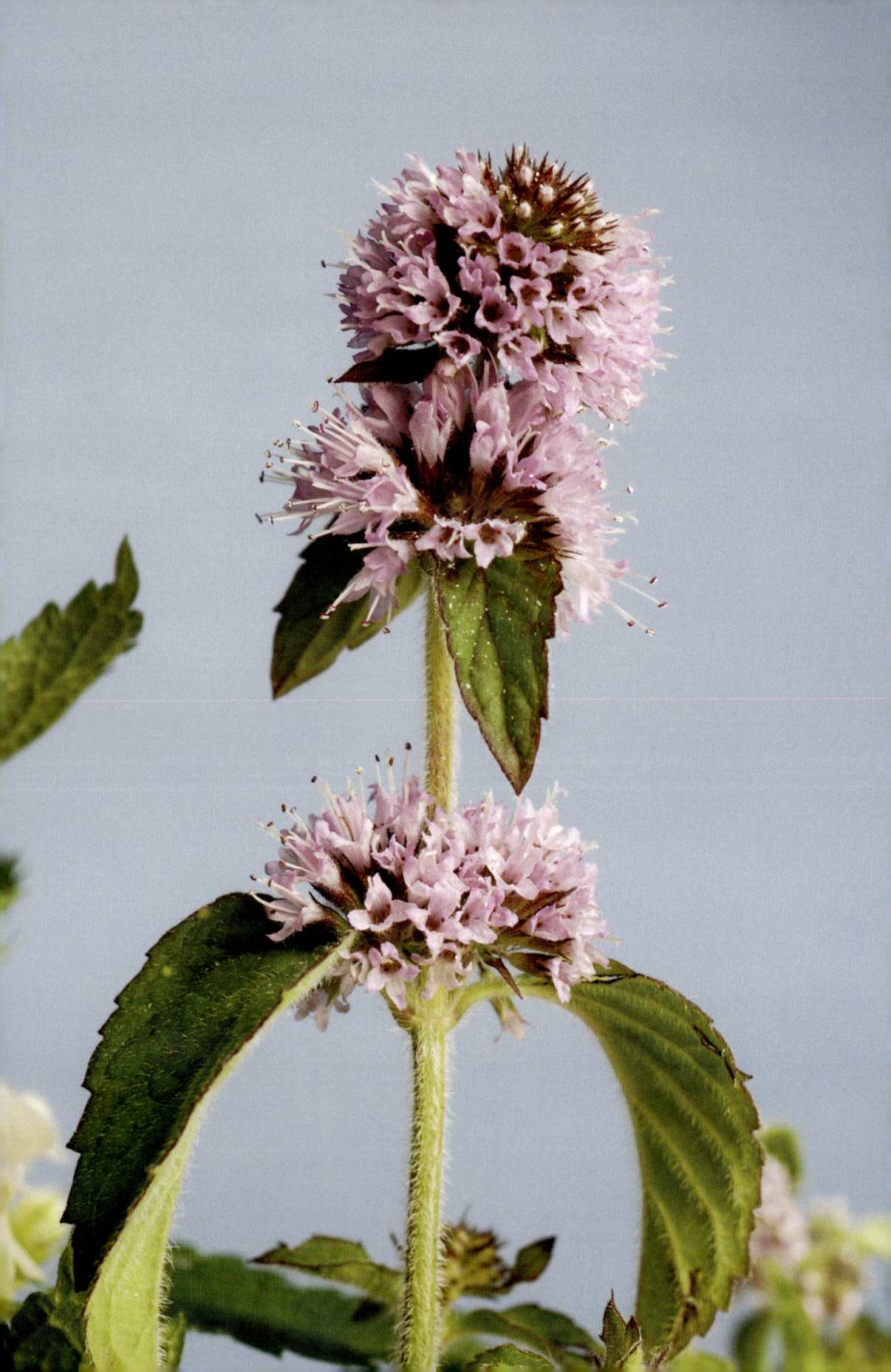

Mentha piperita: Peppermint

The Flower of Refreshment

Then went I forthe on my rigolt honde
Down by a little path I fonde
Of mintes full and fennel green
– Geoffrey Chaucer (1340–1400)

Other Names: Mint, horsemint, balm mint, brandy mint, curled mint, lamb mint, lammint

Parts Used: Leaves, stems and flowers

There is probably no other herb that can rival the popularity of mint. Spearmint, horsemint, garden mint and pennyroyal all have similar virtues to peppermint, but are milder in taste, smell and medicinal action. They are all members of the Lamiaceae/Labiatae family. Mint has been popular for thousands of years. The ancient Egyptians grew it for cooking, medicines and perfumes. Hieroglyphics found on temple walls and remains found in tombs dating back to 3,000 BC show that mint was favoured by them as a ritual perfume and was incorporated into their sacred incense called 'Kyphi'. The ancient Chinese and Japanese were equally fond of it and the Japanese have records of menthol extraction from peppermint dating back 2,000 years.

The ancient Greeks made energising and revitalising oils and perfumes from mint. These were apparently used by athletes to rub into their muscles to enhance performance. The Greeks and Romans added mint perfumes to their bath water to scent their bodies and they were used as a restorative much as the Victorians used smelling salts. Sprigs of mint were woven into crowns used at Greek and Roman religious ceremonies. The Hebrews used to strew mint over the floors of their synagogues for its cleansing and refreshing aroma.

Garlands of mint were thought by the Romans and Greeks to enhance clarity of mind, concentration and inspiration. The name *mint* comes from the Latin 'mente' meaning thought, in reference to the Romans' respect for mint as a brain tonic. The Roman historian Pliny recommended that those who study should bind their head in a crown of plaited mint as it delighted the soul and so was good for the mind. He said, *"The very smell of mint restores and revives the spirit just as its taste excites the appetite."* This actually meant all appetites as mint was considered an effective aphrodisiac. In fact, the ancient Greeks actually forbade their soldiers to take mint during wartime in case its aphrodisiac properties distracted them and reduced their courage. The Arabs have certainly appreciated mint for hundreds of years and drunk mint tea to enhance virility and as a symbol of friendship and love. The English herbalist Gerard said, *"The smell rejoiceth the heart of man"* and that it was *"a good posie for students to smell"*. In the language of flowers, mint represents eternal refreshment.

Meat used to be kept for months by wrapping it in gauze medicated with peppermint oil. The Arabs have long carried mint to ward off flies that carry dangerous germs, while it was used as a specific to ward off rats and mice.

Herbal Remedy and Aromatherapy Oil

With it refreshing taste and penetrating fragrance, mint is one of the most commonly used herbs in the world. It is wonderfully versatile and makes a good adjunct to almost any floral prescription, to mask the less pleasing tastes of other flowers and as a digestive to improve their digestion and absorption. All species of mint can be used as medicines, but the most effective and aromatic mint is peppermint. Peppermint is so called as it has a particularly pungent smell and peppery taste, and it is both cooling and warming, depending on how and where it is used. Its intense taste and smell are provided by the volatile oils (including menthol, menthone, pulegone and carvone), and it also contains antioxidant and anti-inflammatory flavonoids, rosmarinic acid and tannins, as well as other constituents including phytol, carotenoids and coumarins.

Peppermint has a strong affinity with the brain and nervous system and also the digestive tract. Its powerful volatile oils particularly menthol, the well-known ingredient of over-the-counter decongestant remedies, vapor rubs, cough drops, toothpastes and throat lozenges, give it that stimulating and penetrating action. This has an invigorating effect, it awakens the senses, increases focus and concentration and can help with the digestion and assimilation of information and knowledge. Simply rubbing a leaf between your fingers and smelling its penetrating aroma clears the head, decongests the airways and refreshes the mind. When you need to keep the mind alert or feel sleepy after lunch or just want to maintain your concentration, try drinking strong mint tea or take a sniff of peppermint oil and put it to the test.

The volatile oils have an antispasmodic and analgesic effect and make peppermint veritably one of the best herbs for relaxing muscles throughout the body, especially in the gut, and for providing pain relief in headaches, joint and muscle pain, abdominal pain, menstrual pain and asthma. Peppermint also has a mild sedative effect, useful for calming anxiety and tension. The volatile oils have antibacterial, antiviral and antifungal actions, and can be helpful in treating *H. Pylori*, *Salmonella enteritidis*, *E. coli*, TB, *Herpes simplex* and *Tinea* (ringworm) as well as *Candida albicans*.

Peppermint is a renowned remedy for the digestion. It stimulates the flow of digestive enzymes, enhances appetite and digestion and promotes absorption of nutrients. It is excellent for settling the stomach and can be used to relieve nausea and travel sickness as well as vomiting, wind, bloating and colic. It is specific for inflammation and irritation of the digestive system, and can be used to treat heartburn, indigestion, gastritis and enteritis. Its powerfully relaxant effect on smooth muscle can effectively relieve pain and spasm in stomach aches, colic, hiccoughs, constipation, IBS and diarrhoea. The tannins help protect the gut lining from irritation and infection and may have a protective effect on the gut wall, which could be helpful in Crohn's disease and ulcerative colitis. Azulene, one of the components of the volatile oil, has an anti-inflammatory and anti-ulcer effect in the gut which could provide further help. The bitters account for its traditional use for liver problems and gallstones.

The antimicrobial volatile oils with their antibacterial, antiparasitic and antiviral properties, are helpful for combatting unfriendly microorganisms in the gut and help to maintain a healthy gut flora. This action, combined with the tightening effect of the tannins in the gut wall, makes peppermint a good remedy for disturbances of the gut flora and leaky gut syndrome, and all the problems that stem from this.

Taken as a hot infusion, peppermint improves the circulation and has a warming effect. Its stimulant action makes a good general tonic to recharge vital energy and dispel lethargy. Its warming effect can be helpful in cold weather to improve blood flow to the periphery of the body, but equally well it can be cooling in hot weather by dispersing heat; its diaphoretic action disperses blood to the surface of the body and causes sweating, helping to bring down a fever. Hot peppermint tea makes an excellent warming remedy to ward off and relieve winter ailments like colds, catarrh and coughs, as well as chest infections. It has a decongestant action to augment it antimicrobial effects. A few drops of peppermint oil in hot water makes a good inhalant for colds, catarrhal congestion and sinusitis. The combination of its antispasmodic and decongestant effects can be helpful in the treatment of asthma and wheezing.

Externally the refreshing and stimulating effect of mint is followed by a cooling and numbing effect which can be felt on the skin. Peppermint oil added to massage oils cools hot, aching muscles and swollen feet. It is a powerful analgesic, and when the fresh bruised leaf is applied, or the oil added to liniments, it relieves general aches and pains.

Peppermint infusion or tincture makes a useful antiseptic gargle for sore throats and a mouthwash for gum infections and mouth ulcers. As an analgesic it can relieve toothache, sunburn and earache. When made into a tincture, or the essential oil is diluted in alcohol, peppermint is effective for ringworm, *Herpes simplex*, athlete's foot and scabies. It can also be used to relieve pain in neuralgia and headaches.

Homeopathic Remedy
Mentha piperita, like the herbal remedy and aromatherapy oil, is refreshing and revitalising, good for mental dullness in the morning. It has an affinity with the respiratory tract, relieving dry, painful coughs aggravated by cold and smoke, flu, dry and painful throats and earache. It also helps digestive problems, notably colic and wind. It relieves pain in the neck, in shingles, toothache, earache and headache.

Flower Essence
Peppermint helps those who feel sluggish, lethargic and mentally cloudy or apathetic, often with digestive or metabolic imbalances. Such people may crave food which then makes them feel sluggish or sleepy; peppermint improves digestion and absorption and frees energy, helping to keep the mind alert and clear for higher purposes. It helps to dispel mental laziness and poor concentration and awakens the mind. It is an excellent remedy for students.

Growing
There are about 20 true mints. Mints thrive in partial shade to full sun. They like moderate to high amounts of water and are not particular about what kind of soil they grow in. They are perennials and tend to grow in colonies. Plant mint where you don't mind it spreading, as it has a tendency to take over.

Cautions
Peppermint oil should always be used diluted and should be avoided in pregnancy. Do not use on babies or small children. Avoid peppermint in infants and young children as well as patients with hiatus hernia. Avoid excessive use of peppermint if you have blockage in the bile ducts or gallstones. Do not use neat peppermint oil directly on the skin. Serum levels of medications may be increased as the herb inhibits several cytochrome liver enzymes. May inhibit breastfeeding and iron absorption.

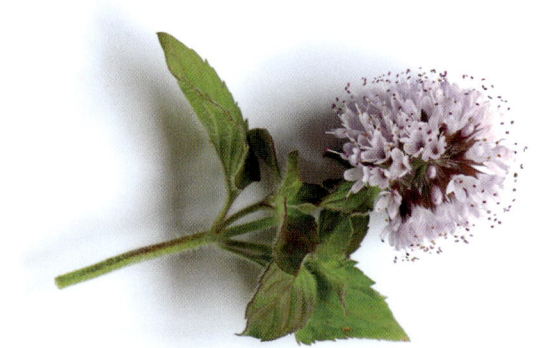

Recipes

Scent your bath water with a few drops of diluted peppermint oil and just feel its restorative effects.

Try a cup of peppermint or spearmint tea after a meal if you suffer from wind.

For travel sickness, try sucking extra strong peppermints or sip peppermint tea from a flask as needed.

If you feel tired after lunch, falling asleep over your desk at work, or nodding off in a chair, drink a strong cup of peppermint tea or inhale a little peppermint oil and you'll simultaneously improve your digestion and reawaken the senses.

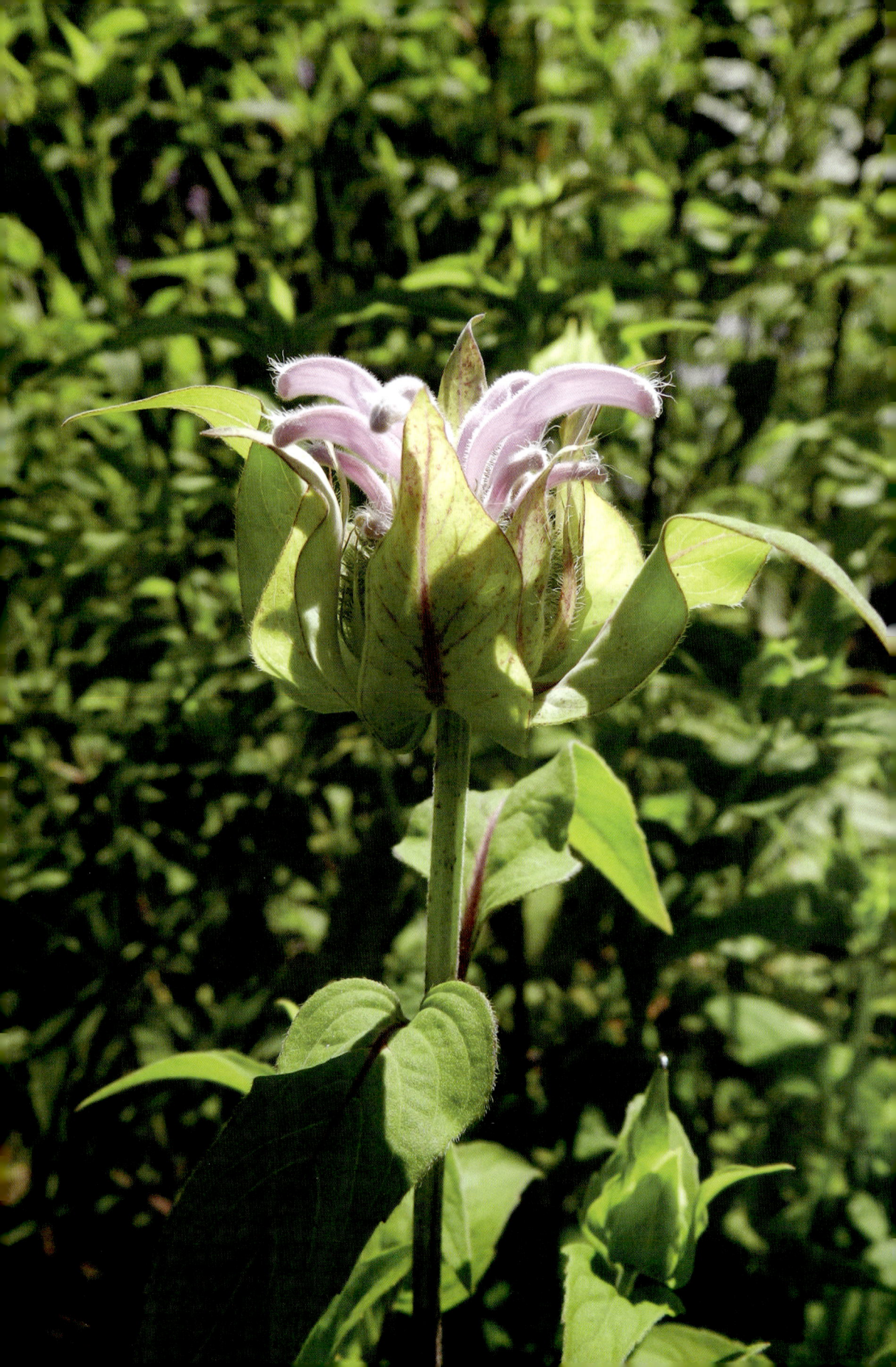

Monarda fistulosa: Wild Bergamot

The Flower of Good Fortune

For the sake of some things
That be now no more
I will strew rushes
On my chamber-floor,
I will plant bergamot
At my kitchen-door
– Edna St. Vincent Millay (1892–1950)

Other names: Firework flower, wild oregano, bee balm, Eastern bee balm, bergamot, monarda, sweet leaf, horsemint, golden melissa, Indian nettle

Parts used: All parts, including the root

Wild bergamot is a perennial wildflower belonging to the mint family (Lamiaceae/Labiatae), native to North America. It is found growing wild in dry meadows, clearings and the edges of woodland on limey soil from Canada to Mexico.

It has unusually shaped flowers called *'firework flowers'* that come in shades from lavender to deep purple. They bloom throughout the summer with a spicy fragrance that is loved by bees and other pollinators which explains its name *bee balm*; it produces a good source of honey. Its name *bergamot* comes from its lovely aroma that is said to be reminiscent of the bergamot citrus fruit. It can grow up to about four feet tall.

Since wild bergamot is a North American native plant, there are no written records going back thousands of years as with European herbs. It is thought that after the Boston Tea Party, when English tea was tossed overboard to protest against the high taxes imposed by the British, the colonists used *Monarda* instead to make their tea. They blended orchard fruits, native and garden plants such as monarda, goldenrod, chamomile and spicebush and made home brews which were called 'Liberty teas'.

The *Monarda* plant was named after the Spanish physician and botanist, Dr. Nicolas Monardes of Seville Spain (1493–1588). He had people bring plants from North America to Spain, and wrote about them in his book *Joyful News – Botany of the New World*. When the seeds were sent across the Atlantic and grown in Europe, *Monarda* was given the names of 'golden melissa' and 'Indian nettle'. There are actually several species of *Monarda* that can be used similarly, but wild bergamot (*Monarda fistulosa*) has a more spicy and hotter action than the common garden variety, red oswego (*Monarda didyma*). Wild bergamot is also called 'wild oregano' as it has a very similar taste and smell, as well as medicinal benefits, to those of oregano. In the language of flowers, *Monarda* symbolises compassion and sympathy.

Wild bergamot was highly valued by Native American tribes for its culinary and medicinal uses. The Cherokee, Lakota, Hopi, Pueblo, Spanish Americans and Tewa all used it as food, and it was often dried and stored for use in winter. The Apache and Iroquois also made a tea from the leaves, while other tribes used it for seasoning and preserving meats.

Wild bergamot also has a tradition of medicinal use. Several of the Native American tribes apparently used the leaves to relieve headaches by placing wads of leaves in the nostrils or made them into poultices to apply to the head. The leaves were also used as teas to relieve colds and chest infections and added to warm baths to soothe and treat infections in babies. They were used to treat stomach pains and other digestive disturbances including cholera. When the leaves were wrapped in cloth they were used as a poultice for skin problems such as acne and fungal infections, for muscle spasms, sore eyes and fevers as well as to stop bleeding. They were popular for using in ceremonial sweat lodges as they have a diaphoretic (sweat producing) effect. Wild bergamot was considered to be an excellent reproductive tonic and was given as a gift to young women to regulate and improve their cycles.

Herbal Remedy
The whole of wild bergamot has a combination of aromatic, pungent and bitter tastes given by the abundance of volatile oils including the antioxidant and antimicrobial phenols thymol, eugenol, carvacrol, limonene, gamma-terpinine, geraniol, rosmarinic acid and cymene. These account for most of its medicinal action. Carvacrol has been shown to have antimicrobial, antitumour, antispasmodic, analgesic, anti-inflammatory, antiparasitic and insecticidal actions. Wild bergamot also contains formic, acetic and butyric acids, thymohydroquinone and a crystalline red colouring matter.

Like other members of the mint family such as lavender, lemon balm, rosemary and oregano, wild bergamot has both stimulating and relaxing/sedating actions, as well as both warming and cooling qualities. Just inhaling the penetrating aroma of either peppermint, rosemary or wild bergamot can invigorate you when you feel tired and sluggish, but also relax you when feeling stressed and anxious. Taken in hot infusion, these lovely members of the mint family can stimulate the circulation and cause sweating which helps to bring down fevers, but when taken cool, they can also they can relieve heat and inflammation and ease pain.

In the female reproductive system, wild bergamot's stimulating action increases the circulation to the pelvis and this can be helpful in painful periods, bringing on delayed periods and regulating contractions during childbirth. Its diuretic effect helps reduce fluid retention and with its antimicrobial and anti-inflammatory actions, it can be helpful in cystitis with severe burning and inflammation, urinary tract infections and irritable bladder.

Wild bergamot is a wonderful herb for treating infections. It has antibacterial, antiviral and antifungal actions effective against infections including *E. coli, Staphylococcus aureus and Klebsiella pneumoniae*. Thymol is the most active constituent of the volatile oils in wild bergamot and it is used as a stabiliser in pharmaceutical products and as an antibacterial and anti-fungal to prevent deterioration. It is used in many leading brands of mouthwash.

In the digestive system, wild bergamot stimulates the flow of digestive enzymes and improves digestion and absorption of nutrients. Its antimicrobial volatile oils help combat unfriendly gut bacteria, further helping digestion and absorption and helping to clear toxins from the gut that can be implicated in so many health problems. It is excellent for treating systemic *Candida* and other unfriendly gut microorganisms that contribute to dysbiosis and cause gastro-enteritis and diarrhoea. Its volatile oils, especially thymol and carvacol, make it a good remedy to treat hookworm and other parasites. Its relaxing antispasmodic effect helps to regulate peristalsis and relieve wind and bloating. It can be helpful in nausea and indigestion as well as acid reflux, as it helps the food eaten to pass downwards. The antioxidant actions of the phenols may have a hepatoprotective effect, protecting the liver from free radical damage caused by toxins, drugs and alcohol.

In the respiratory tract, the antimicrobial volatile oils, especially thymol, make wild bergamot a great remedy for infections including colds, flu, fevers, tonsillitis, laryngitis, ear and chest infections including whooping cough. It makes a great preventative cold and flu remedy in combination with elderberries. The antispasmodic action of wild bergamot, attributed to thymoquinone, can relax the bronchial muscles and help open the airways in tight irritating coughs and asthma.

Wild bergamot has a gentle effect on the nervous system, calming anxiety and lifting the spirits. It can be given for many stress-related symptoms

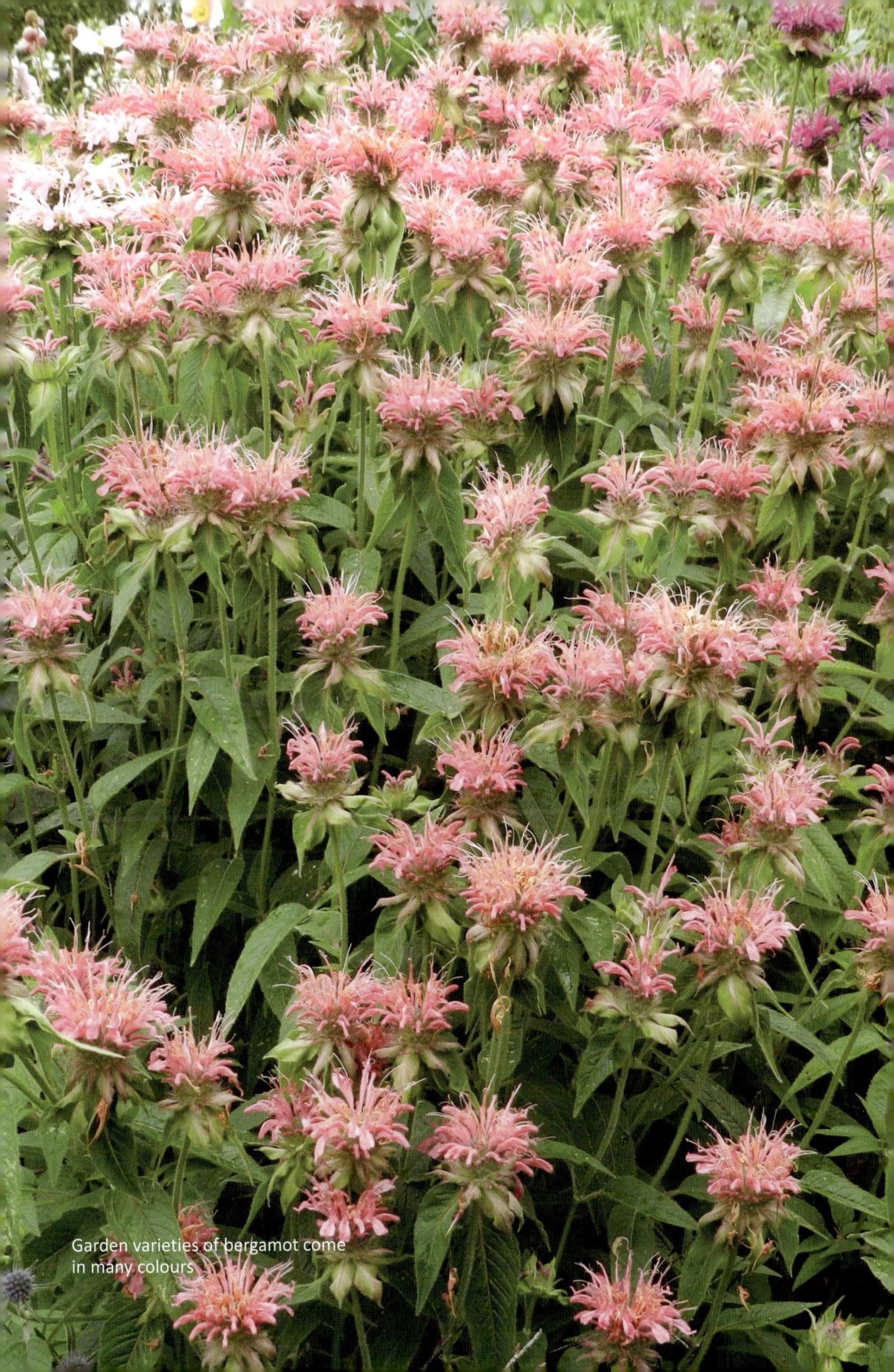
Garden varieties of bergamot come in many colours

including restlessness, nervous tension and insomnia, and it could be helpful in low moods including seasonal affective disorder (SAD) and disorders such as Meniere's disease and tinnitus. The antispasmodic action of wild bergamot can help relax the arteries as well as the smooth muscle of the heart, which could be helpful in high blood pressure and nervous palpitations. Its analgesic effect can be used to reduce nerve pain as well as headaches, arthritis and back pain. Its antioxidant effect may also help to protect the nervous system from free radical damage and the effects of the ageing process. It may have potential anticancer action attributed to the phenols, particularly carvacrol.

Externally the leaves can be made into an antiseptic mouthwash for bleeding gums, mouth ulcers and thrush and a gargle for sore throats. Infusions can be used as a steam to loosen phlegm and clear the airways. An infused oil makes a good massage oil for tight, sore or achy muscles and the tincture can be added to hot water as a foot soak for tired feet. An infusion or dilute tincture can be used to speed healing of wounds and reduce inflammation in skin problems such as eczema. Its antimicrobial action can combat MRSA (methicillin-resistant *Staphylococcus aureus*). The crushed leaves can be used as a poultice or in a salve for burns, scrapes or rashes.

Aromatherapy Oil
Wild bergamot oil is highly fragrant and pungent and, like the herbal remedy, has antibacterial, antiviral, antifungal and anti- inflammatory actions. With its lovely warming, relaxing and uplifting effect, it is a lovely oil for the nervous system, ideal to use when feeling low, anxious and stressed. Like the herbal remedy,

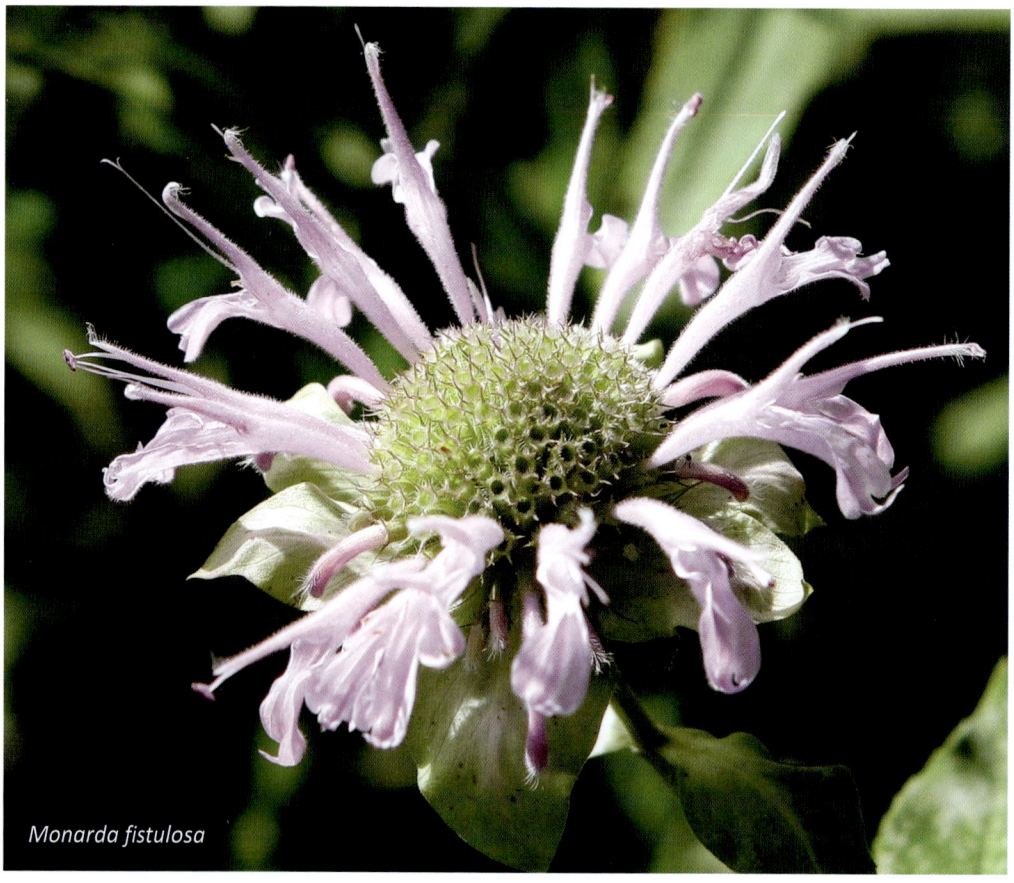

Monarda fistulosa

wild bergamot oil has antibacterial, antiviral, antifungal and anti-inflammatory actions and is a lovely oil for the nervous system.

When applied to the skin, it can combat infections that give rise to acne, boils and abscesses as well as ringworm and athlete's foot. It can speed healing of cuts and wounds and help prevent infection. It also has a rubefacient effect, bringing blood to the surface and causing reddening. This can be helpful in relieving pain in muscular aches and pain, arthritis and neuralgia. A few drops in a carrier oil, such as sesame, can be massaged into the abdomen to relax tension and spasm that causes period pains and abdominal colic.

When diluted in a carrier such as coconut oil, wild bergamot oil makes an effective remedy for seborrheic dermatitis. The essential oil is an effective insect repellent and can repel the yellow fever mosquito *Aedes aegypti*; this is attributed mainly to thymol, carvacrol and eugenol.

Edible Uses
The flowers and leaves can be used in salads and make really pleasant aromatic teas. The leaves can be eaten raw as well as cooked and used to flavour soups, stews and casseroles, in fact they could go well in almost any vegetable, fish or meat dish. The flowers make lovely decoration for garnishes and for deserts, muffins, breads and cakes. You can make infused oils and vinegars with the leaves and petals to use in vinaigrettes for salads and infused honeys for sore throats, coughs and colds.

Growing
Wild bergamot is easily grown in ordinary garden soil preferring alkaline soil, in either sun or partial shade. It grows well from seed and takes between 10 and 40 days to germinate or can be propagated by root division in the spring. It can suffer from a powdery mildew, especially in damp conditions.

Cautions
Due to its stimulating effect on the uterus and its blood-moving characteristics, avoid wild bergamot in pregnancy. Also avoid in thyroid problems. It might cause sensitivity to sun.

Recipes

Wild Bergamot-infused Honey
1 part chopped or crushed fresh flowers and leaves
3 parts raw or unpasteurised honey
Cover the herb with the honey and store in a dark cool place for at least 6 weeks.

Add a teaspoonful to hot water for soothing sore throat and for coughs and colds or use it as an antiseptic dressing for fungal infections and burns.

Calming and Decongestant Tea
Mix equal parts of dried wild bergamot, elderflower, catnip, thyme, mint and yarrow.

Take a teaspoon of the dried herb mixture for each cup of water, place the herbs in a teapot and pour over boiling water.

Leave to infuse for ten minutes and then drink a cupful every two or three hours to bring down a fever, clear catarrhal congestion in colds and respiratory infections and promote calm and restful sleep.

Wild Bergamot Tincture
Fill a jar nearly to the top with leaves, flowers and/or washed roots.

Fill the jar to the top with vodka or gin, making sure the plant is completely covered with liquid.

Put a tightly fitting top on the jar, label it clearly with the name and date and leave in a cool dark place for at least three weeks.

Check it daily to make sure there is no plant material above the liquid level.

When the colour has gone from the plant, after about a month, it is ready to strain off. Press through muslin, discard the plant and store in a dark glass bottle. It is now ready to use.

The essential oil should not be used undiluted without testing on small area on skin.

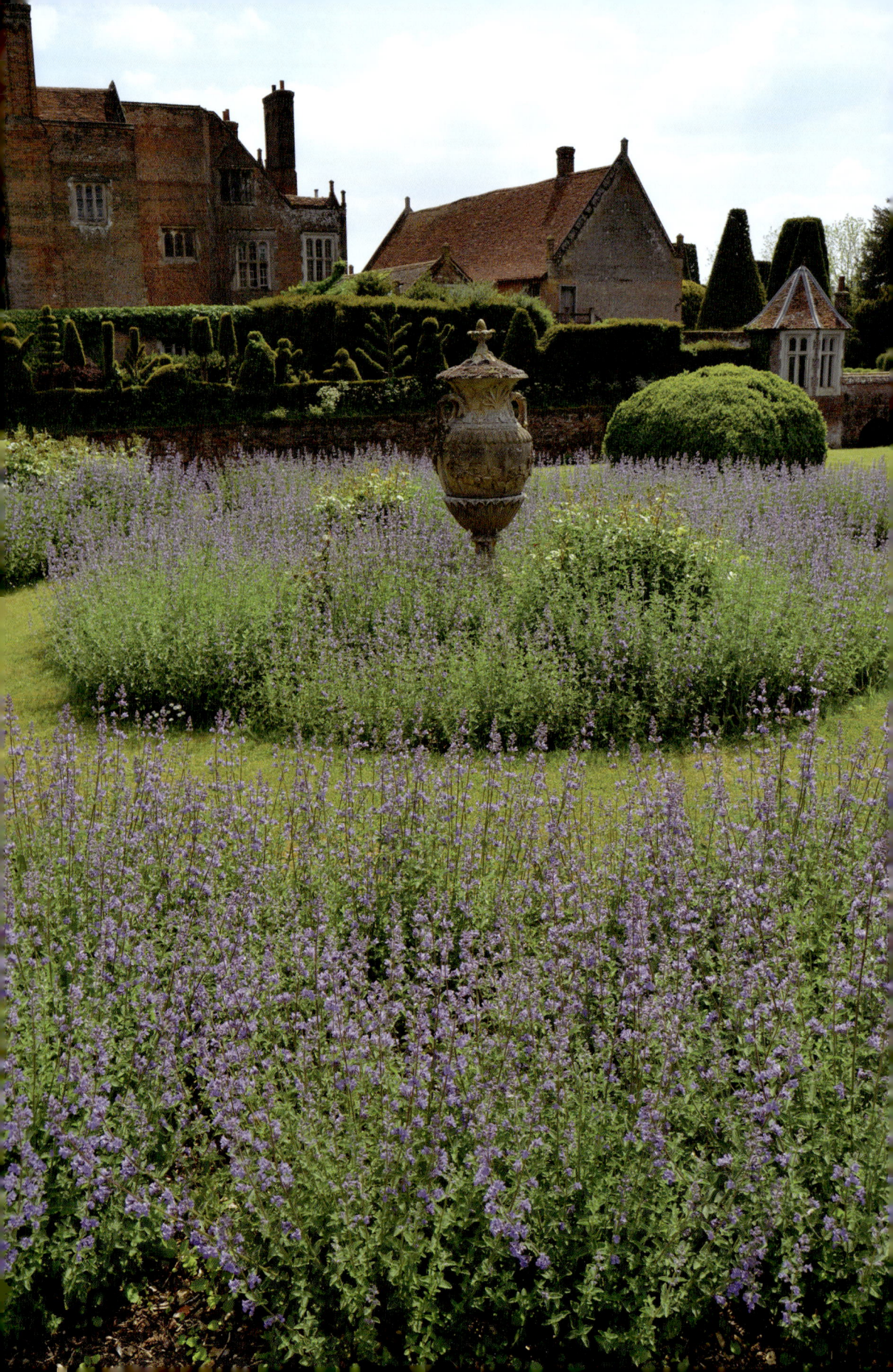

Nepeta cataria: Catnip, Catmint
The Flower of Cats

*If you set it,
the cats will eat it,
If you sow it,
the cats don't know it*
– Philip Miller (1691–1771)

Other Names: Catnep, catmint, catswort, cataire, catrup, catwort, nip, nep and field balm

Parts used: Leaves, stems and flowers

Catnip or catmint derives its name from the well-known fact that cats love its minty scent. They sniff, then chew the plant, then rub their faces on it and roll over and rub their bodies on it, clearly deriving some kind of pleasure. It used to be said that they recognised its medicinal virtues. Other mammals and insects can also be affected by it. It is hard to grow in a garden where cats roam as it will be eaten to the ground unless well protected, but apparently only if it is transplanted into the garden as a plant. If grown from seed, cats are said to leave it alone.

Catmint belongs to the *Nepeta* genus and is related to mint and pennyroyal in the Lamiaceae/Labiatae family which consists of over 200 plants. It gets its name from the city of Nepete, now known as Nepi in Etruria, which was the centre of Etruscan civilization before the rise of Rome. The cultivated variety of *Nepeta* is familiar to gardeners as a lovely herbaceous edging plant which blooms in early summer. It is excellent for attracting pollinators to a garden and often planted for this reason. The wildflower is found in fields and hedgerows on chalk or gravel soil in Europe, North Africa, North America and temperate Asia.

Catnip leaves and flowers have been used as a medicine for many centuries for poor appetite, intestinal cramps, indigestion, to cause sweating, to induce menstruation and as a sedative. The Roman diarist Pliny said, *"Nep also is powerful against Serpents, for the smoke and the perfume of this herb they cannot abide, but will flie from it: which is the cause that such as bee afraid of Serpents strew Nep under them in the place where they mean to repose and sleepe."*

The leaves and flowers have been valued for their relaxing properties, but the root may have a different effect according to Mrs Bardwell in the Herb Garden, *"Before the use of tea from China, our English peasantry were in the habit of brewing Catmint Tea, which they said was quite as pleasant and a good deal more wholesome. It is stimulating. The root when chewed is said to make the most gentle person fierce and quarrelsome."* Perhaps this refers to the stimulating and tonic properties of the plant. It was planted around houses to keep out rats, as they are said to hate it.

Culpeper said that catnip was ruled by Venus, perhaps because it has an affinity with women. According to John Pechy in *The Compleat Herbal* of 1694 *"Tis hot and dry. 'Tis chiefly used for obstruction of the Womb, for Barrenness, and to hasten Delivery and to help Expectoration"* and according to John Parkinson's 1629 *Paradisus Terrestris*, *"Nep is much used of women, either in baths or drinkes to procure their feminine courses."* Parkinson also said that it was used *"to help those that are bruised by some fall or other accident."* The dried leaves have been smoked to relieve respiratory ailments, and a poultice has been used externally to reduce swelling. Catnip plants were taken to North America by the European colonists and several Native American tribes adopted it and used it to treat muscle cramps and to ward off and treat infection. In the early 1900s, the flowering tops and leaves were still used to induce delayed periods.

Herbal Remedy

It is interesting to wonder why cats love this plant so much and what this tells us about how it could be helpful for us. Not only do they chew it and rub themselves on it, they also make certain sounds that suggest sexual pleasure or hallucinations. Some think that catnip is an aphrodisiac, but the reaction is independent of sex and neutering has no effect on cats' responses. Clues might be found in the constituents of catmint. Aromatic catnip contains volatile oils including citronellol, geraniol, citral, linalool, pulegone, thymol and nepetalactone which constitutes 70-99% of the essential oil. It also contains bitter principles, tannins, terpene, acetic acid, valeric acid, carbohydrates, glycosides, flavonoids, vitamin C, A and K, iron, manganese and potassium. Nepetalactone, the main ingredient of the volatile oil that gives the leaves and flowers their penetrating smell, triggers pleasure, perhaps even hallucinations, when ingested or inhaled by cats. Nepetalactone is similar to the valepotriates found in the sedative herb valerian. In the 1960s catnip was used as a natural high and hallucinogen when smoked in place of or with marijuana.

Catnip's relaxing effect can be used to reduce tension and anxiety and lift mood. It can also ease restlessness and agitation. It can be used for insomnia as well as stress-related symptoms such as tight muscles, headaches and nausea. It is considered a good remedy for babies and children, to calm them into a relaxing sleep and stop nightmares. It has analgesic properties which can be used to ease tension headaches and soothe pain.

Catnip is also a good remedy for respiratory infections; taken as a hot tea it stimulates the circulation, increases sweating and brings down fevers. It acts as a decongestant for catarrh and can be taken frequently at the first signs of colds and flu. Catnip can also helpful in bronchitis and asthma. It was used historically for whooping cough and eruptive infections including measles, chickenpox, scarlet fever and smallpox, and it was smoked to relieve respiratory ailments such as asthma, cough and bronchitis. This could be explained by the fact that it contains volatile oils with antimicrobial activity against fungal infections and bacteria including *Staphylococcus aureus*. Catmint also has antioxidant and anti-inflammatory actions.

The relaxant effect of catnip is also felt in the digestive tract where it relieves tension and colic, wind and pain. Catnip can be used to calm griping from stress or gastro-enteritis and for nausea, motion sickness and diarrhoea. With its astringent tannins, it toughens up the lining of the gut and helps to protect it from infection, irritation and inflammation and makes a good remedy for gastritis, diarrhoea and inflammatory bowel problems as well as leaky gut syndrome. In the past it was considered a good remedy for babies with wind or colic, teething pain or trouble sleeping.

More recently catnip is used for its antioxidant actions, scavenging free radicals, and particularly in relation to its effects on blood sugar. When taken in an alcohol extract, it lowers blood sugar and fats by its effect on carbohydrate-metabolising enzymes (α-amylase, β-galactosidase and α-glucosidase) and has the ability to normalise liver function and inhibit lipid synthesis associated with diabetic complications. This means it can play an important part in the treatment and repair of liver damage caused by raised blood sugar in diabetes.

Catnip's relaxant effects are also felt in the uterus. It can be used to relieve period pains as well as tension or stress prior to a period. It can also stimulate uterine contractions and be taken for irregular, delayed or suppressed periods. It may help during childbirth and afterwards to expel the placenta. Catmint has a diuretic effect, increasing urination and decreasing water retention.

Externally, a hot infusion makes a good antiseptic inhalant for sore throats, colds, flu and coughs, a decongestant for catarrh and sinusitis, and a relaxant for asthma and croup. The tannins speed tissue repair and staunch bleeding of abrasions and cuts, they aid healing of burns and scalds, piles and insect bites, as well as inflammatory skin problems.

Homeopathic Remedy
Cataria is mainly used as a remedy for babies or children for colic and abdominal pain. The baby or child may be seen to draw their legs up or twist their body around in pain. It is also recommended for nervous headaches, anxiety, crying, even hysteria. It is similar in action to Chamomilla.

Aromatherapy Oil
Catnip oil is used in aromatherapy to promote relaxation and calmness and can be added to massage oil blends, oil burners and used for inhalation. It can create a relaxing environment, especially if combined with other relaxing oils such as lavender and this can be helpful at night to ease tension or anxiety and aid sleep and a feeling of wellbeing. It can help relieve stress-related problems such as headaches, muscle tension and pain as well as abdominal pain from wind.

Catnip is also used as an antimicrobial and antiseptic for infections and as a decongestant for colds, coughs and catarrh. It is highly regarded as a mosquito repellent, which is attributed to nepetalactone, also responsible for catnip's attraction to cats. It could be combined with citronella to keep insects away. It is best avoided in baths, even when diluted, as it could irritate the skin.

The Flower Essence
Catnip as a flower essence is also calming and can be helpful in building confidence and enhancing social skills. It is a good remedy for easing changes in life such as moving schools, house or job, as it helps us to make good relationships and friends. It can be helpful for anyone who is shy in new or unfamiliar situations or not speaking up when feeling excluded, bullied or under pressure from peers. Catmint can enable you to feel empowered to go out into the world and be yourself or follow your dream for adventure without feeling fearful. It can engender ease in relationships so that you can be free of anxieties about exclusion, and is also helpful in intimate relationships. It allows you to feel safe, even joyful.

Edible Uses
Catnip's leaves and flowers have an aromatic mint-like flavour. They can be added raw to salads, used for decoration in sweet and savoury dishes and used in vegetable dishes, soups and stews. They make lovely light aromatic teas.

Growing
Propagate by sowing seeds in spring, take softwood cuttings in spring, or divide the plant in late summer. Prefers well-drained soil and full sun. Grows up to 3' (90cm) high and flowers June – Sept. Protect the plant from cats if necessary. It makes a good companion plant, deterring insects and beetles, and is loved by bees.

Related plants: *N. mussini* – cultivated variety of this attractive Labiatae, familiar to garden lovers as a lovely herbaceous edging plant which blooms in June with lilac-blue flowers.

Cautions
Catnip may cause headaches and digestive upset in some individuals. May cause drowsiness. Avoid in pregnancy. Increases sedation; caution with alcohol, other sedatives and anticonvulsants, barbiturates, benzodiazepines and insomnia drugs (tricyclic antidepressants). Also, some over the counter cough and cold mixtures that contain diphenhydramine or doxylamine. Avoid with hepatotoxic drugs (eg. Tetracycline, Statins and Acetaminophen, Methotrexate, antifungals).

Excessive sleepiness may occur if Nepeta cataria is taken with hops, St. Johns wort or valerian. Avoid in individuals if allergies or hypersensitivities to the Lamiaceae family are known.

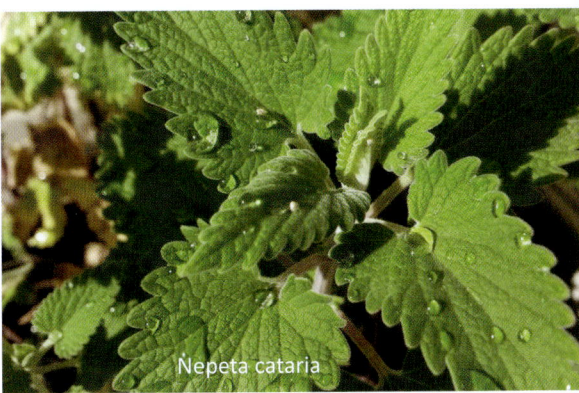
Nepeta cataria

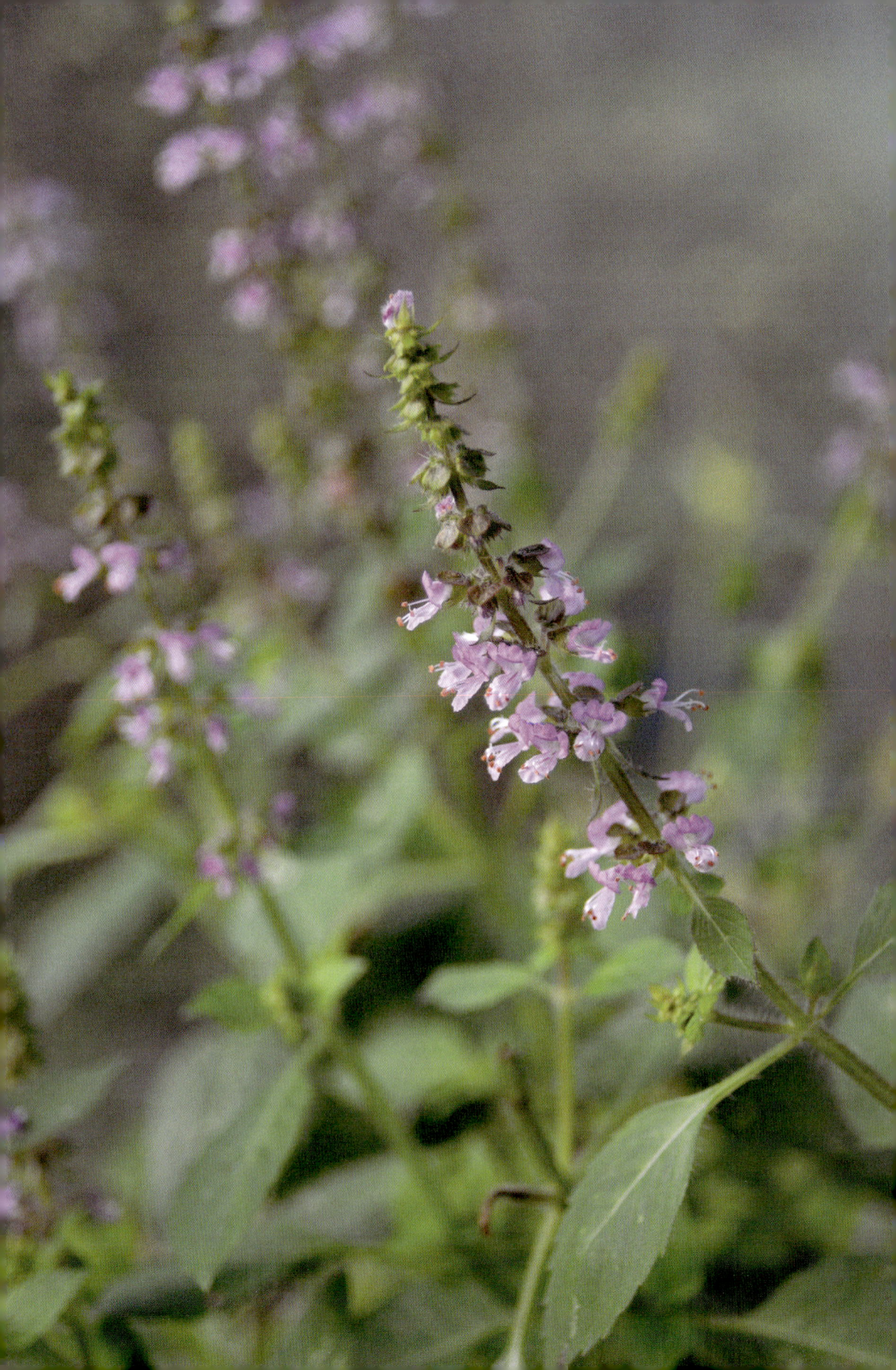

Ocimum tenuiflorum/sanctum: Holy Basil, Tulsi

The Flower of Vishnu

Just by touching Tulsidevi one's body becomes pure.
By praying to her, all diseases practically become removed.
If one waters her or makes her wet,
The fear of Yamaraja (death personified) is destroyed
 – From the Skanda Purana

Other Names: Krishna tulsi, tulsi, sacred basil, tulasi, elixir of life, queen of herbs, goddess of Vrindavan, green holy basil, Indian basil, kala tulsi, rama tulsi, red holy basil, sacred basil, hot basil

Parts Used: Leaves, stems, flowers and seeds

Basil is the collective name for the plants of the genus *Ocimum* in the Lamiaceae/Labiatieae family. Sweet basil (*Ocimum basilicum*) is a tender annual native to tropical areas of Africa and Asia and has been grown throughout the Mediterranean for hundreds of years. It is loved for its exquisite taste and fragrance, probably best described as sweet and pungent with something of a hint of clove – it definitely deserves a place on the menu in Paradise. We are probably most familiar with sweet basil through its use in the kitchen. Holy basil or tulsi (*Ocimum tenuiflorum* formerly *Ocimum sanctum*) is one of the most sacred plants in India, dedicated to Vishnu and Krishna. It is used more medicinally than sweet basil and has more significance for its spiritual uses. It is holy basil that will be described here.

For thousands of years, holy basil has quite possibly been the most revered medicinal herb in the world. Native to India and South-East Asia, holy basil is a short-lived perennial herb or small shrub reaching a height of almost two feet, often grown as an annual. The leaves are green or purple and highly scented, the stems are green but sometimes have a purple tinge and it has a linear spike of violet flowers. The name *basil* comes from the word 'basilisca' or 'basilikon' meaning royal, either because it was considered the queen of herbs, or because in India it was held sacred to Vishnu the preserver, one of the gods of the Hindu trinity.

Holy basil is also sacred to Lakshmi, a consort of Vishnu, who was transformed into '*Tulasi*' or '*Tulsi*' the holy basil. Each year in a festival that lasts for five days before the full moon in mid November, Tulsi is ceremonially married to Krishna, who was an avatar of Vishnu. In every courtyard the plant is surrounded by ghee lamps and there are offerings and prayers made, and in some parts of India there are also fireworks displays to mark the occasion. This ritual is called the *Tulsi Vivaha* and it marks the beginning of the annual marriage season in India. In India a garland of tulsi leaves is still the first offering to Lords Vishnu and Krishna as part of the daily ritual. The name 'Tulsi' in Sanskrit means the incomparable one. In one story, when Krishna was weighed in gold, all the ornaments of His consort Satyabhama could not outweigh Him, but a single tulsi leaf placed by his consort Rukmini was able to tilt the scale.

Maybe another explanation of holy basil's royal title is that in Hindu myths even the king of death gives way before this holy shrub. Going back to the idea that basil deserves a place on the menu in Paradise, it is fascinating that basil has been associated for thousands of years with immortality. In Europe, a basil leaf is traditionally laid on the chest of the dead, so that it will open the gates of heaven for them. Likewise, in Egypt basil is scattered over graves and in ancient times it was used for embalming the dead. In Greece, basil is a symbol of mourning and was also believed to be the antidote to the venom of the 'basilisk', a fabulous reptile who could kill with just its breath or a glance, so it helped to escape from the clutches of death.

The ancient scriptures of India including the 'Puranas' and the 'Vedas' mention its spiritual importance. According to the 'Gandharva tantra', places that promote inspiration, reflection and concentration to enhance spiritual awareness and devotion include *"grounds overgrown with Tulsi plants."* One such place is the Tulsi Manas Mandir temple at Varanasi, where Tulasi is worshipped along with other devas (demi-gods and goddesses). Vaishnavites, followers of Vishnu, revere Tulasi and make offerings of the plant to Lord Vishnu. They also wear beaded necklaces made in places of pilgrimage and temple towns from the stems of holy basil. Another name for tulsi in the Gaudiya Vaishnava tradition (of the International Society for Krishna Consciousness or the Hare Krishna movement) is 'vrindadevi' meaning the goddess of Vrindavan. In this tradition, the many forms of Vishnu or Krishna are seen as expressions or incarnations of the one Supreme God, the primordial being (*adipurusha*) Sri Krishna.

The root of holy basil is a symbol of religious pilgrimage; the branches represent divinity and the crown symbolises an understanding of the scriptures. The root is made into beads which women wear around their neck and arms, and the seeds and stems are made into rosaries and believed to give the protection of the Divine by cleansing the aura and strengthening immunity. In India holy basil is frequently grown in courtyards of homes, often in a specially built structure with images of the deities installed on all four sides and an alcove for small earthen oil lamp. Some households have several tulsi plants to form a 'tulsi-van' or 'tulsivrindavan', a little forest of tulsi particularly those of the worshipers of Vishnu (Vaishnavism). It is also grown inside on windowsills to purify the air. Wherever tulsi is planted is considered a place of peace, piety and virtue. In the Christian tradition, it is said that tulsi grew around the place of Crucifixion and it is also mentioned in Shiite writings.

For thousands of years in traditional Ayurvedic and Unani systems of health and herbal medicine, tulsi has also been highly valued as a medicine too and known as 'the Queen of herbs.' It is mentioned by Charaka in the Charaka Samhita, the central teaching of Ayurvedic medicine, and in the ancient Rigveda. With its highly aromatic and bitter tastes, it is regarded as an elixir of life and believed to promote longevity.

Herbal Remedy
With its 'sattvic' qualities, holy basil has long been respected for its inspiring ability to promote wisdom and intelligence, perception and clarity as well as joy and contentment. It increases energy, vitality, immunity, fertility, longevity and joie de vivre. It aids meditation and supports our spiritual lives. These wonderful qualities are related to some extent to its array of constituents which include flavonoids, saponins, fatty acids (myristic, stearic, palmitic, oleic, linoleic and linolenic), volatile oils (including eugenol, carvacrol, linalool, methylchavicol, borneol, camphor, geraniol, nerol, estragole), triterpenes, tannins, sterols, ursolic acid, rosmarinic acid and polyphenols. They are reflected through its antioxidant, anti-inflammatory, cardioprotective, antimicrobial, immune-enhancing and adaptogenic effects and its beneficial effects on digestion.

In Ayurveda, holy basil is renowned as a rejuvenative, uplifting and strengthening in mind and body. As an adaptogen, it has the ability to increase our resilience to the stresses of modern living of all kinds – mental, emotional, physical and environmental. The polyphenols and flavonoids (particularly rosmarinic acid, apigenin and propanoic acid) have antioxidant and anti-inflammatory actions and as they protect the body from free radical damage and oxidative stress, they help reduce risk of cardiovascular disease, degenerative conditions of the nervous system, diabetes and cancer.

Holy basil enables us to maintain the balance – psychological, physiological, immunological and metabolic – that plays such a crucial role in safeguarding health. It can help to protect us from illness and the declining health that accompanies ageing. It has the ability to

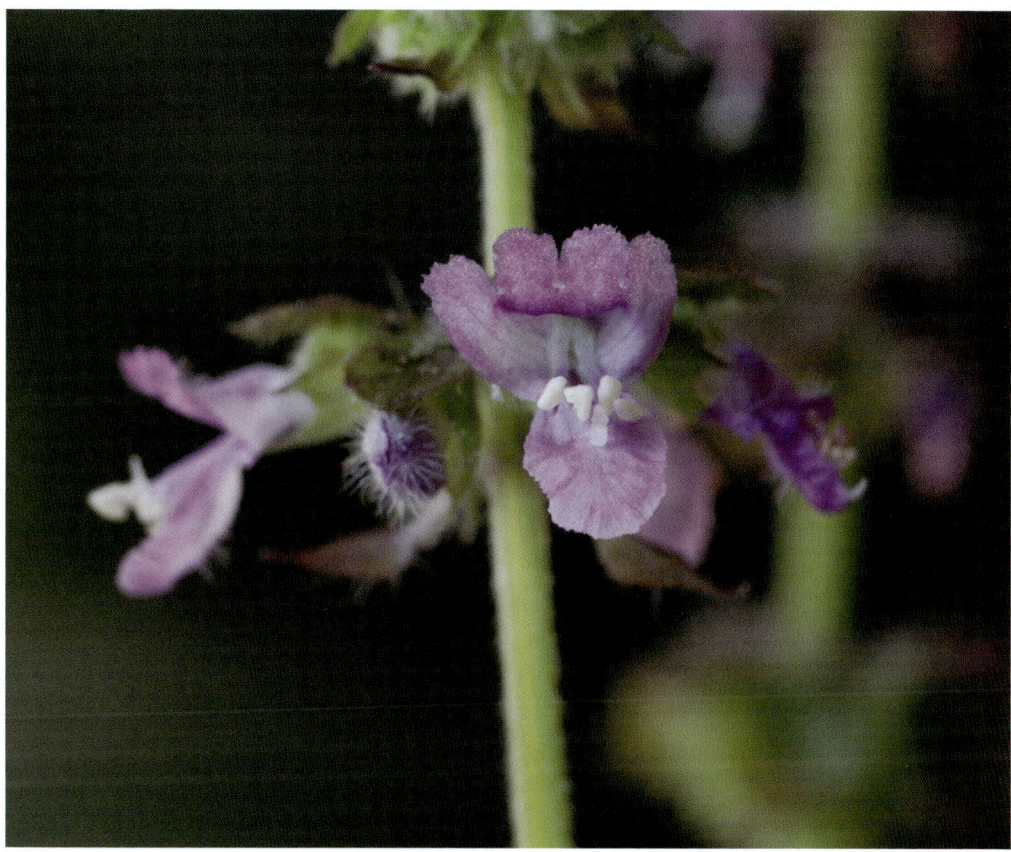

balance hormones such as cortisol (the stress hormone), improve brain function, boost the immune system, reduce inflammation, improve energy levels and have a generally supportive effect on systems throughout the body. With its adaptogenic actions, the leaves and the seeds of holy basil can support the immune system by modulating immune responses. They can increase while blood cell count and enhance their activity, scavenging and destroying harmful bacteria, foreign particles and dying cells. They also increase immune-enhancing compounds including interferon-gamma and interleukin-4 and have an antihistamine action. These immunomodulatory effects may be related to holy basil's remarkable ability to counteract stress and its effect on GABA, the anti-anxiety hormone.

Its antioxidant and anti-inflammatory actions can inhibit prostaglandin production, and this can be very helpful for people with joint pain, inflammatory arthritis and fibromyalgia. Many compounds in the leaves (including eugenol, cirsilineol, isothymonin, isothymusin, apigenin, cirsimaritin and rosmarinic acid) can inhibit COX-1, which is involved with the production of prostaglandins that contribute significantly to inflammation. Holy basil can also be helpful for pain relief in headaches and migraine, whether related to sinus pressure, high blood pressure or infection. The camphene, cineol, carvacrol and methyl chavicol have decongestant, sedative, antimicrobial and analgesic properties.

Holy basil has the ability to lower blood sugar and remedy diabetes and metabolic syndrome, possibly through its anti-inflammatory effect and by increasing insulin production and reducing insulin resistance. Since holy basil helps to protect against metabolic stress, it can also help with weight loss and lower harmful

(LDL) cholesterol and triglycerides and raise good (HDL) cholesterol levels. It can protect the heart and arteries against free radical damage, particularly when it is related to stress and high cortisol levels.

Tulsi is a wonderful herb for the nervous system. As well as enhancing resilience to physical and emotional stress, it is refreshing and reviving when feeling tired, dispelling lethargy and clearing foggy mindedness, while it is also calming when feeling tense or anxious. It helps clear the mind, improve concentration and sharpen the memory. It is particularly helpful when focusing on work, studying for exams or preparing for meetings or teaching as it reduces intellectual fatigue and calms exam nerves. It can be used for a variety of stress-related problems including mild depression, insomnia, neuralgia, back pain, headaches, migraine, indigestion and irritable bowel syndrome.

In the digestive system, the volatile oils including eugenol, carvacrol, linalool, nerol and camphor, give holy basil its pungent taste and warming properties, which improve digestion and absorption of nutrients. It contains nutrients including vitamins C and A, minerals calcium, phosphorus, zinc, iron, protein, as well as chlorophyll and many other phytonutrients and its digestive properties aid the absorption of these as well as the efficient digestion, absorption and use of nutrients from food and other herbs. Its muscle-relaxant actions help relieve stress-related symptoms such as stomach cramps, spasm, wind and bloating, while its appetising and digestive effects improve appetite and can be used to treat nausea and vomiting, abdominal pain, diarrhoea and constipation.

Holy basil helps to regulate metabolism and can be used to reduce weight in obesity. Its antimicrobial and antiparasitic actions against unfriendly micro-organisms in the gut including worms, parasites and *Candida,* help to re-establish a healthy gut flora. They combat stomach and bowel infections that are associated with diarrhoea and dysentery, including cholera. Holy basil also has a mild laxative effect, it increases the production of protective stomach mucus and has anti-ulcer activity, reducing the effect of excess acid, alcohol or irritating drugs on the stomach lining. It can be used to treat hyperacidity, dyspepsia, gastritis and peptic ulcers. Chewing basil leaves, drinking the tea or even just smelling a leaf of basi,l is an excellent remedy for children's stomach aches and travel sickness.

In the reproductive system, holy basil relaxes muscles and reduces pain. It can be used to relieve period pain and the pain of contractions during childbirth. In China, holy basil is used to relieve spasm and promote the circulation before and after childbirth. It may have a reversible effect on fertility by decreasing sperm count, mobility and motility. Its antimicrobial action can be helpful for treating infections in the urinary and reproductive tracts.

In the respiratory system, holy basil's decongestant properties help to clear not only excess mucus, sinus congestion and chronic catarrh, but also the lethargy accompanying it that can dampen the spirits and fog the mind. It is excellent for clearing bronchial congestion, sinusitis, coughs, chest infections, colds, sore throats, ear infections and flu including H1N1 viruses (swine flu), especially when taken as a hot infusion. Its diaphoretic action brings blood to the surface and promotes sweating, helping to clear toxins and bring down fevers. With its expectorant and relaxant actions and its ability to protect against histamine-induced spasm in the bronchial tubes, holy basil is helpful in the treatment of whooping cough, asthma and rhinitis.

Holy basil has antimicrobial activity against a range of micro-organisms including bacteria such as *E. Coli, Staphlococcus aureus, Klebsiella, E. coli, Proteus* and *Mycoplasma tuberculosis* as well as fungi such as *Candida albicans* and *Aspergillus* spp. The leaves and seeds have been used with black pepper for malaria and may have an antiviral effect against viral hepatitis. The high linoleic acid content of the oil in the seeds could contribute towards its antimicrobial activity particularly against *Staphylococcus aureus, Bacillus pumius* and *Pseudomonas aeruginosa*. In India, Holy basil is traditionally grown in courtyards, partly for spiritual purposes but also because its aroma is said to purify the atmosphere. The plant gives off ozone, an unstable form of oxygen that helps to break down chemicals and dispel disease carrying organisms such as viruses, bacteria and insects.

The leaves and seeds of holy basil may also have anticancer actions and an ability to suppress the development of cancer cells by inhibiting the metabolic activation of carcinogens (factors that promote the development of cancer). Holy basil can also be helpful for people who have cancer; it may be able to alter gene expression, the genetic changes that occur in the development of cancer cells; it can promote apoptosis which is important to the immune system as it eliminates potentially cancerous and virus-infected cells. It can also inhibit the formation of new blood vessels that bring nutrients and oxygen to a tumour to enable it to grow, called angiogenesis, and it can inhibit metastasis, the spread of cancer to other parts of the body.

Holy basil may provide significant help to people having to undergo radiation therapy by reducing the unwanted side effects. The antioxidants can protect healthy cells from free radical damage caused by toxicity, including that from radiation and chemotherapy, and protect the heart from damage caused by chemotherapy. Two

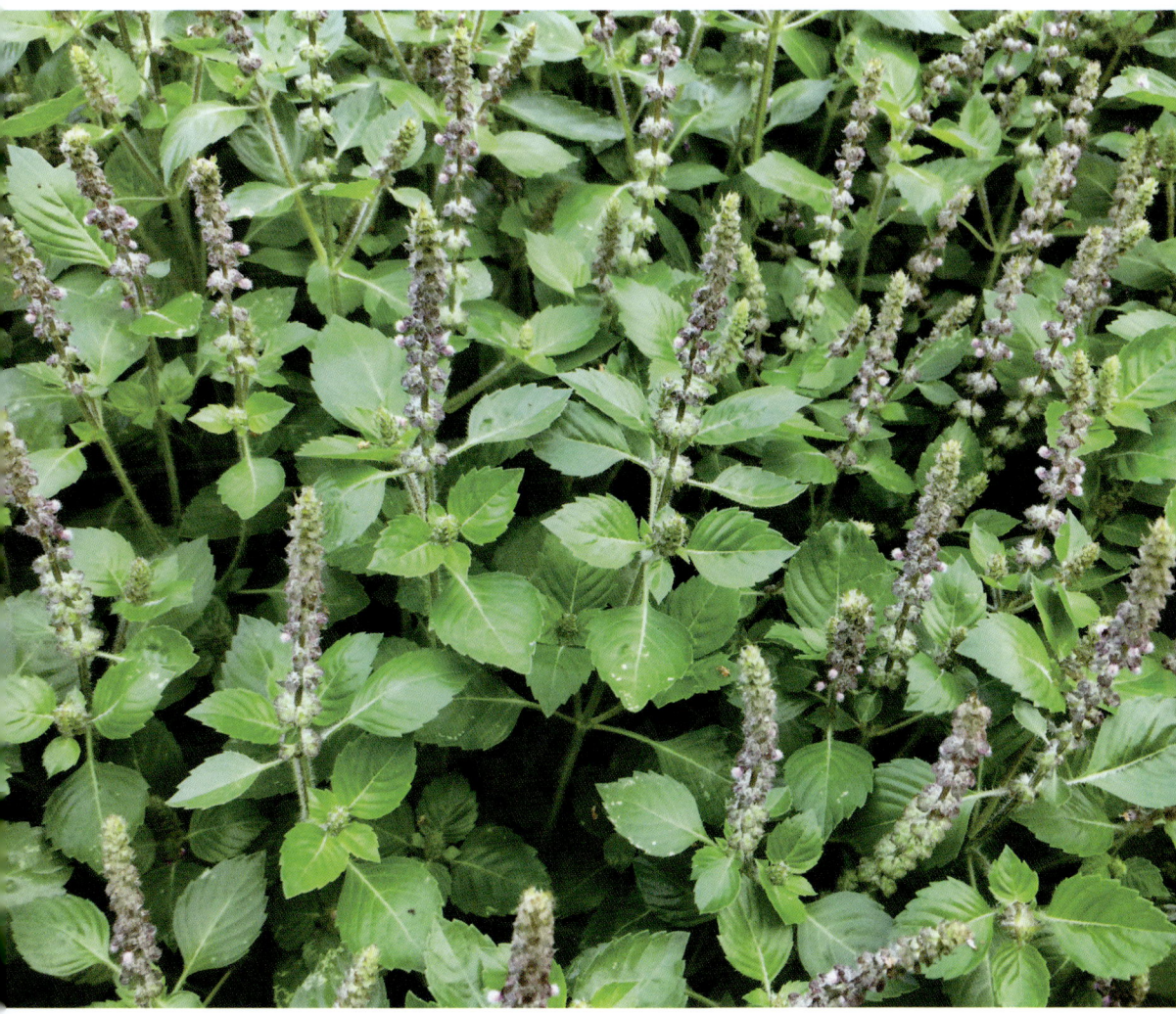

flavonoids in the aerial parts called orientin and vicenin may protect against radiation-induced chromosomal damage in white blood cells (lymphocytes) caused by radiation therapy and improve post-radiation recovery. This protective action is related to holy basil's ability to enhance enzyme systems in the liver that detoxify and cleanse the blood of damaging substances.

Externally you can rub bruised leaves directly onto minor cuts and grazes to speed healing and prevent infection. You can also use infusions, dilute tinctures or creams of holy basil to apply to allergic rashes such as eczema, infections such as athlete's foot, ringworm and acne, and to cuts and wounds to speed healing, reduce formation of keloid scars and prevent infection. They can also be applied to insect bites and stings to reduce irritation and inflammation. An infusion makes a good lotion to bathe inflamed eyes and an antiseptic mouthwash for bleeding gums and mouth ulcers.

Aromatherapy Oil
Holy basil oil is generally called tulsi oil. Its wonderfully penetrating, sweet and pungent aroma helps to calm and strengthen the nerves, clear and stimulate the mind and lift the spirits. It is refreshing and reviving when feeling tired and yet calming when feeling tense or anxious. It is particularly helpful for those studying for exams as it relieves intellectual fatigue and exam nerves. It can be used for many stress-related problems, such as headaches, migraine, exhaustion, indigestion, nausea, muscle and back pain and neuralgia. A few drops of tulsi oil added to the bath at night helps soothe away the stresses of the day and relax you into a good night's sleep.

When feeling tired, weak and vulnerable, basil is strengthening and revitalising and when vulnerable to infection, its antimicrobial properties can help protect against illness. In diffusers and used as inhalation, tulsi oil can clear congestion and reduce headaches in fevers, colds, coughs and flu. Diluted in a carrier, the oil can be massaged into tired, aching muscles and painful joints and it makes a good insect repellent. With its antiseptic and anodyne properties, it has been used diluted as ear drops for earache and can be applied to the head to ease headaches.

Tulsi oil has antibacterial and antifungal actions and can help to keep the skin clear of spots and treat ringworm, athlete's foot, acne, boils and abscesses. Used regularly diluted in a carrier oil, it is soothing and softening to the skin and keeps it youthful looking. It can be a useful anti-inflammatory remedy for allergic rashes and itchy skin conditions.

Homeopathic Remedy
Ocimum canum is prepared from the leaves of Indian basil and is used predominantly for urinary problems. It treats prolapse, engorged breasts, pain on breastfeeding and vulval irritation as well as fevers and arthritis, vomiting and diarrhoea.

Flower Essence
As a flower essence, tulsi has a harmonising, balancing and strengthening effect, enhancing our resilience to daily stress on physical as well as more subtle levels. It could be seen as a spiritual energy tonic. It can help us to integrate our spiritual lives with our material every day lives and find a balance between the two. It connects us to the deeper parts of ourselves so that we can reconnect to love when feeling out of sorts. It helps us to have clarity about our deeper purpose or *dharma* in life. Its *sattvic* qualities of engendering love and compassion, wisdom and gratitude shine through.

Edible Uses
The leaves and flowers are edible and taste pungent and warming with a hint of bitterness. They make a lovely refreshing summer drink when infused in cool water. They can be used in teas and cooking, and some people eat the leaves raw added to salads. The fresh aromatic leaves of holy basil can be chewed or made into a herbal tea. In India, it is used as an alternative to coffee.

Growing
Holy basil is very easy to grow. Sow the seeds in the spring or summer in pots in the greenhouse or directly just under the soil and they should germinate within two or three weeks. Seedlings should be planted out or thinned to about 30cm to 60cm apart. It prefers full sun, fertile soil and regular watering. Since Holy basil is tender it

could be grown as an annual or brought in for the winter before the frosts. In its native tropical Asia, it could live for a decade or more.

Cautions
Avoid during pregnancy and breastfeeding. It could have an antithyroid action. Do not take essential oil internally. Avoid with anticoagulants as it may slow blood clotting time and avoid with thyroid medications. Diabetics should monitor their blood glucose levels carefully. May deplete glutathione levels in liver. Avoid paracetamol or other glutathione depleting medications. Holy basil should not be used by people who are trying to conceive because it may cause uterine contractions and negatively impact fertility. Stop use at least two weeks before and two weeks after surgery.

Recipes

Holy basil is delicious in teas and can also be taken as juice.

It is often combined with ginger, black pepper and honey, especially when used to treat coughs, upper respiratory infections, asthma and indigestion.

Tulsi Tea
You can make holy basil tea using the leaves and flowers, fresh or dried.

Place 2–3 teaspoons of holy basil in a cup of boiling water. Let it steep for 5–6 minutes.

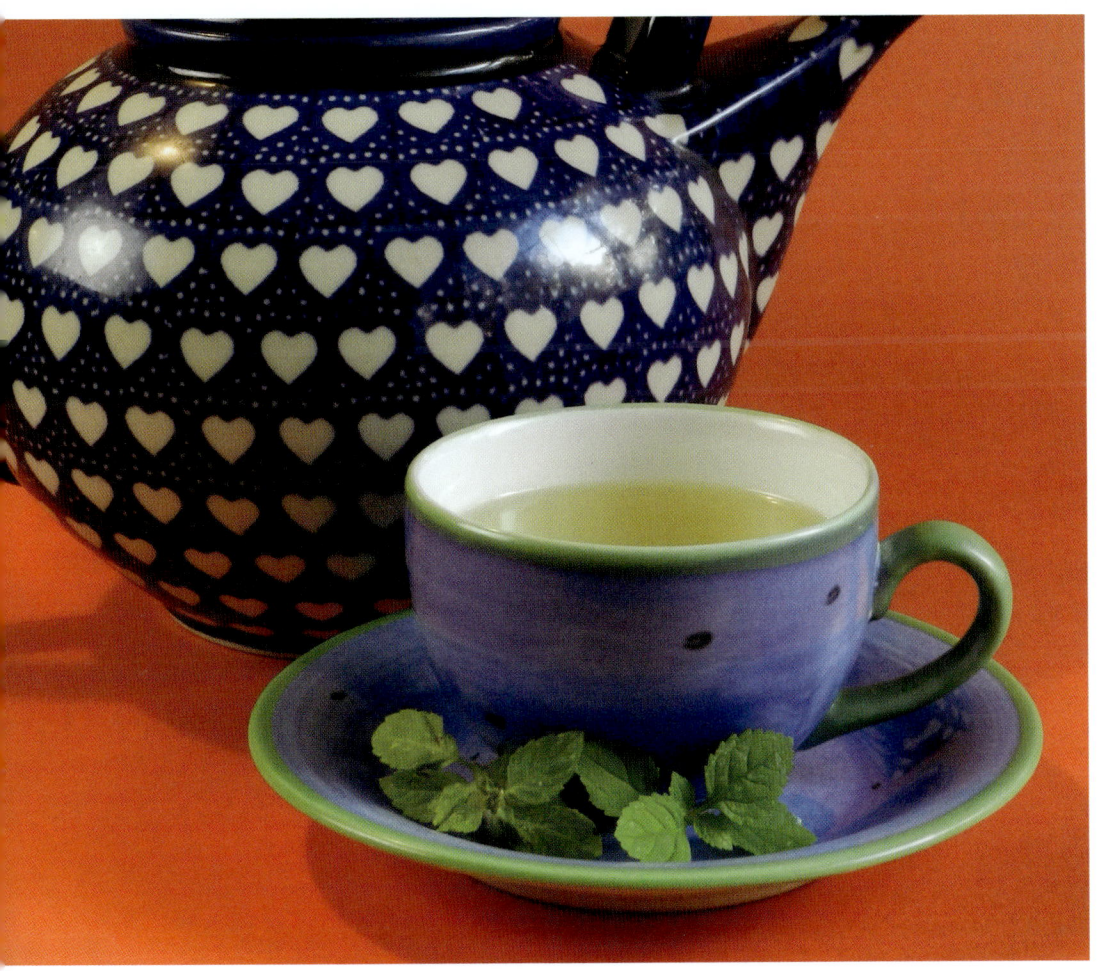

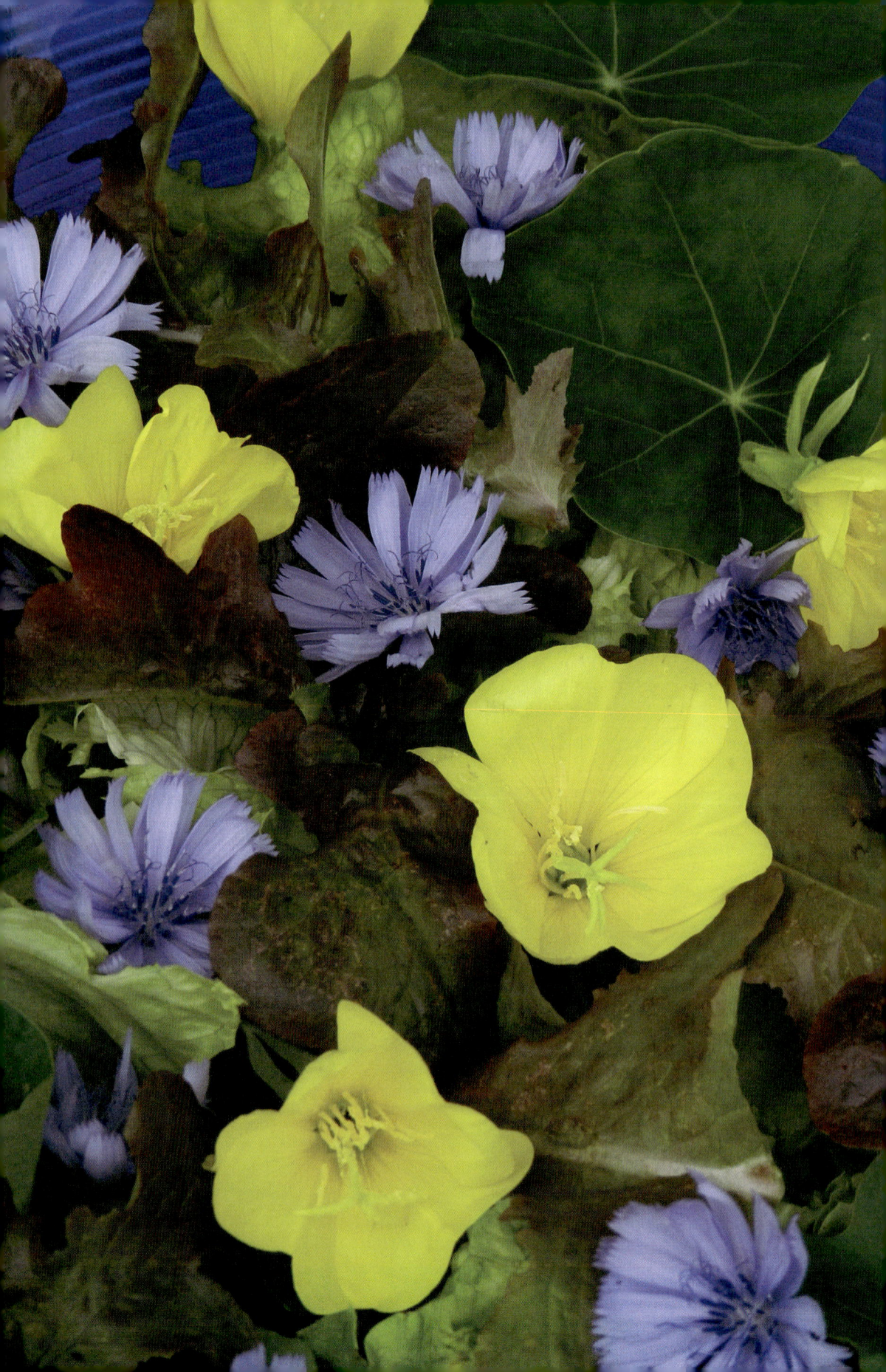

Oenothera biennis: Evening Primrose

The Flower of Silent Love

A tuft of evening primroses,
O'er which the mind may hover till it dozes;
O'er which it well might take a pleasant sleep,
But that 'tis ever startled by the leap
Of buds into ripe flowers.
– John Keats (1795–1821)

Other Names: Sundrop, king's cure all, large rampion, tree primrose, night willow herb, cure all, fever plant, great evening-primrose, scabish, scurvish, tee primrose, Spanish rampion, Rapunzel celery, German rampion, suncups, key to the night sky, nightlights, lazy girls, dim candle, sleeping virgins

Parts Used: Oil from seeds, leaves, stems, flowers

Evening primrose is a tall elegant plant with large fragrant, cup-shaped yellow flowers that only live for a day and generally open at dusk (or on very cloudy days), attracting the night-flying moths and insects which pollinate them. It is a member of the Onagraceae family and comes originally from North and South America; it was brought to Britain via the famous botanic gardens in Padua in Italy in 1614. It has lemon-scented leaves and flourishes happily throughout Europe and can be seen growing wild on disturbed ground all over Europe and North America. A biennial with a sturdy taproot, evening primrose grows to about 8 feet tall and flowers in its second season. It has many common names including 'scabish', 'king's cure-all', 'fever plant', 'night willow herb' and 'German rampion' which could relate to its resemblance to other plants such as rosebay willow herb and rampion (which is a type of campanula), or to its historic reputation as a panacea.

The renowned Swedish botanist called Carl Linnaeus (1707–1778) named evening primrose *Oenothera biennis,* but it is not clear why. *Oenothera* could mean smelling of wine from the Greek 'oinos' meaning wine and 'thera' meaning hunt, in reference to its power to stimulate a desire for wine or to mitigate the effects of over-indulgence. In ancient Greece, there was another plant with this name, a hairy kind of willow herb (*Epilobium*) that also belongs to the evening primrose family, so there could have been some confusion. The second name *biennis* relates to its two-year life span.

The remarkable and beautiful sight of the flower bud opening into the bright yellow, four-petalled, vanilla-scented flower about half an hour after sunset, has inspired many an artist and poet. It is said that Renaissance plant lovers may even have postponed their visits to the theatre till after the plant's magnificent performance. The Europeans had many different names referring to the night-time habit of evening primrose and the fact that the flower only lasts a day including 'key to the night sky', 'nightlights', 'lazy girls', 'dim candle' and 'sleeping virgins.' It was seen as a symbol of the transient nature of life or a sign of heavenly love, as illustrated in the poet C. F. Bürger's words, *"When the night has rewarded all who are tired with sweet slumber, I stealth off to the cottage where my sweetheart lives."* In the language of flowers, evening primrose symbolised both inconstancy and silent love.

The Native Americans valued evening primrose as an edible wild plant. The young leaves were eaten raw in salads or cooked as greens. The seeds were eaten by native Americans in Utah and Nevada. English settlers took the seeds back to Britain in the seventeenth century, after which it was grown there and in Europe as a vegetable. The nutty flavoured, fleshy taproots which develop at the end of its first year, were boiled like parsnips and the seeds were used as a substitute for poppy seeds. In Catholic countries in Europe, it was dedicated to the patron saint of pigs, St. Anthony and called 'jambon de St. Antoine' (St. Anthony's ham) and then 'ham root', 'edible root', 'wild stalk', 'Spanish rampion', and 'Rapunzel celery'. In 1863 a cultivated variety developed by German gardeners was taken back to North America where it became known and loved as 'German rampion'.

The Native Americans have long used evening primrose medicinally in an incredibly varied way. The Ojibwa made a poultice from the crushed leaves for bruises, cuts and sprains, the Cherokee used an infusion of the leaves for obesity and a decoction of the root for haemorrhoids. The south-western Navaho cooked the roots and rubbed their arms and legs with them to give them strength when carrying heavy loads and the Iroquois chewed the seeds against laziness. Young women waiting to be married wore the flowers in their hair at festivals. The Payute chewed the flowers and seeds and then rubbed them on their bodies and moccasins before going deer hunting, to attract the deer while at the same time repelling snakes.

The Shakers applied the leaves and roots to the skin to promote healing of wounds and drank teas of the leaf and root to settle upset stomachs. European settlers learned about the values of evening primrose and began using it as medicine in the eighteenth century. The leaves were cooked with honey to make a cough elixir and tea made from the flowers was used for coughs, bronchial spasms and stomach and intestinal cramps. Much of this knowledge and use was somehow lost, but in the 1980s British researchers took an interest in medicinal properties of the oil from the seeds.

Herbal Remedy
A vast amount of research has been done on the medicinal effect of the oil extracted from the seeds, which has made evening primrose one of the most widely recognised natural remedies. The whole plant contains fatty acids and antioxidant and anti-inflammatory compounds, phenolic acids and flavonoids. It also contains tannins, mucilage, resin, bitters and potassium. The seeds are rich in essential fatty acids, notably gamma linoleic acid (GLA), linoleic acid, oleic acid, palmitic acid, stearic acid and omega 6 fatty acids as well as sterols, polyphenols, proteins, carbohydrates, minerals, and vitamins. The roots contain tannnins and sterols including sitosterol, oenotheralanosterol A and B. It also contains triterpenes and carbohydrates including arabinose, galactose, glucose, mannose and glucuronic acid.

The oil is a good source of omega 6 fatty acids which are vital for healthy functioning of the immune, nervous and hormonal systems. Gamma linoleic acid (GLA) is an essential fatty acid formed in the body from cis-linoleic acid, which comes from foods, and converted into series 1 prostaglandins that regulate various functions in the body and help to prevent inflammatory problems. GLA is found in breast milk and sperm. In some people this conversion is hampered, particularly if they are elderly, eat a poor diet overly high in saturated fats and lacking in magnesium, they smoke or drink excess alcohol. It can also occur as an inherited tendency. A deficiency of prostaglandins is involved in many health issues including cardiovascular, hormonal and skin problems. Evening primrose oil is one of the few oils that contain GLA and provides an excellent way to remedy such problems.

Linoleic acid plays an important role in the proper functioning of the skin. It helps to prevent the skin from peeling and the loss of water through the epidermis (the outermost layer of skin that provides a waterproof barrier and creates our skin tone), and it improves skin softness and elasticity. A deficiency of linoleic acid can cause a deterioration in the protective function of the epidermis.

Evening primrose oil helps maintain normal hormone balance and is helpful in symptoms of PMS including mood swings, depression, irritability and bloating. It may be that some women experience PMS because they are sensitive to normal prolactin levels in the body. GLA converts to a substance in the body called prostaglandin E1 that is thought to help prevent prolactin from triggering PMS. Evening primrose is also helpful in menstrual irregularities and

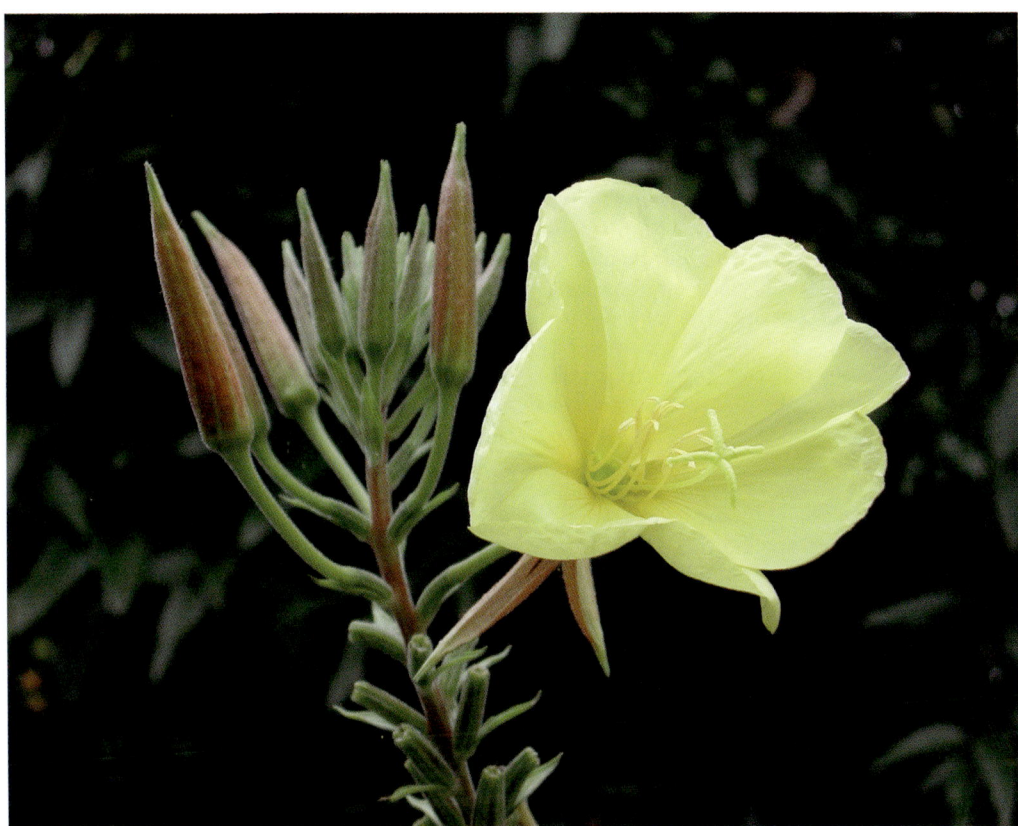

breast problems including fibrocystic breast disease and breast pain, as the GLA helps to balance hormones, reduce inflammation and inhibit prostaglandins that cause cyclical breast pain. Since acne is related to over-production of sebum due to hormonal imbalance, evening primrose is well worth using in this instance. It increases the fat content of breast milk when lactating and is also an effective remedy for menopausal problems including hot flushes and night sweats.

Evening primrose is a rejuvenating herb, increasing energy and vitality and enhancing immunity. It is a great herb for using in any inflammatory problem. Its linoleic acid and gamma linolenic acid (GLA) reduce inflammation because they act as precursors of anti-inflammatory eicosanoids and prostaglandin 1, and they reduce the production of free radicals. This antioxidant action may slow tumour growth and have a protective effect in the cardiovascular system. Evening primrose oil reduces high blood pressure, lowers harmful cholesterol levels and helps prevent blood clots and coronary artery disease.

GLA is helpful in treatment of allergies including atopic dermatitis, eczema, asthma, migraine, as well as metabolic disorders including diabetes and metabolic syndrome. It helps combat viral infections and with its anti-inflammatory actions, it can be helpful in the treatment of inflammatory bowel problems, joint problems and chronic fatigue syndrome as well as autoimmune problems including rheumatoid arthritis, scleroderma, psoriasis, multiple sclerosis and Sjogren's syndrome.

Evening primrose has a mildly sedative effect and makes a good remedy for nervous indigestion and colic, as native Americans well knew. It is well worth using for ADHD and hyperactivity in children. Its benefit to the nervous system could be helpful in the treatment of multiple sclerosis and in diabetic neuropathy. The antispasmodic effects of evening primrose oil can be put to good use in the respiratory system to relieve problems such as asthma and paroxysmal coughing as in whooping cough. Evening primrose oil has a remarkable ability to benefit the liver. It can counteract the effect of alcoholic poisoning and encourages regeneration of a damaged liver. It can be helpful during withdrawal from alcohol and in alcoholic depression and may be a useful herb for weight loss, especially for those with a family history of obesity. The outside part of the flower stems and the leaves are highly mucilaginous. They can be taken to soothe irritated conditions of the digestive tract and to treat diarrhoea.

Externally the oil can be applied to painful arthritic joints and skin eruptions, and a poultice of the leaves can be applied to burns, bruises and sore throats. The outside part of the flower stems and the leaves are highly mucilaginous and can be boiled and used as a lotion to soothe skin eruptions. Evening primrose oil can be used directly on the skin or in creams and salves to relieve the itching and redness of skin conditions such as eczema and psoriasis, and to speed healing of wounds. Massaging the oil into the skin could also be helpful in PMS.

Homeopathic Remedy
Flowers, leaves and stems of Oenothera biennis are used in homeopathic preparations to treat watery diarrhoea that passes without effort and is accompanied by exhaustion. There may be abdominal and other cramps. The symptoms also indicating Oenothera include dizziness, light-headedness, great weakness, numbness and pricking of the skin, fluttering in the heart, and fever with rigors.

Flower Essence
The flower remedy *O. hookeri* is recommended for people who feel rejected or unwanted, often due to childhood problems; perhaps they lacked proper emotional support or love or did not bond closely with their mother during infancy. Such people tend to avoid close emotional contact, intimacy and committed relationships, due to fear of rejection. Evening primrose helps to heal feelings of rejection and feeling unlovable and enables one to be more open emotionally and to form deeper relationships.

Edible Uses
All parts of evening primrose are edible. The young leaves and flowers can be added to salads and the leaves can be cooked like spinach and used in omelettes, fritattas or rice dishes. They may need to be cooked in several changes of water to reduce their bitterness.

Evening primrose is a biennial and in the first year when it only produces a few leaves, the fleshy root can be boiled or roasted as a vegetable and tastes a bit like a parsnip. The seeds can be roasted and sprinkled on top of breads, added to cereals and soups or used as garnishes in place of poppy seeds.

Growing
Propagate by sowing seeds in summer in well-drained soil and full sun. During the first year it produces a rosette of bright green leaves and in the second year it grows up to 4' (120cm) high and flowers from midsummer to mid-autumn. It selfseeds easily and is frost-hardy and long lasting; once established in a garden it will come back year after year.

Cautions
Avoid in epilepsy. It can occasionally cause upset stomach, nausea, diarrhoea, loose stools and headaches. Since evening primrose oil has blood thinning properties, it may increase the chance of bleeding during or after surgery or in people with bleeding disorders. May rarely cause allergic reactions. Avoid with antipsychotic and anticoagulant drugs, phenothiazines and anticonvulsants. May affect fasting insulin and blood sugar levels. Diabetics should monitor blood glucose levels carefully.

Recipes

Nourishing Body Oil
4 teaspoons avocado oil
2 teaspoons evening primrose oil
2 teaspoons vitamin E oil
15 drops lavender oil
15 drops geranium oil

Mix the ingredients together into a bowl and pour into a sterilized bottle. Massage a small amount into the skin as required.

Origanum majorana: Sweet Marjoram

The Flower of Honour

Here's flowers for you; hot lavender, mints, savory, marjoram;
The marigold.
– William Shakespeare, The Winter's Tale

Other Names: *Majorana hortensis* /majorana, sweet marjoram, knotted marjoram

Related species: *Origanum vulgare*: oregano/wild marjoram, *O. onites*: pot marjoram

Parts Used: Leaves, stems and flowers

There are several different marjoram plants, all members of the Lamiaceae/Labiatae family and highly aromatic. They are loved by cooks from all over the world, particularly the Greeks, Turks and Italians. Sweet marjoram (*O. marjorana*) is the most sweetly scented and very attractive with its grey-green leaves and white flowers. It is tender to frosts, so in temperate climates it is only half-hardy. It comes originally from Cyprus, North Africa, south west Asia and southern Europe particularly Portugal, but will grow happily in most sunny places in well-drained

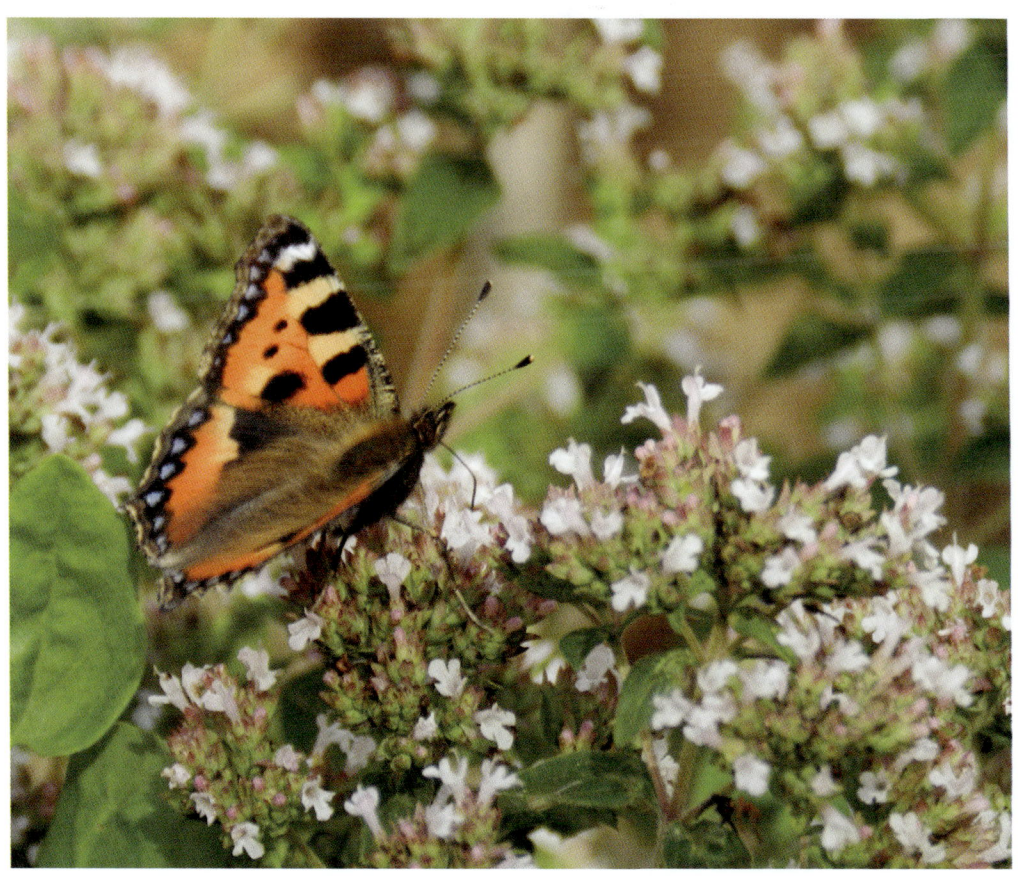

soil. Wild marjoram (*O. vulgare*), also known as oregano, like pot marjoram (*O. onites*), has a sharp warm flavour. All kinds of marjoram have similar healing properties although the more sun the plant has, the greater the concentration of essential oils and so the more powerful and aromatic it is.

Marjoram is one of the most ancient and versatile healing flowers. The botanical name *Origanum* comes from the Greek words 'oros' for mountain and 'ganos' for joy, making joy of the mountain which conjures up a lovely picture of wild marjoram carpeting a mountainside and scenting the warm air. In Greek mythology marjoram is the creation of Aphrodite, while in Roman myths it was a flower of Venus and sacred to her. It was used in rituals in her honour and by young people looking for love and romance. A symbol of honour, love and fertility, marjoram was woven into wreaths for crowns to bestow good fortune and long life on newlyweds in both the Greek and Roman traditions. In the language of flowers, marjoram was said to symbolise consolation.

For the ancient Greeks, marjoram comforted the bereaved and was planted on graves to help the dead sleep in peace. If found growing wild on a grave, it augured well for the happiness of the departed in the next world. Marjoram was also associated with Thor and Jupiter and was said to invoke their protection against thunder and lightning. English dairymaids would hang it in the dairy or near pails of new milk, to stop it from curdling in thundery weather.

The Greeks also used marjoram extensively in medicine, notably to nourish the brain and the digestive organs, for narcotic poisoning, convulsions and dropsy.

Many centuries later in England, John Gerard wrote in his *Herball* (1636) *"Organy or wilde marjerome cureth them that have drunk opium or the juice of black poppy, or hemlocks, especially if it be given with wine and raisins of the sun."* He also said *"Organy is very good against the wambling of the stomache, and stayeth the desire to vomit, especially at sea"*. In Tudor and Stuart times, marjoram was valued for its pungent aroma as a strewing herb and to protect against disease and infestation.

Marjoram has a long history of use to comfort the heart. In medieval monasteries, monks grew marjoram in their herbariums for use as an anaphrodisiac and to benefit *"nervous problems,"* and John Gerard recommended it *"for those who are given to over-much sighing"*. The spicy juice made an aromatic furniture polish, the oil a fragrant hair tonic and the dried leaves were used to make snuff and tobacco as well as stuffing for sleep pillows and sweet bags to smell and keep you in good health. Apparently, Turkey is the largest producer and exporter of oregano herb and oil to world markets.

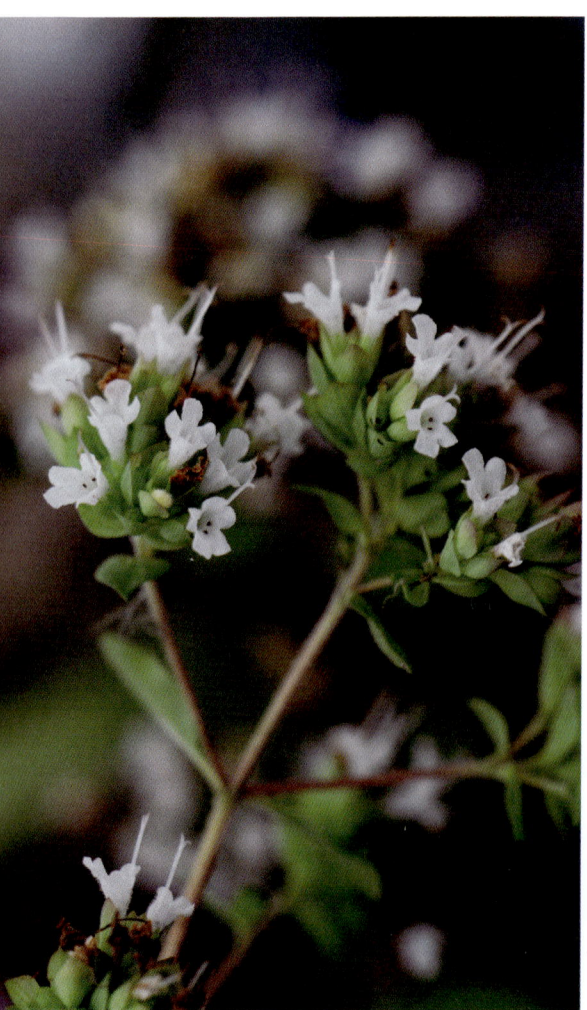

Herbal Remedy and Aromatherapy Oil
The volatile oil in sweet marjoram that gives its combination of pungent and bitter tastes and its wonderfully uplifting aroma is made up of more than 50 different constituents. It includes terpinenes, sabinenes, linalool, borneol, thymol, carvacrol, carnosol, geranyl acetate, citral, estragole, eugenol and cis-sabinene hydrate; the latter is probably mostly responsible for the sweet aroma. It also contains phenolic compounds including rosmarinic acid, methyl rosmarenate, caffeic acid, cinnamic acid, carnosic acid, labiatic acid, chlorogenic acid and quinic acid as phenolic acids, and flavonoids such as ferulic acid, apigenin, luteolin, quercetin, arbutin and methylarbutin. Other constituents include tannins, steroids, triterpenoids (oleanolic acid, ursolic acid), protein and vitamins A, E and C.

The essential oils in marjoram, particularly thymol and carvacrol, have effective antimicrobial effects. They can combat bacteria including *Mycobacterium tuberculosis*, *Staphylococcus aureus*, *Aspergillus* spp, viruses such as *Herpes simplex* and fungal infections including *Candida*. Marjoram has a beneficial effect on the gut flora, helping to combat pathogenic micro-organisms and in this way improves digestion and absorption of nutrients, enhances general immunity and brain function. These antimicrobial actions combined with its digestive benefits make marjoram an excellent remedy for treating a range of digestive problems. It enhances appetite, digestion and absorption and helps to clear toxins from the gut. Its antispasmodic and warming properties help relieve indigestion, calm wind and colic, reduce nausea, and relieve diarrhoea as well as constipation. Oil of oregano has become popular for combatting unfriendly gut bacteria and is active against bacteri, fungi as well as parasites including *Blastocystis hominis*, *Entamoeba hartmanni* and *Endolimax nana*.

With its warming, strengthening, immune-enhancing, relaxing and brain-enhancing actions, marjoram is a wonderful rejuvenative for the later years of life. Its antioxidant constituents help to minimise damage from free radicals and protect the body from the impacts of ageing. This can have far reaching implications to health, protecting against degenerative problems such as arthritis, problems affecting the nervous system such as Alzhiemer's, diabetes, inflammatory problems, lowered immunity and other conditions. Marjoram can improve memory and concentration and increase resilience to stress. In the cardiovascular system, the presence of antioxidants notably rosmarinic acid, tocopherol and flavonoids, helps minimise damage from free radicals and protect the arteries from inflammation and degeneration. Marjoram has antimicrobial as well as immune-enhancing effects, it can reduce inflammation and may restrain the development of certain cancers.

Rosmarinic acid which is also found in other herbs such as holy basil and rosemary, has an anti-inflammatory effect that has been compared to orthodox drugs in terms of pain relief. It can be helpful in poor circulation, chilblains, arthritis and gout.

Marjoram has an affinity with the respiratory tract and helps to protect against winter infections, particularly as it has warming properties, enhancing vital energy and stimulating the circulation of blood and lymph. Its antimicrobial properties help to fight off infections such as colds, flu, sore throats, tonsilitis, coughs, chest infections and *Herpes*. Taken as a hot tea, marjoram can bring down fevers and acts as an effective decongestant. Should coughs and colds develop, marjoram can be used to clear phlegm, soothe coughs and relieve sinusitis and fevers.

Marjoram has long been respected for its ability to calm unwanted or inappropriate sexual desire and to ease loneliness, bereavement and heartbreak. It is comforting to those who have recently lost someone they love and has a long history of use to comfort the heart. We know from history that it was grown by monks in medieval monasteries for use as an anaphrodisiac and as Gerard said, *"for those who are given to over-much sighing."* In aromatherapy, it is used particularly for its emotionally warming and calming properties for lonely people, and those who live alone, perhaps bereaved or heartbroken after ending a close relationship. It is comforting to those who have recently lost someone they love. Marjoram's relaxing effect will help to relieve mental stress as well as physical tension and can be helpful for treating stress-related problems such as insomnia, restlessness, anxiety, depression, indigestion, colic, headaches, migraine, period pains, PMS, lethargy, dizziness, poor concentration and memory.

As an antiseptic diuretic, marjoram relieves fluid retention and hastens elimination of wastes including uric acid from the body, making it a good remedy for urinary tract infections as well as gout. It has also been used to treat problems of the reproductive tract. By stimulating the circulation to the pelvis, it is a good decongestant for accumulations such as fibroids and cysts.

Externally, the warming and relaxing properties of marjoram oil, when diluted in a carrier oil such as sesame, can be felt when massaged into stiff, painful joints, aching and tense muscles, sprains and strains. Apply dilute essential oil or tincture to fungal infections (ringworm, athlete's foot), stings, bites, infected cuts and wounds. A mouthwash can be used for mouth infections. The dilute essential oil can also be used as ear drops for earache and ear infections.

Homeopathic Remedy
Origanum marjorana has an affinity for the reproductive system, and can be used to remedy sexual over-excitement, inappropriate sexual desires, or both. Like the herbal remedy and aromatherapy oil, the homeopathic remedy also helps people who are alone, not involved in a close relationship and thus feel unable to express themselves as they would want to sexually.

Flower Essence
Marjoram is comforting, calming, soothing and greatly supportive in times of grief, sorrow, and vulnerability. It helps one let go of fear of being vulnerable, of being alone, and helps one to be more self-reliant and find inner strength.

Edible Uses
Marjoram is highly popular in Mediterranean and North American cookery. The delicate, warming, thyme-like flavour of the leaves and flowers makes it a very versatile and really tasty addition to many different dishes including salads, vegetables, pasta, tomato-based dishes, stuffings, meats, game, poultry and pulses. It can be used both fresh and dried, but the dried is always stronger tasting. Chop the leaves and add at the end of the cooking time.

Recipe

Anti-inflammatory Tisane
1 part golden marjoram
1 part nettle
1 part meadowsweet
½ part feverfew

Place the fresh herbs in a teapot. Pour on boiling water. Leave to infuse for 10–15 minutes. Drink one cupful three times daily before meals and use as a foot bath at night.

Growing
Propagate by sowing seeds under glass and plant out in late spring, once all danger of frost has passed. Alternatively, take stem cuttings in summer or divide the root in autumn and overwinter in a frost-free area. Prefers light well-drained soil and full sun. Grows up to 10" (25cm) and flowers in late summer to early autumn.

Related plants
O. vulgare: wild marjoram/oregano. Hardy.
O. onites "aureum": oregano with golden foliage. Hardy. *O. onites*: Greek oregano. Hardy.
O. dictamnus: dittany of Crete
O. x. marjoricum: Italian oregano. Half hardy.

Cautions
The essential oil may irritate the skin if used undiluted. Avoid in pregnancy and known allergy.

Oregano does contain naringin and naringenin, chemical constituents contained in grapefruit juice, which has been reported to cause alterations in the metabolism of some drugs. Use with caution in individuals on medications metabolised by the CYP3A4 pathway. May reduce iron absorption.

Passiflora incarnata: Passionflower

The Flower to Passify the Spirit

> *There has fallen a splendid tear from the passion-flower at the gate. She is coming, my dove, my dear; She is coming, my life, my fate; The red rose cries, "She is near, she is near;" And the white rose weeps, "She is late;" The larkspur listens, "I hear, I hear;" And the lily whispers, "I wait."*
> – Alfred Lord Tennyson (1809–1892)

Other names: Passion vine, purple passionflower, water lemon, wild passionflower, lemon fruit, apricot vine, maypop

Parts used: Leaves, stems and flowers

Passionflower is a fast-growing climbing vine with one of the most intricate and stunningly beautiful flowers in the plant kingdom. It is native to the southeastern United States and Central and South America. Its lovely name comes from the Spanish conquistadors who took over Mexico and Peru in the sixteenth century. It was sent to Pope Paul V from a mission in Peru in 1605 because in the remarkable design of the flower they saw various symbols of the Passion of Christ, the period of time between the Last Supper and Christ's crucifixion. The corona in the center of the flower and its petals was thought to resemble the crown of thorns worn by Jesus on the crucifix and the stamen and pistil formation resembled the cross.

Passionflower is a member of the Passifloraceae family and one of at least 500 known species. *Passiflora incarnata* is the one generally used in medicine. *Incarnata* can be translated as 'embodied' perhaps relating also to Christ, God incarnate. Its amazing flowers are white and purple-tinged, it can grow to a height of up to 30 ft (9 m) and prefers subtropical, frost-free climates. Purple passionflower (*P. edulis*) has often been confused with *P. incarnata*. Both bear fruit but *P. edulis* is the main source of passion fruit or 'maypops', which are orange-yellow edible fruits filled with sweet soft flesh and seeds. Native Americans such as the Cherokee of the southern Allegheny mountains cultivated passionflower

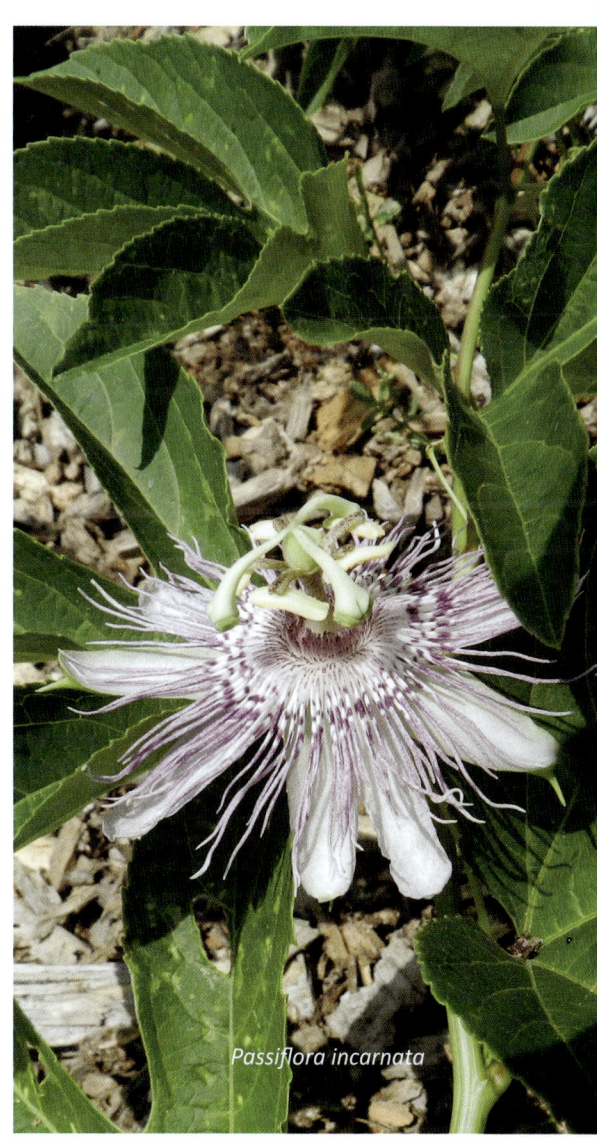
Passiflora incarnata

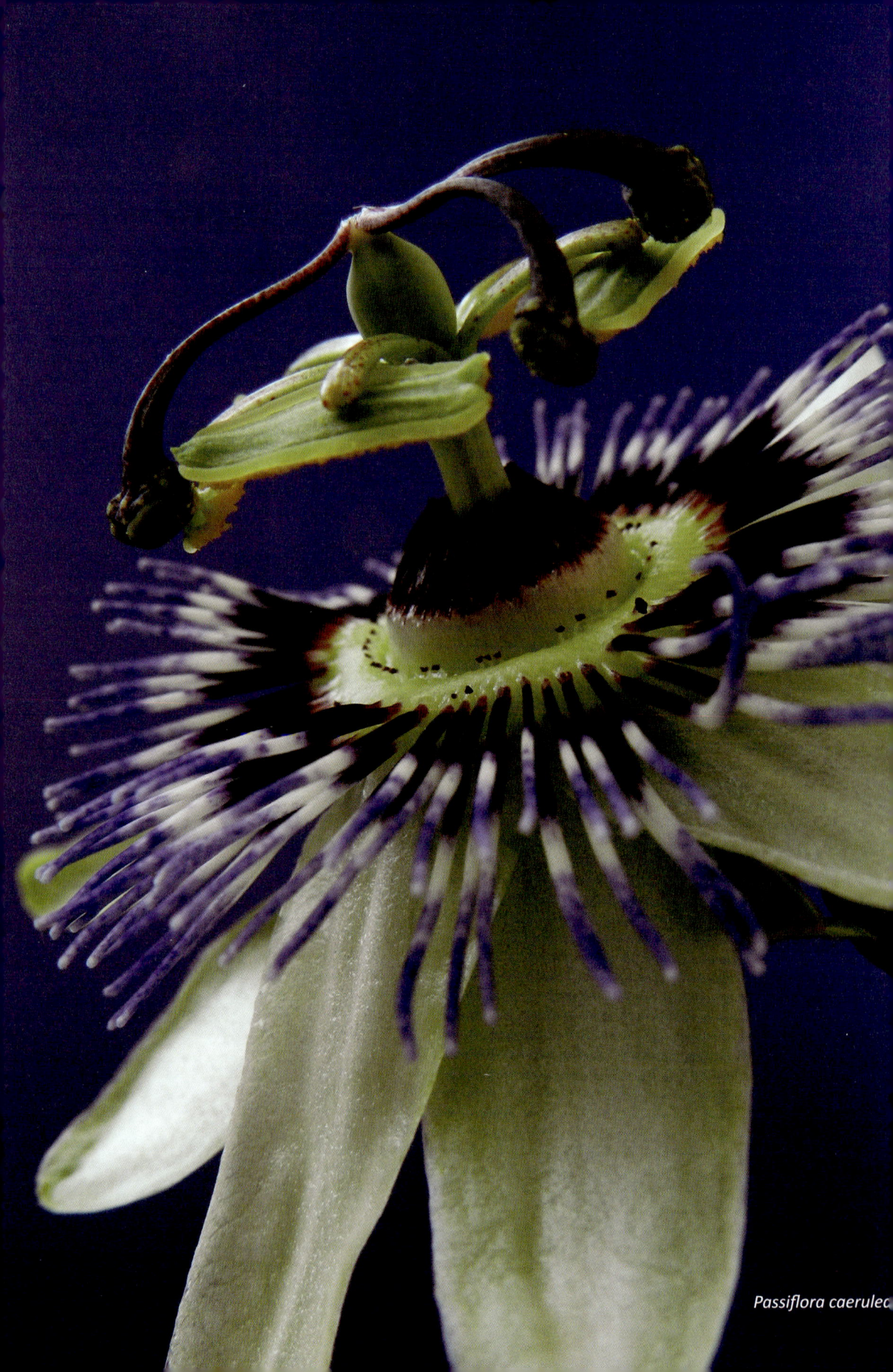
Passiflora caerulea

for its delicious fruit that combines both sweet and sour tastes.

The Spanish explorers learned about the benefits of passionflower from the native Peruvians and the Aztecs of Mexico. It was highly valued as a sedative and once in Europe and North America it became a popular folk remedy for insomnia, anxiety, restlessness and agitation. It was also used for a variety of other conditions including epilepsy, diarrhoea, neuralgia, asthma, whooping cough, seizures, painful menstruation, haemorrhoids, infections, boils, wounds, earaches, indigestion, worms and liver problems. The fruit has been used to flavour certain beverages.

Because of passionflower's use as an anxiolytic to reduce anxiety, and its reputation as a reliable remedy to relax body and mind, the Germans apparently attempted to use one of its its ingredients called harmine as a truth serum during World War II. It was thought to be able to relax you enough to induce a euphoria-like state.

Herbal Remedy
The flower and the vine of passionflower make a wonderfully relaxing remedy for all sorts of nervous conditions. Its ability to calm anxiety and aid sleep can significantly improve the quality of life and increase resilience to stress. It contains flavonoids including apigenin and luteolin, vitexin, isovitexin, kaempferol, quercetin and rutin. It also contains indole alkaloids including harman, harmine, harmaline and harmalol as well as coumarin derivatives, cyanogenic glycosides, amino acids (including GABA), fatty acids (linoleic and linolenic), gums, maltol, volatile oil and phytosterols (stigmasterol).

Passionflower is one of the best tranquilising herbs for chronic insomnia, whether from overwork or exhaustion, aiding the transition into a restful sleep and allowing you to wake refreshed and alert in the morning. It is completely non-addictive. For best results, it is better to take passionflower during the day as well as before retiring for bed.

As both a sedative and antispasmodic, passionflower can calm the nerves, ease anxiety and soothe restlessness and agitation. It can be used for fear and panic symptoms including nausea, trembling and palpitations. It relaxes tension, twitching and cramp in the muscles, and reduces pain as in back pain, headaches, neuralgia and shingles and can be used in Parkinson's disease. It may have an anticonvulsant action which could be of benefit in epilepsy and it may be helpful for low libido and in opiate withdrawal.

Its sedative effects may be attributed to the indole alkaloids such as harmane, harmaline and harmol or they could be related to flavonoids such as apigenin, luteolin and scopoletin. In addition, passionflower contains or affects the metabolism of gamma-amino butyric acid (GABA), a chemical the brain makes to help regulate mood and anxiety and reduce pain. It may be that passionflower can modulate the GABA neurotransmission system in the brain and counter neurotransmitters that cause excitement, thus having its calming effect. This may play a part in the possible anticonvulsant action of passionflower and its benefit in epileptic seizures.

Passionflower can be thought of in any symptoms related to tension and anxiety including headaches, high blood pressure, poor digestion, nausea, painful wind, colic and period pains. The antioxidants in passionflower are likely to have an anti-inflammatory effect, which may explain some of its benefits. Because passionflower has a cooling rather than heating effect generally, it can be thought of in any overly fiery emotion such as anger, frustration, low self esteem, intolerance and irritability. Its cooling effect can also be helpful in menopausal symptoms including hot flushes, headaches, depression, insomnia, mood swings and anger, if taken over a few weeks. It can also improve concentration by reducing exam nerves and may be of benefit in attention-deficit hyperactivity disorder (ADHD).

In Europe passionflower is often used in combination with hawthorn to ease digestive spasms associated with gastritis and colitis. Other members of the *Passiflora* genus might help treat stomach problems including stomach ulcers. These include *Passiflora foetida* which is more commonly known as *stinking passionflower* and *Passiflora serratodigitata*. Both also have antioxidant actions. It is possible that passionflower has potential as a chemopreventive for cancer; it is thought to inhibit an early antigen of Epstein-Barr virus, which suggests that it may also inhibit the growth of cancerous tumours.

Passionflower can relax tension throughout the arterial system and can be used to reduce stress-related high blood pressure and ease nervous palpitations and arrhythmias. Its relaxing effects in the respiratory system relieve tension and spasm, making it a useful remedy for irritating and nervous coughs and asthma.

Passionflower is often used in combination with other sedative plants including hops, valerian, lavender and St John's wort. It is an ingredient in many over the counter (OTC) sedatives for relieving insomnia and anxiety. It has been endorsed by several important European research organisations as a sedative and aid to sleep and approved by Commission E for the treatment of nervous unrest. The standardised sedative tea formula approved by the Commission E contains passionflower and valerian root as well as lemon balm. The European Scientific Cooperative on

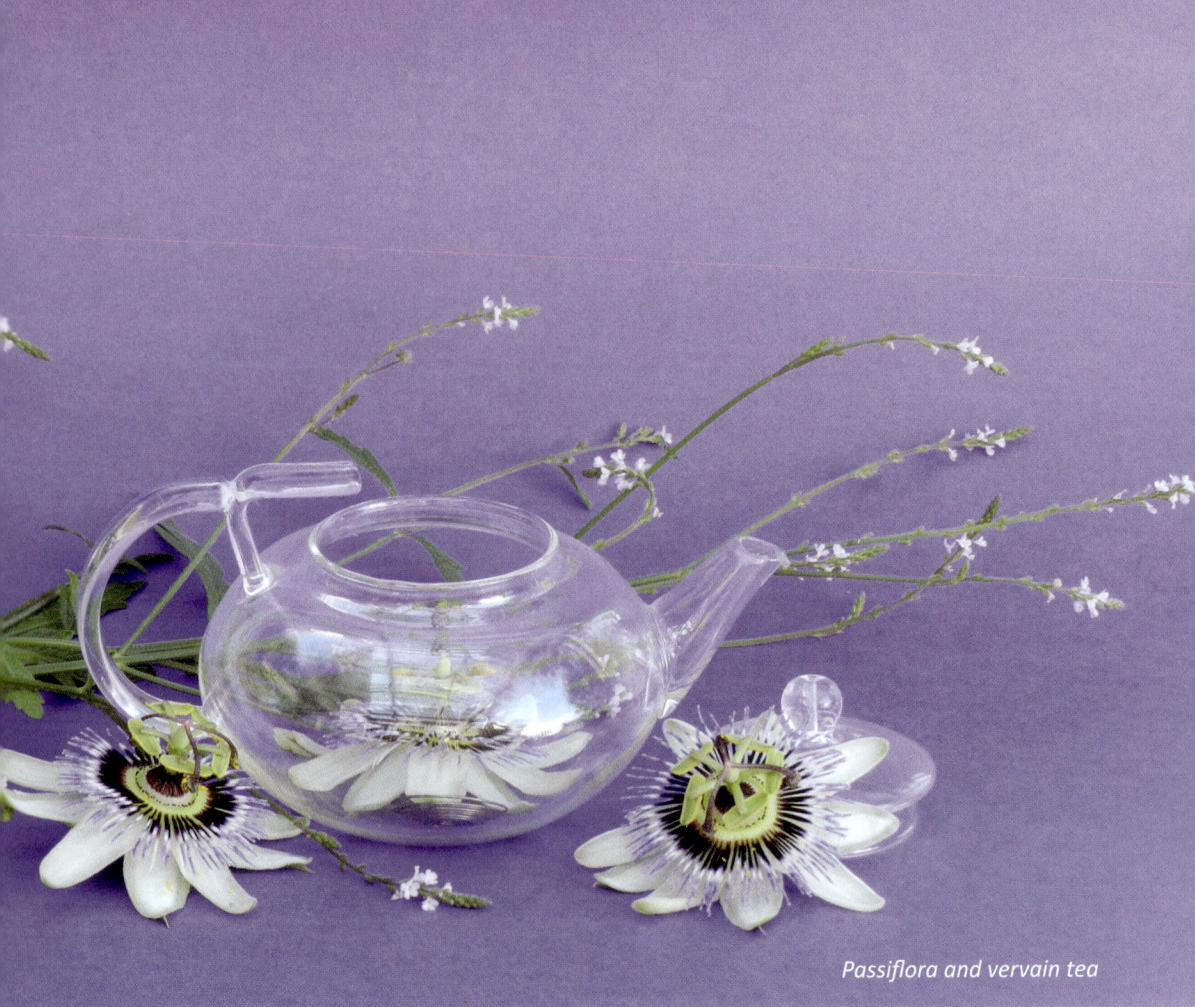

Passiflora and vervain tea

Phytotherapy (ESCOP) has approved it for use in tension, restlessness, and insomnia associated with irritability.

Externally a compress of passionflower can be used as an anti-inflammatory and pain killer. It can be applied to bruises, burns, skin problems, haemorrhoids, inflamed eyes and used to ease pain in toothache and earache.

Homeopathic Remedy
Passiflora is used similarly for symptoms characterised by restlessness, agitation, over-excitement, pain and spasms as in cramps and whooping-cough. It is indicated in insomnia particularly when resulting from exhaustion, anxiety, overwork and a night-time cough. In children, insomnia could be associated with teething, worms, pain and asthma.

Passiflora is also used for hysteria, violent headaches, a heavy feeling in the stomach after eating, wind and belching, and to help withdrawal from opiates such as morphine. It can be helpful in delirium tremens, convulsions in children and neuralgia. It has a quieting effect on the nervous system.

The Flower Essence
Passionflower helps us get in touch with our inner selves, also called our *Christ consciousness*. It eases tensions within and calms the spirit and is said to open the throat and heart chakras. The throat chakra is associated with taking responsibility for our personal needs and for nourishing our inner self. The heart chakra is the centre through which we love. The more open it becomes, the greater our capacity to love an ever-widening circle of life.

Edible Uses
Passionflower can be enjoyed as a relaxing tea, and tastes good when blended with chamomile, lemon balm, rosemary, vervain or other relaxing herbs. The tea can be drunk through the day and added to the bath at night, especially to soothe fractious children into a restful sleep.

The exotic flowers can brighten any meal! They could add a decorative touch to salads and the petals floated in summer drinks. The fruit from *Passiflora edulis* also called '*wild apricots*' can be eaten raw or made into deserts, jams or wine.

Growing
Propagate by sowing seeds in spring, by layering, by taking cuttings in September, or by dividing runners in autumn. It thrives in relatively poor sandy, slightly acidic soils and needs good drainage, full sun and a place to climb. Can reach 30' (10m) and flowers through the summer and bears fruit in early autumn.

Cautions
Avoid in pregnancy and breastfeeding, and in liver or kidney disease. May decrease intestinal motility. Avoid with anticoagulants, Warfarin, salicylates, MAOIs, thyroid medication and sedative medications. Do not take passionflower with monoamine oxidase-inhibiting antidepressants.

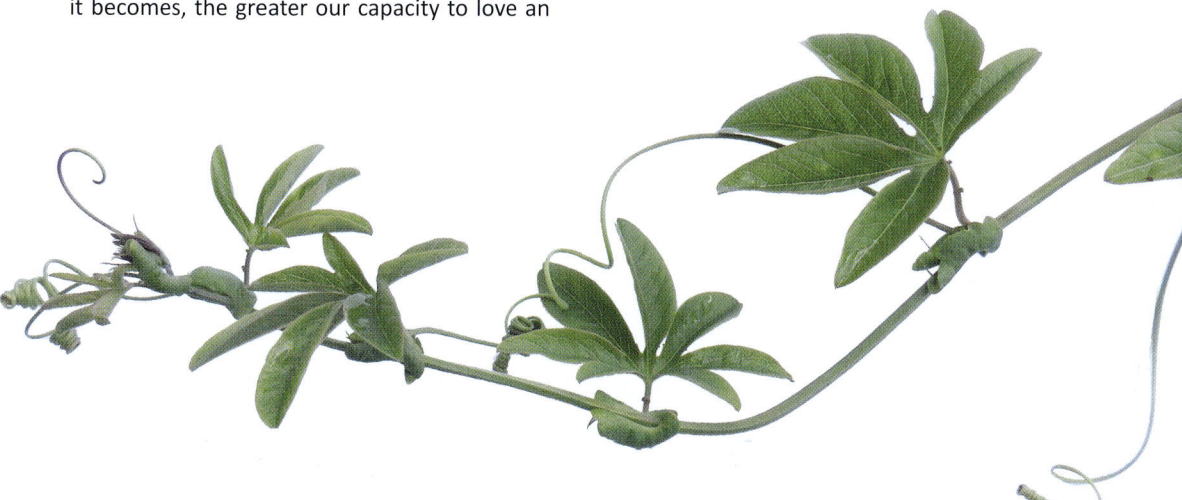

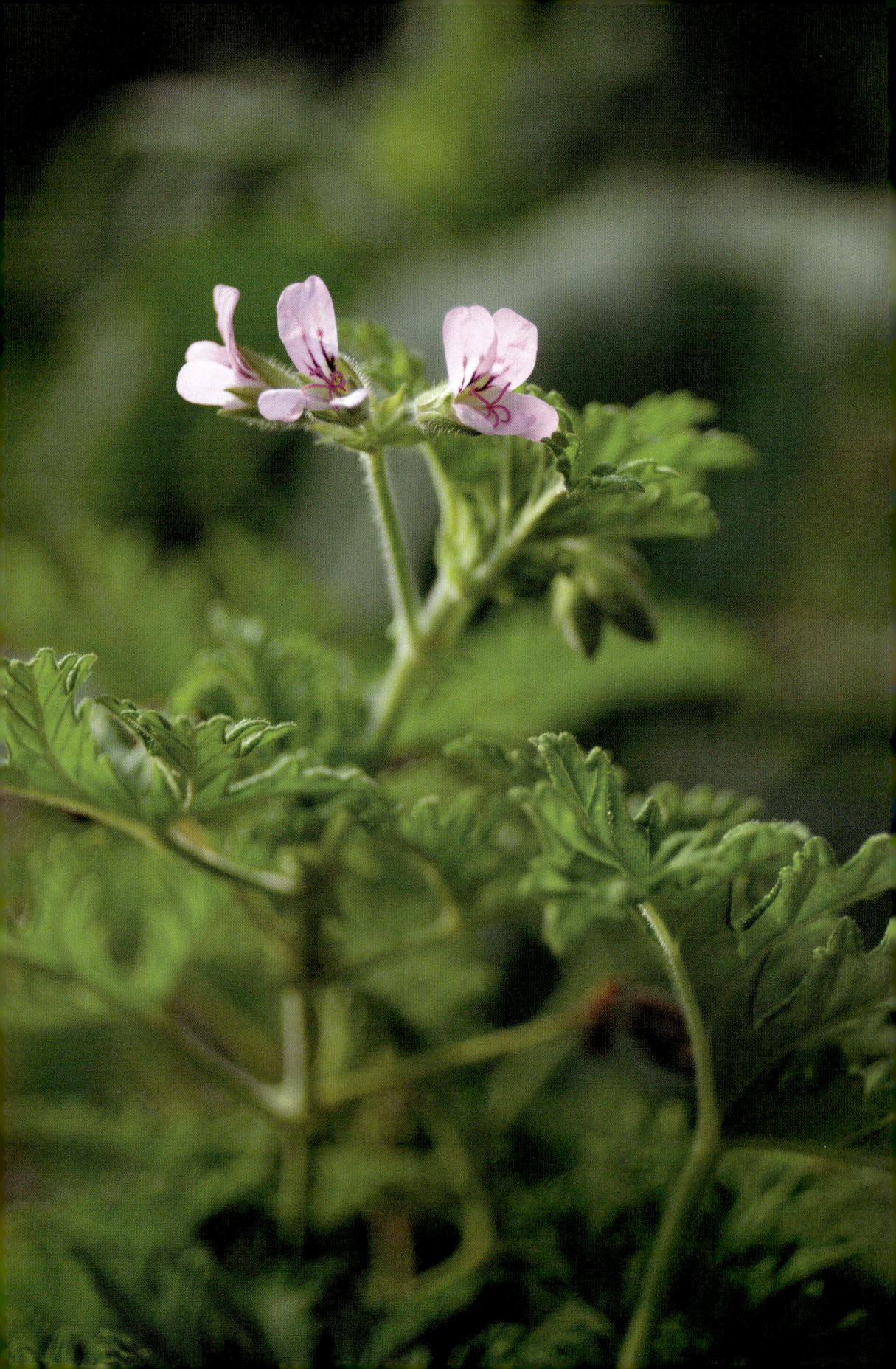

Pelargonium graveolens: Rose Geranium
The Flower of Consistency

The air was fragrant with the breath of flowers
That nodded to each other from costly vases
Scattered through both apartments;
And, before one of the windows,
Rose a bronze stand containing china jars
Filled with pelargoniums, in brilliant bloom
– Augusta Evans (1835–1909)

Other names: Sweet scented geranium, old fashion rose geranium, rose-scent geranium, scented pelargonium, flower of consistency

Parts used: Leaves, stems and flowers

Rose scented geranium is an exquisitely fragrant shrubby plant, related to the cranesbills and belonging to the Geraniaceae family. It is native to South Africa and grows about a metre tall, with small pink flowers, and flourishes in a warm, dry climate. Although perennial, it is not hardy in temperate climates, but can be grown indoors. The flowers and leaves are highly popular as scent and flavouring in food preparation, while the leaves and essential oil are widely used in perfumery and herbal medicine. The name *Pelargonium* comes from 'pelargos' meaning stork.

According to an old Arab legend, rose scented geraniums are descended from the mallow. One day when the prophet Mohammed was washing his shirt in a stream, he hung it out on a mallow plant to dry in the sun. The humble mallow was so honoured by this, that it blushed and turned a deep pink colour and was transformed into the elegant geranium with its highly perfumed leaves.

Pelargoniums were introduced to Europe in the 17th century when naturalists, plant collectors and ship surgeons sailed on trade routes around the Cape of Good Hope and brought plants back from their voyages. Their bright flowers, variety of colours and the beautiful scents from their leaves, from almond to lemon, nutmeg and rose, captivated gardeners and made them so popular that by Victorian times they could be found in almost every English summer's garden. Scented pelargoniums were also grown indoors in greenhouses, in manor halls, on cottage windowsills and in pots strategically placed in homes so that their scents would be released when brushed by the long skirts of ladies as they passed by.

In the Victorian language of flowers, rose-scented geranium meant 'preference', nutmeg-scented heralded an 'expected meeting' while the lemon-scented suggested an 'unexpected meeting'. They were described as plants best used 'for enchantment' and were used in pot pourris, ointments and cooking at this time. They have since been hybridised all over the world. They reached North America with the early colonists who had little access to spices and so used scented pelargoniums as flavouring for foods. Geraniums have been called the 'flower of consistency' as they have the ability to lift spirits, bring joy and balance the emotions. They have special significance in Poland, where they are considered a symbol of hope and a protector of the home.

The roots, leaves and flowers of rose geranium have been used as medicine in European, Chinese, Iranian, African, Indian and Arabic traditional systems. They have been used for their antiseptic, anti-inflammatory, astringent and sedative properties and were made into remedies to treat malaria, gastro-intestinal problems including dysentery, uterine disorders, cancer, to staunch bleeding including that related to menstruation and haemorrhoids, for insomnia, heart problems and to soothe sore muscles.

In African bush medicine, pelargoniums have been used for their astringent, antifungal, anti-inflammatory, antiseptic and styptic (stopping bleeding) properties. The medicine men in Sotho and Zulu tribes made a paste from the crushed leaves to staunch bleeding, heal wounds and resolve abscesses, and they used decoctions of the roots to bathe patients with fevers. Roots were also chewed or powdered and mixed with food.

In the mid-1800s, the French discovered they could match the scent of rose oil with essential oils distilled from rose scented pelargoniums including *Pelargonium radens*, *P. graveolens* and *P. odoratissimum*, and they are still used today in aromatherapy, cosmetics and perfumery all over the world as complements or substitutes for the more expensive Attar of rose (rose absolute). Nowadays the major production of geranium oil takes place in China and the Middle East especially Egypt and Morocco.

Herbal Remedy

The leaves, stalks, flowers and root of rose scented geranium can all be used as medicines. They have antioxidant, anticancer, astringent, nervine, anti-inflammatory, antibacterial, antifungal and acaricidal (against house mites) actions, mostly attributed to the presence of the volatile oils, terpenoids and flavonoids. Antioxidants have an ability to protect the body against damage caused by free radicals which contribute to problems such as cardiovascular problems, diabetes, cancer, Alzheimer's disease,

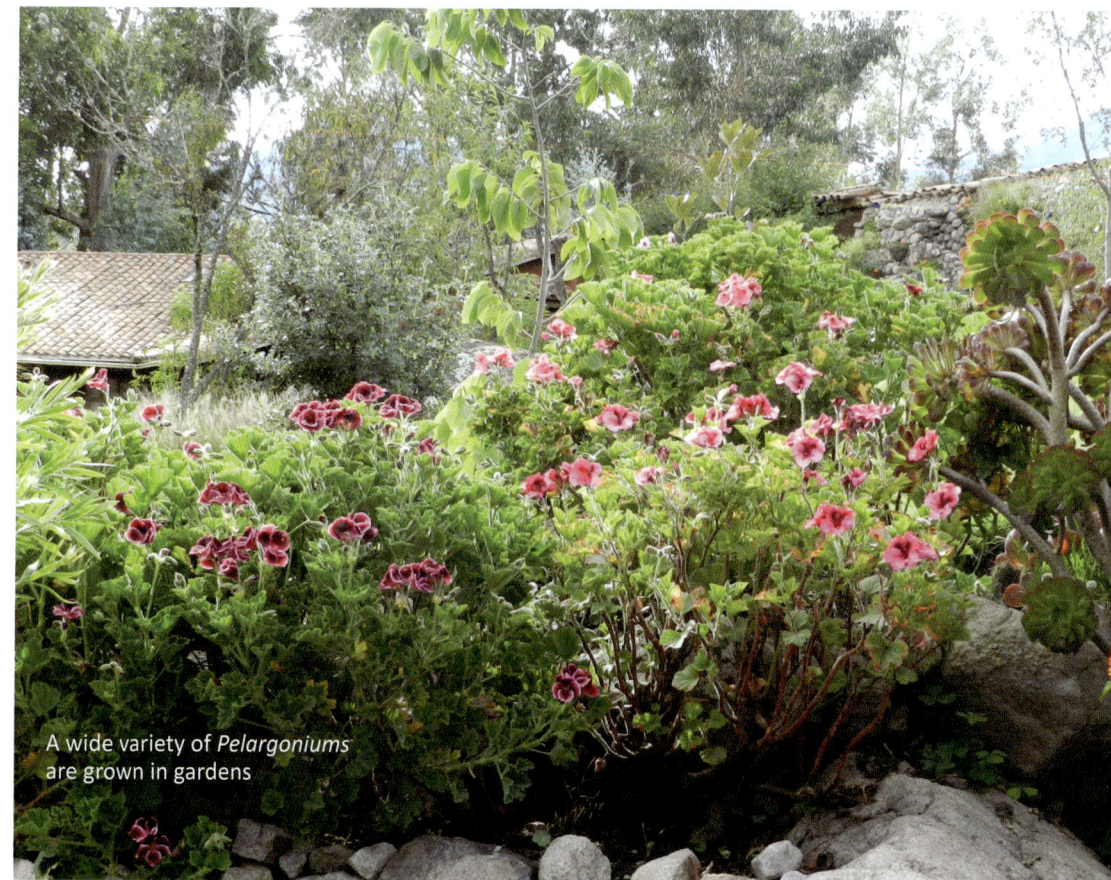

A wide variety of *Pelargoniums* are grown in gardens

Parkinson's disease and many facets of the ageing process. In the cardiovascular system, rose geranium can improve the circulation, stimulate the lymphatic system and is helpful for detoxification. It can be helpful in raised cholesterol, atherosclerosis, high blood pressure, varicose veins, haemorrhoids and fluid retention.

Rose geranium is a wonderful herb for the nervous system. Its relaxing and sedative effects can calm anxiety, lift depression and ease nervous symptoms such as restlessness, anger, frustration and emotional upsets and insomnia. It could be helpful for overcoming addiction. It is well worth using to treat stress-related problems including headaches, stomach aches, menstrual cramps and debility. With its antioxidant and anti-inflammatory properties, rose geranium is highly recommended for treating problems related to inflammation and pain including headaches and neuralgia, as well as neurodegenerative diseases such as Alzheimer's, multiple sclerosis, Parkinson's disease and amyotrophic lateral sclerosis (ALS), where neuroinflammation is involved.

Rose geranium has a beneficial effect in the reproductive system and an ability to balance hormones; it is a lovely herb to treat premenstrual and menopausal problems and with its balancing effect on the emotions, it can ease mood swings and PMS. It can also reduce congestion in breast tissue that causes breast pain or tenderness in the premenstrual phase of the cycle; this could be related to the diuretic action of the plant which reduces fluid retention. Rose geranium can also be helpful in the treatment of acne as it is related to an imbalance of hormones including oestrogen, progesterone and insulin and the overproduction of sebum by the sebaceous glands. The relaxing effect of the volatile oils in rose geranium can help ease stress and anxiety associated with labour and childbirth.

With its astringent tannins, rose geranium can tone up lax muscles which could be useful in prolapse, and it helps to dry up excess secretions such as catarrh and diarrhoea. The tannins also have a styptic (stopping bleeding) action which is useful in nose bleeds and other bleeding problems including heavy periods.

The antioxidant actions of rose geranium may have an effect on male fertility by helping to protect the sperm against free radical damage from toxins. In the last fifty years or more, the average sperm count has almost halved and the incidence of abnormal sperm has risen, and this has been related to toxins in the environment. Treatment with rose geranium may be able to reverse this damage and improve the quality of the sperm.

In the gut, the relaxing effects of rose geranium can be helpful in stress-related problems such as stomach aches, wind, bloating, colic, diarrhoea as well as constipation. Its aromatic volatile oils help to improve digestion and balance metabolism and can be used for overweight and obesity, nausea, diarrhoea, dysentery, gallbladder problems such as gallstones, liver problems and gastric ulcers. The high concentrations of tannins known as oligomeric proanthocyanidins may contribute to its ability to curb diarrhoea, but its antimicrobial action against bacteria that can cause food poisoning, such as *Baccillus cereus*, *Salmonella enteritidis* and other pathogenic gut microbes, could also be helpful in this instance.

The antioxidant effects of rose geranium can also be helpful in the prevention and treatment of diabetes. The development and progression of diabetes is related to oxidative stress caused by high blood sugar which generates free radicals. The volatile oils in rose geranium have the ability to reduce oxidative stress by preventing the generation of free radicals, and in this way, they help to prevent the development of diabetes.

Rose geranium is a great herb to support the immune system. This is largely attributed to the volatile oils that give rose geranium its exotic fragrance. The aerial parts in particular have antibacterial actions against many bacteria including *Staph. aureus, Proteus vulgaris, Staph. epidermidis* and *Enterococcus faecalis*. They also have an antifungal action which is particularly effective against *Candida* spp. as well as *Malasezia* species which are thought to be the underlying cause of a skin problem known as pityriasis versicolor (PV).

Rose geranium makes an excellent remedy to prevent and treat a wide range of respiratory infections including colds, sore throats, tonsilitis, ear and chest infections. It is one of the first herbs to consider at the beginning of colds and coughs to prevent chest infections. It is active against many bacteria that affect the respiratory system, including *Mycobacterium tuberculosis* which causes TB and *Mycobacterium intracellulare* which is implicated in chest infections, affecting people with compromised immunity such as those with HIV. Its antifungal action against *Aspergillus* infections that can also affect people with low immunity means that it can help combat lung infections and allergies caused by this.

With its antioxidant and anti-inflammatory constituents, rose geranium may well be a valuable anti-cancer herb. It could improve the immune cell count of cancer patients having chemotherapy and/or radiotherapy and help to prevent low white blood cell count and immune impairment that usually occurs during cancer therapy. It has potential antitumour activity against precancerous changes of the cervix and leukaemia cells which is attributed to the volatile oils.

Externally rose geranium can be used as an antiseptic, anti-inflammatory and astringent to treat wounds, burns, bruises, eczema, varicose veins, chilblains and haemorrhoids. An infused oil can be gently applied to the skin to relieve nerve pain (neuropathy), especially pain following shingles. Some people also use it topically as an astringent beauty aid to tighten and lighten the skin.

Rose geranium can be used in infusions or dilute tinctures to stop bleeding and prevent infection from grazes, cuts and wounds. It has broad-spectrum antimicrobial activity which may be attributed to the coumarins and phenolic acids. An infusion of rose geranium is good used as a skin toner and antiseptic for excess sebum production which causes spots, greasy skin and acne; its antimicrobial actions combat infections such as *Staph. aureus* which cause boils and abscesses, while its strong antifungal effect is an effective treatment for ringworm and athlete's foot. Used on the breasts, geranium-infused oil can reduce swelling and engorgement and makes a good remedy to prevent and treat mastitis.

Aromatherapy Oil
The delightfully fragrant essential oil extracted from the leaves has very similar uses to the herbal remedy with analgesic, antimicrobial, antioxidant and anti-inflammatory properties. It is a wonderful oil for the nervous system and is used in diffusers and massage oils as a relaxant, sedative and antidepressant to relieve tension, anxiety, nervousness, low moods, stress and fatigue. The high concentrations of citronellol in the essential oil have the ability to inhibit nitric oxide production, which can reduce inflammation and cell death in the brain. This may be of great benefit to people with neurodegenerative diseases that include neuroinflammation like Alzheimer's disease, multiple sclerosis, Parkinson's disease, and amyotrophic lateral sclerosis (ALS).

Diluted in a carrier oil such as sesame and massaged gently into the affected area, geranium's anti-inflammatory and analgesic properties can help pain management and can reduce nerve pain as in postherpetic neuralgia (a complication of shingles). It can also reduce pain in arthritic joints and muscle tension. Massaging with dilute geranium oil or adding a few drops to the bath, can be helpful in oedema and leg and foot swelling related to it, as it has a diuretic effect. Its anti-inflammatory effect is helpful here too.

Geranium essential oil is a great remedy for the skin, and when added to carrier oils or creams it is helpful in acne, boils, abscesses, allergic and inflammatory skin conditions such as psoriasis and eczema, as well as skin infections including ringworm and head lice. It is an effective insect repellent and deodorant. It can help stop bleeding, combat infection and speed healing in cuts and wounds.

Geranium essential oil has effective antimicrobial properties, effective against multiple bacterial strains such as *Staph. aureus*, *Salmonella enteritidis*, *Bacillus subtilis* and *Pseudomonas aeruginosa*. The oil can be used to treat vaginal infections as it is active against bacteria including *Atopobium vaginae, Gardnerella vaginalis, Bacteroides vulgates, Streptococcus agalactiae, H2O2-producing lactobacilli, non H2O2 producing lactobacilli* and *Candida* spp., it can also be applied locally to cervical cancer.

The antimicrobial action of rose geranium is used in the food industry to extend the shelf-life of foods, drinks, pharmaceutical and cosmetic products as many pathogens that cause spoilage and deterioration are fungi and bacteria. Rose geranium is active against fungi including *Fusarium oxysporum, Aflotoxin flavus, H. oryzae* and *T. viride*, as well as bacteria including *Bacillus subtilis*, which causes rot in potatoes.

Rose geranium oil may also be effective as a fumigant for house mites which cause allergies and have been implicated in sudden infant death syndrome. Exposure to house dust mite allergens can cause broncho-constriction and inflammatory reaction of the airways that causes the airways to swell and impede air flow. Most houses are co-inhabited by dust mites *Dermatophagoides farinae* and *D. pteronyssinus*. The acaricidal activity against dust mites of the essential oil is mostly attributed to geraniol and β-citronellol.

Flower Essence
Geranium flower essence is for those who feel down and depressed, lacking colour in their life. Geranium helps to lift the spirits and to bring joy and happiness to daily activities. It is also helpful for those who need strength and motivation to bring plans and projects into action. It helps to get things started in a well-ordered way by providing the energy and clarity that is needed.

Edible Uses
The fresh leaves are lovely simply infused to make a tea. The flowers make charming decoration for salads and fruit salads as well as cakes, biscuits and desserts. The rose-scented leaves can be added to oils and vinegars to add flavour and interest.

Growing
You can sow the seed as soon as it is ripe in a greenhouse or store it and plant it in the spring. It germinates best with a minimum temperature of 13 degrees C. This usually happens within 2 weeks but can take months. Plant seedlings in pots outside in early summer and take them indoors in the winter if you live in a temperate zone, as they are not hardy. You can also grow rose geranium successfully from cuttings; taking them in early summer works best.

Cautions
Rose geranium essential oil should be avoided in pregnancy and breastfeeding. It may cause skin sensitivity if used neat on the skin and can irritate the eyes.

Recipes

Infused Rose Geranium Oil
Fill a glass jar about halfway up with olive or sesame oil and add rose geranium leaves, making sure they are completely covered.

Seal the jar tightly and place it on a sunny windowsill for about a week. Strain the oil through muslin into a different glass jar and throw the leaves away. Add fresh leaves and repeat the process. Leave for another week.

You can continue this process another two or three weeks, as each time it will make a stronger oil.

Pour the infused oil into a tightly fitting bottle and store it in a cool, dry place. It should keep for about a year without deteriorating.

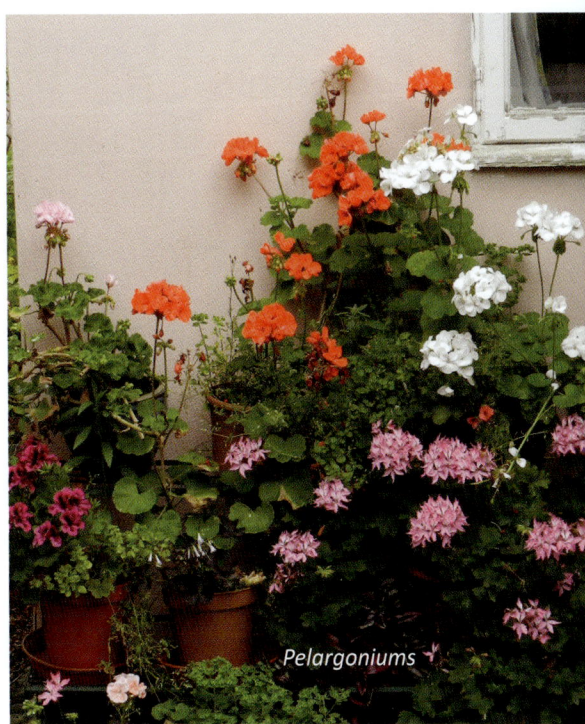
Pelargoniums

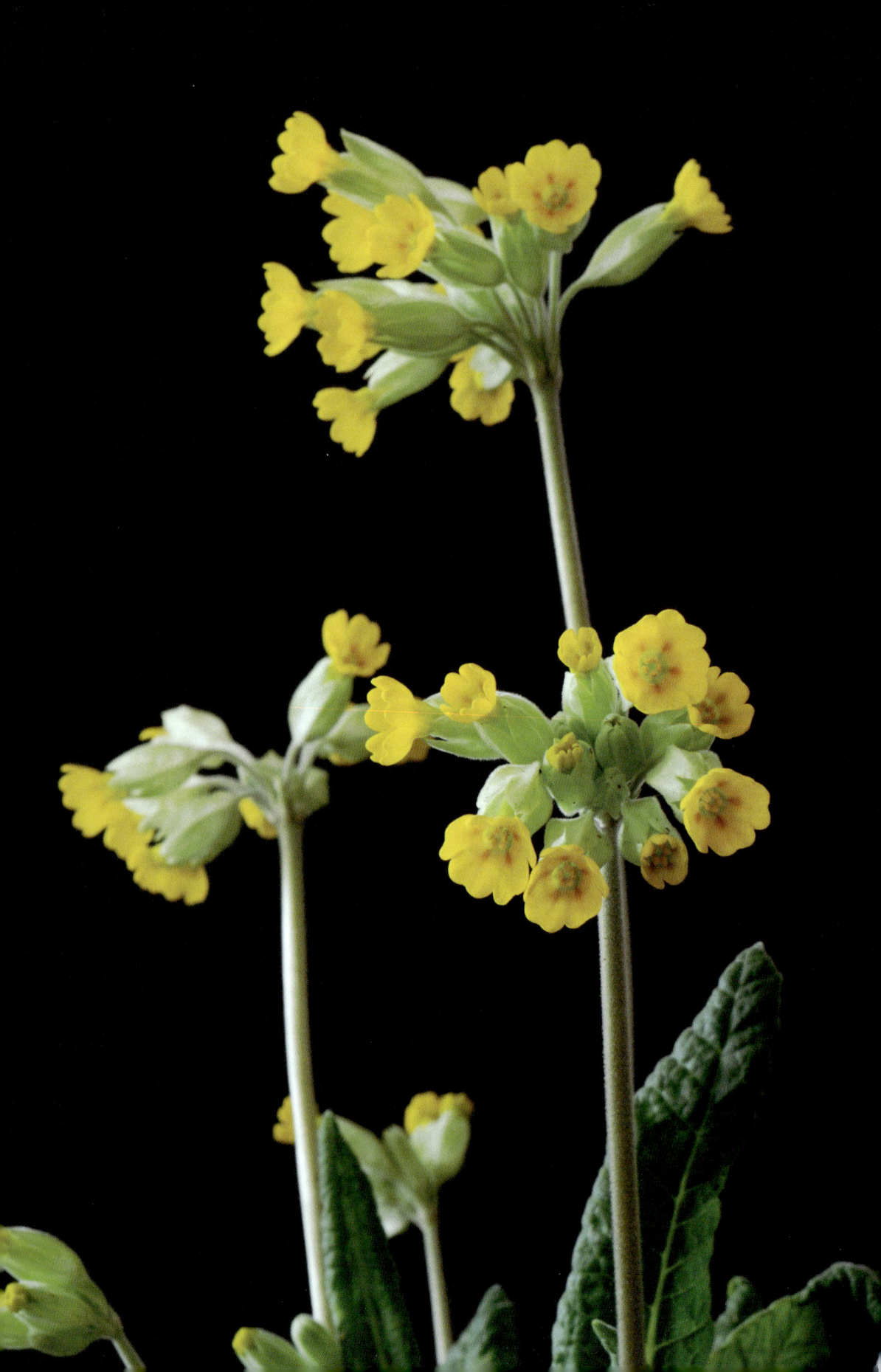

Primula veris: Cowslip

The Flower of Keys

Whilst from off the water fleet,
Thus I set my printless feet,
O'er the cowslip's velvet head,
That bends not as I tread
– John Milton (1608–1674)

Other names: Keyflower, palsywort, herb Peter, Peterkeys, Peterwort, Peterkin, key of heaven, fairy cups, petty mulleins, crewel, buckles, plumrocks, mayflower, password, artetyke, drelip, our Lady's keys, arthritica, herba paralysis.

Parts used: Flowers, leaves, root.

This pretty cousin of the sweet primrose has fragrant, bright yellow flowers with little orange spots that hang in clusters like a bunch of keys. It is a perennial member of the Primulaceae family and can be found growing wild in nutrient-poor grasslands and meadows and at the edges of woodlands throughout Britain, Europe and Asia. It was believed that cowslips were the favourite flower of the nightingale, which apparently only sang where cowslips flourished. While it was once a common feature of the countryside in spring, the charming cowslip has become rare because of over-picking and the use of herbicides – it is now a protected plant. The flowers have certainly been picked in enormous quantities in the past, as the many recipes for making wine, mead and cordials, syrup and vinegar, pickles and conserves, cheese, cakes, tarts, creams and puddings from the 17th to 19th centuries show.

Cowslip flowers threaded on a string and bunched tightly into a ball made a 'totsie' which was tossed to and fro in a game. Girls used these balls as a love oracle, throwing them from one to another saying: "*Titsy, Totsy, tell me true, who shall I be married to?*" Cowslip flowers were apparently a valued ingredient of love potions used by Saxon women. The petals were collected in the morning before the dew had dried on them and placed in a pot with fresh rainwater and left all day in the sunlight. The flower essence was then sprinkled on the pillow of their sweetheart, whose heart was expected to melt within the following month! The plant was exchanged by courting couples and the flowers sold on the streets of London for good luck.

In Norse mythology, the cowslip was dedicated to the goddess Freya, the key virgin. The flowers were believed to open the lock to her treasure palace, hence the old name 'keyflower'. Freya was the ruler of fate, the stars and the heavens and she was a symbol of sexual love (her other name Frigg has descended into slang). The god Odin is said to have learned all his magic and divine powers from the goddess Freya.

With the coming of Christianity, cowslips were dedicated to the Virgin Mary and called 'Our Lady's keys'. They were also linked to St Agatha and St Bertulf as they were said to represent the keys held by Mary Mediatrix to the store houses of heavenly grace. Their appearance was said to resemble a bunch of keys which would open the gates of heaven, so they were also named 'Peterkeys', 'Peterwort' and 'Peterkin' as well as 'key of heaven', and dedicated to St Peter to whom Jesus had promised the keys to the gates of heaven. The name *cowslip* comes from the belief that cowslips grew up wherever a cow left a cowpat and so they were called 'cuslyppe' or 'cuslop', the old English word for cow dung. It then became 'cowslop' and a little later cowslip.

A garland of the flowers was hung around the necks of cattle to increase milk production. Another maybe preferable name for cowslip is 'fairycup' as fairies are supposed to like nestling in the drooping bells of cowslip flowers. Shakespeare mentions cowslips many times and said they were so beloved by Englishmen that they considered the flowers were favourites of the fairies.

Where the bee sucks, there suck I,
In a cowslip's bell I lie
– William Shakespeare, The Tempest

In Russia its name 'pervo-tzuet' means first flower of spring and cowslips are indeed one of nature's first signs of renewed life unfolding, to reveal treasures as yet unknown. In some traditions, girls would exchange posies of cowslips in May as a symbol of trust and friendship.

In the past, cowslip flowers were in great demand for home remedies particularly for strengthening the nerves and calming the mind, relieving restlessness and treating insomnia. Culpeper recommended cowslip for "*all infirmities of the head coming of heat and wind, as vertigo, false apparitions, phrensies, falling sickness, palsies, convulsions, cramps, pains in the nerves, and the roots ease pains in the back and bladder. The leaves are good in wounds and the flowers take away trembling. Because they strengthen the brains and nerves and remedy palsies, the Greeks gave them the name Paralysio*", hence its old name 'herba paralysis'.

John Hill, a sixteenth century English composer, actor, author and botanist, who wrote an illustrated botanical compendium called *The Vegetable System*, said that when boiled in ale, the powdered roots of cowslips were used with success by country folk for giddiness, wakefulness and nervous troubles like those remedied by the flowers. In some old herbal the root was called '*radix arthritica*' from its use as a remedy for muscular rheumatism. According to Mrs Grieve in her 1931 *Modern Herbal*, a tea of the flowers was commonly used "*to ease paines in the head and is accounted next with Betony, the best for that purpose.*" A syrup was taken as a remedy for palsy (paralysis), hence its alternative name 'palseywort'.

Cowslip was considered a very beneficial remedy for the skin. Parkinson recommended cowslip water to cleanse the skin and clear spots and wrinkles, and an ointment was made from the flowers and used as a beauty aid. Culpeper said they "*taketh away spots and wrinkles of the skin, sun burnings and freckles*" and aid "*beauty exceedingly*". According to the doctrine of signatures, the freckles on the petals denoted the flower's value for removing blemishes and freckles on the skin. Shakespeare thought so when he said,

In their gold coats spots you see,
These be rubies: Fairy favours,
In those freckles lie their savours.

Perhaps this is why for some the cowslip flower is a symbol of grace and beauty. Certainly, the beautiful cowslip has been the inspiration for many a poet.

Herbal Remedy
Today cowslip root and flowers are still used as a relaxing and sedative remedy for nervous tension, anxiety, insomnia and as a general tonic to the nervous system. Cowslip is rich in antioxidant and anti-inflammatory constituents. It contains flavonoids (including astragalin and catechin), flavonoid aglycons (apigenin, quercetin, kaemferol), flavonoid glycosides (cinarozid, rutin, hyperozid), phenolic glycosides (primverin and primulaverin), triterpene saponins and glycosides (including primulaveroside and primveroside containing salicylates) and volatile oils.

Both the root and flowers are excellent for stress-related problems such as anxiety, tension, headaches, muscular aches and pains and nerve pain, and have a reputation for lifting the spirits and dispelling depression. They are cooling and anti-inflammatory and have been used traditionally for nervous problems associated with excess heat and congestion such as irritability and hysteria, inflammatory and painful nervous conditions such as neuralgia and neuritis, as well as vertigo. Cowslip also has a reputation for improving memory and increasing resilience to stress. The flowers are recommended for over-activity and sleeplessness particularly in children.

Cowslip is a popular remedy for the respiratory system. Both the flowers and the root are used to treat coughs, bronchitis, chest infections, whooping cough, mucus congestion and chronic catarrh. Cowslip root is particularly high in saponins which account for much of the plant's expectorant action and its ability to liquify mucus to make it easier to clear. Cowslip's combined soothing and sedative actions can soothe dry, irritating coughs and induce restful sleep, very useful when hacking coughs can disturb a good night's sleep. The flowers have antispasmodic and anti-inflammatory properties which make them useful in the treatment of asthma and other allergic conditions.

Cowslip also has antimicrobial actions, excellent to help fight bacterial, fungal and viral infections including influenza strains; its antioxidant and anti-inflammatory actions are helpful here. The flavonoids, notably rutoside, have strong antioxidant as well as antimicrobial and anti-inflammatory activities, the phenolic compounds and salicylates also play their part.

Taken in a hot infusion, cowslips are used to bring down fevers and to clear congestion and inflammation in colds, flu, sore throats, coughs and catarrh. They make a good remedy for babies, children and the elderly alike. By bringing blood to the surface of the body, cowslips relieve heat and also bring out eruptions, explaining why cowslips were an old country remedy for children's measles.

Cowslip may also have benefits for the cardiovascular system. The antioxidant and anti-inflammatory actions of the flavonoids, phenolic compounds and salicylates help to protect the heart and arteries from oxidative stress caused by free radicals, to reduce inflammation of the artery walls and the build-up of atheromatous

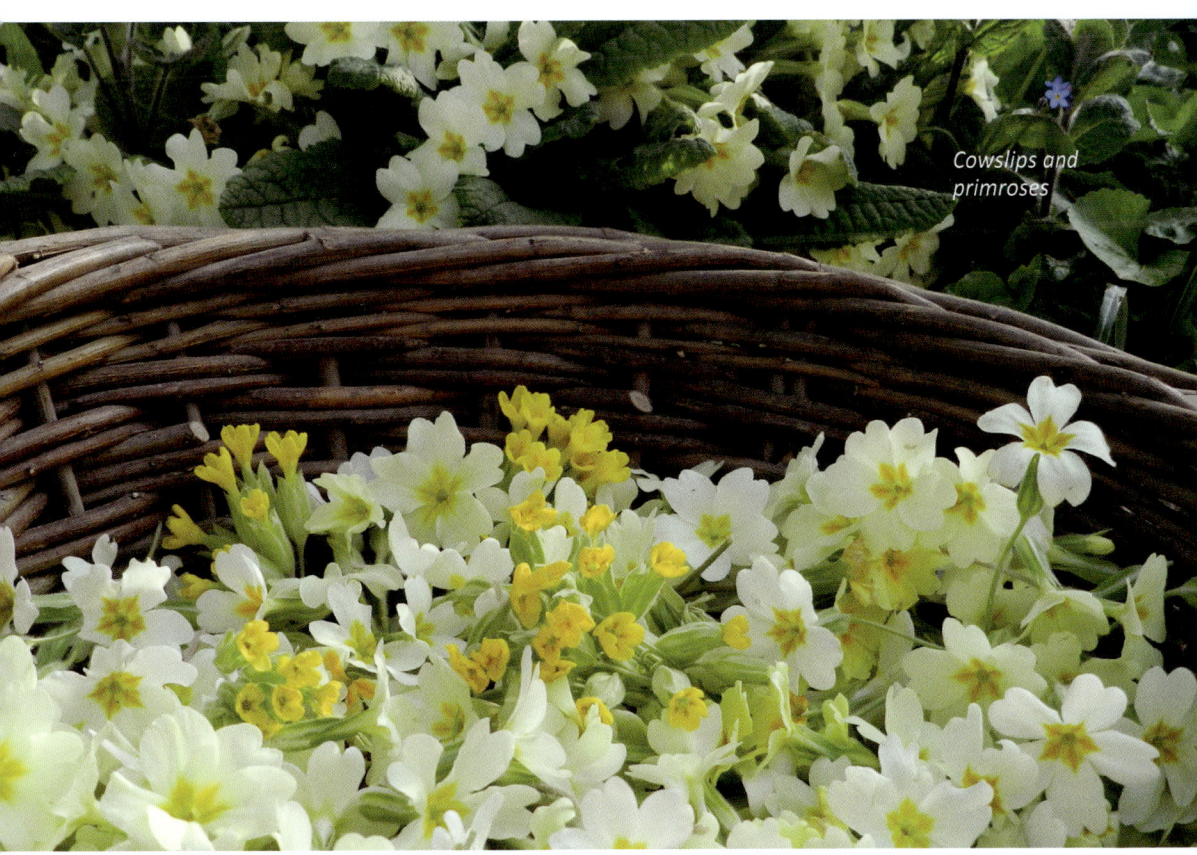

Cowslips and primroses

plaque. The flavonoids such as rutin have a strengthening effect on the arteries. Altogether cowslip has a cardioprotective effect, helping to prevent blood clots, regulate blood pressure and normalise the contractions of the heart, helping to avert cardiovascular problems including heart failure. The diuretic effects of cowslip may add to its hypotensive effect in high blood pressure. The salicylates also in the root have an anti-inflammatory action, particularly useful for swollen joints in arthritis and gout.

Externally, cowslip flowers can be used in lotions and ointments for skin problems such as eczema, spots and acne, and with their cooling and soothing effects, to relieve sunburn. A maceration of cowslip flowers was once a popular poultice to apply to bruises, to draw out infection and speed healing of the skin.

Homeopathic Remedy
The same themes run through the homeopathic use of cowslips in Primula veris. It is prescribed wherever there is heat and for symptoms characterised by burning. The remedy has an affinity with the nervous system, and is useful in headaches, migraine, vertigo, tinnitus, anxiety and febrile excitement. Primula veris is specific for *"threatened apoplexy (stroke) arising from psychic depression"* (Clarke) and cerebral congestion associated with neuralgia, and headaches which are associated with heat in the face and are better from pressure.

Primula is also used to relieve hot burning skin conditions, such as eczema, itching scalps, burning pains in the throat and chest, palpitations, cystitis (where the urine smells of violets), burning in the stomach with a tendency to vomiting and diarrhoea. It is also indicated in burning in the joints, particularly the right shoulder joint, and stiff neck and back. The symptoms tend to diminish in the open air, but are worse from stooping, movement and being indoors in stuffy rooms.

Flower Essence
A relative of the cowslip, the oxslip (Primula elatior), which is very similar in appearance, is used as a flower remedy. Oxlips were well known to the ancient Greeks and called 'dodekatheon' meaning plant of the twelve gods when used in a remedy with twelve constituents as a panacea. The flowers were apparently gathered by the dryads at the new moon and given for melancholy. Cowslip flowers were traditionally woven into funeral wreaths and put on graves and were worn pinned to clothes as a sign of bereavement. As a flower remedy, they can be used to ease the grief of separation or the breakdown of a relationship causing depression, grief, loneliness and feelings of abandonment.

Another relative of cowslip, the primrose (*Primula vulgaris*) is the flower remedy for both unexpressed and unresolved emotions. It is helpful for seasonal affective disorder (SAD) and also for those who have an unrealistic view of love and relationships which can inhibit the development of more grounded, intimate relationships.

Edible Uses
Cowslip leaves and flowers can be eaten raw and cooked and provide us with a source of vitamins and micro-elements in late winter and early spring. The flowers have a slightly citrusy taste and look great in salads and for decoration on almost any dish. The leaves are slightly bitter, but covered in dressing make a good salad ingredient. A tea made with the flowers is pleasant and can be combined with other relaxing or decongestant and expectorant herbs such as chamomile, lemon balm, thyme or oregano.

Growing
Cowslip is easily propagated by dividing the roots of old plants in autumn or raised from seed under glass in trays or in a nursery bed. It self-seeds easily. Cowslip will grow in most soils but prefers chalky soil, and open places or in semi-shade, growing up to 5 – 9" (10–20cm) and flowering in April–May.

Cautions
Cowslip should not be used by pregnant women, or with anticoagulative medications.

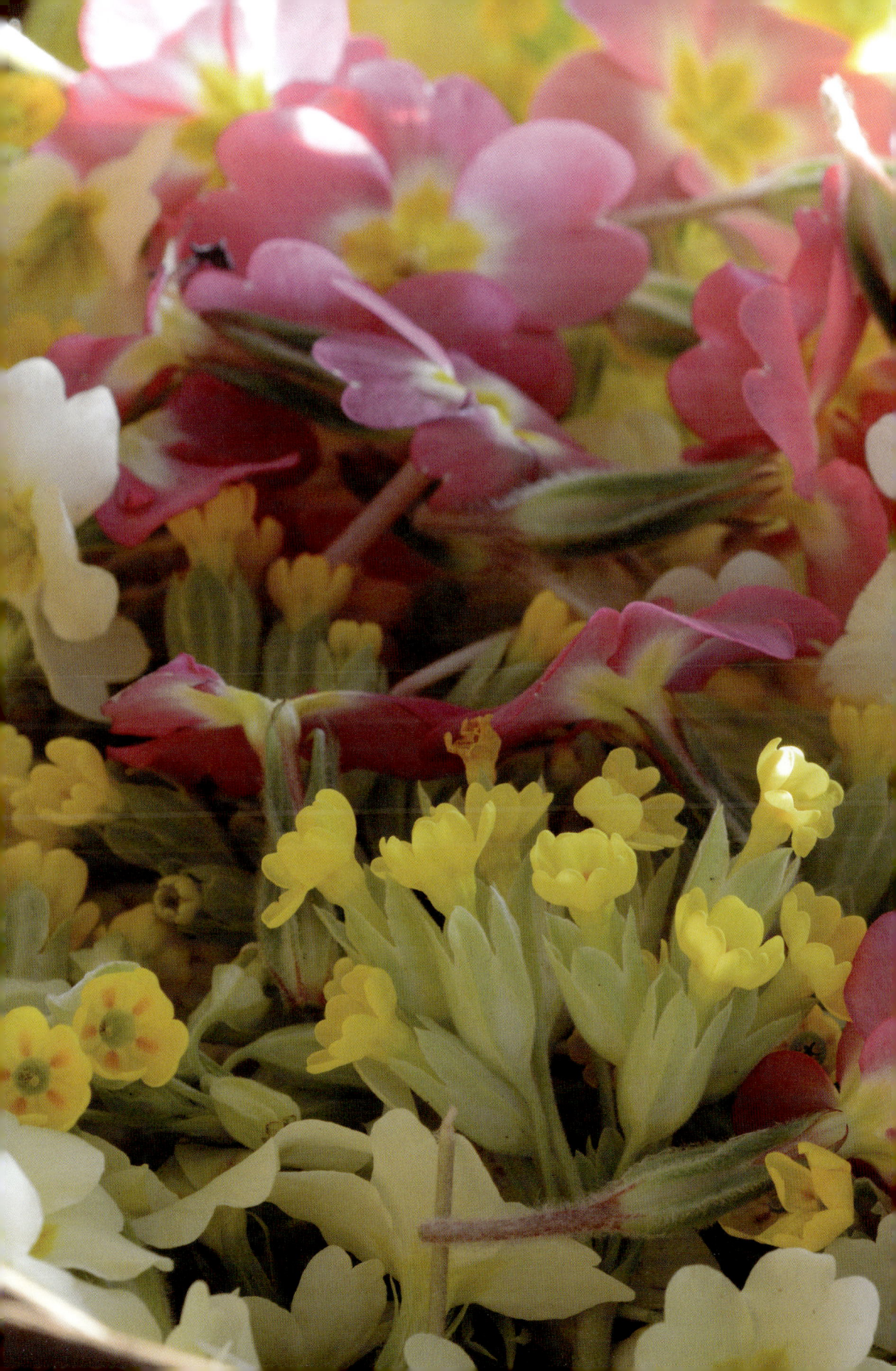

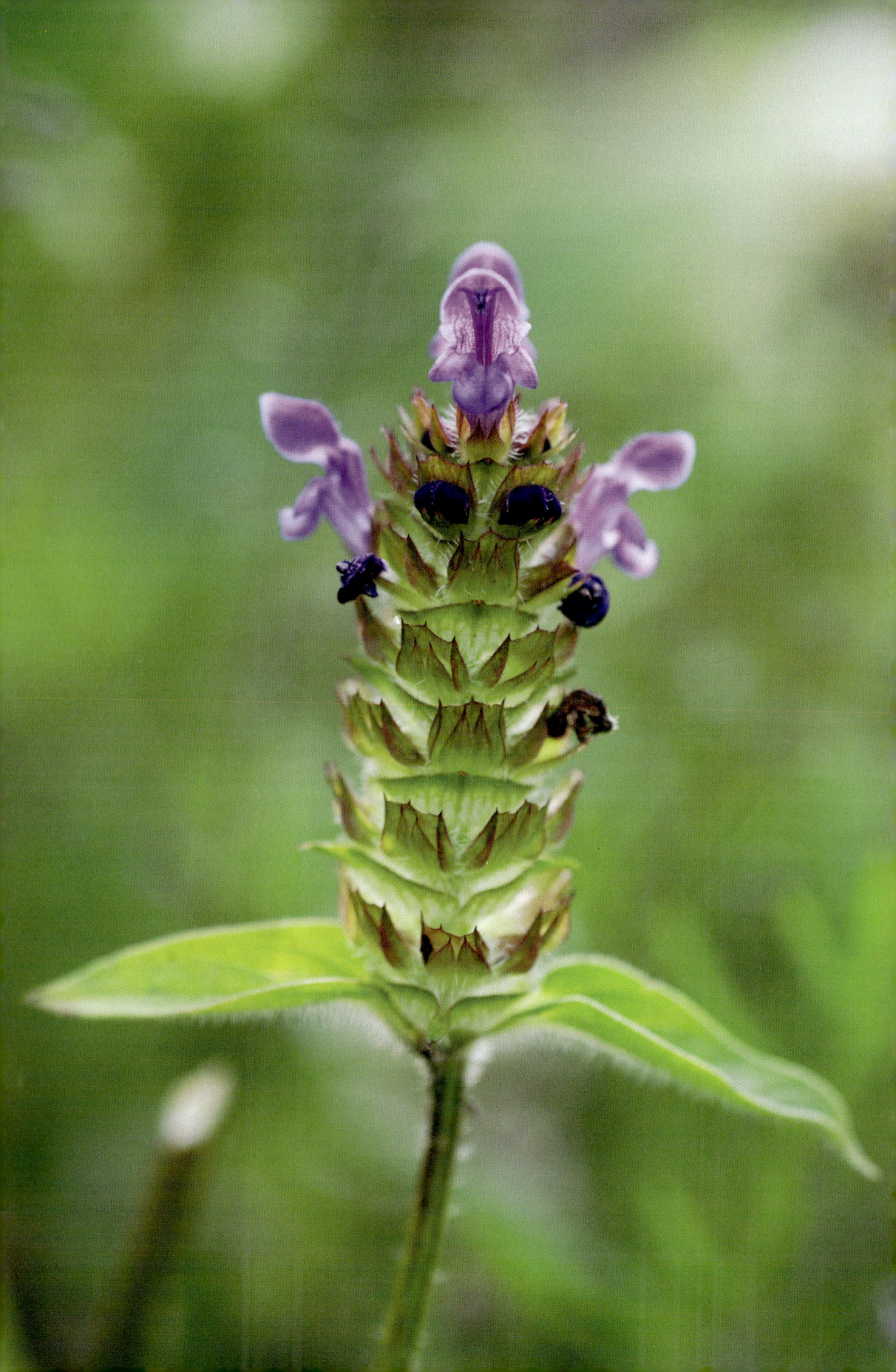

Prunella vulgaris: Self-heal

The Flower of Confidence

*Here is another herb of Venus, Self-heal, whereby when you are hurt you may heal yourself:
It is a special herb for inward and outward wounds*
– Nicolas Culpeper (1616–1664)

Other Names: All heal, woundwort, carpenter's herb, hook heal, heart of the earth, brownwort, blue curls

Parts Used: Flowers and leaves

Self-heal is a pretty little relative of mint, a member of the Lamiaceae/Labiatae family, which can be found growing wild all over Britain and Europe in pastures, woods and clearings and is loved by bees. Self-heal has also been called 'carpenter's herb' and 'hook heal' because the corolla, when seen in profile, is shaped like a bill hook. According to the doctrine of signatures, self-heal was used historically to heal wounds inflicted by sharp-edged tools.

The name *Prunella* was originally 'brunella' or 'brunellen', a name given to it by the Germans as the leaves and flowers were used to treat 'die breuen', which was an inflammatory mouth and throat problem common to soldiers in garrisons.

Self-heal was a popular remedy for throat complaints, because according to the doctrine of signatures, its corolla was seen to resemble a throat with swollen glands. It found its way to North America where it is called 'heart of the earth' and 'blue curls'.

Around the times of Paracelsus (1493–1541), self-heal was considered one of the best herbs to grow for home use and was often known as 'all heal'. The renowned apothecary Gerard said in his *Herball*, printed in 1597, "*The decoction of Prunell made with wine and water, doth join together and make whole and sound all wounds, both inward and outward, even as Bugle doth.*" It was commonly used by country people and labourers for cuts and wounds, and an old saying went "*no-one wants a surgeon who keeps self-heal*". Culpeper, writing in 1616, said that self-heal was under dominion of Venus and explained the name, "*Self-heal whereby when you are hurt, you may heal yourself*". He also said, "*The juice used with oil of roses to anoint the temples and forehead is very effectual to remove the headache, and the same mixed with honey of roses cleaneth and healeth ulcers in the mouth and throat*".

Although largely neglected by modern western herbalists, self-heal is an important herb in Traditional Chinese Medicine (TCM) in which it is known as 'xiakucao', meaning 'weed that withers in summer', as its spikes of purple flowers turn reddish-brown as they dry out during the summer. It is mentioned in the *Shennong Bencao Jing* (a compilation of oral traditions on agriculture and medicinal plants, written around 200 AD and attributed to the mythical Chinese sovereign Shennong, who lived around 2,800 BC). He states that self-heal is used for "*breaking concretions and dispersing bound Qi of the neck.*" In Chinese medicine until today, self-heal has been used for resolving accumulations and masses, particularly in the upper body (the chest, throat, and head).

Herbal Remedy
The combination of astringent, bitter, salty, sweet and pungent tastes in this understated little herb is given by the array of its constituents including bitters, alkaloids, saponins, phenols, tannins, polysaccharides, mucilage, proteins, lipids, volatile oils including rosmarinic acid, camphor and fenchone, caffeic acid, ursolic acid, vitamins (C, B1, K), glycoside (aucubin) and flavonoids (rutin).

In TCM self-heal is classified as bitter, cold and pungent and enters the liver meridian. Its primary effect is to cool 'liver fire' and nourish 'liver blood'. As the liver is connected to the eyes and 'liver fire' can be linked to inflammatory eye problems, self-heal is indicated in painful and dry eyes, inflammatory eye problems such as conjunctivitis, blepharitis and eyestrain as well as glaucoma and hypertension.

Just as its name suggests, self-heal is a wonderful herb with a great ability to enhance our innate healing powers and improve immunity. It is an effective antimicrobial against a range of bacteria and has a potent antiviral action, including activity against HIV and viral hepatitis. This is combined with its immuno-modulatory effect which is attributed to the polysaccharides and can be helpful in lowered immunity, chronic fatigue syndrome and to soothe allergic responses. Self-heal is an excellent remedy for a range of allergic reactions including eczema, asthma, hay fever and urticaria.

With its cooling and detoxifying actions and its supportive effect on the liver, self-heal is used to clear toxins from the system and for resolving inflammation. It is used to treat acne, boils and other inflammatory skin problems. In Chinese medicine, self-heal falls under the 'fire-purging' classification because of its use in treating redness and inflammation of the eyes or infections of the skin. It is added to prescriptions for skin diseases when nodules are present. It can be helpful in hypertension and for treating inflammatory problems including arthritis, gout, skin problems and inflammatory liver problems. Its antioxidant and anti-inflammatory properties are attributed partly to the rosmarinic acid which also may have anti-mutagenic effects, indicating its possible use as an anticancer herb; it may provide a remedy for treatment of lymphoma by suppressing the proliferation of Raji cells.

Self-heal has an affinity with the lymphatic system and can be taken for swollen glands, mumps, glandular fever and mastitis. In TCM self-heal has long been used for resolving accumulations and masses, particularly in the upper body (the chest, throat, and head). It is included in formulae for treating thyroid swellings and breast lumps and it is combined with Isatis root for treating mumps. Its pungency disperses 'stagnant qi' and 'constrained heat' and helps resolve lumps and nodules caused by 'stagnation of liver qi' and 'accumulation of phlegm and heat'.

According to Chinese medicinal philosophy, qi is the energy that flows in the body and governs the movement of blood, lymph, nutrients and toxins into and out of the body. The liver is responsible for ensuring the smooth and regular flow of qi throughout the body and for filtering toxins out of the blood. Symptoms of 'liver qi stagnation' include anger, irritability and frustration, depression, anxiety, stress, a feeling of a lump in the throat and PMS. Pain and inflammation can be caused by a blockage to the flow of qi in the affected part of the body. The pungency of self-heal helps to disperse 'stagnant qi' and 'constrained heat' and to resolve lumps and nodules caused by 'stagnation of liver qi' and accumulation of phlegm (lymph) and heat. Self-heal is widely used in TCM for its anti-tumour properties.

As an astringent and cooling herb self-heal can be taken to soothe the digestive tract during or following an attack of diarrhoea and makes a useful remedy for inflammatory bowel problems such as colitis. The bitters can be helpful in liver and gallbladder problems including viral hepatitis. It is also recommended for gout. Self-heal also shows potential as a remedy for diabetes as it reduces blood sugar and increases insulin sensitivity. The astringent tannins and its cooling effect can help to curb heavy menstrual bleeding.

Self-heal's relaxant properties can be helpful in headaches, particularly when they are related to tension, vertigo, over-sensitivity to light and high blood pressure. Self-heal is used in China for hyperactivity in children and when taken with *Chrysanthemum morifolium,* it is used to treat fevers, headaches, vertigo and to cool 'liver fire'. When taken in hot infusion, the diaphoretic action of self-heal increases sweating and helps reduce fevers. Taken when lukewarm to cool, self-heal has a more diuretic action and clears toxins and excess uric acid via the kidneys and so can be helpful in the treatment of gout. Urosolic acid is a diuretic that also has anticancer properties.

Externally self-heal draws out heat and infection from the skin and with its astringent, antiseptic and vulnerary actions, it makes an excellent wound healer. An infusion or dilute tincture can be applied, or the fresh plant rubbed on to the skin, to stop bleeding from cuts and scratches and reduce swelling from bites and stings, type 1 and 2 *Herpes* lesions, piles, varicose veins and ulcers. Self-heal helps to protect the skin from sun damage and would make an excellent component of sun creams.

A weak infusion can be used as an eyewash for inflammatory eye problems such as conjunctivitis, blepharitis and sties. Tinctures or infusions can be used as astringent gargles for sore throats and mouthwashes for mouth ulcers and bleeding gums. It can also be used in lotions and douches to treat vaginal infections.

Homeopathic Remedy
Prunella is used much like the herbal remedy for healing all types of infections, acute or chronic. It is indicated in low immunity and for people with a tendency to catch infections, or to suffer with chronic problems such as HIV or cancer. Lowered immunity may be linked to a poor sense of self and weak boundaries.

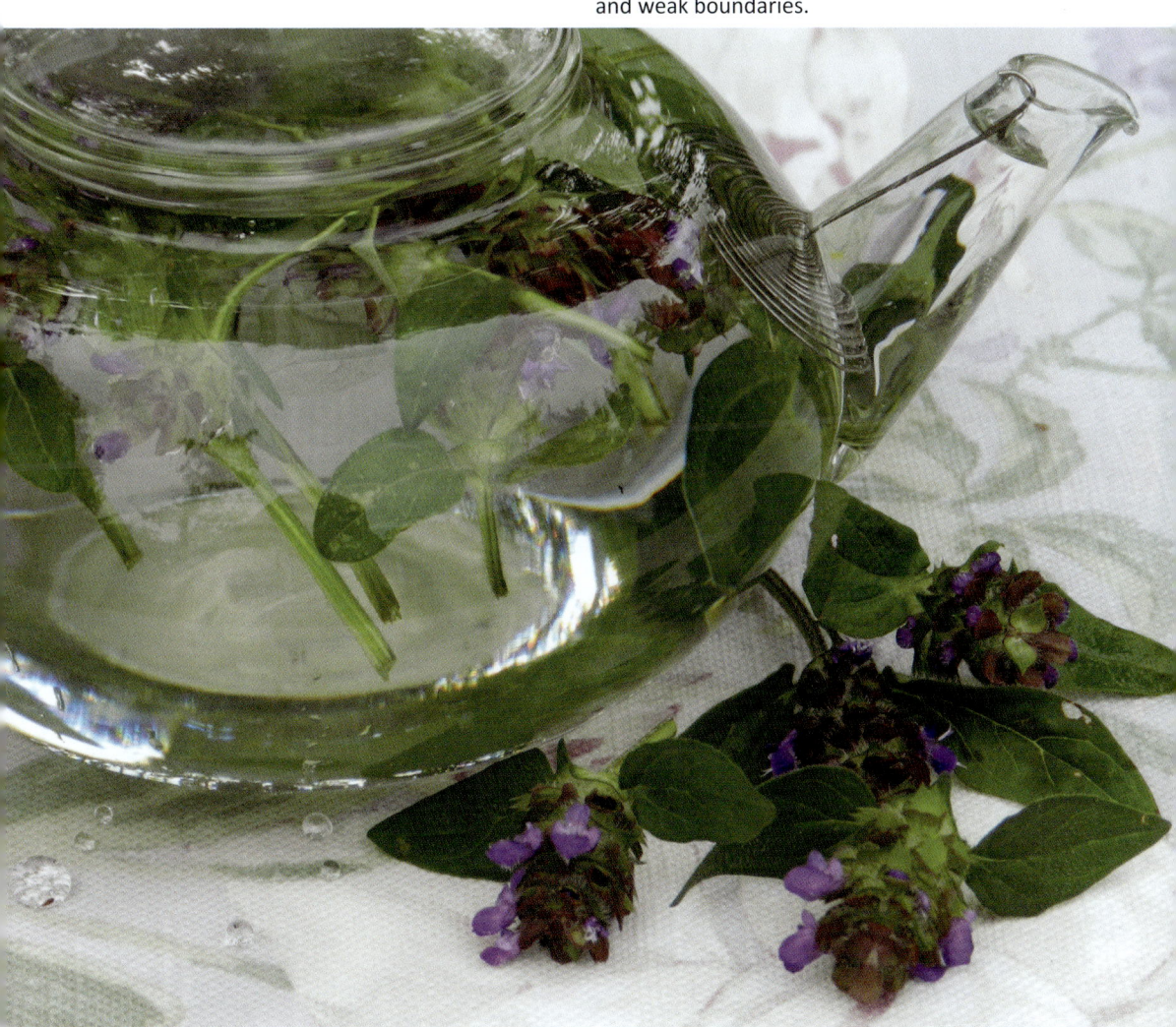

As a remedy to help us heal ourselves, prunella is for those who need to give more love and care to themselves and develop a stronger sense of identity, so they can be more resistant to infection and other illnesses. Like other members of the mint family, it can be thought of for over-excitability of the nervous system, disturbances of the bowels such as colitis and skin problems including *Herpes*.

Flower Essence
Self-heal, as the name suggests, is used to enhance our own healing powers. The body possesses an inherent healing ability, which enables a cut to heal, inflammation to resolve and infection to subside. We are also able to heal ourselves emotionally and we can be healed spiritually.

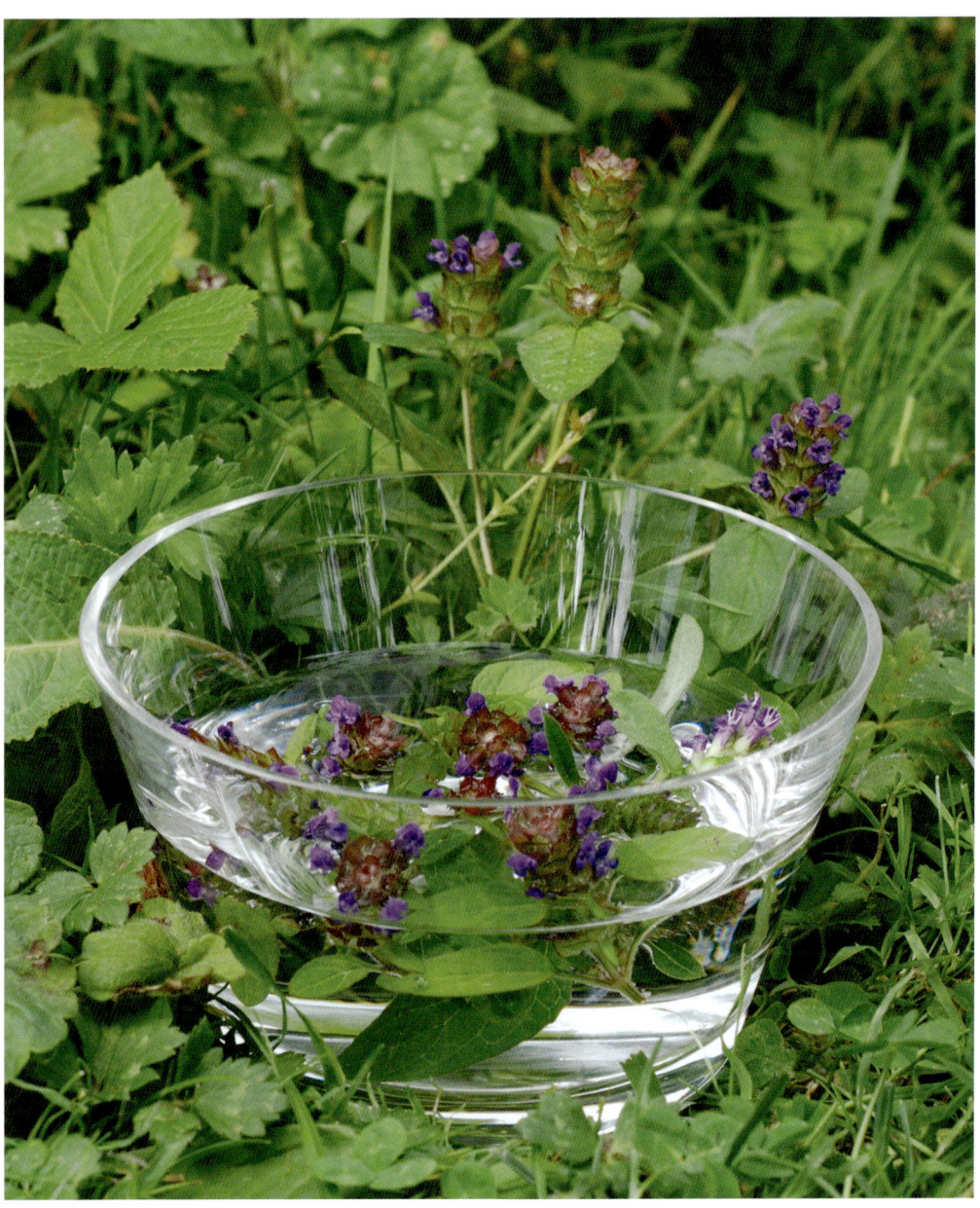

Self-heal increases confidence in our ability to heal ourselves. It is particularly recommended for those who doubt their innate recuperative powers, or who cannot face the responsibility of looking after themselves. They may hand over the responsibility of their physical health or emotional, mental or spiritual welfare to healers, counsellors and gurus.

It may be needed by those who are unwell or unhappy, who have lost belief in their own capacity to be well, by addicts dependent on external factors for their feeling of wellbeing, and for those facing crises in their lives. Self-heal helps to reduce dependence on others, and to inspire motivation and a belief in our own inherent healing powers.

Edible Uses
Self-heal leaves and flowers can be eaten raw, preferably when they are young and taste a bit like lettuce. They can add interest and colour to salads and be used for decorative garnishes. They can also be cooked and added to soups and stews or eaten as greens. They can be used in combination with other more aromatic herbs to make a tisane.

Recipes

Self-heal Salve
450ml of sunflower seed, almond or virgin olive oil
50g of beeswax
A mixture of calendula flowers, chamomile flowers and lavender flowers

Macerate as much herb as possible in 450ml of olive oil and 50g of beeswax for a few hours over a low heat in a *bain marie* (double saucepan). After this time, the constituents will have been taken up by the oil and the mixture can then be pressed through a muslin bag and the herb discarded. When the oil is still warm, it can be poured into ointment jars, where it will quickly solidify.

Growing
Self-heal likes good, moist soil and will bloom in full sun as well as partial shade. It is a mat-forming plant that makes good ground cover in a wild garden and in shady areas along walkways, under taller plants, and in the rock garden. It can often take over lawns!

Cautions
Considered safe if used appropriately. Avoid with insulin and other hypoglycaemic medications (eg. Chlorpropamide). May reduce absorption of prescription drugs and supplements.

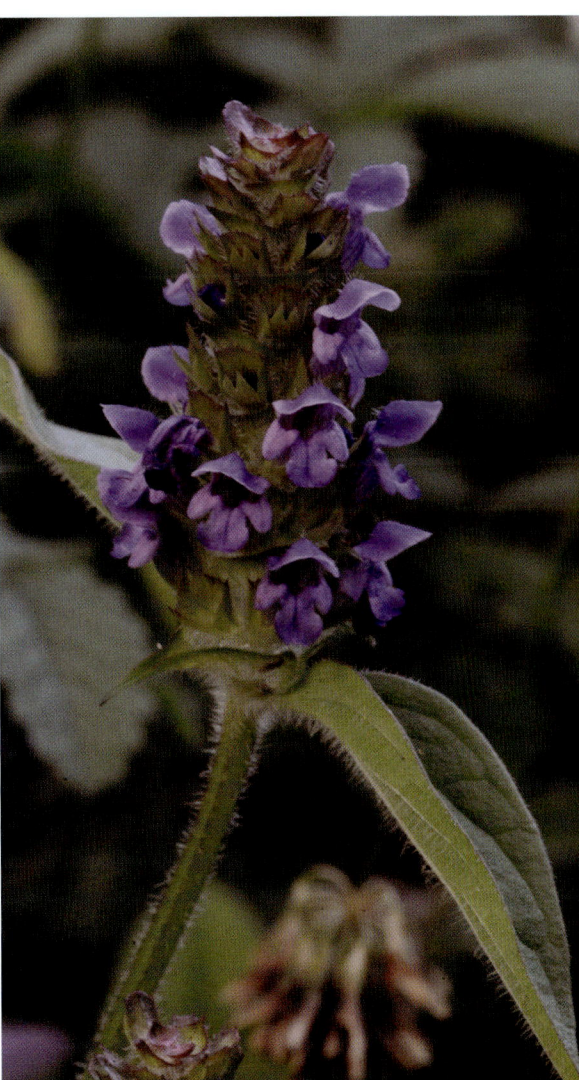

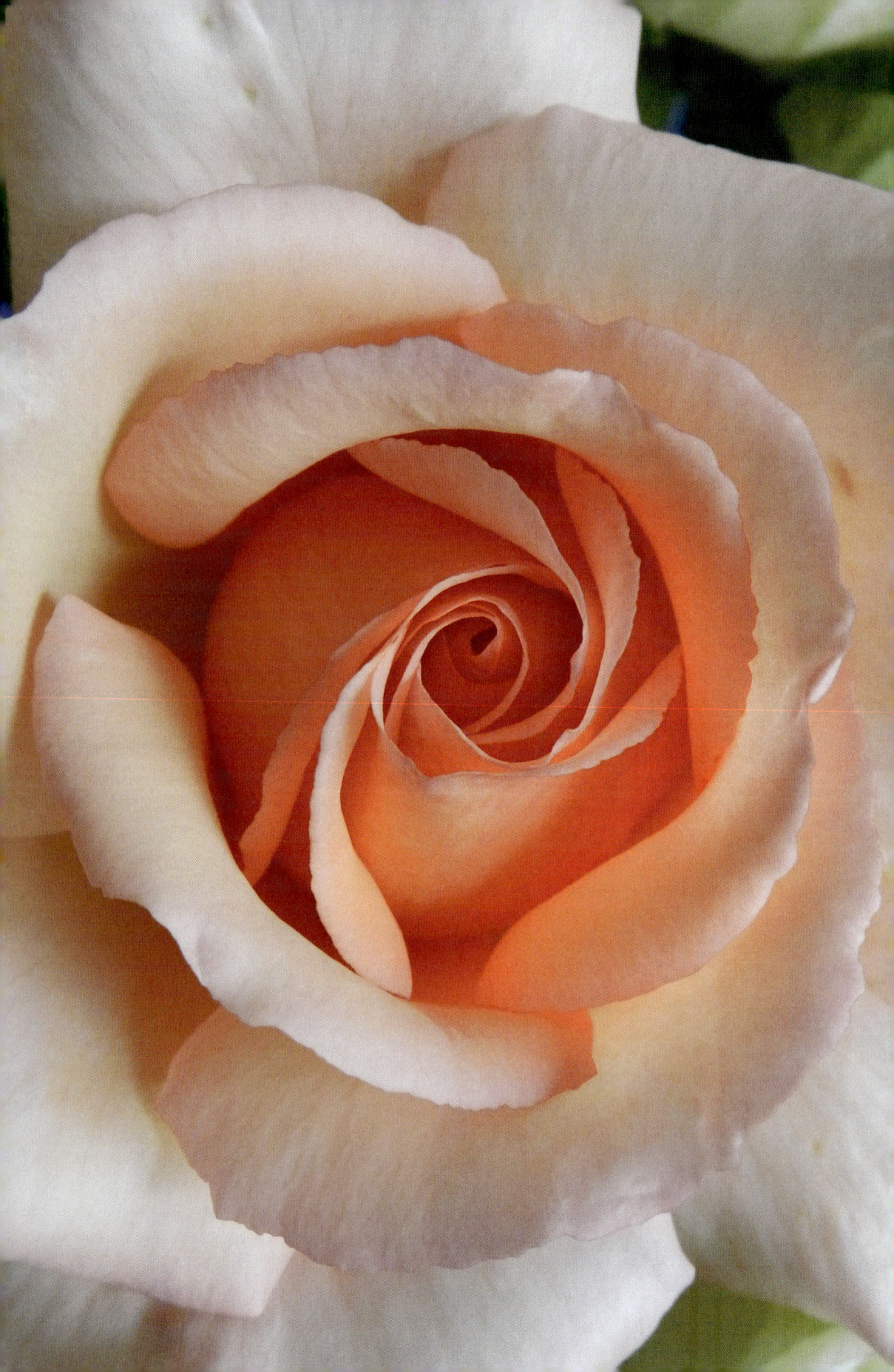

Rosa spp: Rose

The Flower of Love

*This is a holy refuge
The garden of Saint Rose
A fragrant altar to that peace
The world no longer knows*
– Bliss Carman (1861–1929)

Parts Used: Hips, leaves and flowers

This exquisitely beautiful, heavenly perfumed flower, the most sensuous and romantic of flowers, not only inspires love but also enhances well-being and longevity. Clearly, the rose is best known for its ability to heal in the realms of the heart. When we want to express love and affection and cannot find words to convey the depth of our feelings, the rose will do it for us, and this has been the case for hundreds of years, for the rose has long been to artists, poets and lovers alike the symbol of love, beauty and perfection. Its praises have been sung and its beauty depicted in art since the days of the early Greeks; a rose in a Minoan fresco dated 1500–1600BC is probably the *Gallica* rose, often called the *Damask* rose and the one most often used in the apothecary.

The rose has inspired poets and artists for centuries as the symbol of love and beauty. "*My luve is like a red red rose*" said Robert Burns, and Yeats wrote,

*With the earth and the sky and the water, remade, like a casket of gold
For my dreams of your image that blossoms a rose in the depths of my heart.*

The red rose has long been an emblem of physical love and beauty, passion and intimacy, while the white rose has represented divine or spiritual love, the mystic centre of being and the image of a perfect world or paradise. Certainly, the physical perfection and heavenly scent of a rose on a summer's day can transport us to a place of joy and inspiration and can transform a garden into a semblance of paradise.

John Parkinson (1567–1650), herbarist to King Charles I, relates *"Philostratus dedicated the rose to Cupid, whom it doth represent in every part. It is fresh, young and delicate as Cupid, it is crowned with golden yellow hairs, it beareth thorns as darts and leaves as wings, the crimson beauty of the flowers as his glory and dignity, neither the rose nor Cupid keepeth any time, and besides this he calleth the rose the light of the earth, the fair bushy top of the spring, the fire of love, the lightning of the land."*

In Islamic rituals, rosewater is still used to cleanse the body and the spirit before prayer. In India, Hindus bathe the Shiva lingam or phallus with rosewater during the Mahashivratri festival, an annual day of devotion to Shiva which is also celebrated as the day Shiva married Parvati.

The first historical evidence of the rose can be traced back to around 2684BC when the king of Sumeria mentioned the 'trees of roses' he brought back from an exhibition. The birthplace of the cultivated rose was probably Northern Persia, now Iran, from where it was taken to Turkey, Greece, Italy and the rest of Europe. According to Eastern traditions, the original rose was stirred into life by the first rays of the rising sun in the Great Garden of Persia. When a soul knocked at the door of the next world and all material things had to be left behind, only the red rose was allowed to accompany that soul over the threshold. There is a strong bond between roses and the Iranians, who call it 'flower of Prophet Mohammed' because it is said that its perfume reminds them of the prophet; the flowers are used as an aid to meditation and prayer. Rose water is still used today in religious ceremonies in mosques, especially at mourning ceremonies, for its calming and relaxing effect.

The Romans no doubt brought the rose to England as their love of roses was great. Roman emperors would fill their swimming baths and fountains with rose-scented water and sit on carpets of rose petals for their feasts and orgies. The Roman people decorated their banqueting halls with roses and strewed the floors with them to fill the place with their enchanting scent. Brides and bridegrooms were crowned with roses, roses were scattered on the marriage bed, and worn as garlands at feasts, apparently to prevent drunkenness. Rose petals are still used today as confetti at weddings as a symbol of love and happy marriage. Roman ladies would sprinkle themselves with powdered dried rose petals after bathing, brighten their eyelids with rose oil and suck pastilles of rose, myrrh and honey to sweeten their breath. Similarly, the ancient Egyptians used rose body oils and Cleopatra was said to have had her bedroom floor strewn with roses over one foot deep before she seduced Julius Caesar! Roses were associated with joy, merriment and wine (petals were floated in wine cups), but they were also scattered on graves of the dead at funerals and planted on lovers' tombs, perhaps to compare the short span of human life to the quick-fading life of the rose.

Of all flowers, the rose is probably the one most steeped in legend and symbolism, mostly relating to love and beauty. According to ancient Greek myth, Chloris the goddess of flowers one day found the body of a beautiful nymph and asked the help of the three Graces to create a special flower out of the lifeless body of the nymph. The Graces gave the flower joy, brightness and charm. Then she asked Aphrodite the goddess of love to give the flower beauty, Dionysus the god of wine to add a special nectar to create a beautiful perfume to pervade the air and intoxicate the bees, and Zephyr the wind god to blow away the clouds so that the precious flower could open her petals up to the sun. Thus, the rose was born and crowned the Queen of Flowers, dedicated to Venus and the symbol of love. Sappho of Lesbos, the Greek poetess (c.600BC) refers to the rose as the Queen of flowers,

If Jove would give the leafy bowers
A queen for all their world of flowers,
The rose would be the choice of Jove,
And blush the queen of every grove.

Other legends say that the rose was once a Grecian queen whose beauty made the Goddess Artemis very jealous. Apollo the Sun god, Artemis's brother, scorched the Queen with his rays of fire until she was transformed into the flower of our gardens. Stories tell us how the red rose got its colour. The Romans said that Venus blushed when Jupiter caught her bathing and the white rose turned red in her reflection. The Greeks tell how Aphrodite and Persephone were both lovers of Adonis, and when Aphrodite wanted to prevent Adonis from returning to her rival Persephone, she asked Ares the God of war to help. Subsequently Adonis was attacked by a wild boar while out hunting and flying to his aid, Aphrodite scratched herself on a white rose. Red roses sprung up where Adonis and Aphrodite's blood had spilled, and the white roses turned red in sympathy. According to the Persians, a nightingale began to sing when roses first bloomed, and overcome by their heady perfume, it dropped to the earth. Its spilled blood stained the petals turning them from white to red.

In early Christianity, the red rose became the symbol of martyrs' blood and life after death, and the white rose the symbol of innocence and purity, spirituality and virginity, dedicated to the Virgin Mary. At first, the rose was unacceptable to the Christians because of its association with Venus, the goddess of carnal love, but gradually it was taken on as the emblem of divine love and heavenly joy. The rose was depicted in Christian paintings of the garden of heaven, along with the lily and the pink. The perfection of the rose was adopted by poets and artists to symbolise all that was ideal and from paradise, emblematic of the heart or mystic centre of being. The mystics, philosophers and alchemists who founded the secret society called the Rosicrucians in the 15th century had a rose mounted on a cross as their symbol.

The rose is also the emblem of England and the emblem of national union. In the language of flowers, the rose not only means beauty, love and perfection but also unity, particularly of the white rose and the red rose together. In the Wars of the Roses, the white rose was the emblem of the House of York, and the red rose that of the House of Lancaster. After over 30 years of civil war, the two houses were finally bound together in marriage and the two roses were united to form the Tudor rose, which is still used in British heraldry today.

Since those early days, the rose has been extolled not only for its beauty and perfume but also for its medicinal virtues. Greek doctors used the champagne rose as a tonic. Pliny listed 32 medicines prepared by the Romans from roses, including dog roses to cure the bites of mad dogs. Avicenna, the famous Arab doctor of the 10th century, praised the rose and was the first to make rosewater. He used rose jelly to cure spitting of blood. Around the turn of the 16th century, 'otto' or 'attar of roses' was discovered in Persia, now a major ingredient in perfumes and soaps and widely used in aromatherapy.

John Gerard the 17th century herbalist said rosewater was *"good for strengthening of the heart and refreshing the spirits and likewise for all things that require a gentle cooling…it mitigateth the pain of the eyes proceeding of a hot cause, bringeth sleep, which also the fresh roses themselves provoke through their sweet and pleasant smell"*. Culpeper used honey of roses *"in gargles and lotions to wash sores, either in the mouth, throat or other parts, both to cleanse and heal them."* It was also used for abdominal and chest pain, to strengthen the heart, for menstrual and digestive problems and inflammation. Native Americans used a decoction of the root of *Rosa damascena* as a cough remedy for children's coughs. The hips of the wild rose, *Rosa canina*, were found just before the Second World War to contain one of the most abundant sources of vitamin C in the plant kingdom and were made into rose hip syrup, which was rationed in Britain in wartime to ensure children's resistance to infection.

Herbal Remedy and Aromatherapy Oil
Roses, like other members of the Rosaceae family including apple, agrimony and hawthorn flowers, have a combination of bitter, sweet and astringent tastes. In the rose these are provided by its constituents which include ellagitannins and phenolic acids (such as gallic, ellagic, quinine), terpenes, glycosides, flavonoids including kaempferol, rutin and quercetin and anthocyanins (glycosides, such as cyanidins, pelargonidins, and peonidins). Roses also contain carboxylic acid, volatile oils (notably β-citronellol, geraniol, nerol), vitamins (A, C, B, E, K, folic acid), minerals (calcium, potassium, sodium, sulphur, iron) and saponins. Rose hips contain high amounts of vitamin C, B and E, phenolic compounds, carotenoids, flavonoids including anthocyanins, triterpene acids, fatty acids and galactolipids, phytosterols and pectin.

The phenolic compounds in the hips and flowers have a wide range of activities, including antioxidant, anticancer, anti-inflammatory and antidepressant. Their antioxidant actions help to protect against oxidative stress and problems arising from it, including cardiovascular disease, diabetes, high cholesterol and cognitive decline. Roses have an anti-diabetic effect by suppressing carbohydrate absorption from the small intestine and can reduce the postprandial glucose levels, that is the rise of blood sugar after eating.

Rose petals are used for their cooling, anti-inflammatory and antimicrobial properties. They have wide spectrum antimicrobial activities, antibacterial and antiviral actions and enhance the efforts of the immune system against colds and flu and other respiratory problems. The volatile oils have strong antibacterial activity against bacteria involved in pneumonia, urinary tract infections, wound, bone and skin infections and food poisoning including *B. subtilis, Staph. aureus, Salmonella* spp and *B. cereus, Enterobacter* spp., *E. coli, Proteus* spp. and *Klebsiella pneumoniae*.

The hips of the wild rose *Rosa canina* contain one of the most abundant sources of vitamin C in the plant kingdom, which enhances the action of the mucociliary escalator (the little hairs called cilia, which move mucus up and out of the lungs where it can be expelled by coughing or swallowing), and help to prevent chest infections. This action combined with their antimicrobial and decongestant actions brings relief in cold and flu symptoms, sore throat, catarrhal congestion, sinusitis, hay fever, coughs and chest infections. Their antispasmodic effect in the chest helps to relieve coughing and can be helpful in asthma. Roses are an excellent remedy for people who live in polluted cities and tend to suffer from catarrh or chest infections and when feeling tired and run down with lowered immunity. Taken as a hot tea, roses help to bring down fevers and clear heat and toxins from the body that gives rise to skin rashes and other inflammatory skin problems (including *Herpes*, measles and chicken pox).

In the digestive system, the cooling, astringent and anti-inflammatory effect of roses and rose hips can be very helpful in the treatment of gastritis, peptic ulcers, enteritis, diarrhoea and dysentery. Their antimicrobial properties help combat unfriendly bacteria in the digestive tract and re-establish the normal bacterial population of the gut, which is very useful after disruption by antibiotics or a bad diet. The astringent tannins help toughen the gut lining and increase its resilience to infection, irritation and inflammation and can be used to reduce hyperacidity and stomach over-activity causing excessive hunger, thirst and mouth ulcers. Rose petals as well as empty rose hips also help to regulate metabolism and weight. The irritating silky down that fills the spaces between the seeds and the seed case has been used in France and Eastern Europe as a treatment for worms, and by children for itching powder! The delicate aromatic taste of rose preparations makes them useful in medicines to mask the taste of other more unpleasant herbs.

The main affinity that roses have in the body is with the female reproductive system. Their antispasmodic effect can help ease painful periods, while the astringent tannins are very helpful in heavy periods. The hormone balancing effect can help balance hormones and relieve symptoms of PMS. Roses can enhance fertility and are well known for their aphrodisiac powers which can help men and women alike. They truly are the food of love!

When treating gynaecological problems such as period pain, salpingitis, pelvic inflammatory disease, cystitis and vaginal infections such as thrush, rose petal tea or tincture can be taken on a regular basis or alternatively diluted essential oil of rose can be massaged into the abdomen and a few drops can be incorporated into creams and douches. It is important to note that rose should be avoided during pregnancy for it has a mildly stimulating action in the uterus, but makes a lovely uplifting remedy for the last couple of weeks of pregnancy when it will prime the uterine muscles for contraction during the birth. The cooling and hormone balancing effect of roses can be helpful for reducing hot flushes, night sweats and mood changes and emotional difficulties during the menopause.

Rose petals have a diuretic effect, relieving fluid retention and hastening elimination of toxins and wastes through the urinary system. They have been used for infections such as cystitis as well as stones and gravel in the kidneys and bladder. Rose hips have been shown to have anti-inflammatory effects and can be useful for reducing pain and increasing flexibility in osteoarthritis. They have an analgesic effect, attributed mainly to the flavonoids, when the herb or oil is used in a preparation combining water and alcohol such as a tincture.

Rose hips, petals and oil have a restoring effect on the nervous system. With its antioxidant effects, rose has long been used to decrease signs of ageing and improve memory and eyesight. It is possible that roses can have an effect on brain function by promoting nerve regeneration and decreasing the formation of amyloid plaques which contribute to Alzheimer's disease. Taken regularly, rose can calm tension and anxiety, lift the spirits and help relieve depression, dispel physical and mental fatigue, and is the perfect remedy for irritability, low self-esteem, grief and anger. It can be taken to quieten nervous palpitations and last thing at night for insomnia. The flavonoids and terpenes may be responsible for its calming and sleep-inducing effects as they have anxiolytic and antidepressant effects. They may promote sleep through their affinity for the central benzodiazepine receptors or through their effect on GABA, the neurotransmitter that reduces anxiety. This can also be helpful in the treatment of epilepsy. Other components of the

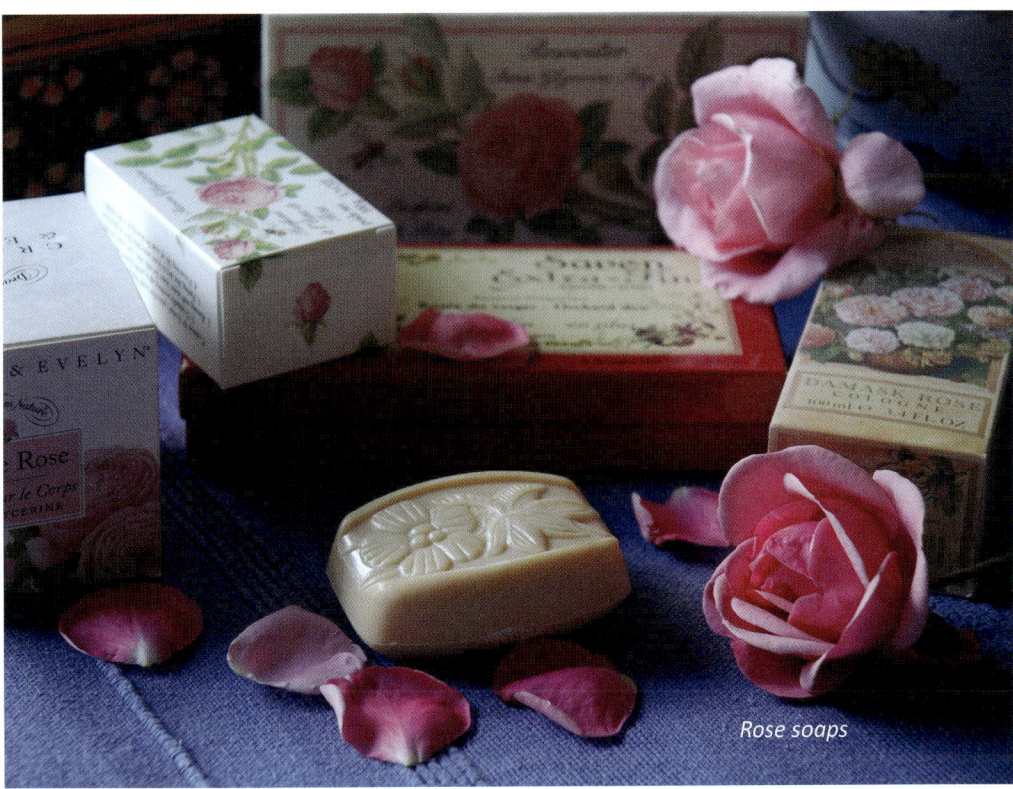
Rose soaps

essential oil including geraniol and eugenol may also have an antiepileptic effect.

You only have to smell a rose to have an inkling of its immense benefit to the world of the emotions. Roses have a particularly healing effect when affairs of the heart and their connection with sexuality give rise to difficult or painful feelings and these emotions contribute to sexual problems like low libido, frigidity and impotence. Rose makes an excellent remedy for those who feel insecure about their sexuality and lacking in confidence in loving, intimate relationships. Rose oil is used in aromatherapy for those who miss love in their lives, who are lonely, bereaved, down hearted, heart-broken, rejected, hurt or despairing, who feel unloved or unlovable. It helps to restore confidence, an ability to give and receive love, and opens us to the joys that love can bring both physically and emotionally. It almost seems miraculous that a simple flower, albeit the *'queen of flowers'* and the most beautiful, can inspire us to recognise not only the beauty of its perfect form, but also to recognise the beauty that lies within us and while a rose may be proffered to us as a token of love, it may also ignite love within us. There is only one way to find out if it works and that is to try it!

Roses have always been associated with beauty and perhaps this derives from their ability to promote beauty within and without. With its antimicrobial and anti-inflammatory effects, rosewater has been used to cleanse and tone the skin, to prevent and smooth out wrinkles, to clear skin blemishes and inflammation such as acne and spots, boils and abscesses. It can be used to bathe sore, tired or inflamed eyes, and also to make eye drops to treat conjunctivitis, dry eyes, and degenerative or allergic eye disorders. It can also be used to promote tissue repair and prevent infection of minor cuts and wounds, and to reduce the swelling of bruises and sprains.

An infusion of rose petals can be used as a mouthwash for mouth ulcers and inflamed, bleeding gums, a gargle for sore throats and a douche for vaginal discharge. Rose oil or ointment makes a good lip salve for dry, chapped lips and an infusion of rose petals in wine or vinegar added to the bath has been used to relieve arthritis and muscle pain. Rose vinegar applied as a compress to the head is a folk remedy to relieve headaches caused by hot sun.

Flower Essence
The rose is the symbol of love. The red rose increases confidence in those feeling insecure about their sexuality and who suffer from feelings of shame or timidity about their bodies. It helps you to open up to love and bring your desires into action.

The white rose is quietly inspiring and strengthening, renewing energy and joy in your life. The white rosebud can be given to infants and children to help them grow up, keeping a sense of heaven on earth.

The wild rose is the remedy of independence. It is traditionally said to mean *'pleasure and pain'* as it brings pleasure to the eyes and heart when found blooming in the wild, but pain from its sharp prickles if you try to pluck it. Wild rose warms the heart and softens the emotions, engendering an easy-going feeling to enhance sensuality.

Growing
Roses can be grown from cuttings taken in late summer. They prefer well drained, moderately fertile soil and sun or light shade. Repeat flowering roses should be deadheaded to stimulate further flower development. Roses can be pruned in either autumn or early spring.

Notable Medicinal Roses

Rosa damascena: Damask rose. The Bulgarian rose "*otto*" oil is said to be the finest in the world.

Rosa centifolia: Cabbage rose/hundred leaf rose. This rose produces the famous Indian attar of roses which is used as perfume, scenting soaps and oils and is official as a medicine in the Indian Pharmacopoeia.

Rosa canina: Wild dog rose

Cautions
Avoid in pregnancy and breastfeeding and kidney disease. May reduce absorption of iron. Avoid using flowers or hips that have been sprayed with toxic chemicals. Remove the irritating hairs from the seeds/hips, before eating them/making a tea from them. Avoid with benzodiazepines, insulin and other hypoglycaemic medicines (eg Chlorpropamide). Patients should monitor blood glucose levels.

Recipes

Indian Rose Syrup and Coconut Milk
Just tasting this sweet nectar is enough to bring joy to the heart. Roses have long been associated with love and all affairs of the heart. They have a wonderfully uplifting and restorative effect and can be thought of whenever you feel tense, anxious, depressed, angry, lonely and upset. They are specifically for those who lack love in their lives. In India, coconut is seen as a gift from the gods to human beings and a token of good luck in romantic relationships.

1 tablespoon rose syrup
250ml coconut milk

To make rose syrup, collect rose petals, weigh them and place in a bowl with an equal weight of sugar. Mash the petals and sugar together, cover and leave overnight. Strain through a fine sieve, pour into clean bottles, and store in the fridge. Stir a tablespoonful of syrup into a cup of coconut milk. Dilute with a little water, if required. The syrup will keep for about a month.

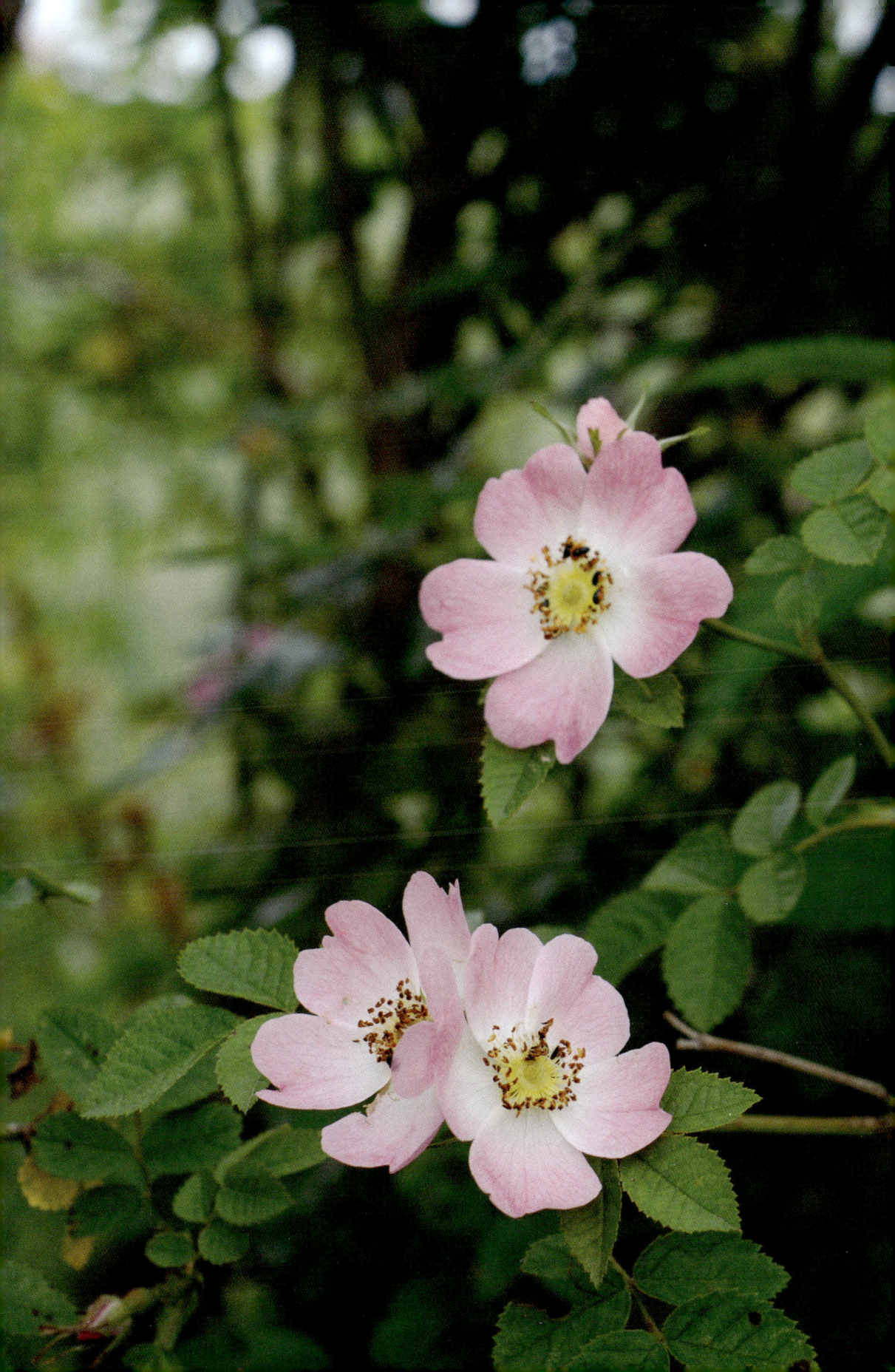

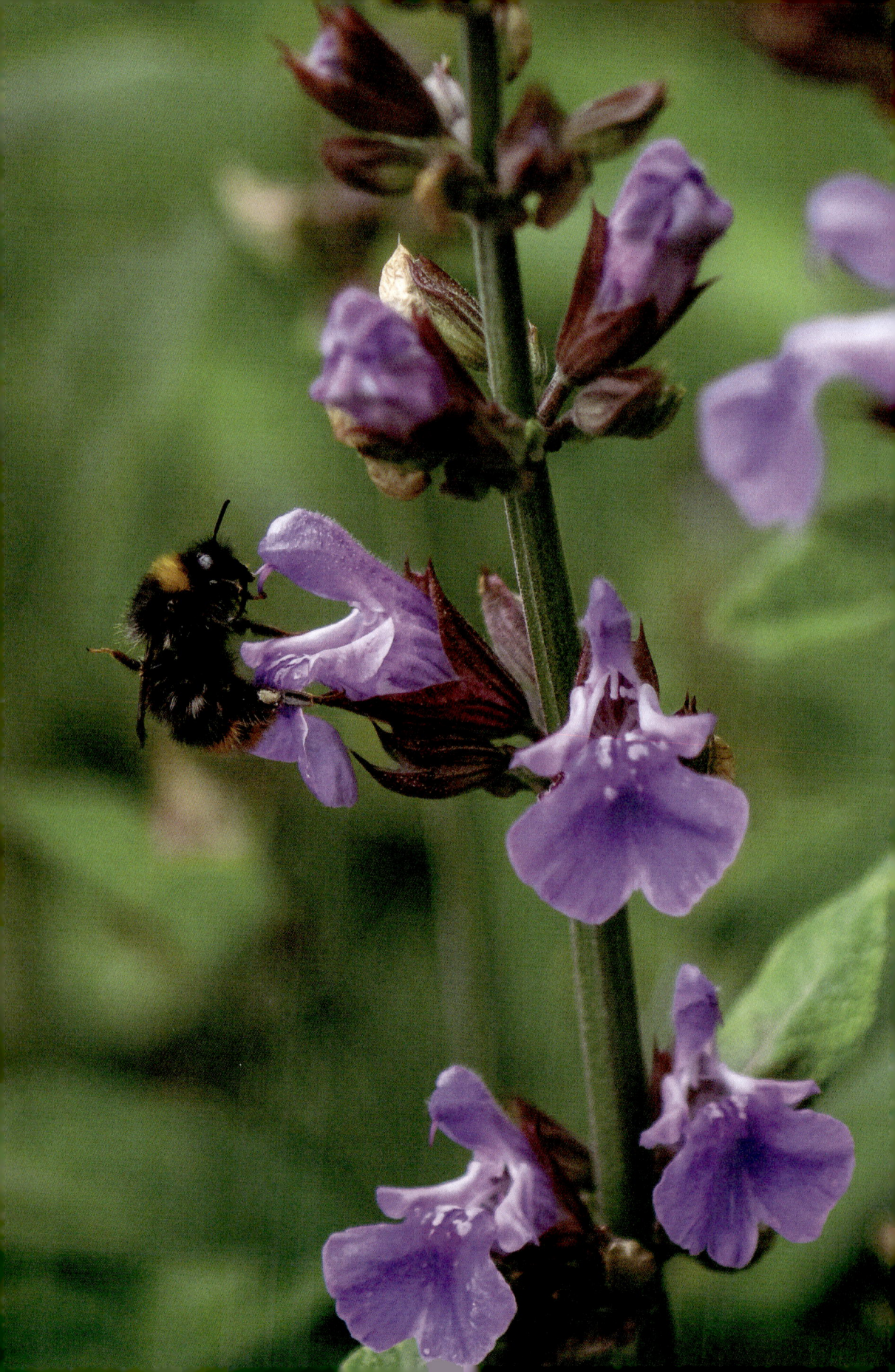

Salvia officinalis: Sage

The Flower of Immortality

In Latin salvia takes the name of safety,
In English sage is rather wise than crafty,
Sith then the name betokens wise and saving,
We count it nature's friend and worth the having
   – The Englishman's Doctor 1608

Other Names: Red sage, purple sage, garden sage, meadow sage, Spanish sage, Greek sage, Dalmation sage, immortality herb, common sage, golden sage, kitchen sage, true sage, culinary sage and broadleaf sage

Parts Used: Leaves and flowers

With its aromatic, soft, velvety leaves and whorls of violet-blue flowers, sage is a popular evergreen member of the Lamiaceae/Labiatae family. It is native to Southern Europe and the Mediterranean, where it can be found growing wild on hillsides and grassland. It is a favourite culinary herb and also a much-loved decorative shrub for the garden in its various cultivated forms.

Sage – the very word suggests wisdom and old age and it is these themes that permeate the use of this wonderful plant in its healing history. Sage is a wonderful brain tonic and rejuvenative and for thousands of years has been believed in many different cultures to enhance mental and spiritual clarity. The word *sage* means wise and the archetypal image of a sage is someone who is old and wise as the old poem from The Englishman's Doctor above says.

The botanic name *Salvia* comes from the Latin word 'salvare' meaning to save or cure. The ancient Greeks considered sage could render us immortal and it became known as 'the immortality herb', perhaps because it was seen to cure so many ills or because it had the power to enhance inner wisdom which goes beyond the realm of our physical form. Certainly, its powerful antimicrobial properties would have been lifesavers in the past when intestinal or chest infections could easily have been fatal. The ancient Greek physician Theophrastus (c. 372–287BC) said it *'drove away the evils of illness and old age'* and the ancient Egyptians revered it as a giver and saver of life and used it for treating the plague. The Romans considered it sacred and prized it so highly that harvesting the leaves was an important ceremony, rather than an ordinary gardening activity. They gathered the aromatic leaves not with iron, but with bronze and silver tools, and harvesters were required to be barefoot, clean and dressed in white tunics. Before it was harvested, sacrifices of food and wine were offered to the gods. Like the Egyptians, they believed sage helped to give as well as protect life, and gave the herb as a fertility remedy to women wanting to conceive.

In ancient Arabic and Chinese healing traditions as well as in Europe in the Middle Ages, sage was a major ingredient in prescriptions for longevity and elixirs of life as it had a wide reputation as a rejuvenating tonic, as the old English saying tells us, *'He that would live for aye should eat sage in May'.* It was considered a brain and nerve tonic to strengthen the mind and the memory, enliven the senses, lift dull spirits, banish lethargy and restore failing virility. It was prescribed for depression, anxiety, nervousness, headaches, insomnia and nervous exhaustion and was given during convalescence and to the elderly to reduce the signs and symptoms of ageing.

In the folk medicine of Asia and Latin America, sage has been used similarly for tremors, convulsions, dizziness, ulcers, gout, rheumatism, inflammation, paralysis, diarrhoea, colds, bronchitis, tuberculosis, haemorrhages and menstrual disorders. Until the discovery of antibiotics, it was given to patients with tuberculosis to prevent sweating and depletion. Several of the native American tribes consider sage to have spiritual properties. They make dried sage leaves into 'smudge sticks' which are cigar-shaped bundles that are lit and wafted around rooms, houses or people to calm and refresh the mind, to purify the atmosphere and remove negative energy.

Herbal Remedy

The distinctive flavour and fragrance of sage is given by its high volatile oil content (which includes cineole, camphor, borneol, thujone, pinene, camphene, caryophyllene, α-humulene and linalool). About 20% of the volatile oil is camphor and this increases as the leaves expand. It also contains diterpenes, flavonoids, polyphenols including rosmarinic acid, caffeic acid, salvianolic acid, carnosolic acid, viridiflorol and ursolic acid, all of which have important parts to play. The flavonoids and polyphenolic compounds have strong antioxidant, free radical-scavenging, antiviral and antibacterial activities. Ursolic acid also has strong anti-inflammatory properties. Antioxidants play a very important role in protecting the body against oxidative stress and free radical damage. These are the cause of many problems as we get older such as diabetes, heart disease, cancer, brain deterioration, arthritis and depleted immunity. Sage has an important role in the prevention and treatment of such problems.

Many might mainly associate sage with sage and onion stuffing which has long been traditional fayre to accompany a rich, rather fatty, Christmas chicken, turkey, duck or goose. This is because sage has a wonderful ability to aid digestion. With its combination of pungent and

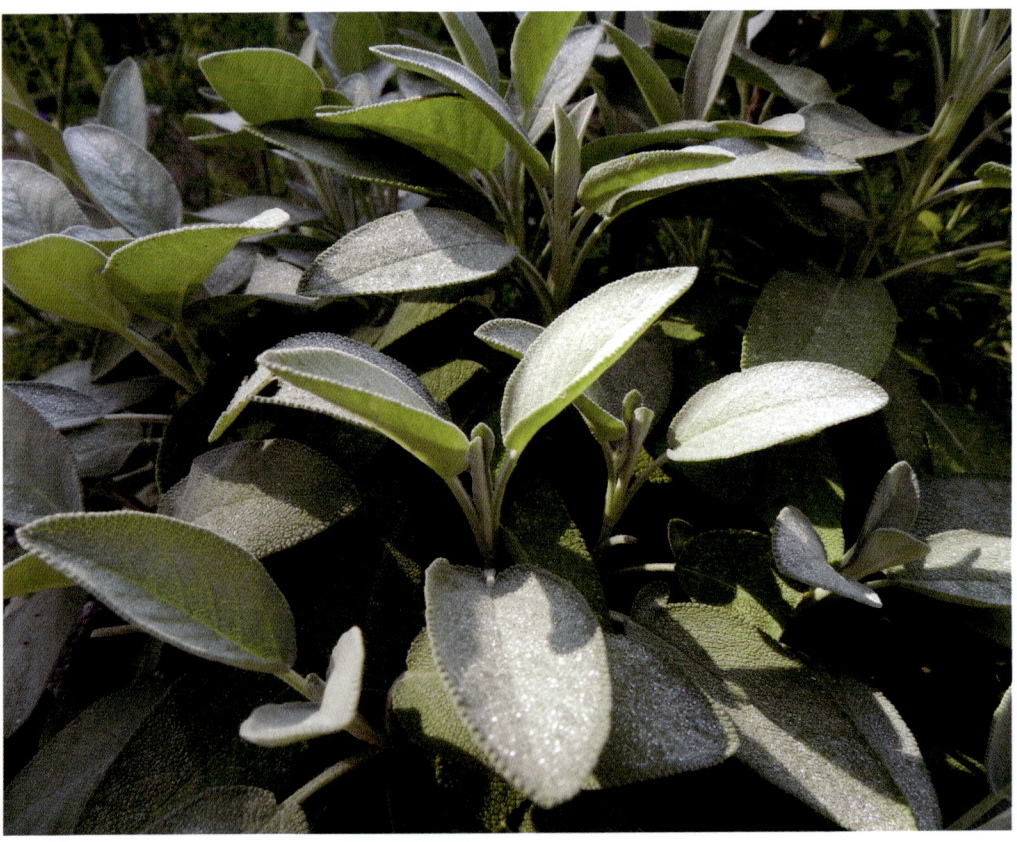

bitter tastes, sage makes an excellent remedy for enkindling appetite and digestion and enhancing absorption. It stimulates the flow of digestive enzymes and of bile from the liver and has a beneficial action on the pancreas. It makes a good remedy for poor appetite, heartburn, indigestion, wind, bloating, nausea and colitis. It is interesting that sage has long been used in cuisine with fatty foods and it was thought that it is because sage helps the digestion of fats. We now know that sage tincture with its diterpenes (carnosic acid and carnosol), actually deters the digestion and absorption of fats (as it inhibits the pancreatic enzyme lipase which breaks down fats) and that it can help to reduce the size of fat tissue, lower weight and prevent obesity.

The tannins give sage its astringent taste and toning effect on the gut lining, they tighten the cell boundaries and help reduce leaky gut syndrome. They are very useful for treating diarrhoea particularly when it accompanies a gut infection or is brought on by stress. In addition, the antispasmodic action of sage inhibits gut motility and relaxes spasm and relieves colic and griping.

Sage can also be helpful in Type II diabetes; it lowers blood sugar levels as it reduces liver glucose production, increases the action of insulin and reduces insulin resistance. It helps to regulate genes involved in lipid and glucose metabolism, it reduces serum lipids and triglycerides and improves the ratio of high density (good) to low density (bad) cholesterol. In this way it can help prevent cerebrovascular and cardiovascular disease. Its beneficial effect on blood lipids may be related to its flavonoid content. Rosmarinic acid for example, can reduce cholesterol and triglyceride levels and rutin can reduce adipose tissue and body weight.

The powerful antimicrobial actions of sage, given by its aromatic volatile oils, would have served well in the kitchen to prevent infection from poultry or meat that was a little 'high' before the days of fridges. They help combat stomach and bowel infections and are helpful for clearing toxins and unfriendly microorganisms from the gut including worms. Sage and in particular the camphor, thujone and 1,8-cineole is effective against bacteria including *Bacillus spp.*, *Enterococcus faecalis* (which can cause a variety of infections, including endocarditis, urinary tract infections, prostatitis, abdominal infections, cellulitis and wound infections), *Aeromonas hydrophila*, *Aeromonas sobria*, *Listeria monocytogenes*, *Enterobacter cloacae* and *Proteus* spp. It also has antifungal activity against *Botrytis cinerea*, *Candida glabrata*, *Candida albicans*, *Candida krusei* and *Candida parapsilosis*.

With its powerful antimicrobial actions, as well as decongestant and expectorant actions, sage is an excellent remedy for treating acute and chronic respiratory infections, including colds, flu, catarrh, fevers, sore throats, tonsillitis, sinusitis and chest infections. It is effective against *Herpes simplex virus II*, *Klebsiella oxytoca* and *Influenza virus II*. Its antiviral activity is attributed mainly to the diterpenoids and the antibacterial action partly to triterpenoids, oleanolic acid and ursolic acid, which can also inhibit the growth of multidrug-resistant bacteria such as *Vancomycin-resistant enterococci*, *Penicillin-resistant Streptococcus pneumonia* and *Methicillin-resistant Staphylococcus aureus* (MRSA). It used to be a favourite remedy for TB and other infections accompanied by night sweats, not only because of its antimicrobial properties but also because it minimises sweating and its debilitating effects. Sage also has anti-malarial effects.

Sage offers possibilities in the treatment of cancer. In cancer, abnormal cells tend to proliferate in an uncontrolled way and in some cases spread to other parts of the body. To be able to do this, the tumours produce a large number of new blood vessels, which is known as angiogenesis. Sage has the remarkable ability to inhibit angiogenesis and ursolic acid may play an important part in this. The sesquiterpenes in sage, notable humulene, could also account for a possible role in the prevention and treatment of lung, kidney and prostate cancer as well as melanoma.

Sage has long been respected as a rejuvenating nerve tonic, promoting brain function, mental clarity and reducing fatigue particularly in the elderly. It has been used for centuries to restore lost or declining mental functions. It reduces anxiety and lifts depression and can improve alertness, memory and concentration in the elderly. The antioxidant and anti-inflammatory properties of sage may help to prevent the development of dementia. Sage is recommended in nervous disorders such as Parkinson's disease, in which case it also decreases excessive salivation, and it is also used to improve mental function in Alzheimer's. In Alzheimer's disease, the enzyme acetyl cholinesterase (AChE) breaks down and inactivates an important neurotransmitter involved in the sending messages in the brain called acetylcholine. The volatile oils in sage can almost half AChE activity and in this way improve memory and cognition. Sage also has the ability to protect nerve cells in the brain against damage caused by amyloid plaques which underlies Alzheimer's. This is attributed to the presence of rosmarinic acid in the volatile oil which has neuroprotective, antioxidative and anti-apoptotic effects against amyloid plaque toxicity. The mood-enhancing effects of sage can be helpful in the treatment of advanced dementia, which can be characterised by moods and agitation.

On a more subtle level, sage is said to be able to clear unresolved emotions from the past which are unconsciously affecting the present and to promote calmness and clarity. Bearing this in mind, people who would like to quieten the mind and practice meditation may find it well worth drinking a cup of sage tea or even burning a few dried sage leaves in their meditation room.

Sage helps to regulate periods and can be used for irregular and painful periods. Its astringent tannins have a drying effect and reduce heavy bleeding and secretions including seminal fluid and breast milk. Its stimulating effect in the uterus can be helpful during childbirth to ease delivery and expel the placenta, but for this reason it should not be taken in early pregnancy. Neither is it recommended while breastfeeding, as it stops the flow of milk, but it could be useful when weaning. Sage is a prime remedy for night sweats either during the menopause or as an accompaniment to debilitating disease including flu, HIV and TB. Sage has a phytoestrogenic action which accounts for its benefit as a remedy for the menopause. Sage and motherwort (*Leonurus cardiaca*) together make a good combination for hot flushes, night sweats and other symptoms of the menopause.

Externally a dilute tincture or infusion of sage makes an excellent antiseptic first-aid lotion for cuts, wounds, burns, sores, insect bites, inflammatory skin problems, ulcers and sunburn. With its powerful antibacterial and antifungal properties, it is excellent for a range of skin infections including spots, acne, boils, ringworm and scabies. It can be included in liniments for painful joints, sprains and swellings. A dilute tincture or tea can be used as a gargle for sore throats and pharyngitis and as a mouthwash for inflamed gums and ulcers. A dilute tincture can inhibit bacteria such as *Streptococcus mutans* and *Actinomyces viscosus* that can contribute to dental caries and *Staphylococcus epidermidis* that is involved in gum disease and can cause infections in wounds in people who have weakened immunity. Sage can also be used as a douche for vaginal infections including thrush. The leaves can be applied to a tooth to relieve pain.

Aromatherapy Oil
Salvia essential oil has very similar uses to those of the herbal remedy. Used in a burner, sage oil can stimulate and clear the mind and has a balancing, uplifting and calming effect. It can promote attentiveness and enhance memory and concentration. Its antispasmodic and anti-inflammatory effects can ease muscular and joint pain, stiffness, backache, arthritis, strains and sprains. It can also be helpful in relieving muscle tightness and spasm associated with coughs, chest and stomach pain and cramps.

Sage oil is a powerful antimicrobial and has a significant inhibitory effect on the growth of bacteria associated with gut, respiratory, urinary and skin infections. These include *Bacillus* spp. involved in infections of wounds, the ears, eyes, respiratory tract, urinary tract and gastrointestinal tract; *Klebsiella oxytoca*, *Klebsiella pneumonia*, opportunistic pathogens that can cause severe infections including pneumonia, urinary tract infection, soft tissue infection and septicaemia; *Salmonella* spp. and *Shigellasonei* which are gut infections that can cause severe diarrhea and vomiting and *E. coli* which can cause symptoms of food poisoning as well as urinary tract infections and pneumonia. When diffused, its antibacterial and decongestant actions can help in respiratory infections, such as colds, sore throats, coughs and chest infections, sinusitis and catarrh.

When diluted in a carrier oil, sage oil can be used topically for inflammatory skin problems and infections such as acne and athlete's foot. Its antimicrobial properties are also useful in minor skin abrasions and injuries such as cuts, wounds, sores and burns. It makes a good ingredient in skin care products to slow and inhibit the appearance of signs of ageing, as its antioxidant properties may help to slow the appearance of wrinkles, fine lines and sagging skin. Sage oil can be used in gargles and mouthwashes when diluted with water and alcohol to a low concentration (1 drop per 10ml of liquid) or a few drops in a bowl of hot water can be used as an inhalation for coughs, colds and catarrh.

Sage oil can also regulate menstrual cycles and related symptoms such as mood swings, fatigue, nausea, and menstrual headaches. It can stimulate contraction of uterine muscles, which can be useful during childbirth, but should be avoided during pregnancy because of the risk of miscarriage. Sage's relative, clary sage, contains a much lower concentration of thujone and shares many of its properties; its use might be preferred when treating women as it is a much gentler remedy. It is a great addition to massage blends during the menopause to reduced hot flushes and night sweats.

Homeopathic Remedy
Sage is used for excessive night sweats, particularly those in TB sufferers when associated with a tickly cough. It is indicated in excessive breast milk and skin problems.

Flower Essence
Sage enhances the capacity for drawing wisdom from experience and is particularly recommended for people who find it hard to find purpose and meaning in life. They may feel resentful about events in their lives, seeing them as ill-fated or undeserved.

Sage is a remedy especially suitable for our later years, for helping to accept what life throws up for us in a calm and detached way. It helps to enhance the wisdom that comes naturally from years of experience. Such wisdom is natural to that end of life, enabling us to be in touch with our spiritual selves, to perceive a higher purpose in life and to experience inner peace. It is a remedy to use during changes and transitions, as it enhances the sage in all of us.

Edible Uses
When using sage in cooking, it is best to use green sage as the taste of purple sage, which is used more medicinally, may be rather overpowering. It is delicious not only in stuffing for poultry, but also as an accompaniment to meat, egg and cheese dishes. Its distinctive flavour can enliven more bland tasting pasta and vegetable dishes and makes delicious herb breads. Try chopping or mincing some fresh green sage leaves and flowers just as they come into bloom and sprinkling them on marrow and other squashes, on potatoes and sweet potatoes, and in bean dishes and tomato soup. With any luck while enhancing your cuisine, it will also enliven your mind, improve your memory, calm your nerves and even bring out the sage in you!

Growing
Propagate by sowing seeds in spring or by taking tip cuttings from spring to autumn. Alternatively, by layering of older bushes. Prefers light, well-drained soil and full sun. Grows up to 2'6" (75cm) and flowers in early summer. To stimulate bushy growth, nip off new shoots. Sage will need renewing every 4– 5 years as it tends to become rather leggy or woody.

Cautions
The normal use of sage is very safe but prolonged use or overdose of the tincture and volatile oil can cause vomiting, salivation, tachycardia, vertigo, hot flushes, allergic reactions and convulsions due to the high content of thujone. Its relative *Salvia lavandulifolia* (Spanish sage) has a similar composition but without the thujone, which would make it more suitable for those concerned

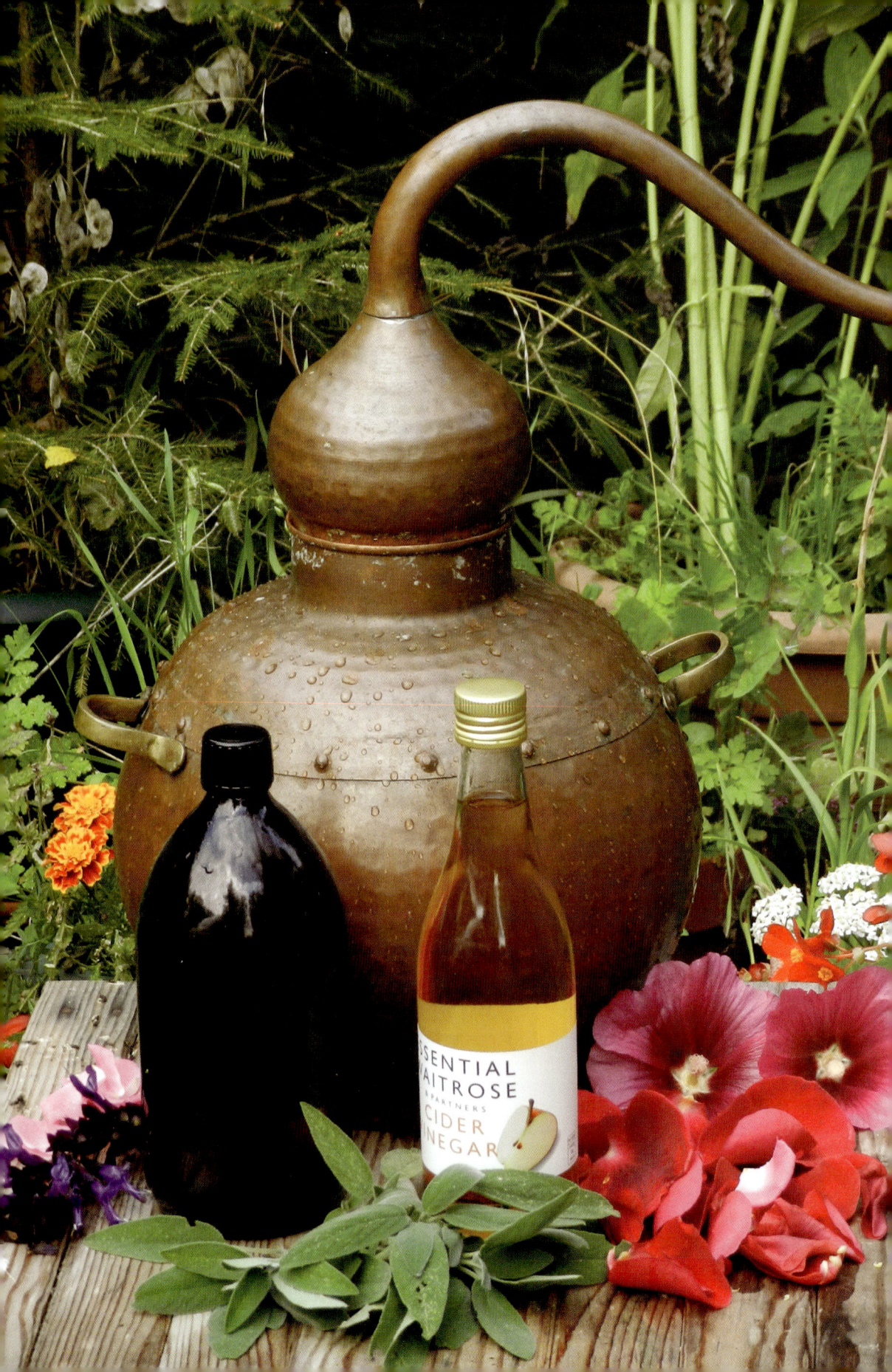

about the excessive usage of sage as a herbal remedy. Avoid in pregnancy and breastfeeding and epilepsy. Avoid with benzodiazepines, insulin and other hypoglycaemics (eg. Chlorpropamide). Patients should monitor blood glucose levels.

Recipes

Antiseptic Mouthwash
Steep a teaspoon or two of calendula flowers, sage and thyme leaves and flowers covered in a cup of boiling water for 10–15 minutes.

Strain and rinse your mouth with the tea morning and night. You can also dip your dental floss in the tea before flossing.

Sage and calendula contain tannins which help to heal sore gums and thyme contains thymol a strong antiseptic essential oil to help combat infection. In fact, several commercial mouthwashes contain thymol.

Hormone Balancing Tea
1 part red sage leaves
1 ½ parts motherwort
½ part lady's mantle
1 part chamomile
1 part rose petals

Add 2 heaped teaspoons of the herb mixture per cup of boiling water to a teapot. Cover and let it steep for 5 to 10 minutes.

Pour the tea into a cup, through a strainer and drink one cupful 3–4 times daily for at least 3 weeks and up to 3 months, to achieve the long-term benefits of the herbs.

This recipe contains herbs which support hormonal as well emotional balance. Motherwort and chamomile are both cooling for hot flushes and are helpful to the liver; sage and rose are also cooling and sage promotes digestion and absorption, helping to deliver vital nutrients to cells, while rose and lady's mantle help balance hormones and enhance mental and emotional equilibrium.

Sage, cayenne, honey and cider vinegar gargle
A handful of sage leaves
A small slice of cayenne pepper or a pinch of dried chilli powder
A pinch of sea salt
100ml boiling water
2–3 tablespoons of honey
2 tablespoons of apple cider vinegar
2 tablespoons of honey

Gargling with sage is a great way to fight off a bacterial infection in the throat. Cayenne is also an excellent antiseptic and analgesic, helping to relieve soreness and pain. Apple cider vinegar is both antiviral and antibacterial.

Place the sage and cayenne in a bowl then pour over the boiling water. Leave it to infuse for 10–15 minutes and then add a pinch of salt which is also great for dispelling infection. Add the cider vinegar and honey and stir well. Gargle with ½ a cupful 3–6 times a day.

Sore Throat Compress
1 part part red sage leaves
1 part calendula petals
1 part plantain leaves

Place equal part of the herbs in a teapot and pour over boiling water. Leave to infuse for 30–60 minutes or until lukewarm to cool. Strain into a bowl and add a few drops of lavender oil.

Soak a thin cotton cloth, such as a head scarf, in the liquid and wring it out gently so it does not drip. Warm your neck area with a warm flannel or by taking a warm shower and then wrap the cotton cloth round your throat, and then cover it by wrapping a wool scarf around your neck and leave it on overnight. You can keep a throat compress on each night (and in the day if you are relaxing at home) until your throat feels better.

These herbs are ideal for an acute throat infection or brewing cold or flu. They stimulate your immunity, help clear congestion in the throat and relieve pain, helping you to sleep more easily and recover more quickly.

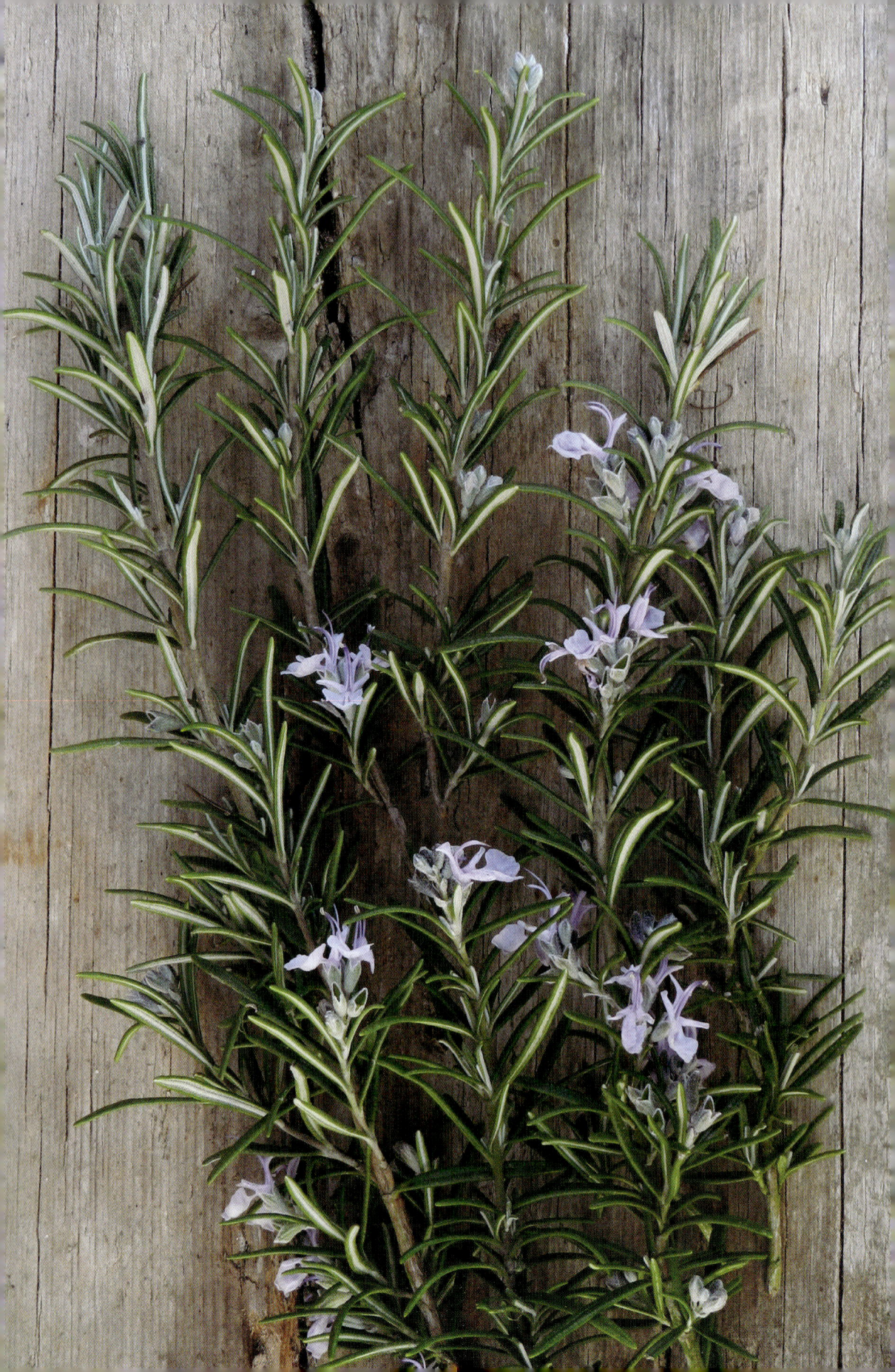

Salvia rosmarinus (Rosmarinus officinalis): Rosemary
The Flower of Loyalty

*There's rosemary, that's for remembrance;
pray, love, remember; and there is pansies,
that's for thoughts*
– William Shakespeare, Hamlet

Other Names: Polar plant, rosemarine, compass plant, compass weed, coronaria, old man, romarin, romarin des troubadours, romero, rose de marie, rose des marins, rosée de mer, rusmari, rusmary

Parts Used: Leaves and flowers

Rosemary is a much-loved aromatic member of the mint (Lamiaceae/Labiatae) family with delightfully aromatic needle-like leaves, found growing wild on dry rocky slopes in the Mediterranean and many parts of Europe, especially near the sea. In fact it derives its name from the sea as *Rosmarinus* means 'dew of the sea'. Rosemary is traditionally the herb of friendship and remembrance and has played an important part in ceremonies associated with marriage, love and death through the ages. It was believed to bring luck and joy, so artisans wove it into royal crowns for kings and emperors, and into posies and veils for brides which explains one of its many names 'coronaria'. It was also a symbol of love and loyalty and sacred to Venus or Aphrodite, the goddess of love who rose from the sea.

Anne of Cleves, the fourth bride of Henry VIII of England, is said to have worn a circlet of gold and precious stones intertwined with sprigs of rosemary, though it did not bring her much luck! It was reputed to have aphrodisiac powers and was often mentioned in the amorous ballads of the Troubadours. It was traditionally known to strengthen the memory, which may explain its use as a symbol of fidelity; in Italy and Portugal, rosemary was traditionally placed in the slippers of the bride and groom so that they would remain loyal to each other. Shakespeare refers to rosemary's association with memory, for Hamlet tells Ophelia, *'Here's rosemary for remembrance .... I pray you love remember'*. A sprig of rosemary was given to mourners at funerals to place in the coffin before it was lowered into the ground, as a symbol of immortality, fidelity and fertility in the next life. The pharaohs of ancient Egypt put rosemary in their tombs, a custom the Welsh continue today. Some say that rosemary was used to protect a man's soul throughout eternity from evil, and so it was placed in the hands of the departed as they lay in their coffin.

Rosemary has been held sacred and valued for its medicinal virtues since at least the time of the ancient Egyptians. It was considered a wonderful tonic particularly to the heart, brain and nervous system. In the days of the ancient Greeks, it was highly valued by students revising for exams and it was customary to wear wreaths of rosemary on the head on such occasions. The Renaissance herbalist of Strasbourg Wilhelm Ryff said of rosemary, *"The spirits of the Heart and entire body feel joy from this drink which dispels all despondency and worry"* and it was worn in a linen cloth tied around the arm to dispel melancholy and make the wearer 'light and merrie'. It was used as a folk remedy for fainting, headaches, nervousness, anxiety, exhaustion, lethargy, depression, insomnia, convalescence and for the elderly. It has been said to cure apoplexy, dim sight, dizziness, drowsiness, drooping spirits, feebleness, palsy, convulsions, and even insanity. John Evelyn said that he found rubbing his closed eyelids with rosemary-infused wine strengthened his sight as well as the rest of his senses.

Rosemary was grown in the early physic and apothecary's gardens; it was a valued remedy for tuberculosis and smoked for coughs and flu or 'la gripe'. Culpeper advised "*Leaves shred small and taken in a pipe, as tobacco is taken, helpeth those that have any cough, phthisick or consumption*" while Gerard wrote: "*If a garlande of the tree be put around the heade, it is a remedy for the stuffing of the head that cometh from coldness.*"

Rosemary was considered a rejuvenating tonic by the early herbalists to the extent that Bankes said, in his Herbal of 1524, "*To smell the scent of the leaves kept one youngly.*" It was the main ingredient of 'Hungary Water', a famous old recipe given to Izabella, the fourteenth century queen of Hungary, by a hermit. Apparently, she was seventy-two and 'infirm of limb and afflicted with gout' and after one year of using the preparation, she recovered her health, strength and beauty so much that the king of Poland wanted to marry her! She had prepared the 'Hungary Water' from alcohol and rosemary flowers and taken one dram once a week and washed her face and limbs with it each morning. Perhaps the power and strength it gave to her explains the old saying 'where rosemary flourishes the woman rules'.

The lovely aromatic volatile oils that lend rosemary its distinctive taste and fragrance are highly antiseptic, and their presence explains the ancient belief that rosemary could protect against pestilence, disease, evil and witchcraft. At one time rosemary tea was brewed by midwives in the delivery room as an antiseptic to protect mother and baby from infection and to sterilise the instruments. In hospitals and sickrooms, rosemary leaves used to be burnt in tubs with juniper berries to fumigate the atmosphere and dispel the foul air of disease and death there and in the homes of the sick. In the streets, ladies of 'delicate health' carried fresh rosemary to disguise bad odours and protect against disease. Rosemary has also been valued for its digestive properties for thousands of years and used to be sold by apothecaries as a hangover cure as well as a remedy for jaundice, 'liverishness', gall stones, gout and arthritis and as a remedy to clear skin problems.

Herbal Remedy

Much of the distinctive taste and smell of rosemary is given by its volatile oils, which include borneol, cineole, pinene, camphor, camphene, terpinol, linalool and limonene. These are responsible for many of the amazing benefits of rosemary including its antioxidant, antimicrobial and potential anticancer activities. It contains other antioxidant compounds including flavonoids (apigenin, diosmetin, luteolin), phenolic acids (rosmarinic acid) and terpenes, as well as tannins, bitters and resins. These help to explain its time-honoured ability to prevent and resolve so many different ailments described by our ancestors.

Rosemary has long been considered a rejuvenating tonic to invigorate the system, with a particular affinity with the nervous system. A steaming cup of rosemary tea, with its combination of pungent and bitter tastes, makes a warming and stimulating start to the day as it is an excellent energiser, helping to enliven and clear the mind, heighten concentration and improve memory. At the same time, its calming effects help guard against becoming stressed by the events of the day. Rosemary has a warming effect throughout the body as it stimulates the heart and general circulation and enhances peripheral blood flow. Its antioxidant effect has a protective effect upon the blood vessels throughout the body; it can be used for varicose veins, tendency to bruising and atherosclerosis. It has an effect on blood platelets and inhibits clotting. In cold weather it makes a great remedy for cold hands and feet and chilblains and can chase away winter lethargy and the blues.

From the story about 'Hungary Water' and many before it, rosemary has gained the reputation of slowing the ageing process, which is proving to be true. It contains antioxidants which help to protect the brain against free radical damage and the ravages of the ageing process, which includes dwindling alertness and a failing memory. The phenolic diterpenes including carnosic acid have a significant effect on memory and concentration, attributed to their antioxidant and anti-inflammatory mechanisms which have neuroprotective effects in the brain. Rosemary appears to be protective against brain damage and to improve recovery which could be useful after a stroke. It is not surprising that rosemary is popular among nervous exam students and interviewees, but it also holds potential for the prevention and treatment of Alzheimer's disease and other forms of cognitive decline. Alzheimer's involves the accumulation of amyloid-beta which causes the progressive death of neuronal cells in the brain, as well as damage caused by free radicals and inflammation. Deterioration of the brain may also be related to the accumulation of metal ions such as copper, zinc and iron in amyloid plaques. As we age, the deterioration of the blood-brain-barrier can allow metals to pass unchecked into the brain. The antioxidant effects of polyphenolic compounds may be partly explained by their ability to chelate iron and other metals and draw them away from brain cells.

Other components of the volatile oils in rosemary can alter brain function and improve cognitive function and alertness. Rosemary has a relaxing and thymoleptic (mood-elevating) effect and can be used to relieve nervousness, anxiety, exhaustion, lethargy, depression and insomnia. By stimulating blood flow to the head, relaxing tense muscles, reducing inflammation, aiding digestion and supporting the liver, rosemary can provide an effective remedy for migraines and headaches of varying origins. It can also protect against the effects of ageing on the eyes and positively promote eye health. Carnosic acid can protect against eye diseases affecting the outer retina including the common eye problem, macular degeneration.

Like other aromatic herbs, the volatile oils that give rosemary its distinctive taste and fragrance have antibacterial, antiviral and antifungal properties. They enhance the function of the immune system and ward off infection. It was because of this that rosemary was believed to protect from pestilence and disease, as well as from evil and witchcraft. The volatile oils and phenolic compounds particularly rosmarinic acid, carnosic acid and carnosol have antibacterial effects against bacteria including *Bacillus* spp., *E. coli, Enterococcus faecalis, Pseudomonas aeruginosa, Staphylococcus aureus* (MRSA), *Micrococcus luteus, Streptococcus thermophilus, Pseudomonas fluorescens, Propionibacterium acnes, Staphylococcus epidermidis* and *Helicobacter pylori*. Rosemary also has antiviral activity against *Herpes simplex* type 1 and 2 and *HIV*. A hot tea can be taken at the first signs of colds, sore throats, flu, catarrh, coughs and chest, stomach and bowel infections. By increasing circulation to the skin and causing sweating, it will bring down fevers. The warming and stimulating effects of rosemary help clear mucous from the head and chest, explaining its old use as a remedy for catarrh, coughs, wheezing, bronchitis and whooping cough. Its relaxant effects help relieve spasm in the bronchial tubes in asthma. It is a great tonic for elderly people with poor circulation, particularly after a debilitating illness such as influenza and pneumonia.

Rosemary has a stimulating effect on the digestion, enhancing the appetite, increasing the flow of digestive juices and relieving wind and bloating. It helps move food and wastes efficiently through the system, removes stagnant food, improves sluggish digestion and helps the absorption of nutrients so that maximum benefit is derived from the diet. Its antimicrobial actions combat unfriendly bacteria in the gut and help to maintain a friendly gut flora thus influencing gut health, immunity and brain function. It helps to protect against *Listeria monocytogenes* and *E. coli*. The astringent tannins in rosemary exert a protective effect on mucous membranes throughout the gut, helping to prevent infection, irritation and inflammation, and explaining its use in diarrhoea. Its antispasmodic action helps relieve wind, colic and griping. Interestingly, rosemary extracts are routinely used as natural antioxidant preservatives to improve the shelf life of perishable foods.

Rosemary used to be sold in apothecaries as a cure for hangovers, and was considered excellent for jaundice, gallstones, *'liverishness'*, and, by cleansing the system of impurities and wastes, for gout, arthritis and as a remedy to clear the skin. It stimulates and regulates the liver and its antioxidant and hepatoprotective actions protect the liver from damage from chemicals, toxins, drugs and alcohol. By enhancing liver function, rosemary helps clear toxins from the system that may account for headaches, lethargy, irritability and general malaise. Rosemary can also have a beneficial effect on blood sugar and cholesterol levels. It may be helpful for those wanting to lose weight as it inhibits pancreatic lipase activity and reduces fat absorption and adipogenesis, the process by which fat cells (adipocytes) develop and accumulate as adipose tissue in the body.

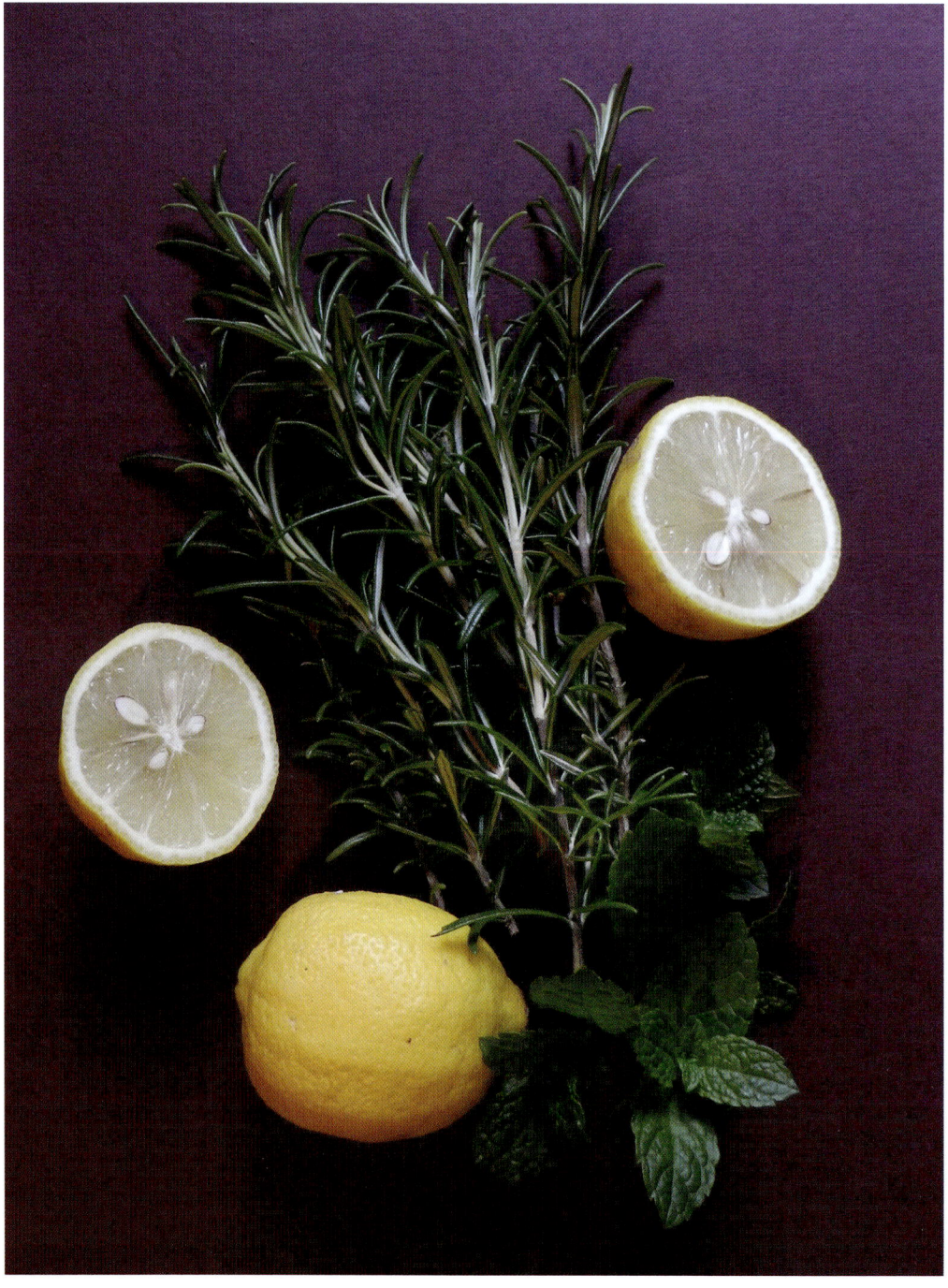

The tannins in rosemary have an astringent effect, which explains its use for reducing heavy menstrual bleeding. Its relaxant effect in the uterus relieves period pains and helps to regulate periods. Rosemary enhances elimination of excess fluid and wastes through its diuretic action. This can be useful in the treatment fluid retention and urinary tract infections.

The antioxidants in rosemary may have further benefit. They may protect the body against the damaging effects of radiation and have anticancer activity. Carnosic acid, the main polyphenol antioxidant in rosemary, may reduce the spread of leukaemia when it is combined with vitamin D. As an anti-inflammatory, rosemary can help relieve pain and swelling in arthritis and gout.

Externally, a bath with a few drops of rosemary oil makes an excellent pick-me-up when feeling tired at the end of the day or simply low, unmotivated or depressed. It is stimulating and relaxing at the same time, so it makes a good early morning bath too. The essential oil diluted in a carrier oil and massaged into the skin is warming and invigorating, and by bringing blood to the surface, it can speed healing and help resolve pain and inflammation in aching or stiff muscles, painful joints in arthritis and gout, as well as sciatica and neuralgia. The oil rubbed into the temples relieves tension and headaches and can be inhaled to dispel drowsiness and increase concentration. A wreath of rosemary was often worn around the heads of students to enhance memory and concentration.

Recipes

To add an extra something to your vinaigrette, try infusing sprigs of rosemary in bottles of balsamic vinegar and virgin olive oil. Add extra ingredients, such as garlic or chilli if you wish. Leave the bottles on a sunny windowsill for two to three weeks to allow time for the flavour to permeate, then strain and add fresh sprigs of rosemary.

Rosemary and Lemon Syrup
½ litre/1 pint rosemary sprigs, gently pressed down in measuring jug
½ litre/1 pint water
juice of lemon
1lb/500gm sugar

Pour boiling water over rosemary in a pot or jug. Cover and leave to infuse for 10 minutes. Strain and add lemon juice and sugar. Heat slowly and stir until sugar is dissolved.

Boil fast for 5-8 minutes, or until the syrup starts to thicken. Remove from heat and when cool pour into jars/bottles. Seal with airtight lids when cold and label clearly. Will keep for several weeks in the fridge.

Rosemary Tea
4 teaspoon dried rosemary leaves
1 pint boiling water
Pour the water over the leaves and leave to infuse for 15 minutes

Mint and Rosemary Mouthwash
Mint and rosemary both combine antiseptic and digestive properties, and when used as a mouthwash help sweeten the breath.

500ml filtered or mineral water
2 teaspoons fresh mint leaves
2 teaspoons fresh rosemary leaves

Place the herbs in a pot and pour over boiling water. Leave to infuse for 20–30 minutes. When cool, strain and use as a mouthwash 2–3 times daily.

This will keep in the fridge for 2 or 3 days. Add 1 teaspoon (5ml) tincture of myrrh if you want to preserve it for a little longer.

Rosemary Salt
Mix a quantity of sea/rock or Himalayan salt with 1.5 times the quantity of fresh chopped rosemary.
If you have a liquidiser, you can blend them for a few minutes.

Spread the salt and herb mixture out thinly on baking parchment and place in a very low oven (150 degrees C, 300 degrees F/Gas 2) with the door ajar, until the herbs are dry. Store in an airtight jar.

Rosemary has long been used in perfumes and cosmetics to enhance the health of the skin and hair. The dilute oil can be massaged into the scalp to check hair fall and condition the hair. Rosemary is frequently used in shampoos and hair conditioners for this reason. It has been used to treat scabies and lice. An infusion of rosemary can be used as an antiseptic and anti-inflammatory lotion for cuts, wounds, sores, chilblains, scalds and burns, insect bites, wasp and bee stings. It also makes a general tonic and beauty aid to the skin to reduce wrinkles and puffiness under the eyes. It can be used as a douche for vaginal infections and as a mouthwash for bleeding gums and bad breath. The fresh leaves can be chewed to sweeten the breath and to combat infection of the teeth and gums.

Aromatherapy oil
The essential oil of rosemary reflects the use of the herbal remedy. It is a wonderful tonic to the nerves, the heart, the circulation and digestion. Its refreshing and invigorating aroma is stimulating, awakening and strengthening, good for tiredness, lethargy, nervous debility, poor memory and concentration and anxiety. It wakens the senses and clears the mind, and has an uplifting effect emotionally, helping to dispel low spirits and depression. It can be used to rekindle energy at the end of a long day, to enhance concentration during mental work, and to help calm the mind during meditation. It is helpful for diminishing of the senses, such as loss of smell or dimness of sight. It also has analgesic properties and helps to dull pain, as in arthritis and neuralgia. It is a rejuvenative oil.

Flower Essence
The colour blue represents heaven and eternity, wisdom and truth and blue or purple is associated with the crown chakra, related to inner peace and ecstasy. The blue-purple flowers of rosemary bring clarity of mind, and peace and balance to the emotions, enabling a meditative state. The remedy increases sensitivity both physically and emotionally and enhances creativity. It symbolises the blooming of higher thought forms in the midst of activity.

Edible Uses
Rosemary is a wonderfully versatile herb and its wonderfully penetrating rather pine-like taste can not only enhance your culinary skills in the kitchen but also aid digestion and benefit your gut flora as well. It blends well with a whole range of rather rich foods such as bread (particularly focaccia), lamb, duck and goose and also goes well with fish dishes, pasta, beans and pulses, mushrooms and leeks. Only use the young tender leaves as dried rosemary can be rather hard and spiky but is fine when used in bouquet garnis to flavour soups and stews. The pretty purple flowers have a more delicate taste and can be used in desserts like pies and crumbles, as well as blended into fruit fools and creams.

Growing
Propagate by sowing seeds in spring or take tip cuttings during summer and early autumn. Prefers a slightly alkaline, well-drained soil, full sun and in a sheltered position as some forms are slightly tender. Grows up to 10' (3m) and flowers in April and May.

To add interest in the garden there are several different varieties of rosemary including *Suffolk blue, Marjorcan pink, Miss Jessop's upright, Prostatus* and *Severn Sea*, and all are effective medicinally and loved by bees. Because they are evergreen, the leaves can be picked all year round.

Established rosemary shrubs can be found at most garden centres, and its attractive foliage and stimulating aroma make it popular amongst gardeners.

Cautions
Avoid in pregnancy. May cause contact dermatitis. Large doses may cause kidney and gastro-intestinal irritation. Since it improves liver detoxification, it may affect the efficacy of some medications. Take away from mineral supplements.

Sambucus nigra: Elder

The Flower of Fairyland

English summer begins with elderflower and ends with elderberries.

Other names: Black elder, common elder, arn, bourtree, boretree, European elder, Judas tree

Parts Used: Flowers, leaves, berries

In early summer, when looking for those fragrant umbels of creamy white flowers to make elderflower cordial and champagne, you never have to go far, for elder grows in abundance all over the English countryside. Part of the reason for this is that historically the elder tree has been considered sacred and magical; in fact, it has been more associated with myth and superstition than almost any other tree. In England, when the masses of fragrant flowers blossom in the countryside, it is a signal that summer has arrived, and when the branches droop with purple-black berries, summer has gone, and autumn is here. A member of the Adoxaceae family, Elder can also be found in profusion along hedgerows, woods and gardens in central and southern Europe, North America and North Africa.

As such a sacred tree, elder has always been treated with great respect. In some traditions, elder is regarded as holy wood and for this reason it is never struck by lightning; witches fear it for the same reason. Elder trees were planted by the back door of English cottages, as it was believed that they had the power to keep out negative influences including witches, lightning and evil.

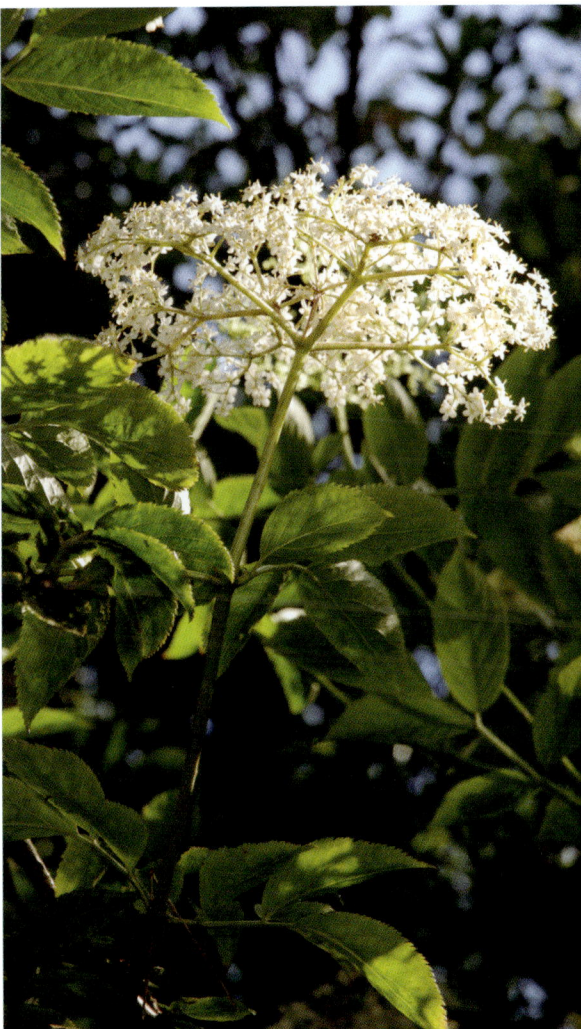

In Russia it was thought that elder could ward off unwanted or evil spirits. These beliefs may have arisen from the traditional use of elder leaves in the kitchen and outhouses to repel flies and other potentially disease-carrying insects. Bunches of leaves were hung by doorways of houses and barns and attached to horses' harnesses. Elder trees also used to be planted near dairies as they were thought to stop the milk from turning. Linen used in the dairy was hung out to dry on elder trees as their aroma helped to deter flies in the dairy. There are other references advising one not to sleep under elder trees as the strong smell of the leaves had a narcotic effect.

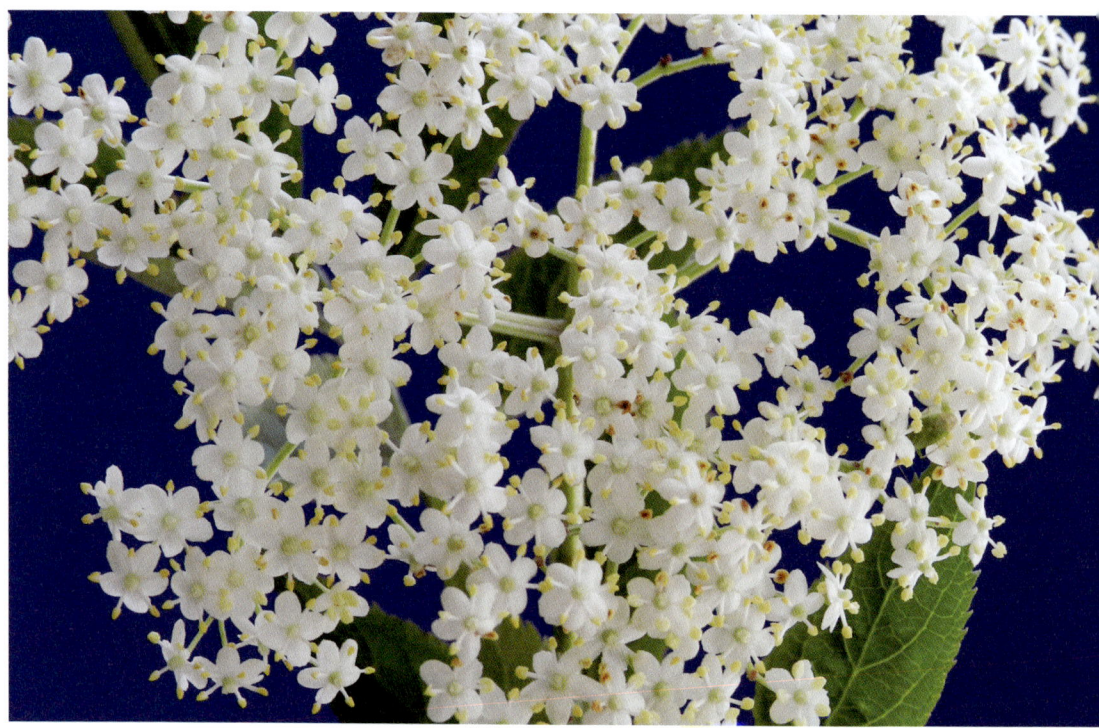

The name *elder* may come from the Anglo-Saxon 'aeld' meaning fire, or from 'ellar' or 'kindler' because its hollow branches were used as tubes to blow through to kindle a fire, like bellows. The wood itself makes a poor fuel as it burns quickly, and its sap makes it crackle and hiss as it burns. It was believed that it was the devil spitting from the fire. Perhaps this is why there are so many superstitions about bringing elder into the house and why in gypsy lore it was taboo to burn it; it is said to be unlucky, and could even cause a death in the family if burnt on the fire. It is supposed to be the tree that Judas hung himself from (hence the name 'Judas tree') and so became the emblem of sorrow and death, and yet the Serbs used to take a stick of elder into wedding ceremonies to bring good luck. In Poland it is customary to bury sins under an elder tree where the tree's power will absorb them. In Russia, it is thought that elder prolongs life and in other traditions elderberries are placed under the pillow to bestow peaceful sleep, and a twig is carried to prevent the temptation to commit adultery. Pregnant women have been known to kiss the tree for good fortune for the baby. Elder branches are hard and polish easily. They have a soft core, making them easy to hollow out, and have often been used to make wind instruments such as whistles and pipes. This explains why some of elder's many common names include 'bourtree' or 'boretree'. Its Latin name *Sambucus* comes from 'sambuke' the Greek musical instrument made of its wood. *Nigra* refers to the colour of the berries. The music made from the wood instruments was said to attract faeries and other spirits. In Denmark there is an old belief that if you stood under an elder tree on midsummer eve, you would see the king of fairyland ride by, attended by all his retinue. In Scandinavian and German folklore, the tree was the abode of the elder dryad or mother, whose permission was vital before the tree was cut down or any part used medicinally. "*Hyldemoer, Hyldemoer, permit me to cut thy branches*" was the request. If permission was not sought, it was feared the dryad would cause harm to home or family.

The whole of the fragrant elder has been valued for so many practical and medicinal uses for thousands of years, it has been known as the 'medicine chest of the people'. Gypsies maintain that the whole plant is beneficial to man, which is another reason why they never burn it. In 1644 the diarist John Evelyn wrote, *"If the medicinal properties of its leaves, bark and berries were fully known, I cannot tell what our countrymen would ail for which he might not fetch a remedy from every hedge, either for sickness or wounds."* It used to be believed by country people that if you carried an elder twig about in your pocket, it would protect you against rheumatism.

In folk medicine, elderberries have been used for their diaphoretic, laxative and diuretic properties and to treat various illnesses including stomach ache, sinus congestion, constipation, diarrhoea, sore throats, common colds and rheumatism. Elderberries used to be popular for making into syrups and wines for preventing and treating coughs, colds and fevers and making into conserves for easing sore throats. Until the end of the 19th century, hot elderberry rob, a cordial made with elderberries and sugar, was sold on London streets on cold winters' days and nights to bring cheer to workers and travellers. Cinnamon was often added to enhance its warming effects. Native Americans also have a tradition of using elderberry for its healing properties and particularly to treat fever and rheumatism.

The leaves, when laid on the temples, have been used as a folk remedy to relieve nervous headaches. They were also used to relieve neuralgia and sciatica. The bruised leaves used to be worn in a hat or rubbed on the face to keep away flies and insects, though this may not be a good idea for those with sensitive skins. They were also used as first aid for cuts, bruises, minor burns, sprains, swollen joints and haemorrhoids.

Despite its relative scarcity in Scotland, parts of the elder tree were used for dying in the Harris tweed industry; blue and purple dyes were derived from the berries, yellow and green from the leaves and grey and black from the bark. The Romans used the berries for dyeing their hair.

Herbal Remedy
Both the elderberries and elderflowers make excellent medicines and have a long tradition of use in herbal medicine to enhance immunity, reduce inflammation and combat infections such as colds and flu. They share many of the same constituents, primarily flavonoids, such as flavonols, phenolic acids, proanthocyanidins and anthocyanins.

Elderflower is rich in antioxidant bioflavonoids, mostly flavones and flavonols, that are known for their antioxidant, anticancer, anti-inflammatory and antibacterial properties. The flowers contained tenfold more flavonols than the fruits and several times more than the leaves. The most abundant flavonols in elderflower are quercetin, isoquercitrin and anthocyanins which have antiviral properties as well. Elderflower also contains large amounts of chlorogenic acids, such as cinnamic acid, which may help with allergies, regulate blood glucose levels and have a laxative effect. It also contains triterpenoids which have analgesic, anti-inflammatory and anticancer effects as well as tannins, essential oils and mucilage.

Elderberry also contains flavonols (quercetin, kaempferol and isorhamnetin), rutin, chlorogenic, crypto-chlorogenic and neochlorogenic acids, ellagic acid, anthocyanins, vitamins A, B, E and C, calcium, iron, sterols, tannins, polysaccharides, and essential oils.

Elder has an affinity with the respiratory system. The flowers are highly valued for their antioxidant content, their antibacterial and antiviral properties and vitamin C which are all great for boosting immunity. They are active against a range of different bacteria as well as human, swine and avian strains of flu viruses. When taken in hot infusion, they make a wonderful remedy to take at the first signs of colds, sore throats, fevers and flu. They stimulate the circulation and cause sweating, which helps to bring down fevers and cleanses the system by promoting elimination of toxins through the pores of the skin. They make a good decongestant remedy for mucus congestion, chronic catarrh and sinusitis. They are traditionally combined with yarrow and peppermint and taken in hot infusions at the first signs of colds or flu and also for catarrh, sinusitis, bronchial catarrh, chest infections and asthma. Their relaxant effect on smooth muscle helps to relieve bronchospasm which is useful when treating asthma. Elderflower also helps alleviate allergies such as hay fever. It contains tannins with an astringent action that helps to dry up runny eyes and noses and this works in conjunction with its anti-inflammatory actions to reduce inflammation and irritation. Elderflower tea is also recommended at the onset of eruptive diseases such as measles and chickenpox, to bring out the rash and speed recovery.

Elderflowers have a diuretic action which is useful for relieving fluid retention and eliminating toxins via the kidneys; this also helps to reduce heat and swelling in the joints. Their antioxidant and anti-inflammatory actions help to protect the joints from damage and also help explain their long use for treating gout and arthritis, especially when the joints are aggravated by cold damp conditions. Their laxative properties also help to clear toxins and wastes from the system.

Elderflowers also have a long history of use as a relaxant to calm the nerves, reduce anxiety and lift depression. A hot infusion at night promotes a restful sleep and is particularly useful for restless or irritable children at the onset of infections, to encourage healing rest and allowing the body to carry out its recuperative work and speed recovery.

Elderflower can help to reduce cholesterol and blood sugar levels. This has been attributed to the flavonoids in elderflower particularly quercetin, which helps to reduce oxidative stress. It also protects blood vessels from damage. Both the flowers and the berries can reduce the accumulation of fat tissue, reduce weight and improve body mass index (BMI).

The berries are rich in antioxidant vitamins A and C and have become renowned for their antiviral properties. They are helpful for combatting many different cold and flu viruses, notably influenza A virus (H1N1) and influenza virus B. Polyphenol compounds from elderberries can directly bind to the virus and inhibit their entry and replication inside the cells of the body and so prevent infection. Phenolic compounds in the form of flavonoids also have the ability to block the penetration and infection by HIV-1

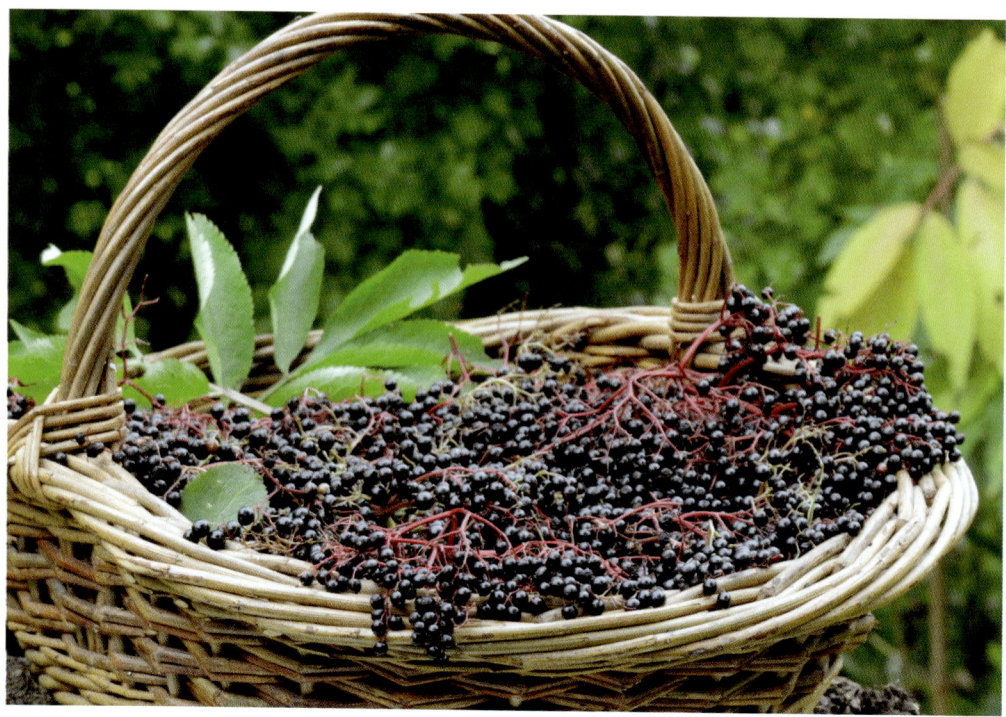

virus. Elderberries also stimulate the immune system and the formation of antibodies against infection. This is attributed mostly to the acidic polysaccharides. Elderberries have antibacterial activity against bacteria including *Streptococci* spp. and *Branhamella catarrhalis* which causes infections of the upper respiratory tract. They also have the ability to activate the immune system by increasing inflammatory and anti-inflammatory cytokine production.

Elderberries are rich in polyphenols and their derivatives anthocyanins and flavonols. Anthocyanins are responsible for the dark purple colour of the fruit. Their medicinal properties are associated with the presence of polyphenols which are powerful antioxidants. Our body uses antioxidants to counteract damage caused to the body by oxidative stress, and thereby help to maintain a healthy immune system, protect the arteries from inflammation and damage, and regulate blood pressure and blood sugar levels.

Elderberries have one of the highest antioxidant actions of all small fruits. They regulate cholesterol and triglyceride levels and can be helpful in the prevention and treatment of diabetes as they can lower blood sugar by increasing the use of glucose in the muscles and increasing the secretion of insulin. They have anticancer activities and may reduce the risk of cardiovascular disease and stroke. They regulate uric acid levels, which is important as an elevated uric acid level can be associated with high blood pressure. High uric acid also occurs in gout, which can also be treated with elderberries. Their anti-inflammatory actions also contribute to their benefit in inflammatory problems including gout and arthritis.

Externally elderflowers can be used for their healing, anti-inflammatory and antiseptic effects. Infusions can be used as lotions and the flowers incorporated into creams for cuts and wounds, burns, bruises, chilblains, sunburn, piles, ulcers and skin problems including eczema and psoriasis. An infusion or dilute tincture makes a good gargle for sore throats and a mouthwash for mouth ulcers and inflamed gums. Distilled elder water makes an excellent toning and cleansing lotion for the face, an eyewash for conjunctivitis and sore eyes and a good remedy for inflammatory skin problems and sunburn. It was popular at one time for preventing freckles. An infusion of the leaves can be used as insect repellent to keep away midges and mosquitoes. Elderflower and elderberry have an antibacterial action against *Staphyloccocus aureus* and could be an effective remedy for MRSA. Liniments of elderflower might help reduce pain and swelling in joints in arthritis.

Aromatherapy Oil
Elderflower essential oil has a rich fruity and floral aroma that has long been used in sacred perfumes, and mythological essences. It has astringent, anti-inflammatory and antimicrobial actions, which makes it a lovely oil to use in skin creams and toners to tighten the skin, combat oiliness and a tendency to pimples, and reduce the appearance of wrinkles. It can also be added to massage blends to ease muscle tension and spasm, and reduce inflammation and pain in arthritis and gout.

Elderflower oil also has a gentle relaxing effect on the mind and can soothe mental tension and anxiety, irritability and frustration and lift the spirits. In burners as inhalations, the antimicrobial and decongestant actions can be helpful to ward off infection and clear mucus.

Homeopathic Remedy
Sambucus acts particularly on the respiratory organs and suits people who are easily frightened or fretful. Such people are prone to anxiety, trembling and restlessness, and their physical symptoms tend to be characterised by spasms. Fright may give rise to suffocative attacks of coughing when the face turns blue, as in asthma, croup or whooping cough. A child may wake suddenly in the night around midnight, crying and unable to breathe.

Like the herbal remedy, Sambucus is used for catarrh, colds and blocked noses, particularly in babies and children, and also for hoarseness with tenacious phlegm in the throat, and for phlegm in the chest. Profuse sweating in the daytime tends to accompany such symptoms. Sambucus will also help relieve fluid retention which causes oedema that may contribute to this excess of catarrh in the system. Other urinary symptoms such as cystitis and nephritis may also call for Sambucus. Fevers, with the skin becoming dry and burning at night, but breaking out in a sweat in the daytime, fevers without thirst, preceded by a dry cough and accompanied by dread of being uncovered also indicate Sambucus.

Flower Essence

The folklore of the elder is echoed in its use as a flower essence. It is recommended for its ability to impart inner strength and to increase self-esteem, making it ideal for times of challenge and change in life, and when in need of courage and fortitude. It helps to calm fears and anxieties and engenders a sense of being nurtured and supported by a strong and stable inner energy.

Elder is an excellent remedy for children as well as adults. As a protective remedy, it is given to people feeling invaded or over-dominated by others or overcrowded by fears and anxieties. Elder stimulates energy, vigour, resilience and joy, and our innate powers of recovery and renewal of energy.

Edible Uses

What could be more blissful on a hot summer's afternoon than to relax in a hammock or chair in the shade of some lovely old fruit tree, and idly while away the hours doing nothing more than sipping elderflower cordial from time to time?

This delicately scented and most refreshing of drinks is so easy to make and provides an excuse, if you need one, for spending another relaxing summer's afternoon in the most pleasant occupation of collecting umbels of the creamy white flowers that adorn the English hedgerows in late June.

Elderflowers can be made into deliciously refreshing summer drinks such as champagne and cordial. They also make an excellent addition to pancakes and fritters, jams, sorbets and cheesecakes.

The delicious juicy berries make a tasty combination with stewed blackberries and apple, and can be eaten for their laxative effect. They are rich in vitamins A and C and used to be made into syrups and wines for preventing

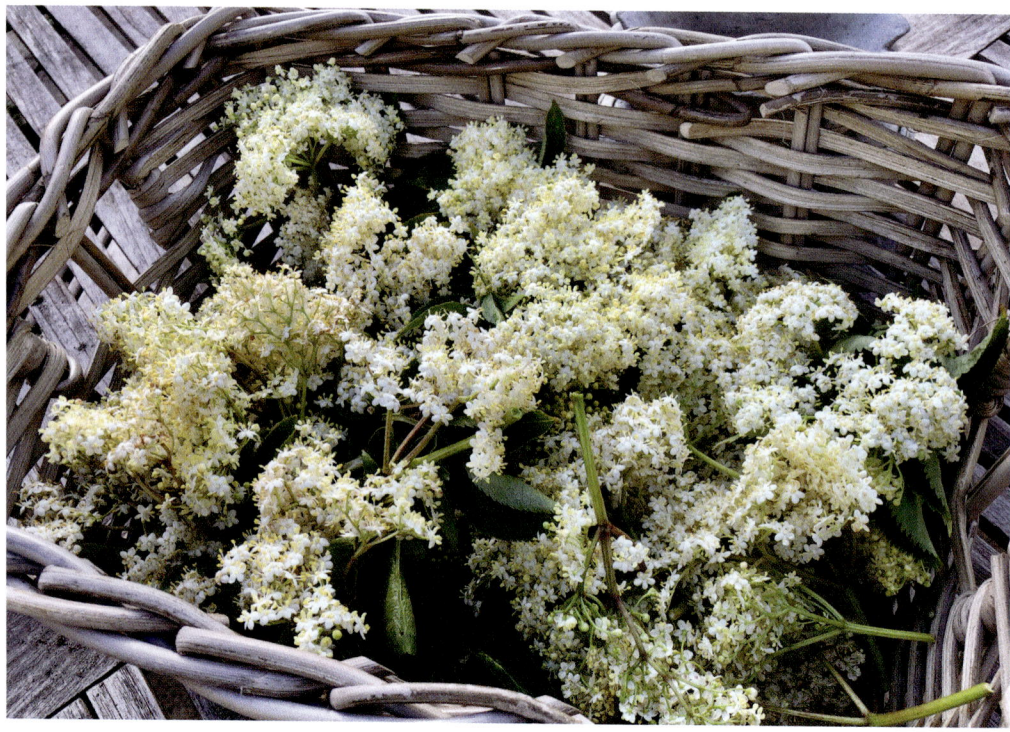

and treating coughs and colds and to bring down fevers, and into conserves for sore throats.

Growing
Propagate by sowing ripe berries in autumn or taking hardwood cuttings in summer or early autumn. Prefers fertile soil, sun or semi-shade, and grows up to 25' (8m), flowering May/June and producing fruit Aug – Nov. Self-seeds easily.

Cautions
Possible interactions of flower and berry products with morphine. Avoid with insulin and other hypoglycaemic medications (eg. Chlorpropamide). Monitor blood glucose levels carefully.

It is best not to eat elderberries raw due to the risk of nausea and other gastrointestinal complaints, so they need to be cooked prior to use. The leaves can cause a reaction on sensitive skins. Avoid use of the root, bark and unripe berries.

Recipes

Elderflower Cordial
This delicately scented cordial makes a light, fruity tasting and wonderfully refreshing drink. One sip and you are transported to the perfection of a warm summer's afternoon in the beauty of England's countryside. The cooling effect of elderflowers is brought about in two main ways. By bringing blood to the surface of the body, heat is released through the pores of the skin, and by their diuretic action, excess heat as well as toxins are eliminated via the kidneys.

1.2 litres water
1.3kg sugar
1 lemon, sliced
25 large elderflower heads
75g citric acid
Sparkling or still mineral water to dilute

Place the water in a large pan and bring to the boil. Add the sugar and lemon and remove from the heat, stirring until the sugar dissolves. Place on the heat again and bring to the boil. Add the elderflower heads and citric acid. Bring to the boil once more, remove from the heat and allow to stand until cool. Strain and bottle in clean bottles with corks. This can be drunk immediately. Stored in a cool place, it should keep approximately 3 months. When serving, dilute with 5 parts water.

Elderflower Rob
This rich dark-red cordial is a storehouse of vitamins A and C, and a delicious syrup remedy for preventing and treating coughs, colds and flu, sore throats and fevers. Cinnamon was often added to elderberry rob to enhance its warming effect.

450g fresh elderberries
450g brown sugar

Strip the berries from their stems, wash and then crush them. Place in a pan with the sugar. Bring slowly to the boil and simmer until a syrup consistency is reached. Pass through a sieve and bottle in clean, airtight bottles. Take 1–2 tablespoons in a cup of hot water regularly as a preventative or at the onset of cold symptoms. This recipe works well with other fruit such as blackberries and black currants.

Scutellaria spp: Skullcap

The Flower of Relaxation

Its soothing influence upon the nervous system conduces to quiet and restful sleep.
– Finley Ellingwood 1852–1920

Other Names: Mad dog weed, mad weed, Virginian skullcap, quaker bonnet, hoodwort, helmet flower, American skullcap, blue pimpernel, blue skullcap, mad-dog skullcap

Parts Used: Leaves and flowers

Virginian skullcap, *Scutellaria lateriflora*, is a pretty member of the mint (Lamiaceae/Labiatae) family and a hardy perennial indigenous to North America. It can be found growing wild in profusion in damp, places, meadows and ditches and by the sides of rivers and ponds. Its Latin name comes from 'scutella' meaning a little cap which the calyx of its little blue flower was said to resemble, hence its common names 'hoodwort' and 'helmet flower'. It was also thought to look like the military helmets worn by the early European settlers. Common skullcap (*Scutellaria galericulata*) and lesser skullcap (*Scutellaria minor*) are found in similar places in Britain and make pretty additions to a herb garden or border.

Traditionally, both the British and the Virginian skullcap have been highly valued for treating excitability, insomnia, epilepsy, convulsions, St Vitus's dance, hysteria, palsy, bites of poisonous insects and snakes and a whole range of other nervous symptoms. In America, Virginian skullcap is also known as 'mad dog skullcap' or 'mad weed' as it was said to cure rabies or hydrophobia, as well as every kind of nervous complaint in humans, even insanity. It was well known among the Cherokee and other Native American tribes as a herb for women, and was used as an emmenagogue and as a ceremonial plant to aid the transition of young girls into womanhood. It was also enjoyed as a remedy to induce visions. While skullcap was held to cure infertility, it was also recommended for people

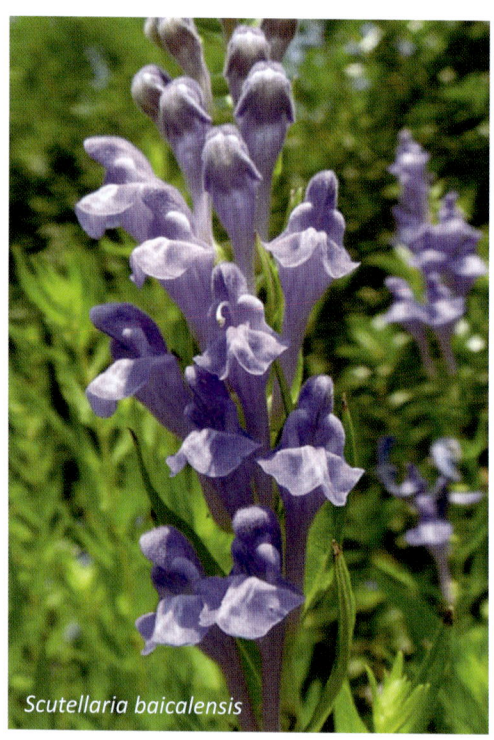
Scutellaria baicalensis

troubled by undue sexual desires. Chinese skullcap (*Scutellaria baicalensis*) is native to several Asian countries as well as Russia. The dried roots have been used for centuries as a Traditional Chinese Medicine in which it is known as 'huang qin'.

Herbal Remedy

Skullcap is rich in nutrients including calcium, iron, potassium and magnesium that are essential to a healthy nervous system and is one of the best nourishing tonics for the nerves – a perfect tonic for supporting us in our busy, stressful lives. It has bitter and astringent tastes and contains flavonoids (baicalin, baicalein, wogonin and lateriflorin), scutellarin, scutellarein, iridoids, volatile oils (limonene, terpineol, cadinene, caryophyllene), lignans, resin, tannins, bitter glycoside, minerals (calcium, potassium, magnesium, silica) and B vitamins.

It is an excellent nervine for reducing anxiety and agitation and can be used for a wide range of nervous complaints, including obsessive-compulsive disorder and panic attacks. Skullcap can improve mood and reduce anxiety by promoting GABA (gamma-aminobutyric acid), a neurotransmitter that helps calm nerves, reduce anxiety, lift mood and aid sleep. Skullcap contains GABA and high levels of glutamine, an amino acid that plays an important role in our response to stress. While GABA may not cross the blood-brain barrier, glutamine does and can be synthesised to GABA and in this way increase the availability of GABA in the central nervous system.

Oxidative stress plays a vital role in neurodegenerative and psychiatric problems; the flavonoids in skullcap have significant antioxidant and anti-inflammatory effects, protecting the brain from free radical damage. Skullcap may help protect against neurological disorders such as Alzheimer's disease, Parkinson's disease, anxiety and depression. It may help rebuild the myelin sheath of the nerve fibres and benefit multiple sclerosis.

Skullcap improves memory and concentration, eases agitation and restlessness and can be useful in ADD and ADHD. It can enhance calm awareness and this way be a great aid to meditation. One of its constituents, scutellarin, enhances the production of endorphins, lifts depression, helps to dispel tiredness and exhaustion and yet promotes restful sleep. Skullcap can be used without fear of dependency to promote sound sleep without unwanted side effects and enable you to feel refreshed and revitalised in the morning.

Skullcap is a great remedy when feeling nervously overwrought or run down and is a good remedy to treat shingles. When taken regularly, it is helpful for breaking addictions, when withdrawing from orthodox tranquilisers and antidepressants as well as caffeine and alcohol. Its analgesic properties can help relieve pain in tension headaches, neuralgia, period pain and arthritis. Its antispasmodic and anticonvulsant actions can relieve twitching muscles, facial tics, chorea, tremors, cramps and palpitations and

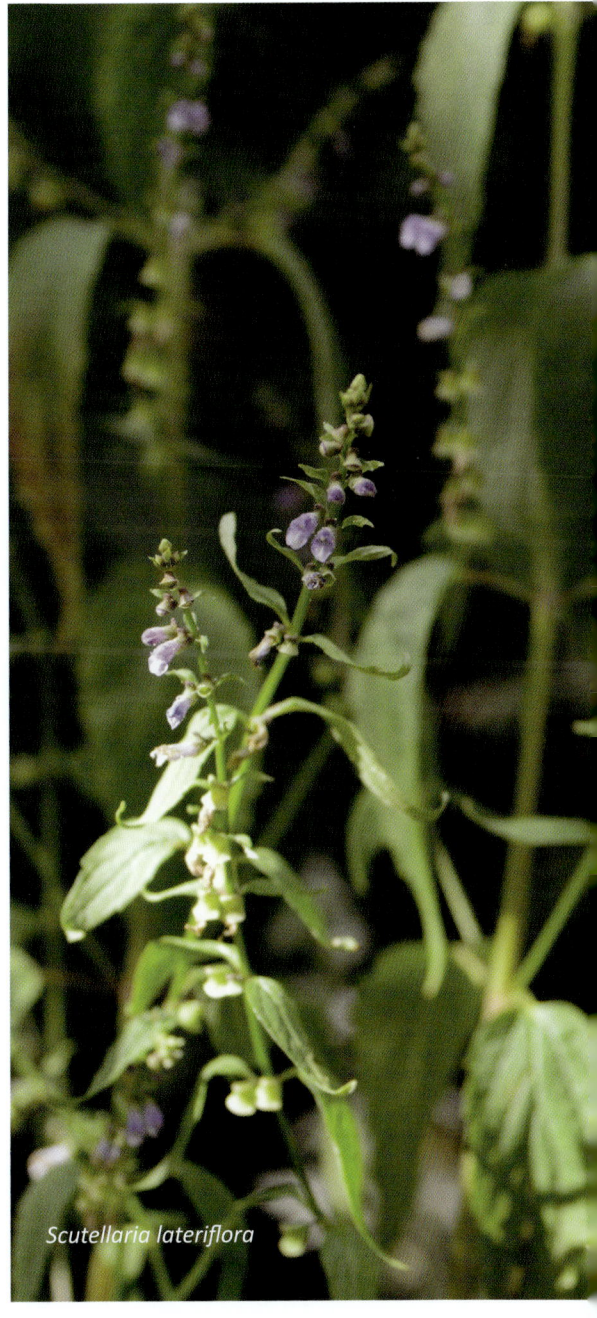

Scutellaria lateriflora

can be helpful in Parkinson's disease, restless leg syndrome and epilepsy (petit and grand mal). By helping to release tension and relax muscles, it makes a good remedy for tight, tense, stiff and aching muscles.

Skullcap can be added to prescriptions for stress-related symptoms including period pain, gut problems (including intestinal spasm, IBS and colitis), asthma, high blood pressure and nervous palpitations. It also acts as an anti-inflammatory and can be used for arthritis, particularly when it is aggravated by stress. The antioxidants in skullcap have a protective effect on the heart and circulation and its antispasmodic action dilates peripheral arteries and reduces blood pressure. When taken hot it can reduce fevers.

When combined with hormone balancing herbs such as vitex and wild yam, skullcap can relieve menstrual headaches and PMS, and when combined with sage, motherwort or both during the menopause it can help relieve menopausal irritability, depression and mood swings. Its antispasmodic action helps ease period pain and pain of endometriosis. Its traditional use for excess libido is worth exploring. Since it can promote menstruation, it should not be given to pregnant women.

With its bitter taste, skullcap has a tonic effect in the digestive tract, enhancing appetite and digestion, and stimulating liver function. It is recommended for stress-related digestive problems. It reduces spasm and colic in the gut, relieves wind and bloating and eases nervous stomach aches. With its diuretic action, skullcap aids elimination of excess fluid and toxins via the kidneys. This is useful for treatment of cystitis and irritable bladder, especially where there is a nervous component.

Chinese skullcap (*Scutellaria baikalensis*) contains similar flavonoids (baicalein, baicalin, wogonin), as well as wogonoside, camphesterol, sitosterol and benzoic acid. The root is used, which has a bitter taste, and its array of beneficial plant compounds include antioxidants which have anti-inflammatory effects and protect cells from free radical damage.

Chinese skullcap is an excellent cooling and anti-inflammatory remedy which is renowned for its ability to treat fevers and allergies including hay fever, conjunctivitis, otitis, food allergies and skin problems such as eczema and urticaria. It enhances immunity, clears heat and inflammation, and combats acute infections and inflammation in the digestive, respiratory and urinary systems. It has antifungal and antiviral actions and is used to treat acute respiratory infections, viral infections (including Epstein Barr, HIV and influenza), sinusitis and asthma. It

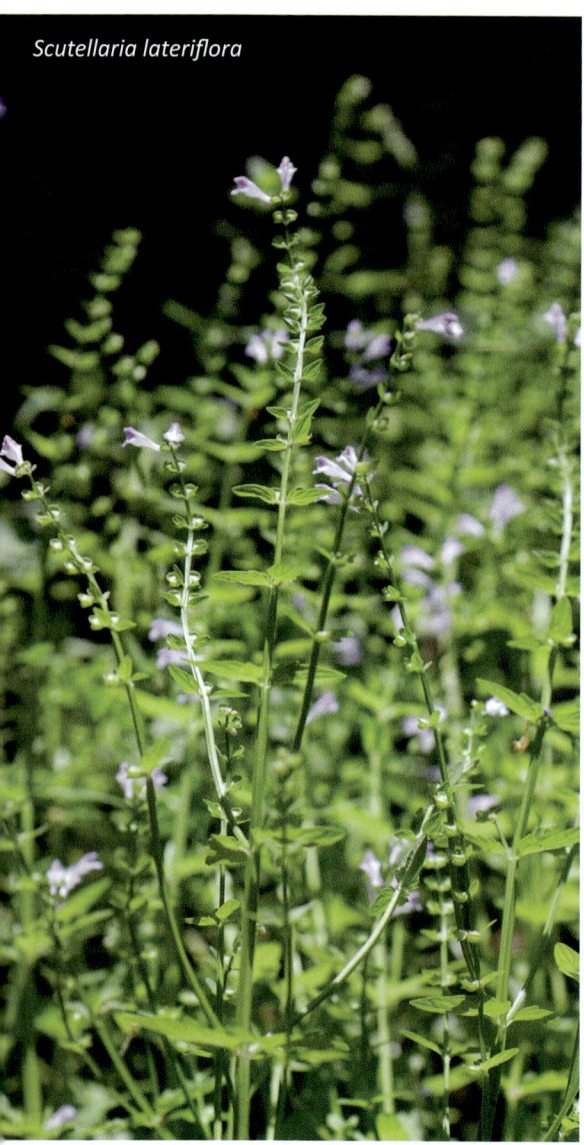

Scutellaria lateriflora

can be helpful in irritation and inflammation in the gut and is used to treat diarrhoea, dysentery and food allergies. It supports the cleansing and metabolic work of the liver and is used for infections and inflammation in the liver and gallbladder.

Chinese skullcap also has a beneficial effect in the nervous system, and is good for treating anxiety, insomnia and stress-related circulatory problems including high blood pressure. Its diuretic and antimicrobial properties can be helpful in urinary tract infections.

Its antioxidants can be useful in inflammatory and autoimmune conditions including rheumatoid arthritis and gout. They may also protect against cardiovascular disease including high cholesterol and atherosclerosis and have the potential to fight cancer, particularly of the prostate, cervix, ovaries and pancreas, and inhibit angiogenesis (the growth of new blood vessels that support the growth of cancerous tumours). It can help to lower blood sugar in diabetes.

Homeopathic Remedy
Scutellaria is a similarly wonderful medicine for a wide range of nervous problems. These include restlessness, excitability, being so tense one is unable to sleep or think, for hysteria, night terrors, heart irregularities and great agitation. It is prescribed for nervous debility after long illness, over-exertion, too much studying, overwork and for symptoms of a nervous breakdown. It is likewise used for epilepsy, convulsions, chorea, delirium tremens, nervousness or spasm in teething babies, and for a range of other stress-related problems including poor appetite, nausea, colic, hiccoughs, globus hystericus, muscle twitching, vertigo, cramps, nervous diarrhoea, frequent and scanty urination and severe headache, mostly at the back of the head.

Flower Essence
Skullcap is used to benefit the nervous system and helps to alleviate the damage caused to the nerves by overuse of caffeine and drugs such as morphine and heroin. It can be used to help withdrawal symptoms from such drugs, and to remedy emotions often linked to drug addiction such as anxiety, low self-esteem, and a feeling of inability to cope with life. It is said to act on the pineal gland, enhancing the secretion of endorphins (natural opiate-like substances) and engendering a sense of physical and emotional wellbeing. Used in massage oils it helps to relax nerves and muscles, and a dab of the flower essence over the medulla oblongata is said to increase psychic healing ability, and to attune one to accepting healing more fully from others.

Growing
To propagate, sow seeds in moist fertile ground in spring once danger of frost has passed or divide the roots in spring or autumn. Likes a sunny position and grows up to 18". Flowers bloom from May to August, gather aerial parts in the summer as flowers bloom, dry and store for later use.

Cautions
In the past, Scutellaria lateriflora has been contaminated with germander (*Teucrium* sp.), a group of plants known to cause liver problems. It is important that skullcap is obtained from a reliable source. High doses may cause giddiness, mental confusion, muscle twitching, irregular heartbeat, and seizures. Avoid during pregnancy and breastfeeding, Avoid with CNS depressants (eg. alcohol, opiates, benzodiazepines, barbiturates, anaesthetics, tricyclic anti-depressants, anticonvulsants).

Avoid *S. baikalensis* in first trimester of pregnancy, avoid with anticoagulants, benzodiazepines, CNS depressants (eg. alcohol, opiates, benzodiazepines, anaesthetics, tricyclic anti-depressants, anti- epileptics), Cyclosporine. Avoid with insulin and other hypoglycaemic medications (eg. Chlorpropamide).

Recipe

Skullcap and California Poppy Tea
Skullcap and California poppy make a great combination for a sleep remedy.

Take a teaspoon of each and place in teapot. Pour over 1–2 cupfuls of boiling water. Leave to infuse for 10–15 minutes and drink a cupful before bed.

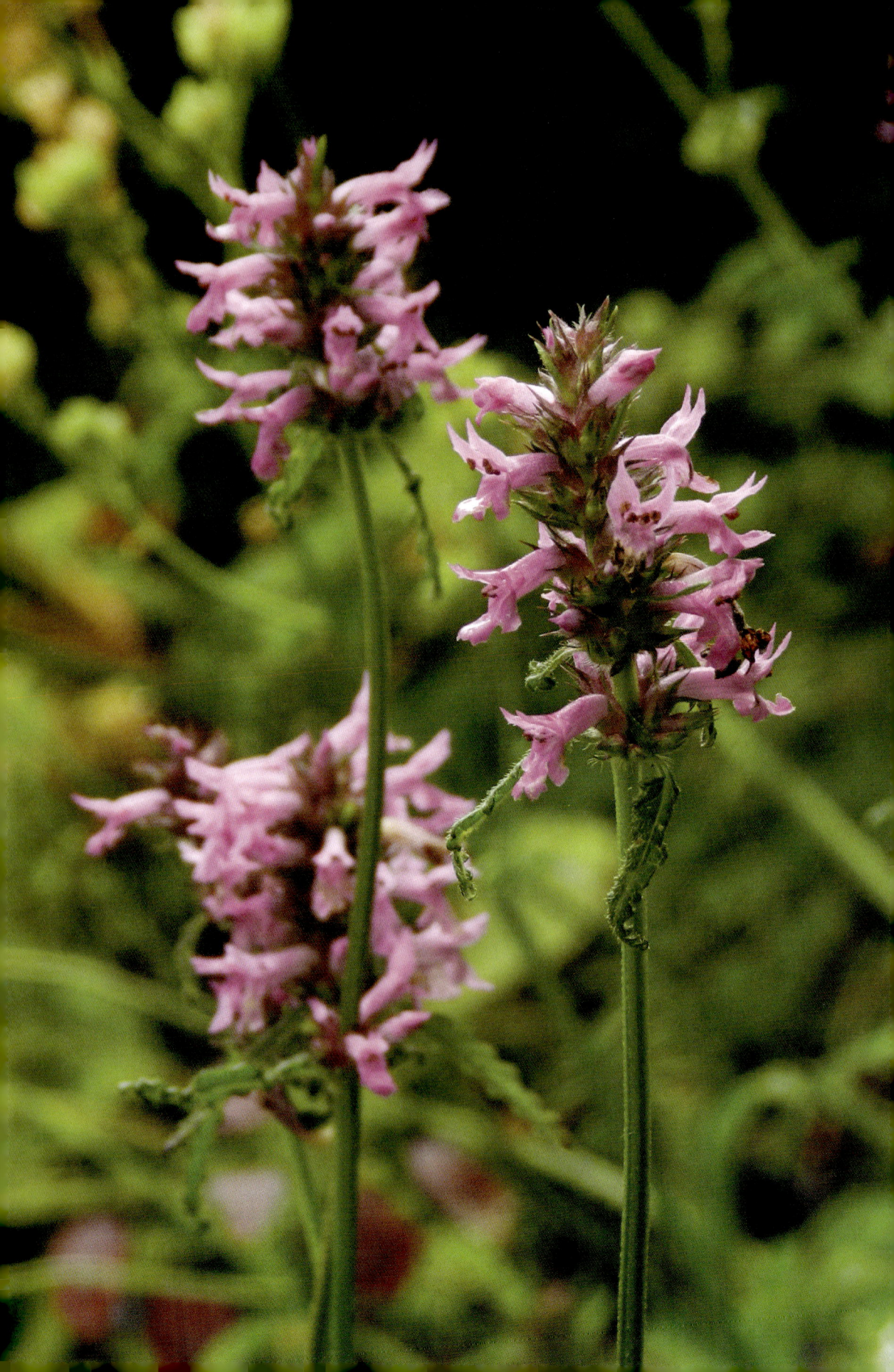

Stachys betonica: Wood Betony
The Flower of Detachment

*Betony, you who were discovered first by Aesculapius
Or by Chiron the Centaur, hear my prayer.
I implore you, herb of strength by Him who ordered your creation,
And ordered that you should be useful for a multitude of remedies.
Kindly help in making these seven and forty remedies*
– Antonius Musa, chief physician to the Emperor Augustus

Other Names: *Betonica officinalis, Stachys officinalis*, purple betony, betony, common hedge nettle, lousewort, wild hop, bishopswort, bitny

Parts Used: Leaves and flowers

Wood betony is a pretty perennial plant with vibrant purple-pink flowers, a member of the mint (Lamiaceae/Labiatae) family and native to Europe. It can be found growing wild in woods and meadows, on heaths and moors and in country lanes. In the Middle Ages, it was grown in the physic gardens of apothecaries and monastery gardens, as it was considered a panacea for all ills. It was valued as a remedy for many ills including jaundice, paralysis, convulsions, gout, fluid retention, headaches, shortness of breath, stitches and pains in the sides and back. It can still be found growing around the sites of ancient monasteries as well as in churchyards, where it was planted for protection against evil. Wood betony was also worn around the neck as an amulet. Erasmus said it sanctified those who carried it about them. It was 'good against fearful visions', while the ancient Greeks held, "*it is good whether for the man's soul or for his body; it shields him against visions and dreams, and the wort is very wholesome.*" It was a religious herb of the Celts.

Few herbs have been more highly praised for their healing properties than wood betony. It has been used in medicine for centuries; it was written about by the ancient Greek physician Dioscorides in the first century AD and was highly praised in Roman times, in fact a whole treatise was written on its virtues by Antonius Musa, chief physician to Emperor Augustus, showing it as a cure for no less than forty-seven diseases. His prayer is written above. Wood betony was described by Roman Pliny the Elder who called it 'ventonica'. This could come from the Vettones, an ancient Iberian Celtic tribe who used it to drive away bad spirits. Two old European proverbs illustrate the high regard in which wood betony was held. The Italians said, "*Sell your coat and buy betony*" while the Spaniards said of a good man, "*He has as many virtues as betony*".

The name *Stachys* comes from the Greek meaning an ear of grain, because the lovely purple flower spike resembles an ear of corn or grain. The name *betonica* comes from the Celtic word 'ben' meaning head and 'tonic' meaning good, as it was considered a good remedy to treat conditions associated with the head. It was taken internally, smoked and powdered and used as snuff for headaches, and when mixed with powdered eyebright, it was used to clear congestion in the head from colds and catarrh.

Gerard said that it protected people from "*the danger of epidemical diseases*" such as the plague, and that "*it helpeth those that loathe and cannot digest their food*". He also says that it cured jaundice, epilepsy, gout, palsy, dropsy, as well as coughs, colds and flu and respiratory problems including consumption.

He recommended taking it with mead and pennyroyal which was "*good for putrid agues*" and said it made a good vermifuge for combatting internal parasites such as worms. He also said it was good for "*obstructions of the spleen and liver*". The juice from the leaves was good for the bites of serpents and mad dogs and for the relief of toothache.

Herbal Remedy
Wood betony has a combination of pungent, bitter and sweet tastes and contains a wide array of constituents – flavonoids including rutin, alkaloids (trigonelline, betonicine, stachydrine), glycosides, delphinidin, saponins, tannins, phenolic compounds including rosmarinic acid, betulinic, ursolic and oleanolic acid, betaine, choline, manganese, phenols and volatile oils (higher in the leaves) containing sesquiterpenes with antioxidant activity.

Wood betony is an excellent tonic to the nerves with sedative and relaxing effects. It is excellent for stress, frayed nerves, hypertension and an inability to relax and is used to relieve anxiety, hysteria, insomnia, depression and lethargy. Its antispasmodic actions help relax tense and aching muscles and have been used traditionally for convulsions and nervous palpitations.

Its antioxidant and anti-inflammatory flavonoids and phenolic compounds play a part in protecting the nervous system from free radical damage. It can be used to relieve pain, particularly nerve pain as in trigeminal neuralgia, shingles and sciatica. It makes a good remedy to improve memory and concentration.

Wood betony has been used for centuries for headaches attributed to a variety of different causes; it relieves headaches related to poor circulation to the head by improving the circulation, those related to a sluggish liver by enhancing the liver's action and those related to tension as it is a relaxant.

Astringent and antimicrobial, wood betony can help clear catarrhal congestion in the respiratory system and help combat infection. The volatile oils have antibacterial activity. A hot tea stimulates the circulation, bringing blood to the surface of the body and helps to throw off fevers, head colds and other infections, and to clear catarrh, sinusitis and coughs.

The flavonoids and glycosides have a hypotensive action helpful in high blood pressure, especially that associated with stress. The antioxidant action of wood betony has been shown to have an anti-inflammatory and cardio-protective effect. It can be used for inflammatory problems including arthritis and gout.

Cooling and relaxing in the gut, wood betony can be used for stress-related digestive problems including nervous indigestion and nausea, heartburn, wind, bloating, colic, diarrhoea or constipation. Bitters in wood betony can enhance appetite and digestion and help to clear toxins including parasites from the gut. The astringent tannins protect the gut lining from irritation, inflammation and infection and make it a good remedy for gastritis, peptic ulcers, leaky gut syndrome, colitis and diarrhoea. It benefits the liver and can be used for a range of liver and gallbladder problems. Trigonelline can lower blood sugar, making wood betony useful to diabetics.

The relaxing and uplifting action of wood betony can be helpful in relieving period pain and PMS, particularly if combined with chamomile. It is interesting that it lowers blood sugar and may be helpful in insulin resistance which is related to polycystic ovarian syndrome (PCOS), as wood betony can be helpful in abnormal uterine bleeding associated with PCOS. It may have a galactagogue action and increase the production of breast milk in lactating mothers. It regulates uterine muscle and can bring on delayed periods. It is cooling and relaxing for menopausal flushes, insomnia and depression.

Wood betony can be used to treat urinary tract inflammation and infection and is good for cystitis and could be useful in acute kidney problems such as glomerulonephritis. With its diuretic action, it aids the elimination of toxins and excess uric acid via kidneys, helpful in gout and arthritis.

Externally the tannins make wood betony a useful astringent to stem bleeding, speed repair and repel infection of cuts and wounds, sores, ulcers, varicose veins and haemorrhoids. A lotion or poultice can also be used for bruises, sprains and strains and to draw splinters and thorns. It can be made into a lotion to beautify the skin.

A gargle can be made for sore throats, laryngitis, and pharyngitis. A mouthwash can be used for gingivitis. The whole plant can also be used as a hair dye, good for giving grey hair a blonde tint. Traditionally it was taken as snuff for nosebleeds and headaches.

Homeopathic Remedy
Stachys betonica is similarly used for problems affecting the head, and for colds and catarrh. It is prescribed for a feeling of fullness in the head and eyes, a heavy sleepy feeling, pain in the eyes and dizziness. These symptoms are relieved in the open air and aggravated by closing the eyes, moving or bending the head, looking at light, reading or thinking.

Flower Essence
Wood betony also relates to the head and is said to enhance the function of the pineal gland, which secretes endorphins, natural opiates which engender a sense of physical and emotional well-being. It helps to bring inner calm and detachment, strengthening the desire for higher principles and goals, and has been used to help resolve conflicts between sexual desires and desires for greater enlightenment. A person using tantric practices, in which sexual energies are potentially transformed into higher spiritual energies, may gain help from wood betony, and the inner calm it brings should support a resolve of celibacy if that is the chosen path. It has been used for people of over-high sexual energy, and for those who are celibate through no choice of their own due to sexually transmitted infections such as *Herpes* or simply being single.

Recipes

A few of the fresh leaves can be added to salads, but they have a mildly bitter taste, so should be finely shredded.

Headache Relief Tea
1 teaspoon dried wood betony
1 teaspoon dried rosemary
250ml of boiling water in a pan
Honey to taste

Put the wood betony and rosemary in a teapot. Pour over boiling water. Cover. Allow to steep for 10 minutes. Strain and pour into a cup and drink; add honey if you wish.

Wood Betony Nerve Tonic
1 bottle white wine
75g wood betony
50g vervain
50g rosemary

Combine the ingredients in a glass jar and leave to macerate for at least two weeks. Take ½ cup to relieve nervous headaches, tension, stress, anxiety etc.

Growing
Propagate by sowing seeds in early spring or by dividing clumps in spring or autumn. Grows 1 to 2' (30 to 60cm) high and flowers in June to September. Prefers fertile soil and light shade.

Cautions
Avoid during pregnancy and breastfeeding. May cause nausea, gastrointestinal cramps, diarrhoea. Caution with hypotensive and anti-diabetic medications.

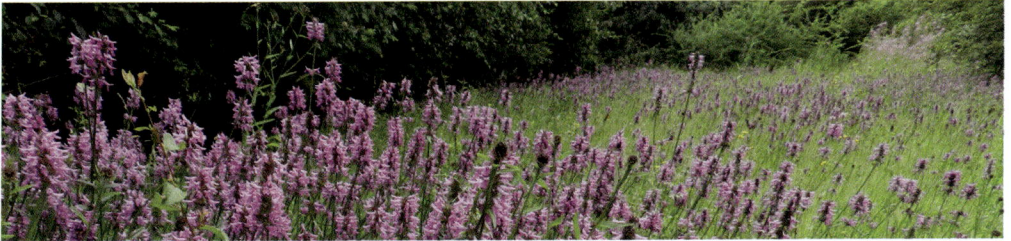

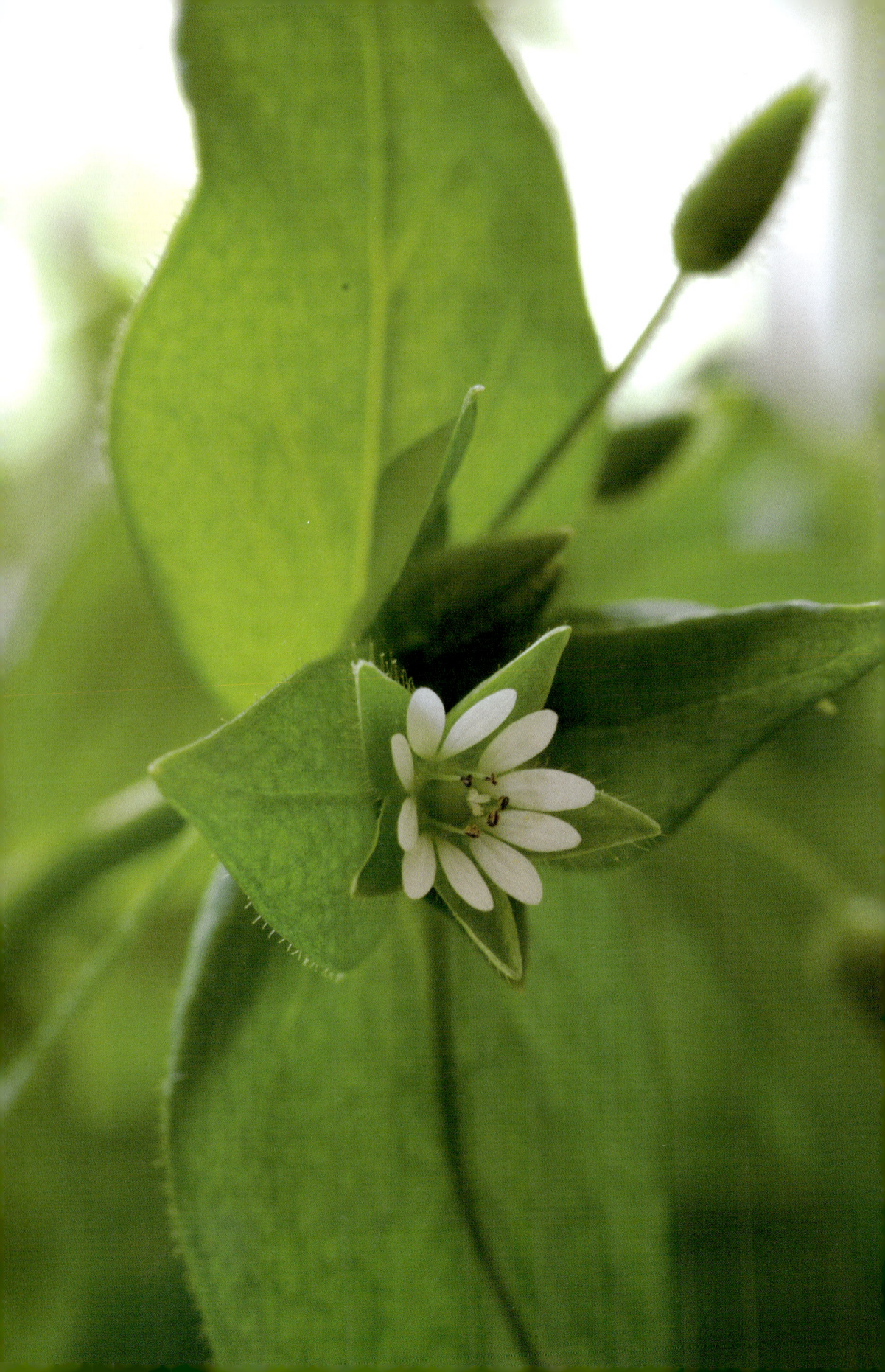

Stellaria media: Chickweed

The Flower of Prediction

It is a fine soft pleasing herb under the dominion of the Moon.
 – Nicholas Culpeper (1616–1654)

Other Names: Starweed, adder's mouth, alsine media, bird's eye, Indian chickweed, mouse ear, bird seed, passerina, satin flower, scarwort, star chickweed, starwort, stitchwort, tongue grass, white bird's eye, winterweed

Parts Used: Leaves and flowers

This sweet little annual with its tiny white flowers is a member of the carnation (Caryophyllaceae) family and is one of the first plants to appear after the winter in temperate regions, heralding the arrival of spring. It used to be called 'winterweed' because it can be found even when there is still frost on the ground. It grows wild in areas following the paths of settlers and provides nutritious greens, rich in vitamins A and C and minerals including iron, copper, potassium and calcium. It is said that sailors used chickweed vinegar to prevent scurvy when fresh citrus fruits were unavailable.

Chickweed's Latin name *Stellaria* comes from 'stella' meaning star, from its pretty white star-shaped flowers that apparently open regularly at nine o'clock in the morning on fine days and close at nine in the evening on summer's evenings. It has been used to predict the weather; if it opens fully into flower there will be no rain for 4 hours, but if the flowers remain shut you will need an umbrella! Its common name *chickweed* refers to the fact that birds and chickens are very fond of it and the seed used to be fed to caged and game birds, so it was also called 'bird seed'.

Chickweed has a long history of use as a nutritious edible green for both humans and animals and was even considered a delicacy. It has been enjoyed since at least the time of the ancient Greeks, it was esteemed as a food as well as medicine in ancient Ireland and was well known throughout Europe as a remedy for gout, constipation and respiratory problems including tuberculosis. It was given as a blood tonic in the spring and during convalescence and to consumptives and undernourished children to build them up. The Swiss used to eat it to strengthen the heart. It was said to improve eyesight, probably due to its vitamin A content, and was used as a remedy for inflammatory eye problems. Culpeper recommended *"The juice or distilled water is of much good use for all heats and redness of the eyes, to drop some thereof into them"*.

Culpeper said chickweed's element is water and called it *"A fine, soft, pleasing herb, under the dominion of the Moon"*. It was valued as a cooling remedy for hot inflammatory conditions, particularly for the skin and has long been used in lotions, ointments and creams and applied fresh to burns and scalds, ulcers, piles and abscesses. It was used for its drawing properties to bring poisons and infections to the surface. Traditionally the plant was chopped and boiled in lard to make a green cooling ointment for piles, sores and other skin conditions and eye problems. Gerard said, *"The leaves of Chickweed boyled in water very soft, adding thereto some hog's grease, the powder of Fenugreeke and Linseed, and a few roots of Marsh Mallows, and stamped to the forme of Cataplasme or pultesse, taketh away the swelling of the legs or any other part"*. It was used by country women to cool the body during fevers.

Chickweed's cooling properties were used internally as well as externally as Culpeper tells us, *"The herb bruised, or the juice applied, with cloths or sponges dipped therein to the region of the liver, and as they dry to have fresh applied, doth wonderfully temper the heat of the liver and is effectual for all impostumes and swellings whatsoever; for all redness in the face, wheals, pushes, itch or scabs, the juice being either simply used, or boiled in hog's grease; the juice or distilled water is of good use for all heat and redness in the eyes ... as also into the ears...."* Rubbed onto arthritic joints it was said to relieve pain and inflammation and an infusion was drunk to promote weight loss.

In European folklore, chickweed was believed to promote fidelity, attract love and maintain relationships. If a sprig of chickweed was carried in your hand, it was said to draw the attention of or ensure the fidelity of a loved one.

Herbal Remedy
This diminutive but resilient plant with its combination of bitter, sweet, sour and salty tastes contains a wealth of nutritious and medicinal ingredients. These include vitamins A, B, C, D and folic acid, minerals including calcium, copper, iron, magnesium, potassium and zinc, gamma-linoleic acid, flavonoids including apigenin and rutin, triterpenoid saponins, phytosterols, coumarins, mucilage and organic acids (carboxylic acids). The saponins have an anti-inflammatory action, as do the flavonoids, which are also anti-allergenic and antimicrobial. They also help the elimination of potentially harmful compounds from the body, including carcinogens. Rutin has also been shown to have potential anticancer properties.

Our ancestors described chickweed as cooling and modern herbalists still use chickweed today as a cooling and soothing remedy for hot inflammatory problems such as gastritis, colitis, acid indigestion, irritable bowel syndrome and excess heat in the liver and gallbladder. Its carminative and mild laxative properties help relieve wind, bloating and constipation. It has an affinity with the respiratory tract, and with its expectorant and soothing effects provided by the saponins and mucilage, it can be given for sore throats, laryngitis, bronchitis, asthma and harsh dry coughs. Taken as a hot infusion it can help bring down fevers, and when taken cool it relieves thirst.

Chickweed's diuretic action reduces fluid retention and helps eliminate toxins, excess uric acid and heat from the system via the kidneys; this could be useful when treating inflammatory conditions such as skin problems, arthritis and gout. The antioxidant actions of chickweed may help reduce inflammation in these cases. Its diuretic action may also be helpful in high blood pressure. As a soothing diuretic, it can be drunk as a lukewarm infusion to relieve cystitis and irritable bladder. Chickweed is used to support the lymphatic system in its cleansing work and by some herbalists to flush deposits of fat including fatty tumours like lipomas from the body and aid weight loss.

Externally chickweed is renowned as a cooling, soothing and healing remedy for the skin and is popular in creams and lotions for inflammatory and itchy skin conditions such as eczema, heat rashes, urticaria, sunburn, boils and spots. Its mucilage has drawing properties so chickweed can be used as a drawing remedy to bring boils and abscesses to the surface. The fresh leaves or a cream can be applied for their wound healing properties to speed tissue repair of fresh cuts and wounds, burns and scalds, piles and ulcers. A cool infusion can be used as an eyewash for inflammatory eye problems and an oil or ointment can be applied to cool hot, inflamed joints.

Homeopathic Remedy
Heat and burning characterise many of the symptoms calling for the cooling and moistening qualities of Stellaria. There are burning pains in the liver area, hot inflammatory eye symptoms, flushes of heat in the face, burning on the lower lip with neuralgic pain and heat and dryness in the mouth. There may also be respiratory symptoms: short, dry, irritating cough, hawking of thick mucus, and a feeling of constriction in the chest.

Stellaria is also used for inflammatory problems, particularly of the joints and the liver. It is indicated by sharp rheumatic or arthritic pains which dart about all over the body. A Stellaria person may be irritable and lethargic, with little energy to motivate themselves to work. They sleep well but wake unrefreshed and are generally worse in the mornings, from warmth, and better in the evenings and in cold air.

Flower Essence
Chickweed is taken for unresolved emotional issues from the past that create tension or insecurity and stop one from entering joyfully into the present. Carrying around such unresolved feelings may affect one's health and energy, and may cause problems such as being overweight, as the body adds protective layers to compensate for feeling vulnerable. Chickweed helps one to let go of the past and relax into the present moment, able to respond freely to whatever arises, without feeling threatened or needing to be in control.

Edible Uses
Chickweed has been regarded traditionally as a delicacy in Europe and eaten in salads or cooked like spinach. It is said to be more tender than any other wild green. It has a light refreshing taste and is highly nutritious with significant levels of vitamins and minerals.

Growing
Chickweed can thrive almost anywhere; it can survive very cold temperatures and needs little water. Its shallow, fibrous roots are easy to uproot accidentally, but the plant will recover quickly if you replant it quickly. It is easy to grow from seed and self-seeds effortlessly in soil with a balanced pH, so it can be a good indicator of the health of your soil. To harvest, snip the leafy tops off and a second crop will be ready several weeks later, in fact it can produce up to six generations in a single year.

Cautions
The leaves contain saponins, excess doses could cause diarrhoea and vomiting. Avoid in pregnancy and breastfeeding.

Recipe

Chickweed pesto
2 cloves of garlic
3 tablespoon pine nuts or sunflower seeds
¼ teaspoon salt
2 packed cups chopped fresh chickweed
½ cup olive oil
½ cup Parmesan cheese

Blend or chop in a food processor and enjoy!

Great with pasta or eaten on crackers or vegetables.

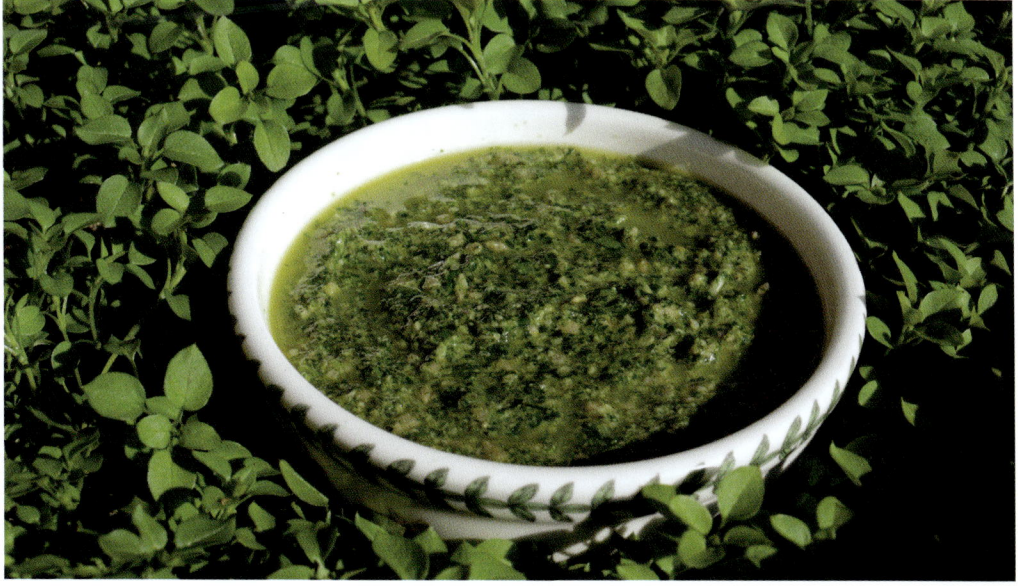

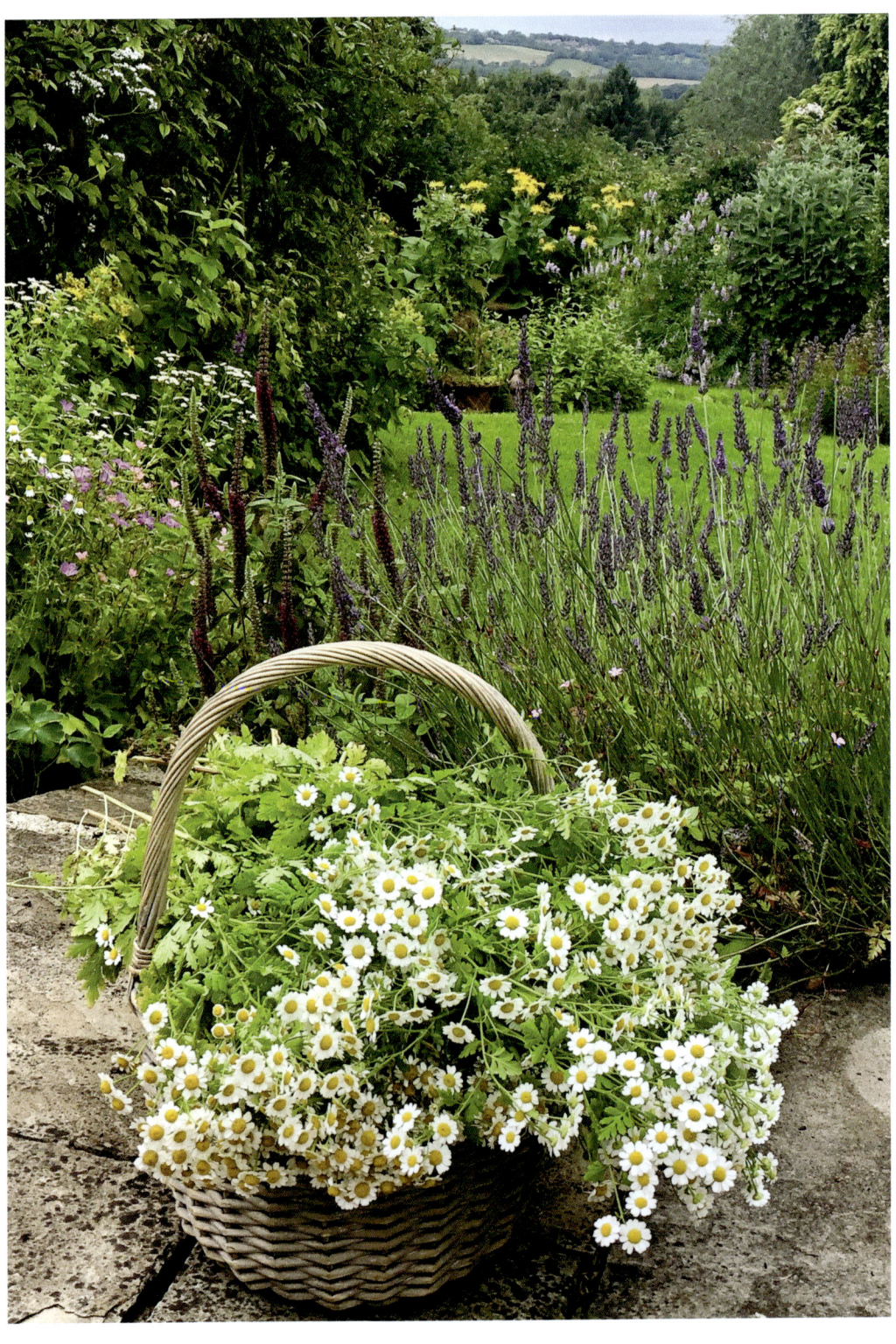

Tanacetum parthenium (Chrysanthemum parthenium): Feverfew

The Flower of Relief

*It is very effectual for all pains in the head coming of a cold cause,
The herb being bruised and applied to the crown of the head:
As also for the vertigo; that is, a running or swimming of the head.
The decoction thereof drank warm,
And the herb bruised with a few corns of bay-salt,
And applied to the wrists before the coming of the ague-fits,
Does take them away*

– Nicolas Culpeper (1616–1654)

Other Names: *Chrysanthemum parthenium*, featherfoil, midsummer daisy, bachelor's buttons, maydeweed

Parts Used: Leaves and flowers

Feverfew is an attractive hardy perennial with aromatic lacy-edged leaves and daisy flowers which are loved by bees. It is excellent in the herb garden or flower borders as its cheerful flowers bloom in late summer when many other flowers have gone over. It is a pretty member of the daisy family, native to south-eastern Europe, Turkey and the Caucasus. Though now in the genus *Tanacetum,* it was previously included in other genera of the Asteraceae/Compositae family, *Matricaria, Pyrethrum* and *Chrysanthemum*. It was called *Matricaria* because of the plant's beneficial relationship to the 'matrix' the Latin word for womb, as feverfew has been used for centuries for a wide range of women's problems. The name 'pyrethrum' comes for the Greek 'pyro' meaning fire, as the roots of feverfew have a hot taste.

One of its common names, 'bachelor's buttons' comes from the tradition of young men who wished to gain the love of a lady by carrying feverfew around in their pockets. The name 'feverfew' comes from the plant's ability to bring down fevers; in one tradition the herbalist had to pick the herb with the left hand and speak the name of the feverish patient while looking behind. It was highly valued in the days of Culpeper and Gerard for relieving ague (malaria), as well as colds and catarrh, menstrual problems and other women's complaints.

Other names for feverfew indicate its usefulness for women. *Parthenium* comes from the Latin meaning virgin and may also come from the use of feverfew in ancient Greece. There was apparently an incident in Greek history when a man who had fallen from the Parthenon during its construction was cured of his head injuries by treatment based on feverfew. Dr John Hill (1808–1885) recommended feverfew for violent headaches and as an antidote for mercurial poisoning. People believed that carrying feverfew along with hyssop and rosemary would protect from accidents, and amulets of feverfew were worn to prevent all afflictions of the head and to keep one's bearings straight so no accident would befall you. It is interesting that today feverfew is a major remedy for head pain.

'Maydeweed' was one of its old country names as it was recommended for a variety of nervous problems and particularly 'hysterical distempers' to which young women were said to be prone. It is interesting that hysteria was commonly ascribed to women and relates to the womb (indicated by words such as 'hysterectomy' for surgical removal of the womb). It was considered ideal for highly nervous people who were oversensitive to pain, and prone to sudden fits of irritability or anger. It was also prescribed for convulsions and for soothing fretful children.

Culpeper said that feverfew is ruled by Venus and *"hath commended it to succour our sisters to be a general strengthener of their wombs and to remedy such infirmities as a careless midwife hath there caused; if they will be pleased to make use of her herb boiled in white wine and drink the decoction, it cleanseth the womb, expels the afterbirth and doth a woman all the good she can desire of a herb."*

Feverfew was also regarded as a magical plant. If a girl who was not a virgin smelled the flowers, she would have an urgent need to pass water and if a pregnant woman smelled them, she would give birth to a red-haired child. It was believed by many that planting feverfew around the home would purify the air and protect against disease.

Herbal Remedy
Feverfew has a bitter taste and a cooling and anti-inflammatory effect. It contains sesquiterpene lactones, flavonoids, volatile oils (camphor, terpene, borneol), tannins, bitter resin, pyrethrin and polyacetylenes. It makes a good digestive remedy, enhancing appetite, digestion and absorption of nutrients and it stimulates the flow of bile from the liver. It supports the liver in its metabolic and detoxifying work, helping to clear heat and toxins from the body and reducing symptoms associated with a sluggish liver such as lethargy, irritability and headaches. It can be used for nausea and vomiting and inflammatory gut problems such as gastritis and colitis. The flowers have been used as a vermifuge to expel worms.

Feverfew's anti-inflammatory properties may be related to its ability to prevent and relieve migraines and headaches. Its sesquiterpene lactones inhibit the release of prostaglandins and histamine and make it helpful in the treatment of allergies including asthma, migraine and hay fever. It can also help relieve inflammatory joint problems including autoimmune problems such as rheumatoid arthritis, as well as inflammatory skin problems including psoriasis.

Feverfew has a beneficial effect on the nervous system with relaxant, anti-inflammatory and analgesic actions and is famous for preventing and relieving migraines and headaches. Its effect on migraines may be related to its antihistamine effect as well as its ability to block inflammatory pathways. The leaves can be eaten fresh every day with food (taken alone they cause mouth ulcers in some people). It may take up to a month for results to be seen. It can also be used to relieve nerve pain, as in trigeminal neuralgia, sciatica and shingles, as well as Meniere's disease and vertigo. It is indicated in oversensitivity to pain, irritability and anger and can be helpful in easing tension, lifting depression and promoting sleep. It may have GABA activity, meaning that it can ease anxiety.

Feverfew has a vasodilatory action, opening the blood vessels, and inhibits blood clotting which may also be helpful in migraines. When taken in hot infusion, it increases sweating and reduces fevers as its name suggests. With its decongestant action, it helps to clear excess mucus and can be used to treat chronic catarrh and sinusitis. Its decongestant effect may contribute to its usefulness in treating dizziness and tinnitus.

Through its ability to relax smooth muscle in the uterus and bring blood to the area, feverfew can be used to ease painful periods and sluggish or irregular menstrual flow. As an emmenagogue, it can be used to regulate periods and promote contractions during childbirth. It was traditionally used for depression or hysteria due to menstrual disorders, so could be helpful in PMS.

Externally, a tincture of the fresh plant can be dabbed on to insect stings and bites to relieve pain and swelling, and a dilute tincture used as a skin lotion is said to repel insects, as well as remove pimples, boils and haemorrhoids.

Homeopathic Remedy
Pyrethrum parthenium is prescribed for a range of nervous symptoms similar to those that

respond well to feverfew when used as a herbal remedy. It is indicated in convulsions, fevers, delirium, twitching, restlessness, loquacity, arthritis and dysentery.

The symptom picture of feverfew is being excited and talking incessantly for hours, lying in bed in a state of stupor or being delirious, a rapid pulse, diarrhoea, passing mucus with blood, pain with diarrhoea, sore tongue, muscle twitching in the limbs, convulsions and restlessness.

Flower Essence
Feverfew is used for headaches and migraines, particularly those experienced by women in a cyclical pattern related to their menstrual cycle. It eases tension and engenders calmness and serenity through times of change.

In our busy fast-paced lives where we push through and forget to listen to our body's needs, feverfew helps us to nurture ourselves when we need to, and to allow a bit more relaxation and flexibility into our lives. It enables us to let go of things, including patterns of behaviour that no longer serve us. This can be helpful when moving through transitions in life such as changing jobs, moving house and letting go of relationships. Feverfew helps to make changes easier as we become more adaptable.

Growing
Feverfew grows in any soil and likes full sun. Propagate by sowing seeds in spring, scattering them on the surface of well-drained soil and watering in. Alternatively, divide the plants in autumn. It self-seeds easily, grows up to 3 feet (90cm) and mainly flowers from July to August.

Cautions
Avoid the herbal remedy during pregnancy. Fresh leaves may cause mouth ulcers. Irritation – skin reactions and mouth soreness/ulcers – have appeared in some sensitive people when they have taken fresh feverfew. Do not abruptly stop taking feverfew if you have used it for more than 1 week as this may cause Stopping feverfew too quickly may cause rebound headache, anxiety, fatigue, muscle stiffness, and joint pain. Do not use if allergic to pyrethrums. Use with caution in individuals with severe ragweed allergy or allergy to members of the daisy and chrysanthemum family. Use with caution in individuals with bleeding disorders. Avoid with SSRIs due to anti-serotogenic activity, and with anticoagulant and antiplatelet medicines such as warfarin (Coumadin) or aspirin. Avoid for a least a week prior to surgery. It may interact with anesthesia.

Recipes

Anti-inflammatory tisane for arthritis and gout
1 part golden marjoram
1 part nettle
1 part meadowsweet
½ part feverfew

Place the fresh herbs in a teapot. Pour on boiling water. Leave to infuse for 10–15 minutes. Drink one cupful three times daily before meals and use at a foot bath at night.

Pain-relieving tisane for headaches and migraine
Using equal parts of rosemary, peppermint, feverfew and meadowsweet, place a couple of handfuls into a teapot, pour over approximately a pint/500ml of boiling water and leave to infuse for 15 minutes. Drink one to two cupfuls every hour or two if necessary, until the pain subsides.

Footbath
You can prepare the herbs as above and leave them to infuse for 24 hours. Pour the infusion into a large bowl, add a little hot water and soak your feet for 15–30 minutes.

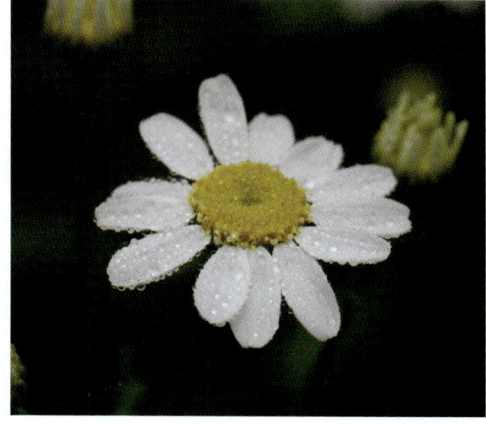

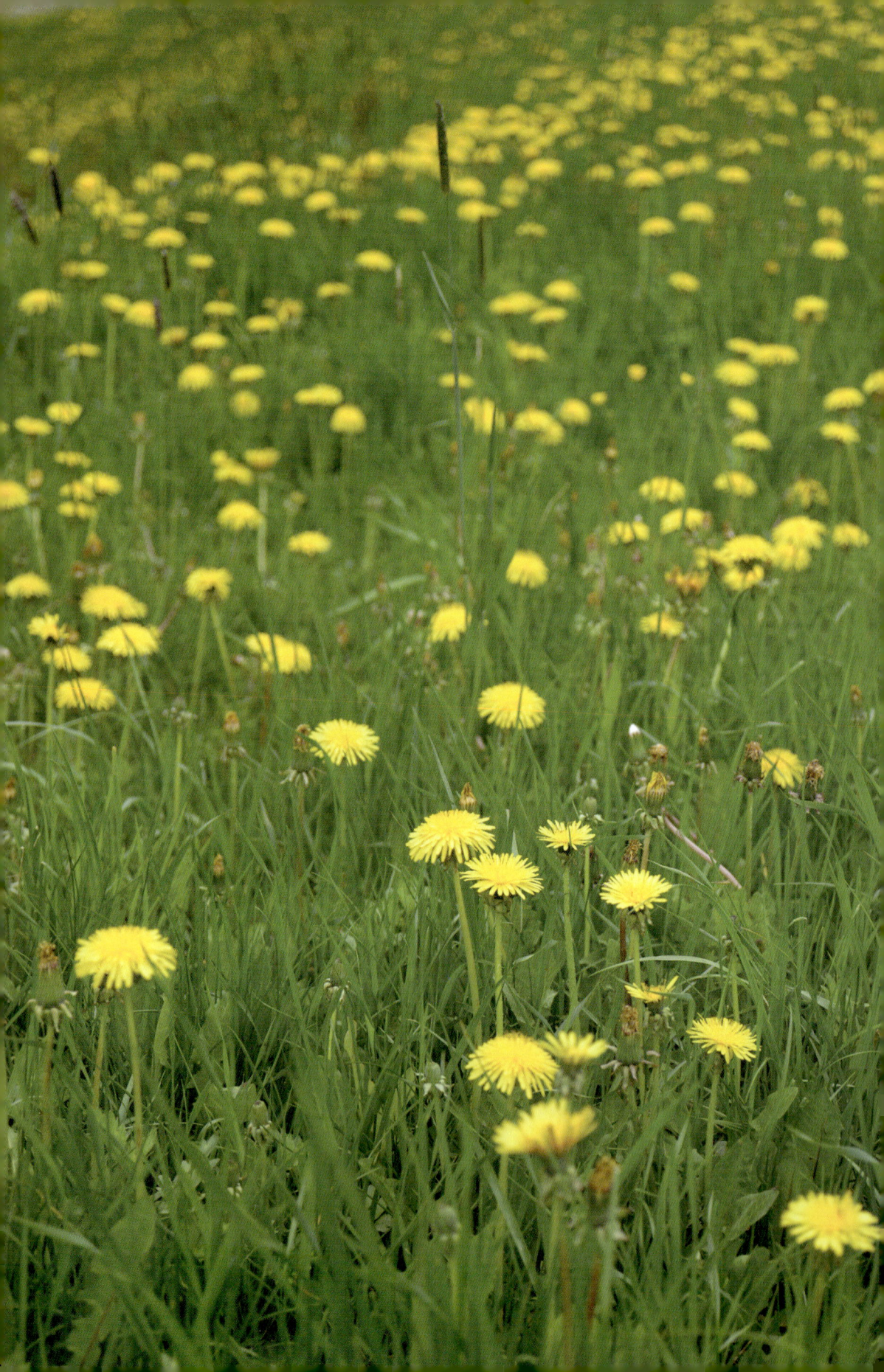

Taraxacum officinale: Dandelion

The Flower of Survival

Leontodons unfold
on the swath turf their ray-encircled gold,
with sol's expanding beams the flowers unclose,
And rising Hesper lights them to repose
– Erasmus Darwin (1731–1802)

Other Names: Faceclock, Irish daisy, lion's tooth, canker wort, wild endive, pee-a-bed, piss-in-bed, piss en lit, blowball, bitterwort, clockflower, devil's milk pail, doonhead clock, fairy clock, fortune teller, sun-in the grass, tell time, tramp with the golden head, piddly bed, yellow gowan and wild endive.

Parts Used: Leaves, root and flowers

This familiar wildflower is a member of the Asteraceae/Compositae family. With its cheerful yellow flower and remarkable resilience, dandelion has been much admired and widely respected as a healing plant for thousands of years. Said to originate in temperate areas of Europe, dandelion was used as a medicine in ancient Greece and was praised in herbals in the Middle Ages. It is found in folklore traditions all over the world.

The name *Taraxacum* is said to come from the Greek word 'taraxo' meaning disorder and '*takos*' meaning pain or remedy, because of dandelion's esteem as a great healing herb. It might also come from the Arabic corruption of the Greek word 'trogemon' meaning edible. The leaves are delicious in salads or cooked like spinach, and highly nutritious, being rich in vitamins C and B, and pro-vitamin A, and minerals, particularly potassium, calcium and iron. The roots can be roasted and ground into a tasty, caffeine-free substitute for coffee. Dandelion was the food with which Hecate entertained Theseus in the Greek myths.

There is a quaint legend about how the dandelion first appeared on the earth. In ancient days when the world was populated by fairies, elves and gnomes, the first humans to arrive caused problems as they could not see these elemental beings and kept treading on them. Some of the sun-loving fairies dressed in bright yellow gowns had nowhere to hide, unlike the gnomes and elves who took refuge behind rocks or under the ground, so they were transformed into dandelions. If you step on a dandelion it will soon spring up again, as it is said to contain the spirit of the fairies.

This accords with the almost supernatural power of the dandelion to survive; when weeded from lawns and gardens they soon reappear. The seed heads bear numerous airborne seeds, easily dispersed in the wind, while their roots are long and tenaciously hold themselves in the ground in any soil. Not surprisingly, the dandelion has come to symbolise faithfulness.

The French name 'dent de lion' meaning the tooth of the lion, from which we get the name dandelion, refers to the toothed margin of the leaves or the fact that the golden flowers resemble the colour of the royal lion and the shape of his open mouth showing its teeth. The number of incisions on the toothed leaves of this perennial plant indicates the amount of sunlight it gets. The leaves are deeply toothed when it has plenty of light and only slightly so when it grows in shady areas and it will only bloom with sufficient sunlight.

In the language of flowers, dandelion means rustic oracle. It was used as a country clock which was fairly precise, as the flowers were said to open at five minutes past five in the morning and close at nine minutes past eight in the evening. Children prefer to tell the time by blowing at the seed heads, the number of puffs needed to blow them all off indicating the hour.

The seed head was also used to find out what your lover was thinking of you; 'he loves me' with one puff of the seed head, 'he loves me not' with the next. It was said that if you whisper the words of love to your favourite person and blow the seeds gently towards him or her, the seeds willcarry the words to your beloved. Children also believed that if they could blow all the seeds off a dandelion in one breath, then their wish would come true. Apparently, witches said that if you rubbed yourself all over with dandelion you would be welcome everywhere and your wishes would come true.

Dandelion was valued by the ancients as an antidote to poisons and it has long been said that if you drink a cup of dandelion tea daily you will never have rheumatism. Traditionally, it has been respected for its ability to promote elimination of toxins and wastes through the liver and kidneys, and in this way cleanse the blood. The leaves are eaten young in the spring as a bitter tonic, to clear the body of wastes from the heavy clogging food and more sedentary habits of winter. Their diuretic properties earned dandelion the country names of 'pee-a-bed' and in French 'piss-en-lit'. Mothers would give their children dandelions to smell on Mayday and hope they would not wet their beds for the rest of the year.

Dandelion roots and leaves were used in Europe to treat liver problems, fevers, boils, eye problems, diabetes and constipation. Native Americans also drank a decoction of dandelion root to treat kidney disease, swelling, skin problems, heartburn and upset stomachs. In Traditional Chinese medicine (TCM), dandelion has long been used to treat stomach problems, appendicitis and breast problems including mastitis and poor milk flow.

The ancient Celts celebrated February 1st as the festival of the White Goddess, whom Christianity later adopted and renamed St. Brigid, and one of her symbols was the dandelion. Dandelion is one of the bitter herbs of the Passover tradition.

Herbal Remedy
This brightly coloured wildflower, and all its parts, is renowned as a gently detoxifying bitter tonic. The leaves are bitter, especially the older they get, and the roots are bitter and sweet and become sweeter with roasting. The flowers are less bitter once the calyx is removed. Dandelion contains sesquiterpene lactones, triterpenes (amyrin, taraxerol, taraxasterol), acids (taraxinic, chicoric, chlorogenic, caffeic acid), carbohydrates, vitamins (A, C, B complex, D and E), minerals (calcium, iron, magnesium, sodium, silicon, copper, phosphorus, zinc, manganese and potassium), phytosterols (sitosterol,

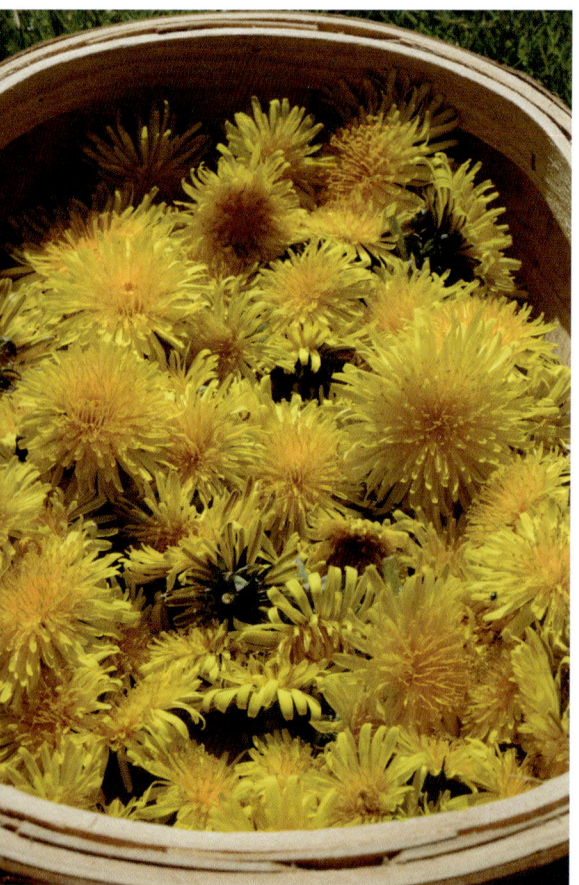

stigmasterol, taraxasterol), flavonoids (apigenin, luteolin, chrysoeriol) and coumarins.

The health-promoting benefits of dandelion can be largely attributed to the presence of the bitter sesquiterpenes and phenolic components which have antioxidant and anti-inflammatory activities. One of the most abundant constituents in the roots, flowers and leaves is the polyphenol chicoric acid, which also has antidiabetic and potential anticancer actions. The flowers are good sources of antioxidants due to rich content of phenolic components including flavonoids, luteolin, coumaric acid and vitamin C.

Dandelion is also one of the richest vegetable sources of beta-carotene, a building block for vitamin A and a potent antioxidant, which protects cells from oxidation and cellular damage. Antioxidants have far-reaching effects in preventing a wide range of problems including cardiovascular disease, diabetes, inflammatory and degenerative problems such as arthritis, diminishing brain function and immunity. The roots of dandelion contain polysaccharides notably inulin, carotenoids (lutein), fatty acids (myristic acid), minerals, choline vitamins, mucilage and pectin.

Today dandelion is still popular as a bitter digestive and liver tonic, for enhancing appetite and promoting digestion by increasing the flow of digestive juices. The bitter taste of both the root and the leaf stimulates the bitter receptors in the mouth and the digestive tract and by reflex this activates the secretion of digestive enzymes and bile from the liver. With its cooling and anti-inflammatory action, dandelion can be used to relieve heartburn and acidity, gastritis and inflammatory gut problems. By increasing bile production and flow, it supports the work of the liver as the major detoxifying organ of the body. The whole plant can be used to treat liver problems including hepatitis, as well as gallbladder infections and gallstones. The terpenoid and bitter sterol components such as taraxacin and taraxacerin may be helpful in this respect. Dandelion can be taken for problems associated with an overworked liver such as tiredness and irritability, headaches and a range of inflammatory skin problems. The root is also mildly laxative. On a more subtle level, like other herbs that work on the liver, dandelion helps to relieve emotional stagnation and can promote expression of repressed emotions such as anger, frustration, envy, resentment and grief. In this way, dandelion helps clear them and prevent further problems. In this sense dandelion is cleansing or purging in mind and body.

Up to 45% of dandelion root consists of inulin, a complex carbohydrate known as a fructo-oligosaccharide, with many beneficial actions particularly as a prebiotic, promoting good bacteria in the gut flora including *Bifida bacteria* and eliminating toxins in the gut. Through their action in the gut, fructo-oligosaccharides stimulate the immune system and help to suppress abnormal cell growth. They can also help to normalise blood sugar levels and prevent obesity as well as osteoporosis. Inulin helps to reduce the tendency to constipation by regulating the gut flora and increasing peristalsis.

Dandelion can help boost the immune system both through the regulation of the gut flora with the help of inulin and through its antimicrobial actions, having antiviral and antibacterial properties; they can help limit the growth of Hepatitis B. One of the tripterpenes called taraxasterol (present particularly in the roots) has anti-inflammatory properties and has antimicrobial activity against *Staphylococcus aureus*. It may help to counteract the development of cancer particularly in the colon, pancreas and liver at various stages.

The antioxidant and anti-inflammatory and actions of dandelion are attributed to the triterpene taraxasterol, the sesquiterpene lactones, phenols, flavonoids, cichoric and chlorogenic acid. They also have hepatoprotective actions, meaning they can protect the liver against damage from free radicals and toxins such as alcohol and drugs and help to prevent fatty liver disease. The antioxidants are also helpful in the prevention and treatment of diabetes since oxidative stress is a prime marker of type 2 diabetes. Dandelion may stimulate the release of insulin in pancreatic β-cells, helping to bring down blood sugar while simultaneously improving the absorption of

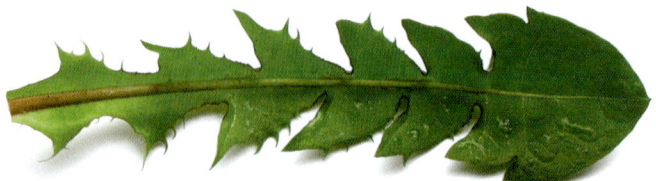

glucose in muscle tissue. It inhibits enzymes that digest carbohydrates which also helps to regulate blood sugar. Chlorogenic acid has the potential to prevent obesity and inflammation and improve insulin secretion and sensitivity. By reducing carbohydrate and fat absorption and regulating their metabolism, dandelion can also be a helpful aid to weight loss.

The increased bile flow promoted by dandelion's effect on the liver can improve cholesterol and triglyceride metabolism as well as the metabolism of hormones. This can be helpful in menstrual problems, PMS and menopausal symptoms and could be valuable in the prevention of osteoporosis. Dandelion is a good source of nutrients that contribute to the maintenance of strong, healthy bones. The leaves contain calcium and vitamin K, both of which are associated with the prevention of bone loss. Inulin, the oligosaccharide in the root, may also support healthy bones through improved digestion and the promotion of healthy gut bacteria.

Dandelion has an affinity with the breasts. The root acts as a galactagogue, promoting the supply of milk in breast-feeding mothers. It is helpful in breast congestion, cysts and mastitis. Dandelion extracts have been used in traditional Native American medicine and Traditional Chinese Medicine for treatment of leukaemia and breast cancer.

Dandelion, particularly the leaf, has a close affinity with the urinary tract and is an effective diuretic, as the traditional names 'piss-a-bed' or in French 'pis-en-lit' tell us. It is an effective remedy for fluid retention, breast tenderness, cellulite, urinary infections and prostate problems. While diuretic drugs leach potassium from the body and require a potassium supplement, dandelion comes complete with its high potassium content, replacing that lost through increased urination. Potassium is a mineral associated with lowering blood pressure, so dandelion could be helpful for high blood pressure both through its potassium content and its diuretic action. A decoction of whole plant is a folk remedy for dissolving urinary stones and gravel. Since dandelion improves elimination of uric acid and has an anti-inflammatory action, it makes a useful remedy for gout. Combined in a tea with celery seed and taken regularly, the leaves and flowers make an excellent brew for arthritis and gout.

Externally dandelion has cooling, anti-inflammatory and antimicrobial properties, excellent for treating inflammatory skin problems and infections such as eczema, acne, boils and abscesses associated with heat and toxicity. An infusion of the leaves and flowers makes a good wash for ulcers and skin complaints, and a lotion for freckles. You can apply the white juice from the fresh stems daily over a few weeks to cure warts.

Dandelion root can increase the generation of new skin cells, which can help slow the aging process. It may help protect the skin from sun damage and keep the skin hydrated and youthful. The flowers are especially valued for their mild analgesic properties, making them an excellent addition to massage oils and liniments for sore muscles, stiff joints or other aches and pains. An infused oil made from the flowers can be incorporated into creams and salves to soothe and heal chapped or cracked skin.

Homeopathic Remedy

Taraxacum is again mainly used for liver and digestive problems. It is specific for liver pain, bilious attacks, gallstones, gastric headaches, jaundiced skin and the associated debility. It is given for poor appetite, flatulence, with the sensation of bubbles bursting in the bowels, for sluggish bowels, for a bitter taste in the mouth and a sore, mapped tongue, where the tongue coating is stripped away in patches leaving sore, raw areas.

Taraxacum, like the herbal remedy, acts on the urinary system and is used for frequency of urination, difficulty passing water and great thirst. A Taraxacum person tends to have profuse night sweats, restless limbs which are painful to touch, and feel worse from pressure. They may have rheumatism or painful joints, tension and stiffness in the back and neck, and shooting pains in the neck muscles. There may be skin problems, such as purulent pimples on the face, with heat and redness. During a fever they may feel thirstless, or worse from drinking, the fingertips may feel cold, and they have a bitter taste in the mouth. They feel hot in the face and the toes and sweat on falling asleep. Generally, they feel worse lying down and sitting, and feel chilly after eating.

Flower Essence

Dandelion suits people who have a tendency to cram far too much into their lives. They are so full of enthusiasm for life that they take on too much and become compulsive 'doers'. They over plan and over-structure their lives in an effort to fit in everything they want to do, and leave little room for relaxation or reflection, until the point is reached where they no longer know how to be quiet or relaxed. They leave little space in their lives for spiritual or emotional expression, and as they push themselves beyond the body's natural capacity, they no longer listen to the needs of their bodies. Such harsh physical demands and unexpressed inner life creates great tension, especially in the muscles of the neck and shoulders.

Dandelion helps to release this tension, allowing the body to relax and emotions to be released and expressed. It can be added to massage oils and used in body work. It enables you to listen more closely to emotional messages and bodily needs and shifts the emphasis from being a human 'doing' to a human 'being'. Energy, activity and enthusiasm become balanced with a sense of inner ease.

Edible Uses

The young leaves, which grow through several months of the year, can be used in teas, salads and steamed as a vegetable or added to stir fries before they grow too large and bitter. Being rich in vitamins, minerals and trace elements, they make a nutritious addition to any meal as well as providing wonderful medicine at the same time. In Greece the leaves are used instead of spinach for making *spanakopita* – spinach pie with filo pastry.

Dandelions have long tap roots that can be pulled up, chopped, dried and then roasted to make a tasty alternative to coffee. They can also be cooked like a root vegetable. The flowers are of course highly colourful and decorative as well as sweet and a bit crunchy. Once removed from the green base, which can be a bit bitter, they can be added to salads, added to vegetable dishes and soups, or used to make dandelion wine.

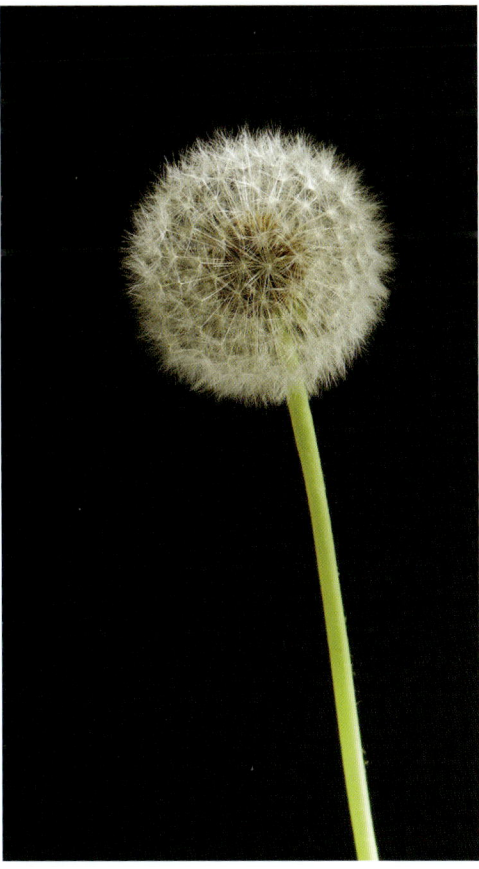

Recipes

Cure for Warts
The old gypsy cure for warts is dandelion juice. A little white sap from the leaves or stalks applied regularly to the wart should make it turn black and disappear.

Cold Infusion to Clear the Skin
Use equal parts of wild pansy, borage, gotu kola, dandelion, lavender, nasturtium, strawberry leaves.

The bright blue star shaped flowers of borage and the sweet faces of the wild pansies lend this recipe eye appeal.

Place equal parts of wild pansy, borage, gotu kola, dandelion, lavender, nasturtium, strawberry leaves in a wide necked bottle or flask.

Fill with spring water, the equivalent of 2 teaspoons of the herb per cup of water. Leave to infuse overnight and use as drinking water for the day. Drink at least 3–4 cups of the water per day to help clear the skin.

Dandelion Flower Infused Oil
Dandelion flower infused oil can be added to creams and salves to soothe and heal chapped or cracked skin, and to massage oils and liniments for sore muscles and stiff joints.

Place dried dandelion flowers in a pyrex bowl and cover with your favourite oil (sesame, sunflower, olive or almond for example). Place the bowl on top of a small saucepan of water as a *bain marie* and place on a low heat for a few hours keeping a close eye on the water level. Top it up from time to time if necessary. Remove from heat and strain the oil by pressing through a fine mesh sieve, and decant into a preferably dark glass bottle and label clearly with the name of the herb and the date the oil was made.

A slower way is to infuse the dried flowers in oil in a dark glass jar and leave for around 4 to 6 weeks, shaking occasionally when you remember to. Then strain. The oils made this way will keep for a up to a year if stored in a cool dark place. Sunlight will cause more rapid deterioration.

Dandelion Flower Salve
100ml of dandelion infused oil
15g of beeswax pastilles

Place the oil and beeswax pastilles in a heat proof bowl and place on top of a pan containing several inches of water like a *bain marie* (the same process as used for making an infused oil).

Place on a low heat and leave until the wax is melted. Remove from heat and carefully pour into jars immediately before it has a chance to solidify.

Leave it to sit until firm. Label clearly with the date and the name of the herb.

Growing
Dandelion will seed itself easily in the garden and can be propagated by sowing seeds in spring, barely covering the seeds, in most soils and full sun. Grows 2– 12" (5–30cm) and flowers from late spring to early autumn.

Cautions
Avoid in obstructions of the bile ducts and gallbladder. The milky latex in leaves can cause dermatitis and if sucked excessively by children may lead to nausea, vomiting and diarrhoea. Caution with diabetics. People who are allergic to chamomile, yarrow or other related plants should use dandelion with caution. Dandelion in excess may adversely affect male fertility. Diuretic properties of the leaf can interact with orthodox diuretics and hypotensives. Root may reduce serum levels of some drugs. Avoid with Lithium, quinolones, insulin, anti-coagulants, anti-diuretic or blood-sugar controlling drugs.

Thymus vulgaris: Thyme

The Flower of Bravery

I know a place where the wild thyme blows, where oxlips and the nodding violet grows
- William Shakespeare

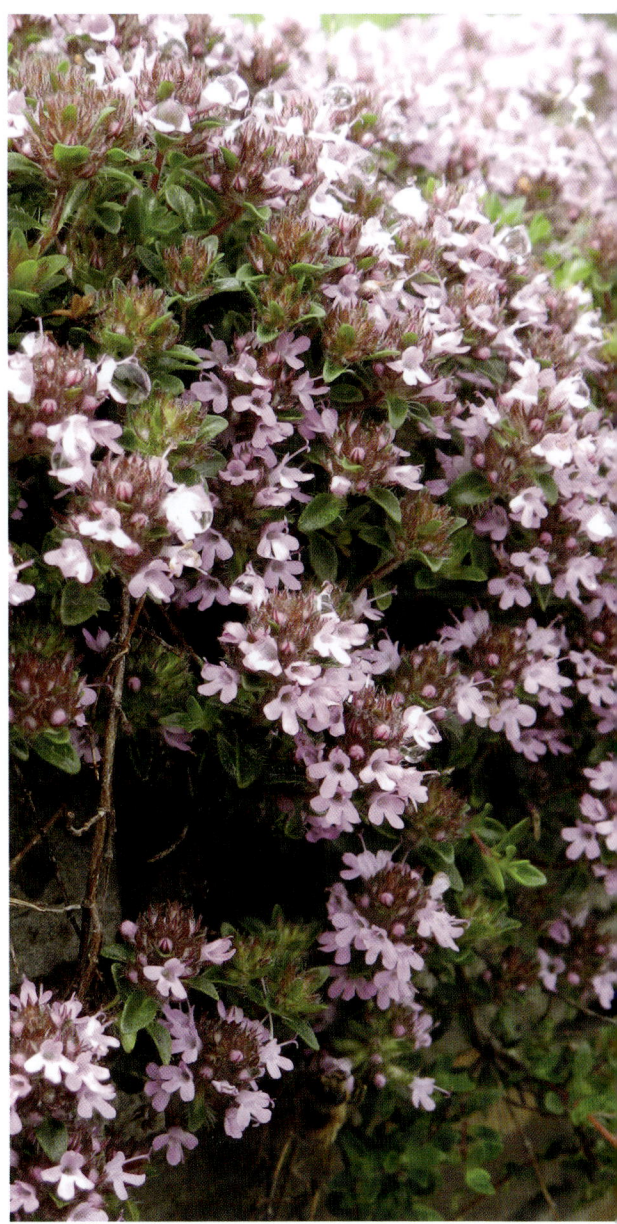

Other names: Common thyme, wild thyme, French thyme, garden thyme, rubbed thyme, Spanish thyme
Also used: *Thymus serpyllum*

Parts used: Leaves and flowering tops

Thyme is a much-loved member of the mint (Lamiaceae/Labiatae) family. It is a small, highly aromatic evergreen shrub native to the Mediterranean where it can be found growing wild on warm, dry, rocky banks and heaths. Thyme is a popular herb for its culinary virtues and in the garden, its cultivated forms with fragrant lilac or white flowers are appreciated for their wonderful aroma that is also loved by bees and impart a delicious flavour to honey.

Since ancient times thyme has been praised for its myriad virtues. According to legend, thyme grew where Helen of Troy's tears fell to the ground. The name *thyme* comes from the Latin 'thymus' which can be traced further to the Greek 'thumos', meaning to smoke or fumigate, as it was made into an incense to drive away insects and infection, or perhaps it means spirit as the Greeks burned it on their altars when making sacrifices to the gods. The ancient Greek physician Hippocrates (460BC to 370BC), the father of Western medicine, recommended thyme for respiratory diseases and conditions. It was used by the Romans as an antidote to poison and they added it to their food to protect against infection. Bundles of thyme were burned in ancient Rome to purify temples and homes and to protect against the plague; thyme was the main ingredient of posies of herbs worn when the Black Death struck in the 1340s and apparently it was used in preparations to apply to remedy blisters that resulted from the plague.

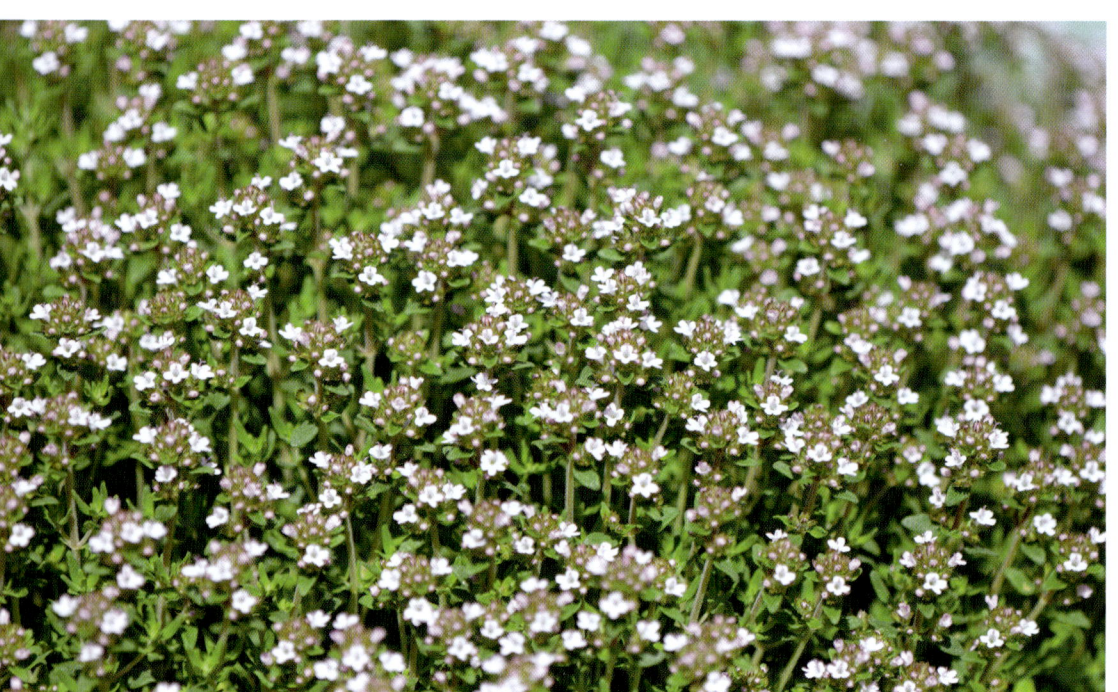

The name *thyme* is also said to come from the Greek 'thumus' meaning courage, because of the plant's strengthening and energising properties. To the ancient Greeks thyme was an emblem of bravery and action, and ladies in medieval England would embroider scarves with a bee hovering on a sprig of thyme to present to their knights when they left for battle to give them courage. Inhaling thyme incense was also thought to evoke spirit or courage and it was thought that if death should befall the knight going into battle, thyme would aid his journey to the afterlife. The ancient Egyptians used thyme as an embalming fluid.

Wild thyme is called *serpyllum* because of its creeping habit and also called 'mother of thyme' in allusion to its therapeutic effect on the womb, which used to be referred to as 'the mother'. Thyme has an affinity for the reproductive tract and because of its reputation for increasing strength and energy, it was naturally thought to be an aphrodisiac and a love herb. It was said to encourage wild times (or thymes!) and made good medicine for those who had had too much of a wild time! Culpeper said that thyme was ruled by Venus. Wild thyme is best known as a bee plant as bees love it; Greek thyme honey is prized all over the world for its wonderful flavour. It was in this connection that wild thyme came to symbolise sweetness. Its delightful fragrance appealed so much to Bacon and the Elizabethans, that it was planted in the garden where its scent would bring constant pleasure when trodden underfoot.

The Romans apparently slept on thyme, inhaling its sweet aroma to cure melancholy, while in other traditions thyme has been used to quell fears, stop nightmares, prevent convulsions and remedy vertigo, ringing in the ears and migraine. The Romans also used thyme to flavour cheese and alcoholic drinks. When the Roman armies came to the British Isles, they brought thyme with them and it became incorporated into local herbal traditions. John Gerard said in his 17th century *Herball*, it was "*profitable for such as are ferfull, melancholicke and troubled in mind.*" Made into a soup, it was said to cure shyness and when inhaled, its aroma was reputed to strengthen the brain and increase longevity. Vinegar of thyme is an old folk remedy which was used like smelling salts for nervous headaches.

Thyme was also renowned for its ability to cure coughs and chest infections. Nicolas Culpeper said that thyme is *"a noble strengthener of the lungs, as notable a one as grows, nor is there a better remedy growing for whooping cough. It purgeth the body of phlegm and is an excellent remedy for shortness of breath. It is so harmless you need not fear the use of it... it is excellent for those that are troubled with the gout and the herb taken anyway inwardly is of great comfort to the stomach."* Thyme has been used since the Middle Ages for a variety of women's problems, particularly infections of the reproductive tract and regulating the menstrual cycle.

A more recent renowned herbalist the French Maurice Mességué also sang thyme's praises, *"From my long years of experience as a herbalist I can appreciate thyme because of its antiseptic qualities; its smell destroys viruses and bacteria in the atmosphere as it destroys infectious germs in the body. I do not know of any infection that cannot be mitigated if treated with this precious herb. It is an excellent weapon against epidemics and much cheaper than other methods of controlling them."*

Herbal Remedy
Thyme has a wonderfully pungent aromatic taste and smell, and warming properties. As a herbal remedy, thyme is most famous as a powerful antimicrobial for both internal and external use and helps to combat bacterial, viral and fungal infections of the respiratory, digestive and genito-urinary systems, such as colds, coughs, flu, gastro-enteritis, cystitis and salpingitis. In fact, thyme is said to be active against at least 120 different strains of bacteria that occur in the mouth, respiratory tract and genito-urinary tract, including antibiotic resistant *Staphylococcus* species including MRSA. The main component of its volatile oil, thymol, has long been used in antiseptic creams, lotions, mouthwashes and toothpastes. Thyme also contains bitters, antioxidant phenols, essential oil (including carvacrol), terpenes and flavonoids (apigenin, luteolin, thymonin, naringenin), saponins, tannins, caffeic acid, salicylate and labiatic acid as well as vitamins A and C, and minerals including copper, fibre, iron and manganese.

Thyme makes an excellent remedy for the respiratory system. It is a favourite remedy for coughs whether caused by nerves and anxiety or an infection such as bronchitis, pneumonia or whooping cough. Its renowned antimicrobial actions can help combat almost any infecting organism in the respiratory tract that causes sore throats, tonsillitis, laryngitis, colds, flu and chest infections. Thymol is in a class of compounds found in plants known as biocides that have the ability to destroy harmful organisms such as infectious bacteria. Together with other biocides, including carvacrol in thyme, it may account for much of the antimicrobial action and its effectiveness in the treatment of acute infection such as bronchitis.

The significant relaxant effect on the muscles in the bronchial tubes (which is also attributed to phenols including thymol and carvacrol) relieves constriction of the bronchi in asthma and whooping cough and quietens the cough reflex, which helps to soothe an irritating cough. In addition, thyme's expectorant action increases the production of fluid mucus and helps shift phlegm – particularly useful for dry, hacking coughs. Its decongestant action, especially when taken in hot infusions, helps to clear congestion and catarrh and is helpful in colds, sinusitis and hay fever or allergic rhinitis. By virtue of its sudorific properties, thyme also helps to increase perspiration and bring down fevers. As a result of the centuries of use and proof of its amazing ability to combat chest problems, backed up more recently by substantial research, thyme is approved by Germany's Commission E for treatment of bronchitis, whooping cough and upper respiratory inflammation.

Thyme has a wonderfully pungent taste and warming properties, just right for dispelling cold in winter. Adding a strong infusion to the bath or drinking a tea or dilute tincture of thyme will stimulate the circulation, help throw off chills and lethargy and act as an exhilarating tonic to the whole system. Its tonic action on the nervous system makes it excellent for physical and mental exhaustion. It also relieves tension and anxiety and when taken regularly can help lift depression. Among the medicinal compounds in thyme, carvacrol exerts a positive effect on mood by increasing levels of the neurotransmitters dopamine and serotonin that regulate motivation, drive and mood.

Thyme makes an excellent digestive herb, enhancing appetite, digestion and absorption and stimulating the function of the liver. Thymol stimulates peristaltic muscle movements so that food is not held in the stomach for prolonged periods of time. Thyme makes an excellent remedy for indigestion, poor appetite, liver and gallbladder complaints. Its relaxing antispasmodic effects (which may be due to the action of flavonoids on calcium ion influx) can be used for relieving wind, intestinal colic and IBS associated with stress. The astringent tannins help to protect the gut from irritation and inflammation and reduce diarrhoea, while the antimicrobial volatile oils combat infections causing food poisoning, gastro-enteritis and dysentery and are active against resistant strains of *Staphylococcus, Enterococcus, Escherichia* and *Pseudomonas* bacteria. A teaspoonful of thyme tincture with castor oil taken half an hour before breakfast is a traditional cure for worms and other parasites. Thyme can help re-establish a normal bacterial population in the bowel which is a great help after taking antibiotics and for disturbances of the gut flora including *Candida*. This impacts greatly on general immunity and brain health and may be related to thyme's possible use to protect against colon and breast cancer.

Thyme has a powerful antioxidant action, attributed to many of its different compounds including phenols, flavonoids, tannins and vitamins, that protects the body against free radical damage. This contributes to a wide range of degenerative problems including arthritis, diabetes, deterioration of brain function, lowered immunity, cancer and many elements of the ageing process. Thyme has an effective anti-inflammatory action possibly by inhibiting prostaglandin synthesis. In the cardiovascular system, thyme can protect the arteries from inflammation and damage and the build-up of atheromatous plaque, which impedes circulation and increases the risk of heart attacks and strokes. The antispasmodic qualities of thyme (especially from the essential oil) help to relax the arteries and this in turn helps to lower blood pressure and ease stress on the heart. Thyme's pungent taste and warming properties stimulate the circulation and can be used to prevent chilblains and the effects of cold in the winter. In the brain, thyme's antioxidant actions can help neurodegeneration that is associated with senile dementia and Alzheimer's.

Thyme acts as a natural diuretic increasing the flow of urine without upsetting the body's electrolyte balance. This helps combat fluid retention and with its antimicrobial essential oils, thyme can be used effectively for treating infections of the urinary tract. It also acts on the reproductive system and can be used for gynaecological infections and for regulating the menstrual cycle. Thyme's relaxant effect can be helpful for painful periods, while its emmenagogue action on the uterine muscles could be helpful just before and during childbirth and for this reason is contra-indicated in pregnancy.

Externally, thyme can be used in liniments and lotions for relieving arthritis and muscular pain. Thyme is known for its antibacterial properties and it makes a great remedy to speed healing and deter infection of wounds, cuts and grazes, wounds, sores and ulcers and to treat acne. It is also good for fungal infections on the skin as well as inflammatory conditions like eczema. Compounds in the volatile oil, notably caryophyllene, camphene and thymol, could be mainly responsible for its antiseptic action.

Thyme tea or oil makes an excellent inhalant for chesty conditions, asthma, colds, catarrh and sinusitis. Bunches of dried thyme can be dried and burned in the way that the ancient Greeks and Romans did, to dispel airborne infection. This can also help to clear the mind and enhance concentration and focus.

An infusion or tincture of thyme makes a good gargle for sore throats, an antiseptic mouthwash and a douche for thrush and other vaginal infections. It can be added to creams to soothe and relieve irritation and inflammation in vulval lichen sclerosis. It can also be used daily for friction of the hair and as a hair lotion, giving it a healthy lustre and stopping hair fall.

Aromatherapy Oil

Thyme produces several oils depending on the soil, climate and altitude in which it grows. The chemo-type that contains a high level of carvarol is a powerful antiseptic, while linalol, geraniol and thujanol chemotypes have much gentler properties and are preferable for home use. Thyme linalol is the only one that is suitable for children.

The use of thyme oil in aromatherapy is very similar to that of thyme in herbal medicine. It acts as a warming stimulant to the circulation, warding off winter ailments such as sore throats, flu, head colds, catarrh, sinusitis, coughs, bronchitis and other chest infections. It is also stimulating to both mental and physical energy, as the ancients said. It is excellent as a tonic in debility, for depression, lethargy, when feeling nervously run down, anxious or under stress as when studying for exams. One of its constituents called carvacrol can affect neuron activity and boost positive feelings of wellbeing. Diluted in a carrier oil, it can be used in massage or bath oil to soothe tired, aching muscles, whilst calming and focusing the mind.

Thyme also energises the digestion, acting as an aperitif and digestive and calming colic and wind. In the chest thyme oil relaxes the bronchial tubes, which is helpful in asthma, and acts as an expectorant. Inhalations of thyme can be used for coughs, chest infections, whooping cough, emphysema and TB. Used as a hair oil, thyme can stimulate the circulation and help prevent hair loss. It can also be used for head lice.

Thyme oil is a good insect repellent. A combination of thymol, alpha-terpinene and carvacrol has the ability to kill the tiger mosquito larvae which is native to tropical and subtropical areas of Southeast Asia and carries West Nile virus, yellow fever, St. Louis encephalitis, dengue fever and Chikungunya fever.

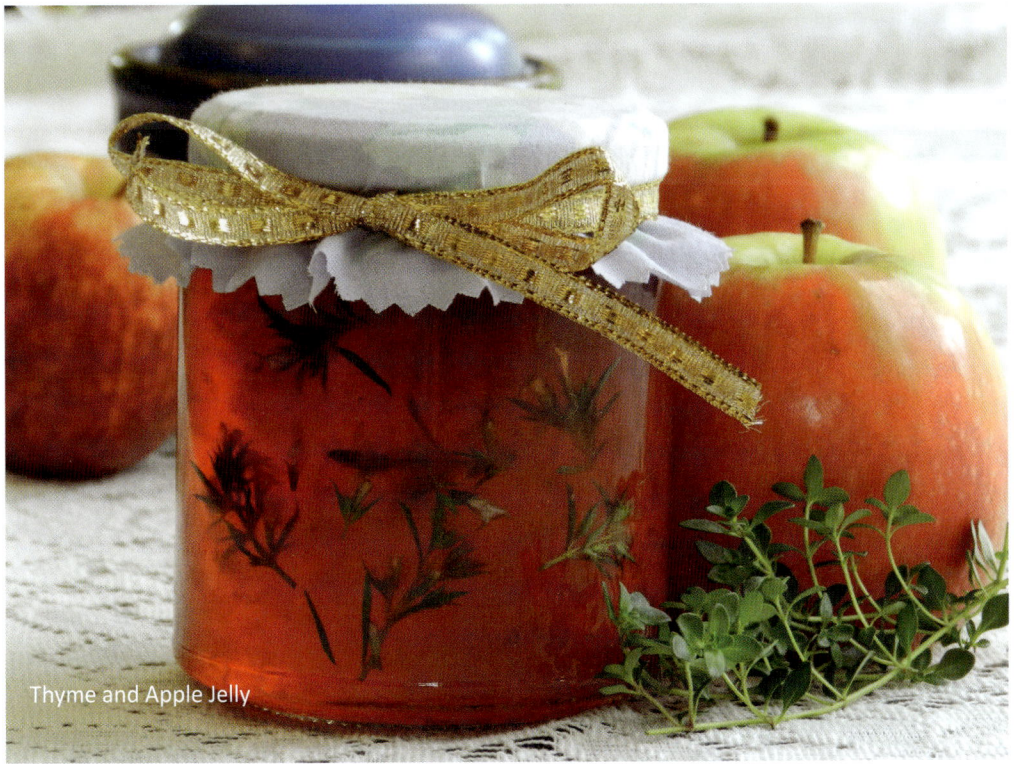
Thyme and Apple Jelly

Homeopathic Remedy
Both thymol, the main component of the essential oil, and the tincture of wild thyme *Thymus serpyllum* are homeopathic remedies. Thymol is specific for hookworms, and for genito-urinary problems. It is prescribed for sexual debility, prostate problems, priapism and nocturnal emission. The symptom picture includes low energy, unrefreshing sleep and lascivious dreams, profuse urination with burning and dribbling indicative of prostate problems, aching in the lower back and irritability. The patient wants his own way and craves the company of others.

Thymus serpyllum is used for respiratory infections particularly in children, for asthma associated with tension, for dry nervous coughs, whooping cough and sore throats. It is also prescribed for ringing in the ears, with a feeling of pressure in the head.

Flower Essence
The use of thyme as a flower remedy is related to the passage of time, and its acceleration. When dabbed on to a wound or cut, or over an area of trauma or disease in the body, thyme is said to speed healing. It has an amplifying effect, increasing strength and courage, and enhancing the body's metabolic processes. It imparts greater physical stamina, making it particularly useful in the elderly. When used in combination with other flower essences, thyme acts to amplify their effects. Thyme the herb has been used since the days of the ancient Greeks to increase energy and longevity. The flower essence similarly increases energy, enhances concentration and the ability to adapt to seasonal change and the passage of time. It is good for people struggling with time, stressed by deadlines, always trying to beat the clock; or for in old age, helping to protect mind and body from the effects of ageing.

Edible Uses
Thyme is a wonderful ingredient of cuisine around the world, particularly in France, Italy and throughout the Mediterranean. Fresh leaves or whole sprigs can be used to flavour soups, bread, vegetable dishes, meat and poultry. Thyme is also an excellent ingredient to use with fish. You could also use thyme to make pesto which can be used as a condiment or try it added to pasta or rice.

Growing
Propagate by sowing seeds in spring, by taking stem cuttings in summer, by dividing the roots in autumn or by layering older plants by mounding. Prefers well-drained, alkaline soil and full sun, and grows prostrate or upright to 12" (30cm), flowering in summer. It is best to clip back after flowering and again in autumn to encourage bushy growth, otherwise thyme can become rather woody. Plants may need replacing after 4–5 years.

Cautions
Avoid large amounts in pregnancy. Avoid essential oil near mouth and nose of infants. Only use thyme oil in small amounts and do not use it undiluted on the skin.

Recipes

Thyme Syrup
This sweet fragrant syrup from Greece makes an excellent remedy for all kinds of cough. Thyme is highly antiseptic and, with its expectorant action, chases away infection and clears congestion from the chest. This is a perfect syrup for children with its smooth, velvety texture and delicious taste.

50g fresh or 25g dried thyme leaves
600ml boiling water
300g runny honey
300g sugar

Place the thyme in a teapot. Pour on boiling water, cover and leave to infuse for 10–15 minutes. Heat the infusion with the sugar in a stainless steel or enamel saucepan. Stir the mixture as its starts to thicken and skim off any scum from the surface. Add the honey and stir. Leave to cool. Pour into a cork-stoppered bottle and store in the fridge.

Take 2 teaspoons, 3 times daily for chronic problems, and every 2 hours for acute conditions.

Tilia europaea/T. cordata: Lime, Linden

The Flower of Grace

And in summer, when you go to sleep,
Put fresh linden leaves on the eyes,
Covering your whole face
To make your eyes clear and clean
– Hildegard of Bingen (c.1098–1179)

Other names: Linden flowers

Parts used: Flowers

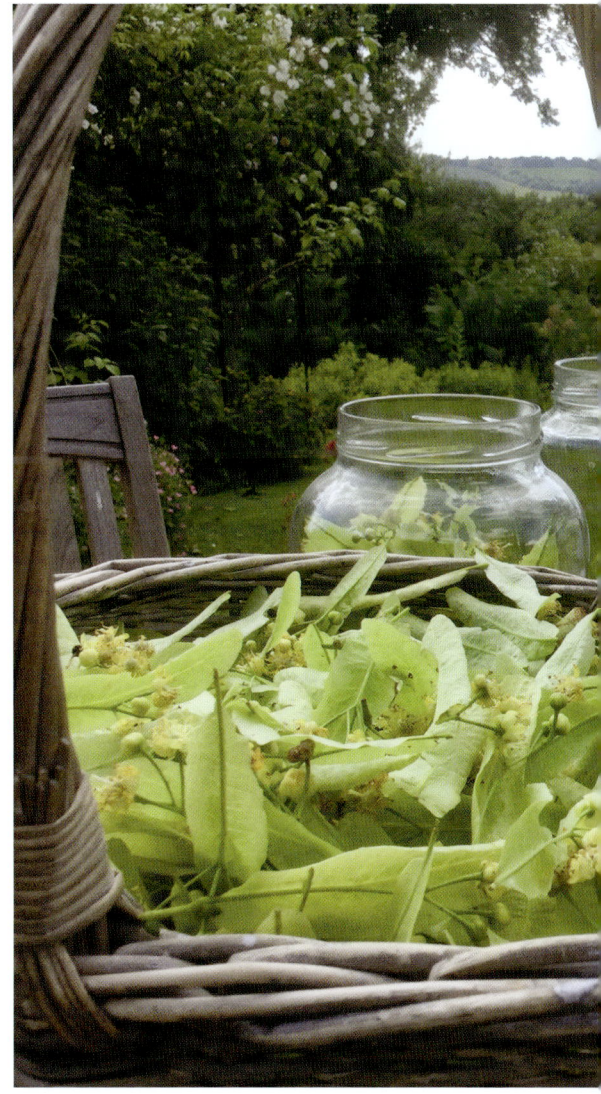

The lime tree, *Tilea europea,* is a handsome deciduous tree with a profusion of creamy flowers that smell like honey and are loved by bees. It is a member of the Malvaceae/Tiliaceae family and native to Europe, W. Asia and North America. It can grow over 100 feet (30m) tall and may live up to 1,000 years. *Tilia cordata,* the small-leaved linden, is native to Europe, eastwards to central Russia and the Caucasus. Its name *cordata* comes from the Latin 'cor' which relates to 'cordis' meaning the heart, referring to the shape of the leaves. It is interesting that lime flower has long been associated with affairs of the heart.

Lime trees are seen in parks and gardens all over Britain and Europe and planted along roads and avenues in town and countryside alike. The lime tree is very resilient and can be cut and trained with little trouble and flourishes even in the smoke-laden atmospheres of cities. The flowers are rich in volatile oils which give it that heady sweet and very relaxing scent, and pleasant taste. Teas made from dried flowers have long been a popular drink in many countries, particularly in France where it is called 'tilleul' and in Italy where it is 'tiglio'. There has been a long tradition in France and other European countries for families to go out collecting lime flowers in the summer and drying them for use through the year. That makes practical sense as it takes a long time to pick the flowers and small leaves. 'Tisane de tilieul', an infusion of lime flowers, was a popular remedy for colds, fevers and restless children. The flowers are loved by bees and lend their sweet aromatic taste to honey. During the Middle Ages, lime trees were often planted around monasteries and castles to provide honey. Lime trees are also valued for their wood and charcoal. The name 'linden' probably comes from the old Norse name of the plant 'lundr' meaning grove or tree. In Britain, linden trees are called lime trees, as lime is probably a corruption of 'lundr'.

The majestic linden tree is an ancient symbol of feminine grace, beauty, happiness, sweetness, peace and love. Certainly, the flowers have a sweet honey-like taste and smell and are loved by bees, but it also relates to stories from the time of the ancient Greeks. In Greek mythology, one of the demi-gods was the sea nymph called Philyra. She was one of the daughters of Tethys, the goddess of the seas and subterranean rivers and Oceanus, the god of the oceans. She was seduced by the cruel god Kronos (also known as Cronos, Saturn or Time) who was caught during their lovemaking by his wife Rhea. He panicked and to escape detection, changed himself into a stallion and galloped off. Philyra was left to give birth to the child they conceived, who was half man half horse, a centaur named Cheiron. Philyra was so ashamed at having given birth to him that she implored the gods not to have to continue living in human form. They changed her into a beautiful lime tree. Chiron grew up at the foot of this lime tree, his mother, and in her tree form she educated him with wisdom and love and the boy grew up to be a wise centaur. Many kings sent their sons to Chiron to be educated under the branches of the big lime tree and the lime became the symbol for abundant love and care. *Philyra* is still the Greek word for lime or linden tree.

Lime trees were sacred to many Germanic and Slavic peoples. In Germany, they were dedicated to Freya, the goddess of beauty, sensuality and fertility. In the Slavic Orthodox Christian church, the wood from lime trees was considered the best for icon painting, as it became very smooth once sanded, and when seasoned it did not warp easily. In Norse mythology lime trees commemorated Odin's wife Frigg, the goddess of wisdom and foreknowledge, and in other countries, lime trees were worshipped as a symbol of knowledge. They were planted as mark trees which were trees grown in geomantically significant sites like crossroads to symbolise the cosmic axis. Lime trees were also planted in turf mazes and pollarded to symbolise 'Yggdrasil' the world tree. In Medieval times lime trees were planted in the heart of many German villages, where matters of justice were settled by the elders, markets were held and marriages and other celebrations took place under their spreading branches. In England the tree was dedicated to the goddess Venus, while Culpeper said it was ruled by the planet Jupiter, representing expansion, learning and wisdom.

The lime tree was also revered for its healing properties. In the Middle Ages, Hildegard of Bingen used the lime tree as a talisman to ward off the plague. She apparently wore a ring with a green stone beneath which were some lime flowers wrapped in a spider's web. Good luck charms were carved from lime wood, partly because it is also an easy wood to carve. In Baltic mythology, the goddess of fate is called 'Laima' and the lime is her sacred tree where she lived and decided peoples' destinies in the form of a cuckoo. Lithuanian women would pray and make sacrifices to lime trees to ask for good luck such as a good harvest and fertility.

Since the Middle Ages, lime flowers have been used as a diaphoretic to promote perspiration, to bring down fevers and as a calming remedy to treat hysteria, convulsions, indigestion and diarrhoea. Some believed you only had to sit under the tree to be cured of epilepsy. The flowers were used for affairs of the heart including palpitations, throbbing headaches, high blood pressure and shortness of breath. They were highly regarded for aiding sleep and allaying tension and anxiety. Hildegard of Bingen recommended *"for those with gout, take the earth, around the root of the linden tree, and bring it into the fire to give it heat. And in the steam bath one pours water over it and bathe so. Do this for nine days, and he will be healed."*

Herbal Remedy
Lime flower tea has a delicious taste, due in part to the aromatic volatile oil found in the flowers that is made of compounds that include farnesol, farnesyl acetate, geraniol and eugenol. It also contains antioxidant flavonoids (rutin, hyperoside, quercitrin, isoquercitrin, herperidin,

quercetin, kaempferol, astralagin) and phenolic acids, eugenol, tannins, anthocyanidins, calcium, manganese, vitamin C and mucilage (mainly arabino-glactans).

For many centuries lime flowers have been used in healing to ease tension and anxiety, calm restlessness and agitation, relieve depression and irritability and induce restorative sleep. An infusion added to a night-time bath can be excellent for excitable children to get them into bed. Lime flower is used for insomnia, especially in children, for recurrent nightmares and is well worth taking for anticipatory nerves, such as before exams or an interview. Maurice Mességué says it is one of the ingredients of his 'tea of happiness' that bring peaceful nights, joyful awakenings and happy days if taken regularly. With their antispasmodic and sedative actions, lime flowers can be taken for any condition associated with stress such as headaches, migraine, period pain, muscle tension, neck, shoulder and back pain and cramp. It can ease digestive problems including wind, bloating, diarrhoea, constipation, heartburn, indigestion, stomach aches and colic. *Tilia cordata* has been used to relieve sinus headaches and migraines, insomnia, stress and panic disorders.

The lime tree grows slowly and steadily and lives for centuries. It is said it can prolong the lives of others through these therapeutic actions, if they can learn its lesson of moderation and regular, steady progress. Lime flowers may well help us in our quest for longevity. With their antioxidant flavonoids, anthocyanidins and phenolic compounds combined with their relaxant effects, lime flowers make a good remedy for the cardiovascular system, protecting it from the effects of ageing, as our ancestors well knew. Their antioxidant and anti-inflammatory effects combined with their relaxant effect protect the walls of the arteries from free radical damage and help prevent raised cholesterol, atherosclerosis, clots and coronary heart disease. They can be used for nervous palpitations and arrhythmias, their antispasmodic action can relax and dilate the coronary arteries and can relieve anginal pain and reduce high blood pressure. They may be helpful in the treatment of other circulatory disorders such as varicose veins, phlebitis, migraine and auto-immune attacks on the vessel

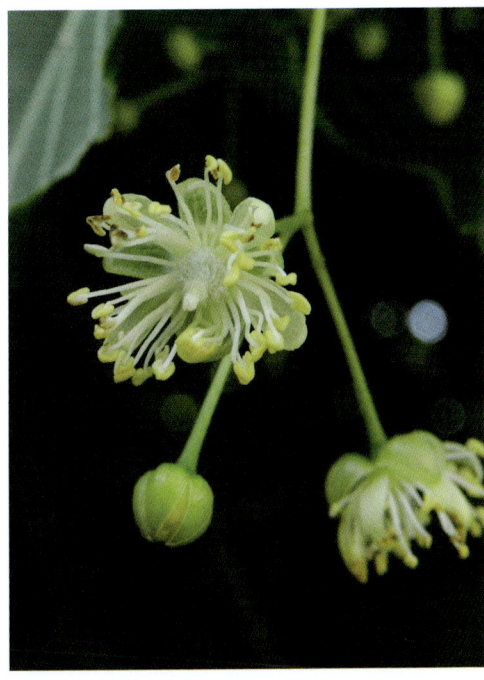

walls, such as arteritis. They have also been used to heal the heart emotionally, to help unblock problems from painful experiences in the past which inhibit the giving and receiving of affection and love, and to enable openness and warmth in relationships.

Taken in hot infusion, lime flowers have a diaphoretic action, increasing blood supply to the skin and promoting sweating. The tea makes an excellent cooling remedy for fevers, which tastes pleasant and is easy to give to children. When the flowers are combined with elderflowers and mint, the tea makes a good decongestant, antispasmodic and soothing expectorant for feverish colds, flu, catarrh, irritating coughs, bronchitis and asthma. The diaphoretic and antispasmodic properties have been attributed to p-coumaric acid and the flavonoids. The flavonoids, particularly epicatechin, and the oligomeric procyanidins have an anti-inflammatory effect and support the traditional use of lime flower tea for treating inflammation and irritation of the respiratory tract in colds, pharyngitis and tonsillitis. The mucilage has a soothing action and can be soothing for harsh irritating coughs and sore throats.

A cool infusion of lime flowers has a diuretic action, clearing fluid and toxins from the system via the urinary system. It can be taken for fluid retention, cystitis, urethritis and frequency due to nerves. Its anti-inflammatory action is helpful in the treatment of arthritis, gout and inflammatory skin problems. It may also contribute to the action that lime flower has in the gut, inhibiting the digestive enzymes that digest carbohydrates, which could help prevent raised blood sugar and blood pressure associated with type 2 diabetes.

Externally lime flower tea makes a soothing and anti-inflammatory lotion for skin problems like acne, spots, boils and abscesses and allergic rashes such as eczema and urticaria. A cooled infusion can be used as a lotion for scalds and burns and an eyewash for inflamed eyes. It also makes an anti-inflammatory gargle for mouth ulcers and added to the bath helps to calm restless children. Lime flowers smell lovely mixed with lavender flowers or lemon balm leaves and are excellent for making sleep pillows.

Aromatherapy Oil
The sweet fragrant essential oil extracted from lime flowers has a similarly relaxing and antispasmodic effect as when the flowers are used as a herbal remedy. It can be added to the bath or used in massage oils to relieve many stress-related problems including anxiety, restlessness, headaches, migraine, muscle tension, pain and spasm. A few drops in the bath or a burner at night helps to promote relaxation and sleep. It lifts the spirits and engenders calm that can be helpful during meditation. It helps to eliminate excess water with its diuretic effect and is good for hot dry or irritated skin problems such as eczema.

Homeopathic Remedy
Tilia is prescribed for muscular tension and weakness throughout the body, vertigo, neuralgia, headaches and migraine and to relieve pain. It is particularly recommended for toothache in children. It will relieve disturbed and restless sleep, with vivid or frightful dreams. As in herbal medicine, Tilia is given for fevers with night sweats, catarrh and colds, sore burning throats and hoarseness, and tickly irritating coughs. It is given for heart pains, palpitations, feelings of pressure in the chest, rapid pulse, and to thin the blood where there is a tendency to clotting. A Tilia person may be depressed, weepy or lovesick, irritable or reclusive and shy. Tilia has a specific use for pelvic inflammation in women and for post-partum infection.

Flower Essence
The flower remedy is closely related to linden's application in healing matters of the heart, when it was a symbol of conjugal love, sweetness, peace and happiness. It is a good remedy for those who have trouble giving and receiving love and affection, because of painful experiences in the past. Linden flower helps to release emotional blocks and engenders warmth and openness. It increases awareness of our connectedness to the rest of humanity, relaxes and softens communication between people and strengthens relationships between loved ones.

Edible Uses
Lime flowers make one of the most delicious and fragrant teas. Its taste is sweet and delicate. To make the tea, simply pour boiling water over the dried flowers, cover and leave to brew for about 5–10 minutes. Generally, use one teaspoon per cup of boiling water; for a diaphoretic and decongestant effect for fevers and catarrh, double the amount. Take a cupful three times a day to ease nervous tension, hypertension, or a cold or flu, or enjoy a cup before bed for a relaxing sleep.

Harvesting
Lime trees flower for a short period around the end of June/beginning of July, so make sure you don't miss the opportunity! The flowers are often fairly high so you may need a step ladder to reach them. Once collected, the flowers can be air dried for couple of days in a warm, semi-dark place, filling the room with a sweet, honey like fragrance – just relax and breathe it in!

Cautions
Large doses may cause nausea and allergic reactions. Dried lime flowers ferment easily and so are best if not kept longer than a year. Take away from mineral supplements and food as they could impair iron absorption.

Trifolium pratense: Red Clover

The Flower of Good Fortune

*Crimson clover I discover
By the garden gate,
And the bees about her hover,
But the robins wait.
Sing, robins, sing,
Sing a roundelay,-
'Tis the latest flower of Spring,
Coming with the May!*
– Dora Read Goodale (1866–1915)

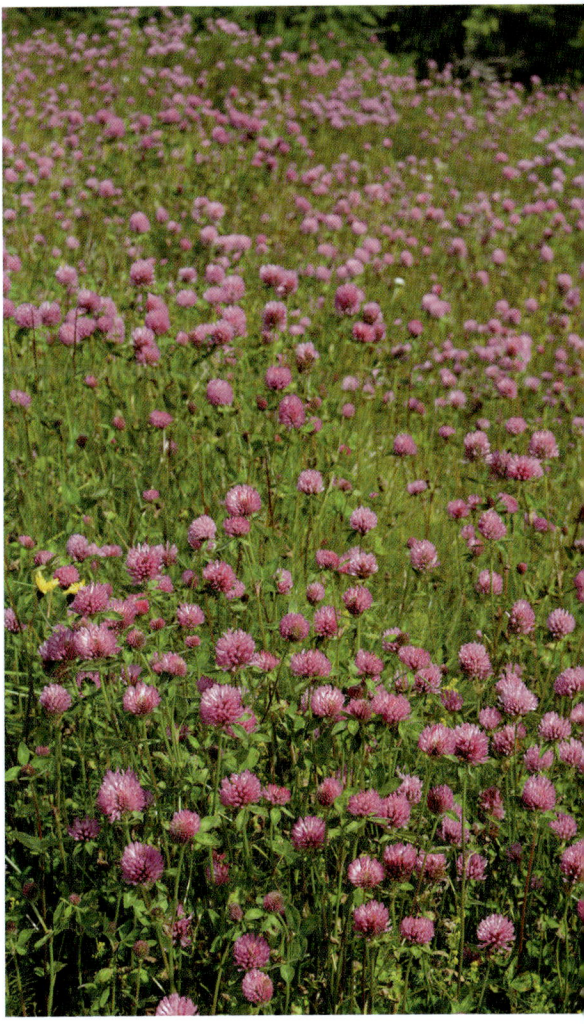

Other names: Purple clover, sweet clover, cow clover, bee bread, trefoil, meadow clover, wild clover, meadow trefoil, cow grass and three-leafed grass

Parts used: Flowers

This attractive cousin of the pea and bean has pretty pink flowers that can be found growing in profusion in meadows, fields and mountainsides, flowering from early summer to autumn. It is a perennial member of the Fabaceae/Leguminosae family, native to Britain, Europe, Asia and North Africa and naturalised in North America and Canada. Clover is familiar to many of us as a good luck charm, particularly the four-leafed clover. It has been considered lucky since ancient times; to the medieval Christians, a four-leafed clover was seen as a symbol of the Holy Cross and a three-leafed symbolised the Holy Trinity. It was believed to be especially lucky for women to whom the three-leafed clover represented the triple goddess: the maiden or young woman, the mother or fertility symbol and the crone of old age and wisdom. The Druids considered red clover to have the power to protect from danger and evil influences, including witches. It afforded psychic protection.

Clover has also been a symbol of fertility and domestic virtue. It is rich in minerals and trace elements and contains nitrogen-fixing bacteria in the root, making it valuable as a feeding crop for cattle. The phrase 'living in clover' alludes to cattle being put to feed in rich pasture. Red clover is still widely cultivated as a fodder crop for animals and it benefits the soil by fixing nitrogen, making it an ideal cover crop for enriching soil fertility for other crops to follow.

Red clover has been used traditionally as a medicine by Asian, European, and native American cultures as an expectorant for coughs and asthma and to treat skin problems including psoriasis and eczema. Russian folk healers recommend it for asthma. According to the doctrine of signatures, the white crescent-shaped markings on the leaves meant that the plant could be used for cataracts.

Red clover has been used traditionally in many parts of the world as a detoxifying herb. Although red clover is native to Britain and Europe, it was not until it became naturalised in North America, and the Native Americans discovered its medicinal benefits, that it became used as a medicine in Europe. The flowers were incorporated into many popular 'Trifolium Compounds' and marketed as blood purifiers to help clear the body of toxins, resolve skin complaints such as eczema and psoriasis and as an anti-cancer remedy in the 1930s. It also used to be smoked as a remedy for asthma. In North America, red clover is the state flower of pastoral Vermont.

Herbal Remedy

Red clover flowers have a combination of sweet, bitter, astringent and salty tastes and contain more than 100 chemical substances. These include tannins, isoflavone phytoestrogens (biochanin A, daidzein, genistein, pratensein, trifoside, formononetin, kaempferol, pectolinarin), phytosterols (sterol, sitosterol), flavonoids, coumarins, essential oils, saponins, phaseolic acid, polysaccharides, galactomannan, vitamins, minerals including calcium, iron, magnesium, sodium, potassium, copper and zinc and salicylic acid.

Red clover flowers are still used as a 'blood purifier' and detoxifying remedy, particularly used for deep-seated, chronic conditions of toxicity. They aid elimination of toxins in several ways. With their diuretic effect, they enhance the elimination of wastes via the urinary system.

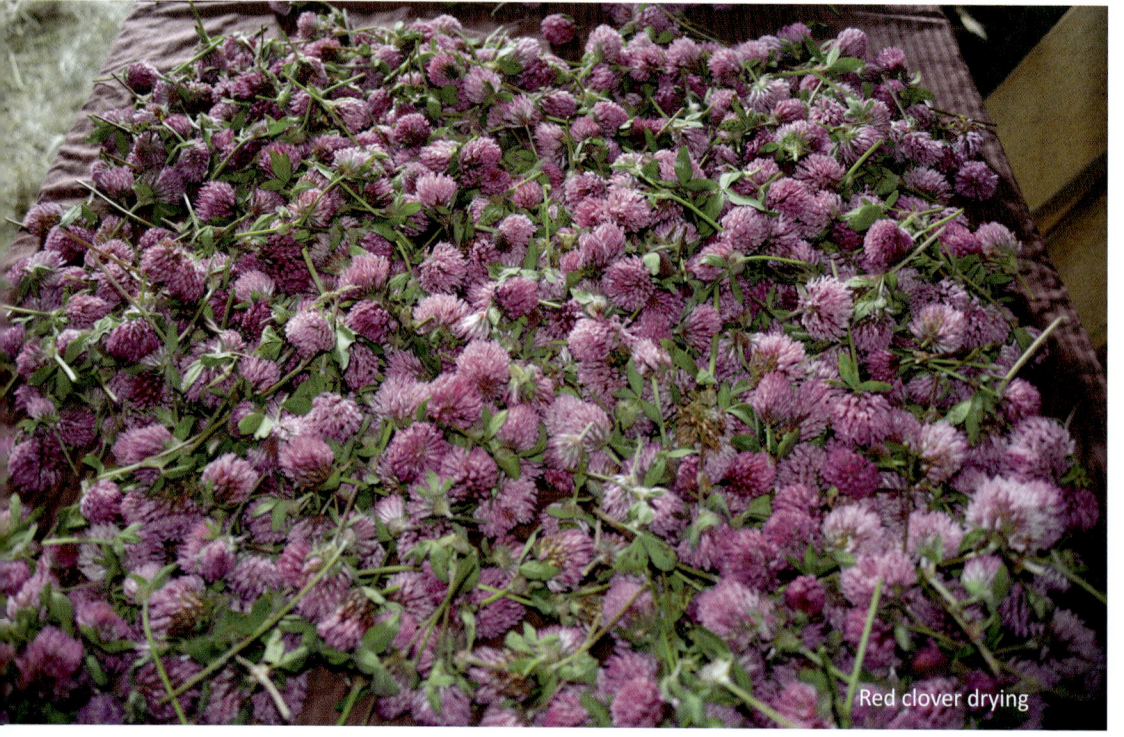
Red clover drying

They stimulate the lymphatic circulation and the liver and support them in their detoxifying work and they also have a mild laxative effect, enhancing clearing of toxins and wastes through the bowels.

With its combination of anti-inflammatory effects partly attributed to salicylic acid and its detoxifying actions, red clover is a popular herb for treating a range of allergic and inflammatory skin problems. These include eczema, psoriasis, acne, rosacea, impetigo and urticaria. It is an excellent remedy for children and may be safely used in childhood eczema. It has relaxant properties, helping to relieve pain as well as tension and anxiety, and can be used for stress-related symptoms such as headaches and muscle spasm. The pain-relieving properties of red clover are likely due to the presence of the anti-inflammatory compounds, eugenol, myricetin and salicylic acid.

In the respiratory system this relaxant effect together with a soothing expectorant action is very helpful in irritating coughs, asthma, bronchitis, spasmodic coughs including whooping cough and other bronchial problems. Since it also helps to clear the skin, red clover is used for coughs during measles, and for children with the eczema-asthma syndrome. It also has antiviral and antifungal properties, excellent for other respiratory infections, including sore throats with swollen glands, colds and flu. When taken as a hot infusion it can promote sweating and help to bring down fevers.

Red clover contains many antioxidant and anti-inflammatory compounds which help to protect against free radical damage and in this way, it may have many benefits to health, especially for women as they get older. Some herbalists use red clover as a deep cleansing remedy for chronic problems such as pelvic inflammatory disease and to relieve heavy or painful periods. Through its beneficial effect in the lymphatic system, red clover can be helpful in cyclic breast pain and tenderness as well as mastitis. Because of its concentration of isoflavone phytoestrogens, particularly daidzein and genistein which mimic the activity of oestrogen, red clover has been used for its ability to alleviate many symptoms of the menopause including hot flushes and night sweats. It can also be useful for insomnia, anxiety, depression and vaginal dryness and for more cosmetic purposes related to its oestrogenic effects such as improved hair and skin texture. Red clover may also be able to increase bone density; the isoflavones may well be helpful in the prevention of osteoporosis as they promote calcium storage in cells and inhibit osteoclast (a type of bone cell that breaks down bone tissue) activity and differentiation.

Red clover may also benefit post-menopausal women in other ways, particularly in relation to cardiovascular health. It can decrease low density lipoprotein (LDL the 'bad' cholesterol) and increase high density lipoprotein (HDL the 'good' cholesterol) perhaps through the ability of beta-sitosterol to reduce the absorption of cholesterol. In folk medicine, red clover has been used to thin and purify the blood. The coumarins in red clover may affect platelet activity and reduce the tendency to blood clots. Interestingly, in Iran, red clover and alfalfa tea is used traditionally with this intention. Red clover has been used in standardised extracts that include specific quantities of the four isoflavones genistein, daidzein, biochanin and formononetin and these have had a beneficial effect in improving heart health in postmenopausal women.

Red clover has a diuretic action, eliminating excess fluid and wastes via the urinary system. It can be used for cystitis and irritable bladder especially when it occurs in post-menopausal women. Its traditional use for arthritis and gout may be explained to some extent by its antioxidant and anti-inflammatory actions. It can be used as a remedy for arthritis particularly in post-menopausal women.

Red clover has a reputation as a remedy for male pattern baldness and it may decrease hair loss and promote hair growth when taken internally as well as applied externally. It is also used to help prevent prostate problems including benign enlargement of the prostate and it can help relieve some of its symptoms including getting up frequently at night to pass water.

Red clover has long been used as a remedy for the treatment of cancer. A variety of compounds in the flowers including biochanin-A, caffeic acid, chlorogenic acid, coumarin, formononetin, genistein and isorhamnetin may have potential anti-cancer properties and the sterol beta-sitosterol can inhibit tumour growth. Red clover is an ingredient in traditional herbal formulas for cancer including Essiac tea and the Hoxsey Therapy and may be helpful in cancers of the breast, ovaries, prostate, lung and lymphatic system as well as melanoma and leukaemia. Flavone glycosides and isoflavones, notably genistein, may inhibit cancer by inhibiting angiogenesis (preventing the growth of the new blood vessels that feed tumours) and the sterol beta-sitosterol may also inhibit the growth of tumours.

Externally an infusion of red clover flowers can be used as a wash for skin problems including eczema, psoriasis, acne, sores and ulcers. A poultice can be made from fresh flowers for insect bites and stings. Their antifungal and antiviral actions can be helpful in ointments or creams for athlete's foot and ringworm and *Herpes*. A cooled infusion can be used as an eyewash for sore eyes and conjunctivitis. An infusion can be used as a douche to relieve vaginal itching and as a wash for sore inflamed nipples. It also makes a good gargle for sore throats and, used as a liniment, it can relieve the pain of arthritis and gout. An oil or lotion could be helpful if applied regularly for male pattern baldness (androgenic alopecia) and may increase hair growth.

Homeopathic Remedy

In homeopathy also, red clover is used for cancer and a range of respiratory symptoms: spasmodic coughs, whooping cough, coughs followed by hiccoughs and chills with a cough at night. It treats sore irritated throats, mucus in the throat with constantly wanting to clear it, and hoarseness. It is also prescribed for hay fever symptoms.

It is also used for chronic skin conditions, tension and headaches with a stiff neck and back which is relieved by heat, and confusion and headache occurring after unrefreshing sleep. Red clover is helpful where there is constipation, great thirst and colicky pains.

Flower Essence

Red clover the flower essence is also a cleansing remedy, a blood cleanser, relating to the psychic properties of the blood where the spiritual self is said to reside. It helps to clear negativity

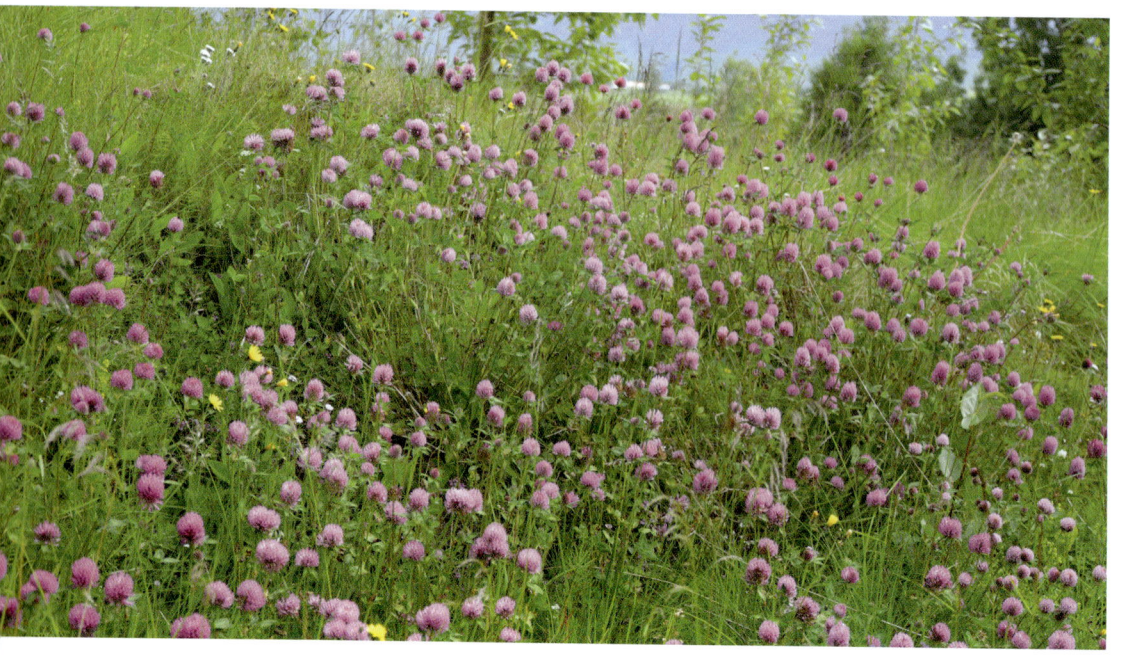

picked up from others and is particularly useful for those who feel susceptible to the problems of others, or to taking on the emotions of those around them. This may occur in crises, such as economic crises or natural disasters, where the reaction of fear, panic, confusion or hysteria can be highly infectious, or during political or religious rallies where crowds can become highly inflammatory, even destructive. The same may occur in emotionally charged work or family situations.

Red clover the flower essence acts as a balancer, helping one to remain centred within despite the storms outside. It instils calmness and clarity and enhances self-awareness.

Edible Uses
The flowers can be used as a colourful garnish and added to salads and fruit salads as they taste pleasantly sweet and slightly salty. They make a nice mild tea that combines well with other more aromatic herbs such as lemon verbena, lemon balm or mint.

Growing
Red clover grows wild in profusion so it is unlikely that it will need to be cultivated. Harvest when the flowers are in full bloom in summer.

Cautions
Avoid in pregnancy, breastfeeding and oestrogen-sensitive cancers and bleeding disorders (due to the presence of coumarins). Caution with anticoagulants, salicylates, Warfarin, oestrogen and oestrogen-like medication, oral contraceptives. Avoid 7 days prior to surgery.

Recipes

Red Clover Lemonade
3 cups of red clover flowers
8 cups water
Juice from 6 freshly squeezed lemons
3–4 tablespoons honey

Simmer the water and flowers together in a covered pan, for 10 minutes. Add honey and leave to steep for a few hours. Strain and add the lemon juice. Enjoy!

Red Clover Syrup
4 cups red clover flowers
4 cups water
4 cups sugar
½ lemon or orange (organic if possible) chopped with peel
1 tablespoon of beetroot or elderberry juice to give it a lovely colour

Simmer flowers and water gently in a covered pan for about 15–20 minutes, then leave to infuse overnight. Strain through a fine sieve or piece of muslin and press the liquid out. Add the sugar and sliced citrus and then return it to a pan and heat slowly, stirring now and again, for several hours or until reduced to a thick, honey-like syrup. Pour into dark bottles and label clearly.

Red Clover Tincture
Place 100g of fresh or 200g dried red clover blossoms in a large glass jar and cover with 500ml of either brandy, gin, or vodka. The alcohol should be enough to cover the flowers. Stir and cover.

Place the mixture in a dark cupboard for three to five weeks. Shake the mixture several times each day. Strain and store in a tightly capped, clearly labelled dark glass bottle. A standard dose is 1–3ml of the tincture three times a day. Tinctures properly prepared and stored will retain medicinal potency for two years or longer.

Red Clover Ointment
Cover as many red clover flowers as possible with 450ml of your favourite oil such as olive, almond or sunflower in a pyrex or heat proof bowl. Add 50g of beeswax and place the bowl on the top of a pan of water as a *bain marie* and leave it on a low heat for a few hours, checking the water regularly to make sure it has not evaporated. After this time the constituents will have been taken up by the oil and the mixture can then be pressed through a muslin bag and the herb discarded. When the oil is still warm it can be poured into airtight ointment jars where it will quickly solidify. Label clearly with the name and the date and store in a cool dark place.

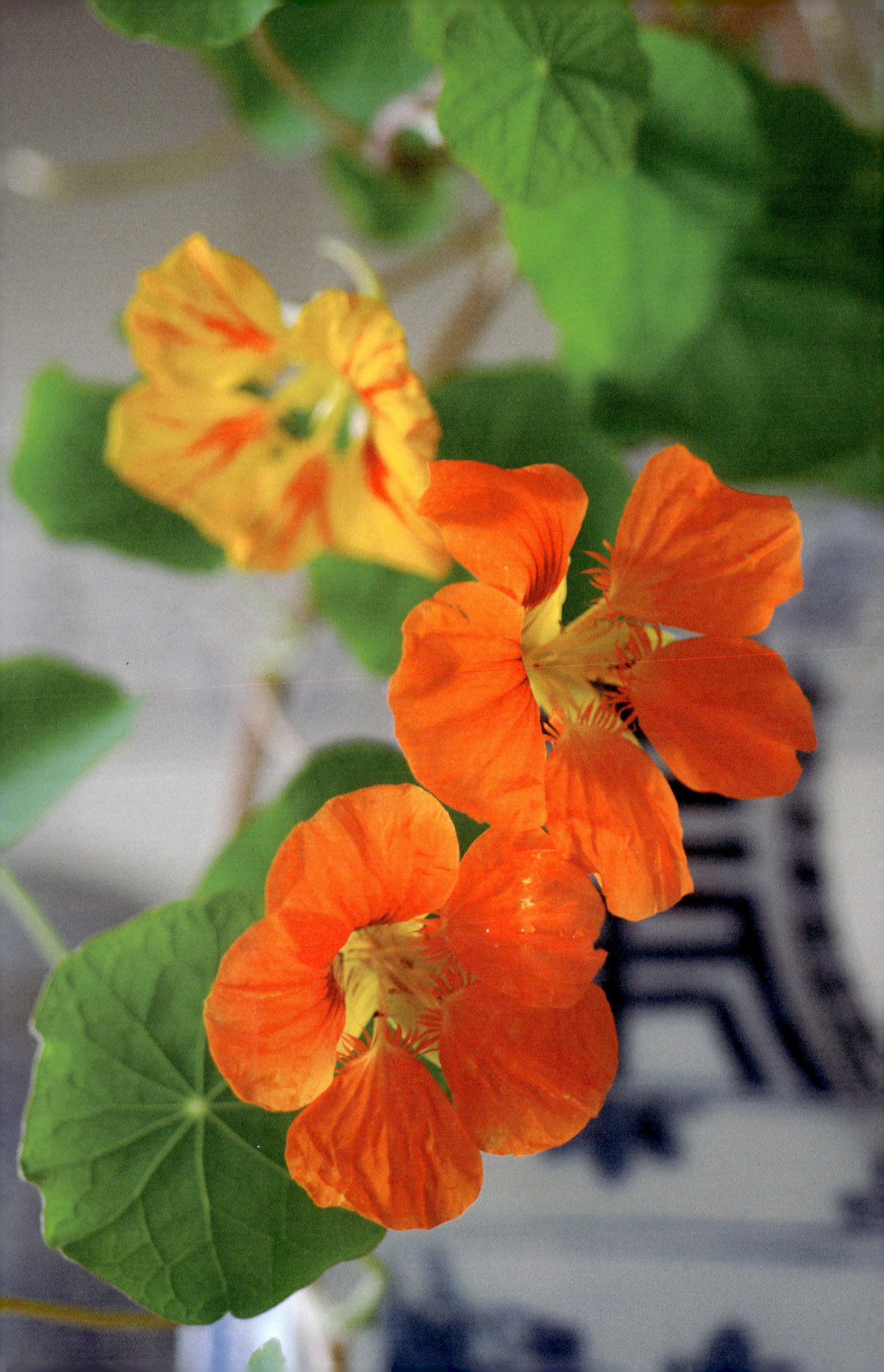

Tropaeolum majus: Nasturtium

The Flower of Patriotism

Shield-like Nasturtium, too, confusedly spread,
with intermingling trefoil fills each bed -
once graceful youths, this last a Grecian swain,
The first an huntsman on the Trojan plain
   – Paul de Rapin (1661–1725)

Other names: Indian cress, garden nasturtium, monk's cress, passionflower, flower of love

Part used: Flowers and leaves

This bright and colourful annual is one of the easiest and most rewarding flowers to grow from seed. Nasturtium is a member of the Tropaeolaceae family and is native to tropical South and Central America, where it is perennial. It was among the treasures brought back from Peru to Europe in the late 15th to early 16th century by the Spanish conquistadores along with the gold of the Incas. The first nasturtium brought was *Tropaeolum minus*, a semi-trailing vine with spurred, lightly scented orange-yellow flowers with dark red spots on the petals and shield-shaped leaves. According to Jesuit missionaries, the Incas used nasturtiums as a salad vegetable and as a medicinal herb for urinary problems and respiratory infections including coughs, colds and the flu.

In 16th century England, nasturtium was called 'blood flower of Peru' and 'Indian cress' because of its similarity to watercress (*Nasturtium officinale*) with its pungent taste and smell. The name *nasturtium* comes from 'nasus tortus' meaning nose-twisting because of its peppery smell. The flower was welcomed as a rare treasure in Elizabethan and Stuart England. John Evelyn recommended the seed for scurvy and described it as *"The most effectual and powerful agent in conquering and expunging that cruel Enemy."* Others used the peppery leaves to prevent scurvy, and the leaves and seeds to supplement the daily diet and add flavour.

Some say that the Latin name *Tropaeolum* was given by the Swedish botanist Carl Linnaeus who thought the flower petals resembled Roman trophy poles called 'tropaeums'. Others say *Tropaeolum* comes from the Greek 'tropaion' meaning trophy. In one story about the origin of the flower, the nasturtium is said to have arisen from the spilled blood of a Trojan warrior, the round leaves being his shield and the trumpet-shaped flower his helmet. In the language of flowers, nasturtium symbolises patriotism.

Herbal Remedy

Nasturtium is not only a versatile and eye-catching ingredient in the kitchen, but also nutritious. The green leaves and flowers are rich in antioxidants and other nutrients, including vitamin C and beta-carotene and a variety of minerals including potassium, phosphorus, calcium, magnesium, zinc, copper and iron which can be easily absorbed by the body. Its peppery taste and smell are given by the volatile oils and it also contains phenolic compounds and acids including gallic acid, caffeic acid and p-coumaric acids and flavonoids; myricetin, quercetin, kaempferol epicatechin and luteolin.

The taste of nasturtium flowers and leaves is both bitter and pungent. Pungency has a warming and stimulating effect in the body. Nasturtium invigorates the digestion, improving appetite, digestion and absorption and its antimicrobial actions help combat unfriendly gut bacteria. This means that nasturtium flowers and leaves are not only a delightful food, but also make a good remedy for poor digestion, reducing stagnation of food in the gut that leads to toxicity and helping to remedy leaky gut syndrome. Nasturtium also increases the circulation of blood carrying the absorbed nutrients around the body to where they are needed. In this way nasturtium promotes health and vitality and a general sense of wellbeing. The bitters in nasturtium are also detoxifying. They stimulate liver, pancreas and gallbladder activity and promote the secretion of digestive enzymes, thereby improving digestion and absorption. The bitters, particularly those in the seeds, stimulate the bowels and ensure the elimination of wastes through this route. Nasturtium also acts on the kidneys and bladder, increasing the elimination of waste products via the urine.

Nasturtium has antioxidant and anti-inflammatory effects on account of the presence of compounds such as anthocyanins, polyphenols, volatile oils and vitamin C. This means that it can help to prevent damage caused to the body from oxidative stress that contributes to many health problems as we get older including cardiovascular disease, arthritis, degeneration of the brain, lowered immunity and cancer. It has an impressively high content of an antioxidant called lutein which is associated with protection against free radical damage particularly in relation to eye and skin health.

Nasturtium has long been used to boost immunity and for its antimicrobial properties. The essential oils such as myristicin, α-terpinolene and limonene found in the stems, the seeds and leaves, and the phenolic compounds, have antimicrobial activity against different bacteria including some strains of *Streptococcus* and antifungal activity against *Candida albicans*. The leaves and flowers also have decongestant properties and can be used as fresh juice or in infusions for colds, hay fever, catarrh, sinusitis, chest infections, asthma and other bronchial problems. Its high vitamin C content is useful as it also enhances immunity and helps to clear the chest by promoting the action of the muco-ciliary escalator (those little hairs in the bronchi which sweep away unwanted substances and thereby protect the lungs). Nasturtium can also be taken for acute urinary tract infections such as cystitis. As a natural antimicrobial, it has the advantage of not destroying the normal bacterial population of the gut in the way that orthodox antibiotics do.

The combination of its nourishing, detoxifying and immune-enhancing properties makes nasturtium a good tonic for those feeling depleted and run down. Being high in iron, it is helpful when feeling tired due to anaemia. Its strengthening effect was used in the past as a rejuvenative and an aphrodisiac, hence its names 'passionflower' and 'flower of love'.

Externally, nasturtium has an old reputation of retarding balding; the tincture of nasturtium leaves, oak bark and nettles was massaged regularly into the scalp. Apparently in India they use the fresh leaves to clean their teeth and gums; this has the benefit of preventing infection while at the same time leaving your mouth feeling fresh. The bruised fresh leaves can be rubbed on to cuts and grazes to speed healing. They can be used as a poultice or compress for bacterial and fungal skin infections. Erucic acid, a type of omega-9 fatty acid, is found in nasturtium seeds and acts as a natural lubricant; it can be used to benefit the skin and hair as it has hydrating and soothing effects.

Homeopathic Remedy
Tropaeolum majus is used for urinary problems, including infections such as cystitis, stones and gravel.

It is indicated for foetid smelling urine and in cases of urinary difficulties of undefined causes. It is also indicated in respiratory and skin infections much like the herbal remedy.

Flower Essence
Nasturtium flower essence, like the herbal remedy, is warming, rejuvenating, refreshing and revitalising. It is particularly recommended for those who feel drained from excess mental activity, such as students and those whose careers demand concentrated intellectual work. Such people may become over-developed mentally and live too much in the head, lacking physical or emotional expression, and divorced from

many of the realities of daily life. Such imbalance may predispose to illness, immune dysfunction, coughs, colds and catarrh. Nasturtium brings balance between intellectual, emotional and physical activity. It restores emotional warmth, physical vitality and earthly practicality.

Edible Uses
The leaves and flowers are both edible, deliciously tangy and nutritious, being rich in iron, vitamin C, minerals and trace elements. The unripe seeds can be pickled with vinegar and spices to make a tangy condiment and garnish, a good substitute for capers. The flowers and leaves add piquancy to soups, and can be mixed like watercress in salads, used to make pesto and salsa verde, added to stir fries, omelettes, used on top of pizzas and crackers, and with their exotic hues of flaming coral, orange, yellow and magenta to decorate almost anything! They also make a pleasant tea.

Growing
Nasturtiums are very easy and rewarding to grow from seed and will thrive best in poor soil. If they are grown in soil that is too rich, they will produce lovely healthy leaves but sadly few flowers. Although perennial in the tropics, in temperate regions they grow as annuals, flowering until the first frosts of autumn. They make excellent companion plants in the vegetable garden to grow with beans as they attract aphids.

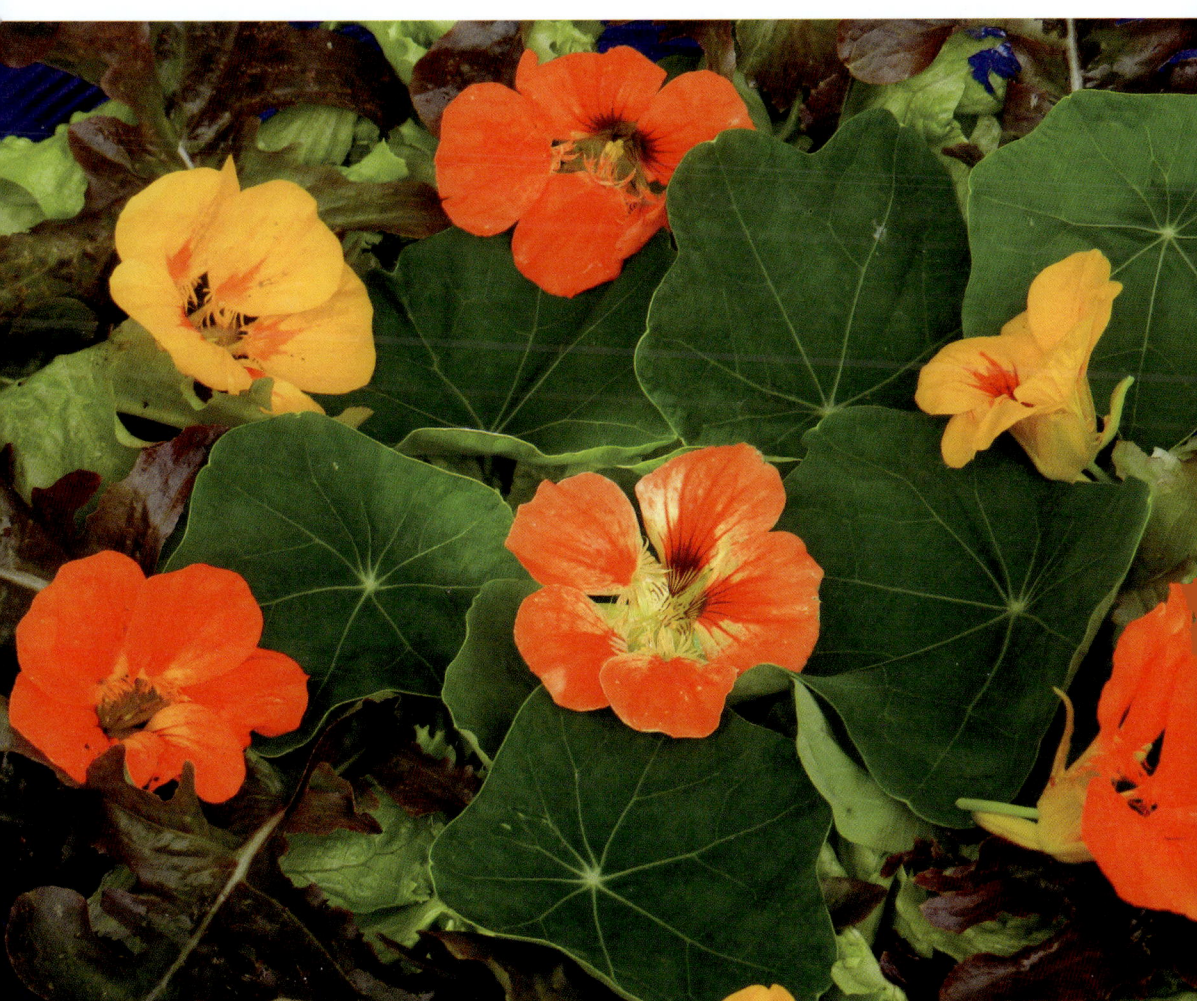

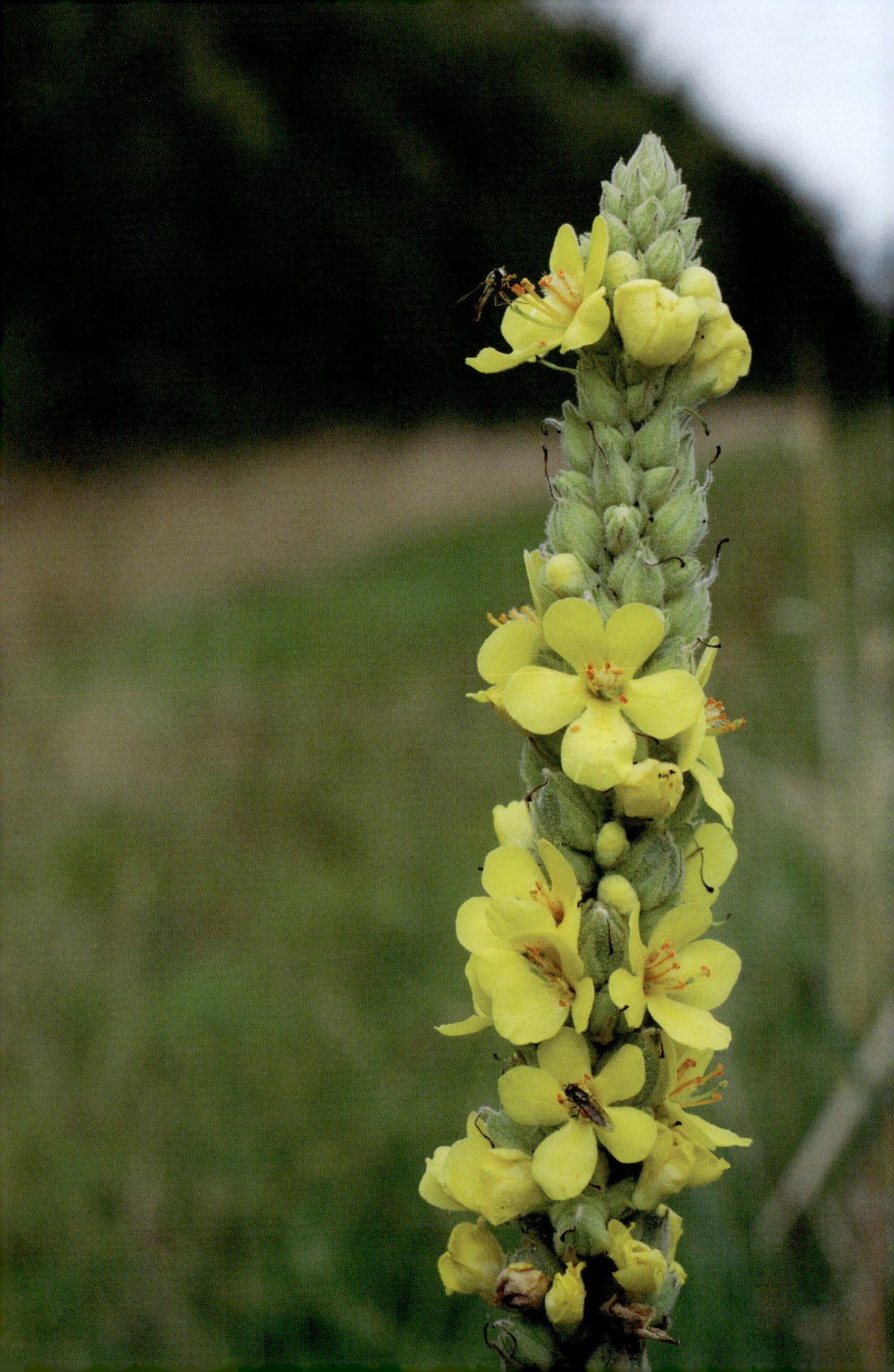

Verbascum thapsus: Mullein

The Flower of Light

> *By thy woodside railing, reeves*
> *with antique mullein's flannel leaves*
> *These, though mean, the flowers of waste,*
> *Planted here in nature's haste*
> *Display to the discerning eye,*
> *Her loved, wild variety*
> – John Clare (1793–1864)

Other Names: Aaron's rod, hag's taper, Jacob's staff, witches' candle, beggar's blanket, candlewick plant, torches, velvet dock, flannel plant, feltwort, shepherd's staff

Parts Used: Leaves, flowers and root

Mullein is an impressive biennial member of the Scrophulariaceae family with tall spikes of yellow flowers, native to Europe, Asia and N Africa. The word *mullein* comes from the Middle English 'moleyne' and the old French 'moleine' and originally from the Latin 'mollis' all meaning soft, as this stately biennial has large soft downy leaves which are covered in little hairs. The name *Verbascum* is probably a corruption of the Latin 'barbascum' meaning a bearded plant, while *thapsus* may refer to the Greek island of that name where the plant originally thrived.

The woolly leaves were once used by poor country people to line their shoes, to keep their feet warm in the winter and to protect them on rough ground, hence the other names 'Adam's blanket', 'flannel plant', 'velvet plant', and 'beggar's blanket'. In the language of flowers, mullein symbolises comfort. This may be because of the comfort it gave to the feet, or for the soothing nature of its action when used medicinally for irritation and inflammation in the respiratory and urinary systems, and its painkilling properties.

Mullein often grows to over 5 feet (1.5 metres) tall and has a solitary upright stem in its second year covered with pale yellow flowers. The stem encloses a thin rod of white pith, which gave rise to such names as 'Aaron's rod' and 'Jacob's staff'. The down on the leaves and stem burn easily when dry and were used as tapers or candles as far back as Roman times, when the plant was known as 'candelaria'.

Since the days of the ancient Greeks, mullein has been used to protect against infection, evil spirits and witches. In the Greek myths, Ulysses was said to have used mullein to protect himself against the sorcery of Circe. In ancient Rome, torches made from mullein were carried in ceremonial processions.

Mullein was grown in monastery gardens to keep out the devil and it was carried on journeys as a talisman of safety. This ability to protect against the forces of darkness was another way mullein was used to provide light, or to light one's path like a candle. It was used in dream pillows to prevent nightmares and hung in doorways for protection. Mullein was also said to be used by witches during their rituals and was called 'witch's candle' and 'Hag's taper'. Candles made from the dried stalks are used in Samhain ceremonies to honour the dead. 'Hag' is a word from Anglo-Saxon 'hoege' or 'hage' meaning 'hedge', so the name 'Hag's taper' may not refer to witches at all but simply to the fact that mullein with its stem of yellow flowers resembled a lighted taper. It was also used in love potions.

In Elizabethan times, mullein leaves were carried to ward off epileptic attacks and water was distilled from the flowers as a remedy for gout. Mullein used to be cultivated widely in Ireland for its efficacy in treating TB and the leaves used to be smoked to relieve irritating coughs. In America, the leaves were used a tobacco substitute and smoked ritually by Native American tribes. They also boiled the leaves and applied them to painful joints and to the head to relieve headaches. It is still believed in some cultures that the smoke from the plant can drive away ghosts from children.

Herbal Remedy
Mullein has a combination of bitter, astringent, sweet tastes and contains flavonoids including methylguercitin, luteolin, hesperedin and verbascoside with antioxidant and anti-inflammatory actions and phenylethanoid glycosides which have anti-inflammatory, antioxidant and antiviral properties. It also contains saponins which have anti-inflammatory, pain-relieving and antitumour properties, iridoid glycosides including harpagoside; harpagide and aucubin (especially in the leaf) with anti-inflammatory actions, polysaccharides (verbascose, heptaose, octaose) and mucilage with soothing prebiotic actions. The volatile and fixed oils have antimicrobial properties. Other constituents include sterones, sesquiterpene acid, tannins, resins and lignan glycosides.

Mullein has cooling and soothing properties and makes an excellent remedy for the respiratory system. The saponins have an expectorant action helping to clear phlegm from the chest, the iridoid glycosides and flavonoids decrease inflammation, the mucilage is cooling and soothing while the tannins help to protect the lining of the respiratory tract from irritation, inflammation and infection and have a drying effect, useful for excess mucous.

Mullein has antibacterial activity against bacteria including *Klebsiella pneumonia, Staphylococcus aureus, Staphylococcus epidermidis* and *Escherichia coli*. It also has antiviral action against *Influenza* viruses A2 and B as well as *Herpes simplex*. These benefits contribute to make mullein a wonderful medicine for almost all respiratory problems, including harsh, irritating and dry coughs, as well as chronic catarrh, sinusitis and hay fever. It is used for irritated and inflamed conditions of the respiratory tract such as sore throats, hoarseness, pharyngitis, tracheitis, bronchitis and bronchiectasis. Its relaxing and painkilling effects in the chest are helpful in tight chests, asthma, croup, whooping cough and pleurisy, while its antimicrobial action is helpful for combatting respiratory infections. It has been used for centuries for pneumonia, bronchitis, and tuberculosis. The leaves used to be smoked to relieve irritating coughs and asthma.

With its antimicrobial properties to enhance the efforts of the immune system to ward off infection and its anti-inflammatory actions, mullein can help relieve pain of swollen glands and mumps. Taken as a hot infusion mullein can also be used to bring down fevers.

Mullein has sedative and analgesic effects, and the seeds have narcotic properties. The dried leaves used to be smoked for mental relaxation. As a pain-killer, mullein can be used for headaches, migraines and neuralgia, and painful inflammatory conditions such as arthritis. The relaxant and analgesic properties, especially of the flowers, help to encourage restful sleep, particularly for those disturbed by coughing and pain.

Mullein is used specifically for pain in the ears and can be applied as an infused oil locally as well as taken internally for catarrhal deafness and tinnitus, ear infections, wax accumulation and head pain caused by congestion in the ears. Mullein can also relieve tension and anxiety and has a history of use for nervous palpitations, heart irregularities, cramp and nervous colic. A decoction of the root was an old remedy to relieve toothache, cramps and convulsions.

Mullein's astringent tannins have a toning effect in the gut, while the mucilage is very soothing, making it useful for treating diarrhoea, particularly when it is related to nerves. With its antimicrobial and vermicidal actions, mullein can be helpful in gut infections, for disturbance of the gut flora, leaky gut syndrome and for treating worms and parasites. Verbascose, an oligosaccharide in the root of the mullein acts as a prebiotic supporting the beneficial bacteria in the gut. The whole plant can be used to treat diarrhoea and dysentery, as well as inflammatory gut problems. As a soothing diuretic, mullein can be used for burning and frequency of urination in cystitis, and for fluid retention. By increasing elimination of toxins and uric acid via the kidneys and with its anti-inflammatory actions, it is useful in treatment of arthritis and gout.

Externally a compress or poultice made with mullein leaves can be applied to painful arthritic joints and aching muscles, and used to speed healing of wounds, burns, sores, ulcers and haemorrhoids. The flowers have antifungal, antiviral and antibacterial actions and can be used for ringworm and other skin infections. The leaves can be applied to the chest for asthma, to the head for headaches and to the throat for sore throats, swollen glands and mumps. Mullein oil prepared from the flowers is an excellent antiseptic and can inhibit skin infections including *Klebsiella pneumoniae* and *Staphyloccocus aureus* and can be used as eardrops or massaged around the ears for earache and eczema of the outer ear.

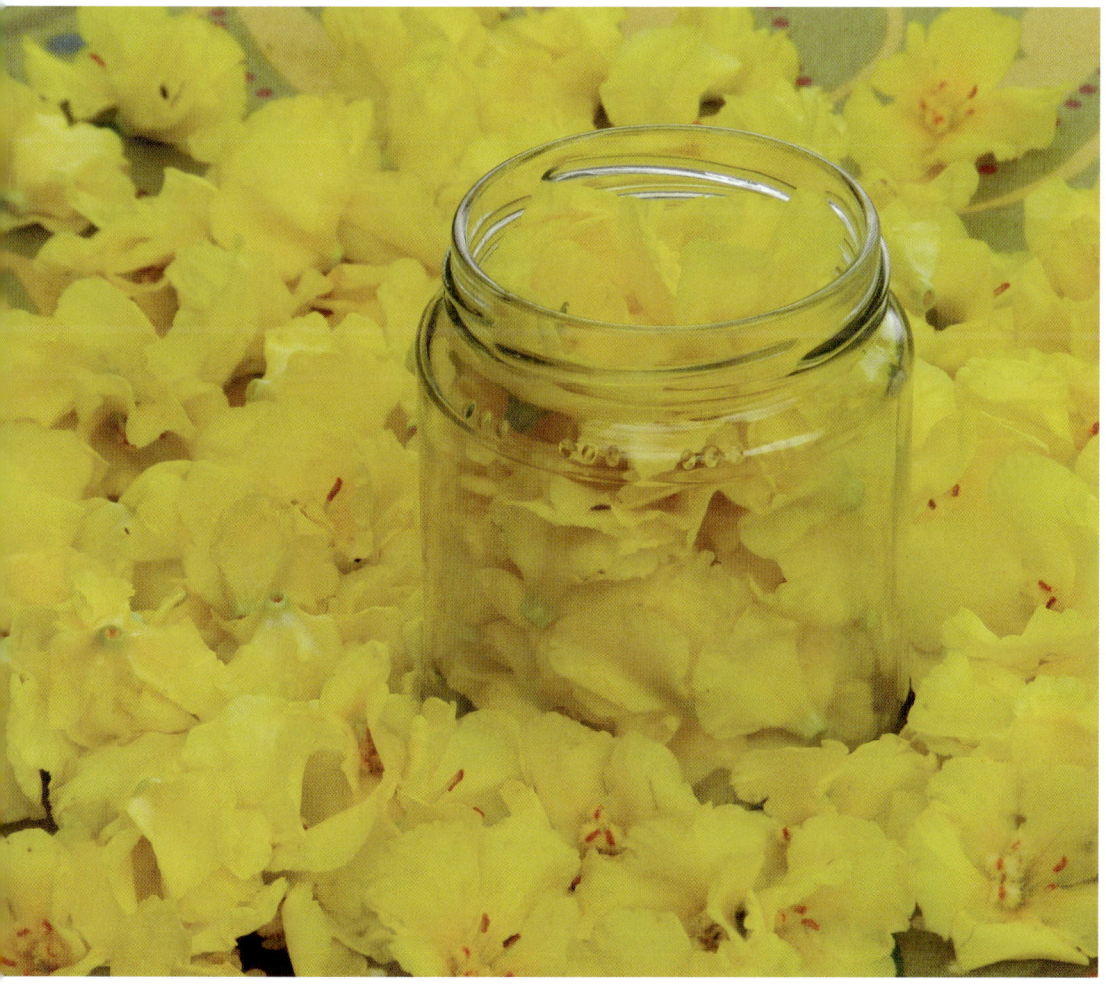

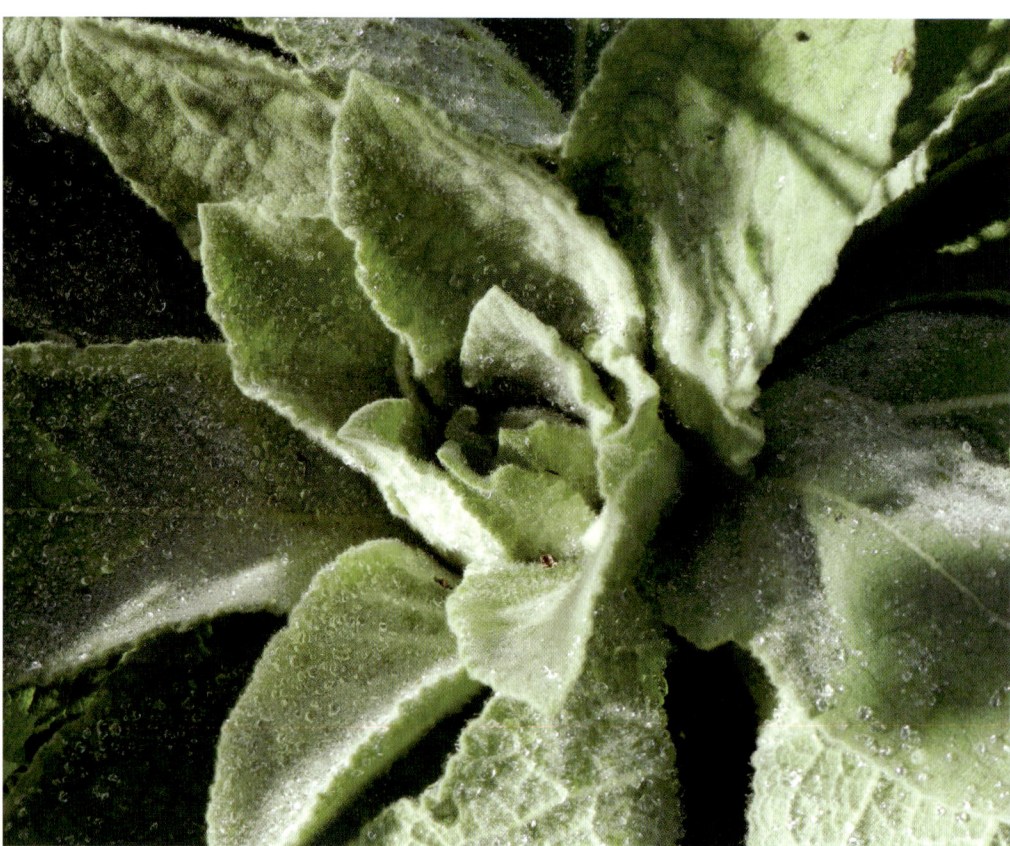

Homeopathic Remedy
As a homeopathic remedy, like the herbal remedy, Verbascum has a pronounced action on the ear, the respiratory system and the urinary system. It is prescribed for deafness as if the ear is blocked, and when getting water in the ears from swimming causes a blocked sensation. It will also relieve pain in the face (it affects the interior maxillary branch of the 5th cranial nerve), and facial neuralgia that recurs periodically, with lightning pain, as if crushed with tongs. It is also for catarrh and colds when associated with neuralgia on the left side of the face. The pain is worse with changes of temperature, pressure and motion, as in talking and sneezing.

Verbascum can also be used for hoarseness, and deep hollow coughs that sound like a trumpet, for tickling in the larynx and chest, catarrh, asthma, colds, nervous coughs, and coughing during sleep.

In the urinary system, Verbascum will relieve cystitis symptoms, burning and dribbling urination, frequency of urination through nervousness, and bedwetting. It can also be used effectively for piles, and irritating conditions of the genitals. A Verbascum person may feel morose or apathetic, suffer from a poor memory, ill-humour, and be easily distracted. They also have lively imaginations.

Flower Essence
Mullein again is the remedy of light, an inner light to guide us along our path. It is also a remedy for uprightness, honesty, moral conscience, particularly for those who feel weak or confused, unable to tune into their inner voice, or who are wrestling with their conscience. It is helpful when needing inner strength to withstand social pressures or trends, tempting one to lie either to oneself or to others, and to help sort out moral values. It can be taken for indecision, to clarify or

hear better your inner voice, or to be guided by your inner light, and thus lead towards a greater fulfilment of your true potential. Mullein helps you to be true to yourself.

Growing
Propagate by sowing seed in autumn in well-drained, fertile soil. Press or water the seeds into the soil. In the first year, mullein grows a large rosette of woolly leaves and the flowers arrive the next season. Self-seeds readily. The plant may attract caterpillars of mullein moth which can devour most of the leaves. Grows 1–6 feet tall (30cm–2m) and flowers June to August.

Cautions
Contact with leaves may cause skin irritation.

Recipe

Mullein Flower and Garlic Oil for Earache
This is a wonderful and effective natural remedy for ear infections, which can be used by adults and children alike. It can relieve the pain quickly and helps combat the infection.

2–3 teaspoons garlic, chopped
2–3 teaspoons dried mullein flowers
Extra virgin olive oil

Place the garlic and dried mullein flowers in a *bain marie*/double boiler. Add enough olive oil to cover the herbs. Warm for 1–2 hours over a low heat, strain through a fine wire mesh strainer or muslin/cheese cloth. Label clearly and store in a tightly covered glass jar in the refrigerator. Transfer into dropper bottles for use.

Warm the oil to body temperature by placing the dropper bottle in a cup of hot water. Put 3 to 4 drops in each ear and massage the outer ear and around the base of the ear with some of the oil. Put a cotton ball gently into the ear to catch the excess oil. Re-apply every 30 minutes or as often as needed for relief in acute infection.

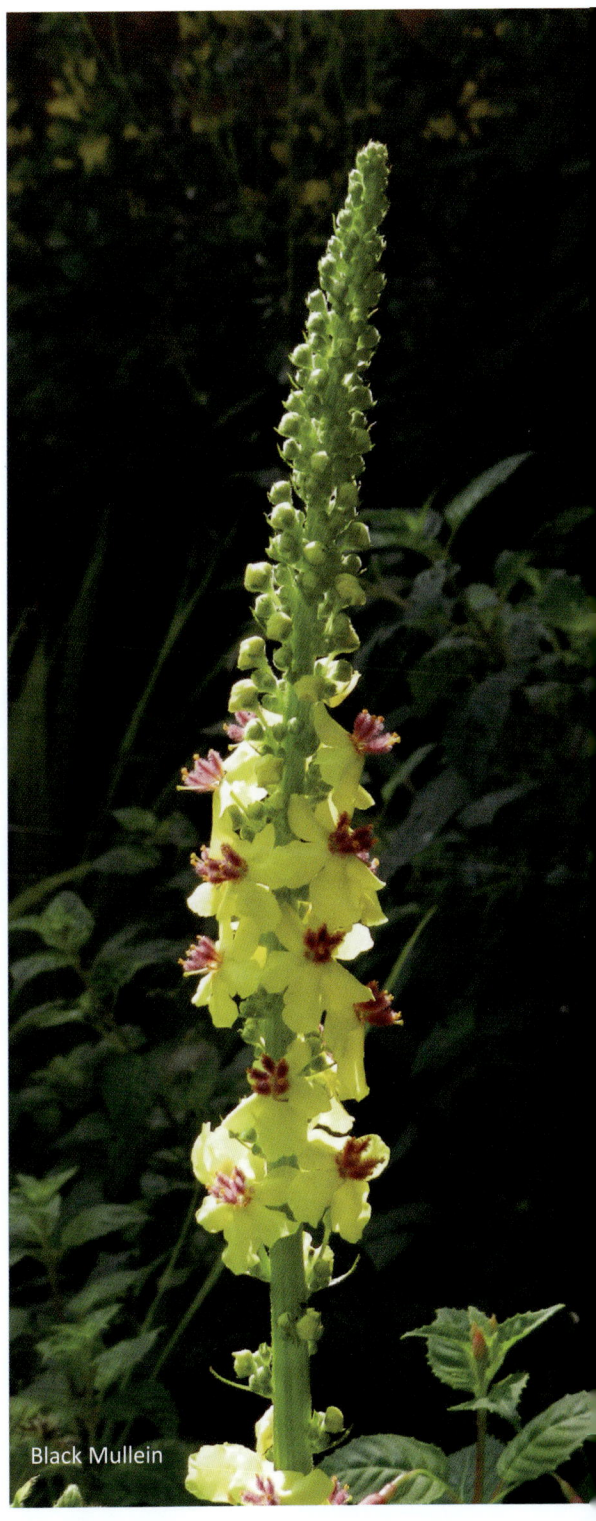
Black Mullein

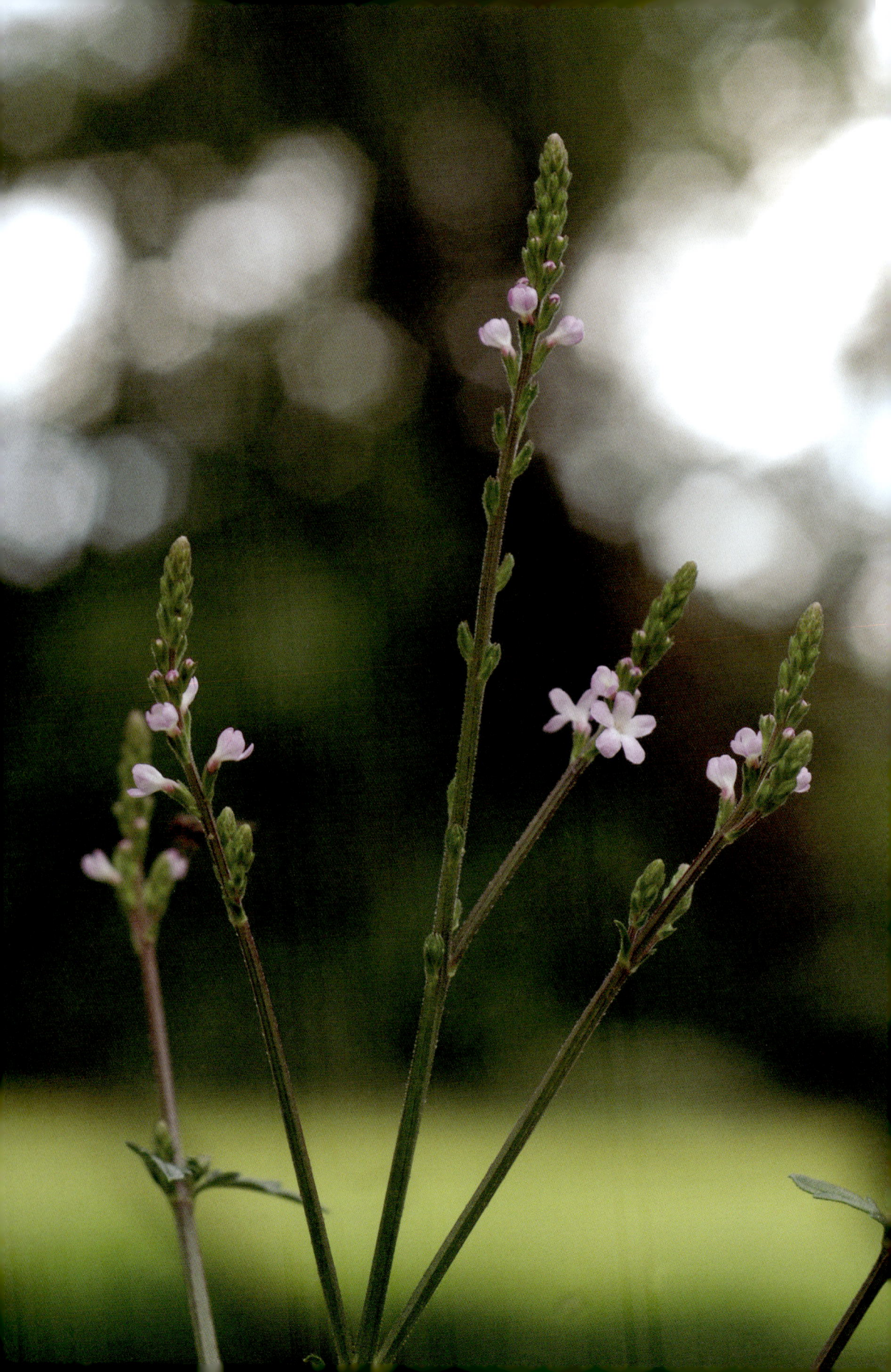

Verbena officinalis: Vervain

The Flower of Magic

Trefoil, vervain, John's wort, dill,
Hinders witches of their will
– Sir Walter Scott (1771–1832)

Other names: Enchanter's plant, herb of enchantment, herb of grace, Indian hyssop, holy herb, simpler's joy, blue vervain, herb-of-the-cross, Juno's tears, pigeon's grass, pigeonweed, wild hyssop, iron weed, wild verbena

Parts used: Leaves and flowers

Vervain is a modest little member of the Verbenaceae family, found growing wild in Britain, central and southern Europe and Asia along roadsides and lanes and on waste ground. It is a hardy perennial with pretty rather understated lilac-coloured flowers on slender spikes and is cultivated extensively in France and other European countries where vervain tea is very popular. Despite the inconspicuous nature of its flowers, vervain was the foremost magical herb of antiquity. It was considered sacred, a wizard's herb for casting spells and a vital ingredient of magic potions. It was important for spells, divination, magic, medicine and for amulets to protect against witchcraft and evil. The Druids cleansed their altars with an infusion of vervain before offering sacrifices, they held it in as high esteem as mistletoe and probably introduced it to the Romans who used it to crown ambassadors and similar dignitaries. The Romans made it into bundles for ritual cleansing and to sweep the altars to the gods, and in honour of this sacred plant, they even held an annual festival called 'verbenalia'.

With the coming of Christianity, vervain continued to be held sacred. It was said to have been discovered on Mount Calvary at the foot of the cross and used to staunch the bleeding from Christ's wounds. It was called 'the holy herb' and was crossed and blessed when gathered. In the Middle Ages, sorcerers and magicians endowed it with miraculous properties – it was believed to heal every wound received in battle and bring immortality to heroes.

At the end of the 16th century Mattiolus wrote, *"Sorcerers lose their senses at the mention of the herb. For they say that those who are rubbed with it will obtain all they ask, and that it will cure fevers, and cause a person to love another, and, in short, that it cures all illness and more besides."* Clearly it was seen as a panacea for all ills, and was used around this time for jaundice, kidney disease, the plague, heart disease, toothache, difficult pregnancies and childbirth. Culpeper said it was excellent for strengthening the womb, and that being hot and dry, it would open all obstructions, cleansing and healing as it went. Other apothecaries prescribed it for jaundice, kidney disease, difficulty in pregnancy, heart disease and the plague. Vervain tea was valued for its calming effect and was used to promote sleep and to treat 'over-enthusiasm' as described in the 1652 book *The English Physician*.

Culpeper also said that vervain was ruled by Venus, and in fact, the Romans had dedicated it to the goddess Venus, calling it 'Veneris Herba' meaning *herb of Venus*. They believed it could reignite the fires of dying love and worked as an aphrodisiac. It was picked by Roman brides to wear at their weddings and was also dedicated to Isis, the goddess of birth. At New Year, the Romans would exchange lucky nosegays of vervain and they also made infusions to sprinkle in banqueting halls to make their guests merrier. Later, in the Middle Ages, vervain entered into the preparation of most love philtres. A child who wore a sprig of vervain was said to be well-behaved, lively, good-humoured and a lover of knowledge.

Not only was vervain a sacred magical herb, and an emblem of love, but it was also a herb of protection. Chaplets of vervain were worn by Roman heralds-at-arms carrying messages of war to give them immunity from the enemy. The herald was called a 'verbenarius' and vervain was believed to ensure a peaceful settlement and used as a flag of truce between warring factions. The physicians of Myddfai recommended warriors to wear vervain to protect them when fighting.

Herbal Remedy
Vervain is a wonderful tonic to the nervous system and is a popular remedy for calming the nerves, easing tension and irritability and increasing resistance to stress. In the past it was famous as a remedy for nervous disorders, to stop nightmares and for epilepsy.

It has bitter and astringent tastes and contains iridoids (verbenin, verbenalin, bastatoside), phenylpropanoid glycosides, essential oils (citral), mucilage, vitamins (C, K), minerals (zinc, potassium, sulphur), tannins and bitters.

It is now known to have neuroprotective effects attributed to the flavonoids and tannins, protecting the brain and nervous system from the damaging effects of free radicals and oxidative stress. It can reduce anxiety and be used at night to relieve insomnia. Vervain may also prevent epileptic seizures, and this is related to the presence of iridoids called verbenalin and verbenin which are thought to have anticonvulsant properties.

Vervain can also be taken to lift depression and for stress-related problems such as headaches, migraines, nervous coughs, asthma, insomnia, high blood pressure and nervous exhaustion. It is particularly good for people who suffer from low self-esteem, workaholics and those who push themselves too hard – driven people who then have a tendency to burn themselves out and suffer from nervous exhaustion, headaches, migraines and inflammatory eye conditions.

Vervain has anti-inflammatory and analgesic effects which are attributed to the iridoid glycosides and it can be helpful in headaches and neuralgia. It also has an antispasmodic action which can ease muscle tension, pain and spasm, particularly when related to excess stress and lack of rest and relaxation. The phenylpropanoid glycosides in vervain have a significant antioxidant action and neuroprotective action, and contribute to improving the resilience of the nervous system and the immune system. The glycoside verbenalin, also known as cornin, may improve brain damage after a stroke by promoting the development of new blood vessels in the brain. This may improve mitochondrial function in the brain; mitochondria are responsible for energy production in each cell and require oxygen to do so. Verbenalin may also protect against the loss of brain cells in Alzheimer's disease by reducing the accumulation of beta-amyloid plaques.

Vervain can be thought of when stress appears to contribute to nervous exhaustion, depleted immunity and symptoms of this including neuralgia, shingles and post viral fatigue. It has antimicrobial actions, and may be effective against bacterial infections including *Staphylococcus aureus*, *Pseudomonas aeruginosa* and *Citrobacter freundii*. Taken in hot infusion, vervain acts as a diaphoretic to increase sweating, helping to clear toxins and bring down fevers.

Vervain's calming effect on the nervous system can be helpful in bringing down blood pressure and for nervous palpitations. Its antispasmodic action can relax blood vessels and improve blood flow through the coronary arteries in the heart and can be helpful in stopping leg cramps. The antioxidant actions attributed to the flavonoids and verbenalin or cornin, help to protect against cardiovascular disease by preventing free radical damage to the arteries and the build-up of cholesterol and its anticoagulant action can help to prevent blood clots.

A good digestive herb, vervain enhances appetite, digestion and absorption. It is particularly good for stress-related digestive problems, cooling heat and inflammation in the stomach and small intestine and relieving heartburn and acidity. The bitters help regulate the liver, making it a useful tonic for problems related to a sluggish liver, including constipation, lethargy, depression, headaches and irritability. It has been used for liver disorders and gallstones and to speed recovery and increase energy during convalescence. The astringent tannins aid the resilience of the gut wall to irritation, inflammation and infection and help to stop diarrhoea, while the anti-inflammatory and antimicrobial effects may help in gastritis and peptic ulcers as well as inflammatory gut problems.

The antioxidant constituents in vervain may provide further benefit particularly in relation to the immune system. The phenylpropanoid glycosides (verbenosides A and B), triterpenoids and essential oils may help inhibit tumour growth and induce the death of cancerous cells. Additionally, citral in the essential oil has anticancer as well as antimicrobial activities and the flavonoids may have an antibacterial action.

In cool infusion, vervain has a diuretic as well as an antimicrobial effect and is used in oedema, cystitis and irritable bladder. It has a long reputation for preventing kidney stones and gravel. By aiding elimination of toxins and excess uric acid via the kidneys, vervain acts to detoxify and this can be helpful in the treatment of arthritis and gout.

Vervain has an affinity for the female reproductive system. It is an effective uterine sedative and tonic and can be used to regulate periods and to ease painful periods. It is used for cramping with bearing down pain, back and thigh pain (in acute cases), endometriosis, threatened or repeated miscarriages and to prepare for labour. It is also a good herb to take during childbirth to regulate contractions. It helps prevent uterine irritability, over-strong contractions, false labour pains and after-pains. Vervain has long been used as a galactagogue to enhance milk supply in feeding mothers and to clear toxins from the milk. Its cooling and astringent properties can help prevent excessive menstrual flow and hot flushes during the menopause. It is a good remedy for

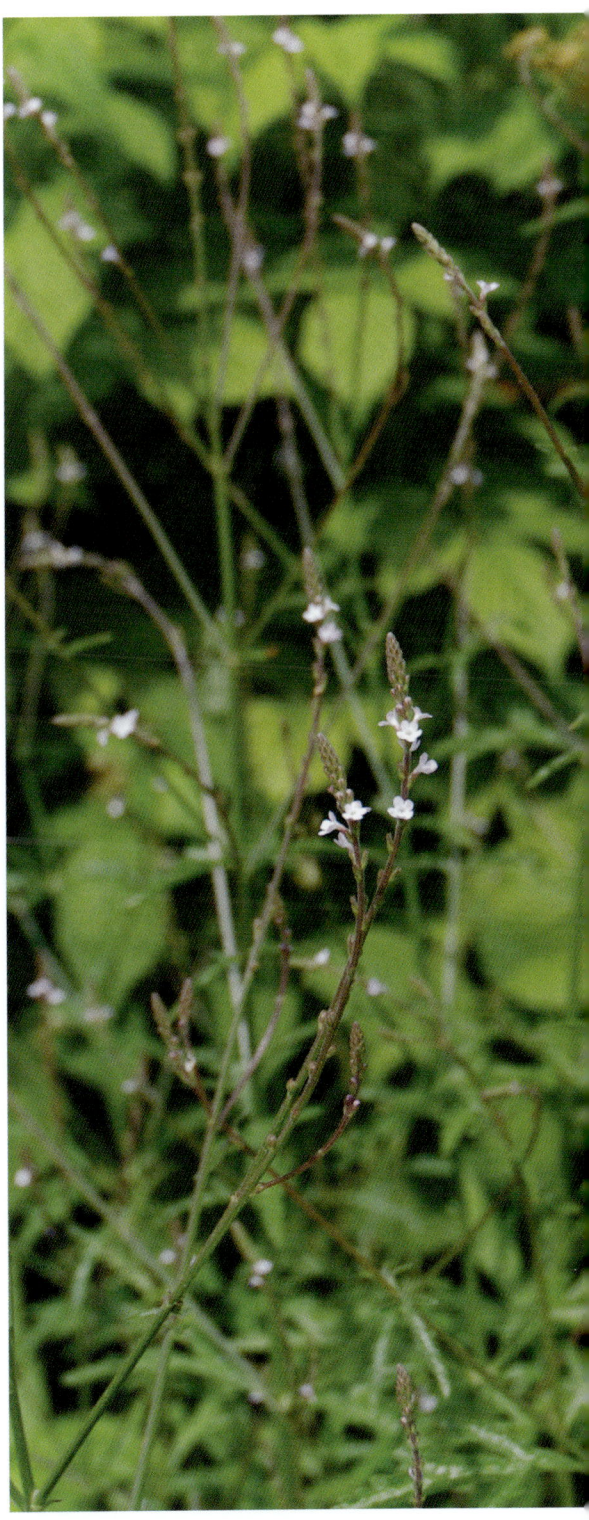

menstrual migraines and can be used for benign prostatic hypertrophy as an antispasmodic.

In Traditional Chinese Medicine, vervain is widely used for clearing heat and toxins, promoting blood circulation and removing stasis, promoting diuresis and clearing dampness. In America, relatives of *Verbena officinalis* are used; *Verbena sticta*, hoary vervain is used for an upset stomach and *Verbena hastata*, also with a blue flower, is helpful in coughs, urinary stones and gravel, worms, bruises and skin problems. The latter had tonic properties and was traditionally used for nervous problems and epilepsy.

Externally, the tannins in vervain make it a useful antiseptic astringent when used as a mouthwash for bleeding gums and mouth ulcers, and as a gargle for sore throats and tonsillitis. As a skin lotion it has antiseptic, anti-inflammatory and analgesic effects attributed to the iridoid glycosides and can be used for skin infections as well as sores and wounds, ulcers, burns and insect bites.

Aromatherapy Oil
Vervain essential oil has many similar uses to vervain as a herbal remedy. It can be used in burners and the bath for colds, coughs, catarrh and other respiratory problems including hay fever and asthma. It has an anti-inflammatory action and can help to reduce inflammation involved in allergies and infections which can cause excess mucus and restrict breathing.

Vervain oil also has an analgesic effect that can be helpful in nerve pain and neuralgia as well as headaches and migraines when used in massage oils. Its anti-inflammatory effects can also help to relieve pain as in muscle or joint pain and also pain caused by injuries such as sprains or strains. Vervain oil can also benefit the brain as described in the use of the herbal remedy.

When applied to the skin in a carrier oil, verbena oil with its antimicrobial actions will help prevent infections in cuts and wounds and speed healing. It can protect against antibiotic-resistant bacteria such as MRSA and fungal infections.

Homeopathic Remedy
The blue vervain, *Verbena hastata,* which is indigenous to America, is employed as a tincture. It is also prescribed for nervous disorders – depression, anxiety, tension, epilepsy, muscle tension and spasm, insomnia and mental exhaustion. It helps to calm over-excitability and brighten mental powers in those nervously run down and exhausted.

Like the herbal remedy, verbena is used to reduce fevers and as a diuretic to clear toxins from the system which contribute to skin problems, and to aid elimination during treatment for TB. It promotes the absorption of blood, and so helps allay the pain of bruises. It is also used for Rhus poisoning.

Flower Essence
Vervain is a Bach Flower Remedy for charismatic people with huge resources of energy, which can be a great inspiration to others. They can be full of enthusiasm and idealism and by radiating their enormous energy, they have a great capacity for leading and healing others.

Vervain people tend to espouse themselves to causes or get involved in charitable works and welfare organisations. Their commitment to their work or ideals can lead them to sacrifice all their energy and time to further their cause. It can take over their lives, and they are unable to rest or relax, feeling the need to win those around them to their viewpoint and expend all their energy in the process. They have enormous willpower and, often being revolutionaries at heart, are prepared to suffer for their convictions. They have great courage and are not afraid to speak out although this, combined with their over-enthusiastic, domineering, overzealous attitude, can actually be detrimental to their cause. Such people are often seen as overbearing, over-intense, even fanatical. They rarely deviate from their firm principles, convinced as they are of the rightness and urgency of their cause.

In this condition, vervain people overuse their energy resources, being constantly on the job, and never giving in to messages from their body or inner selves to rest. This can lead eventually to

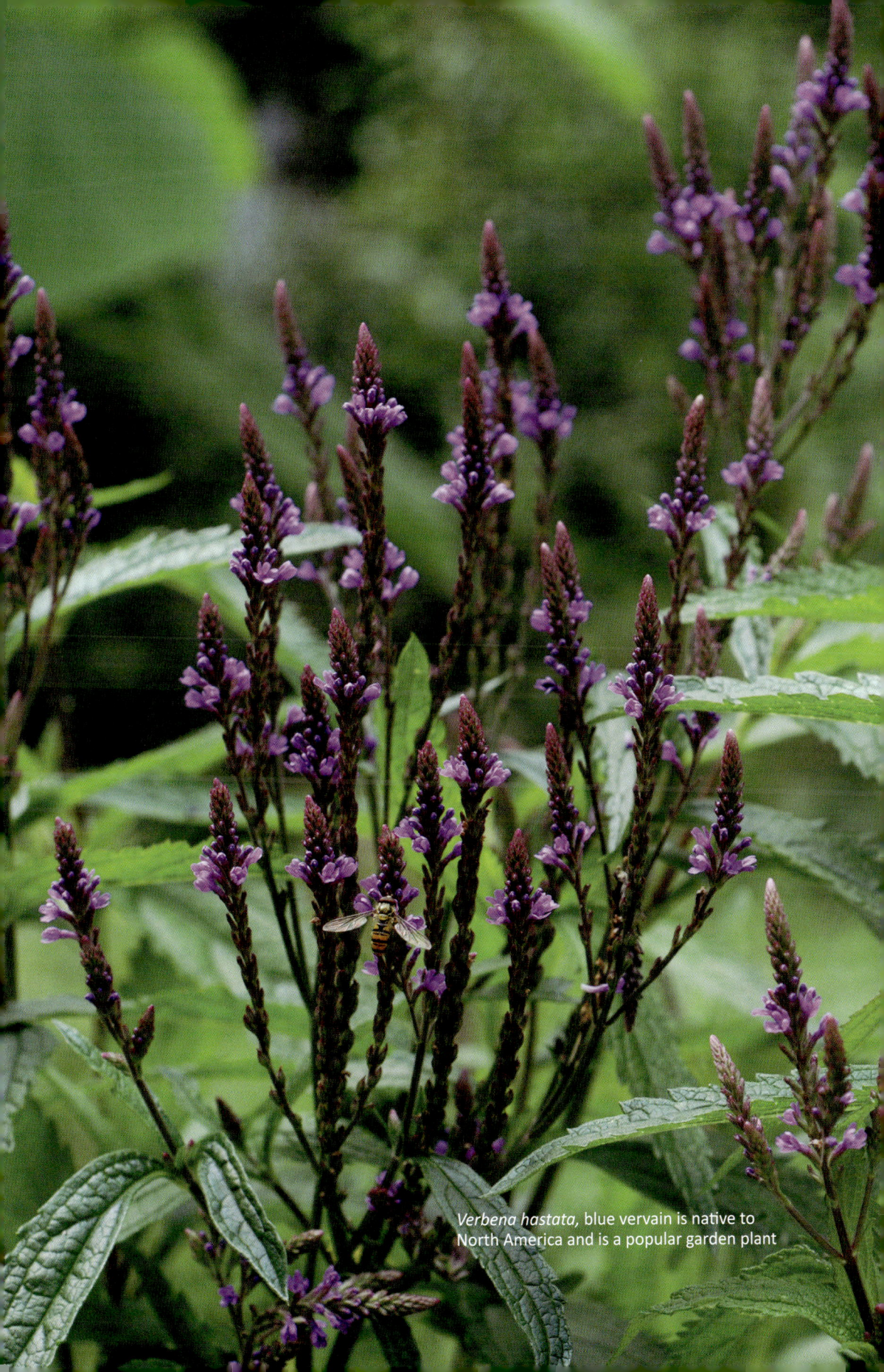

Verbena hastata, blue vervain is native to North America and is a popular garden plant

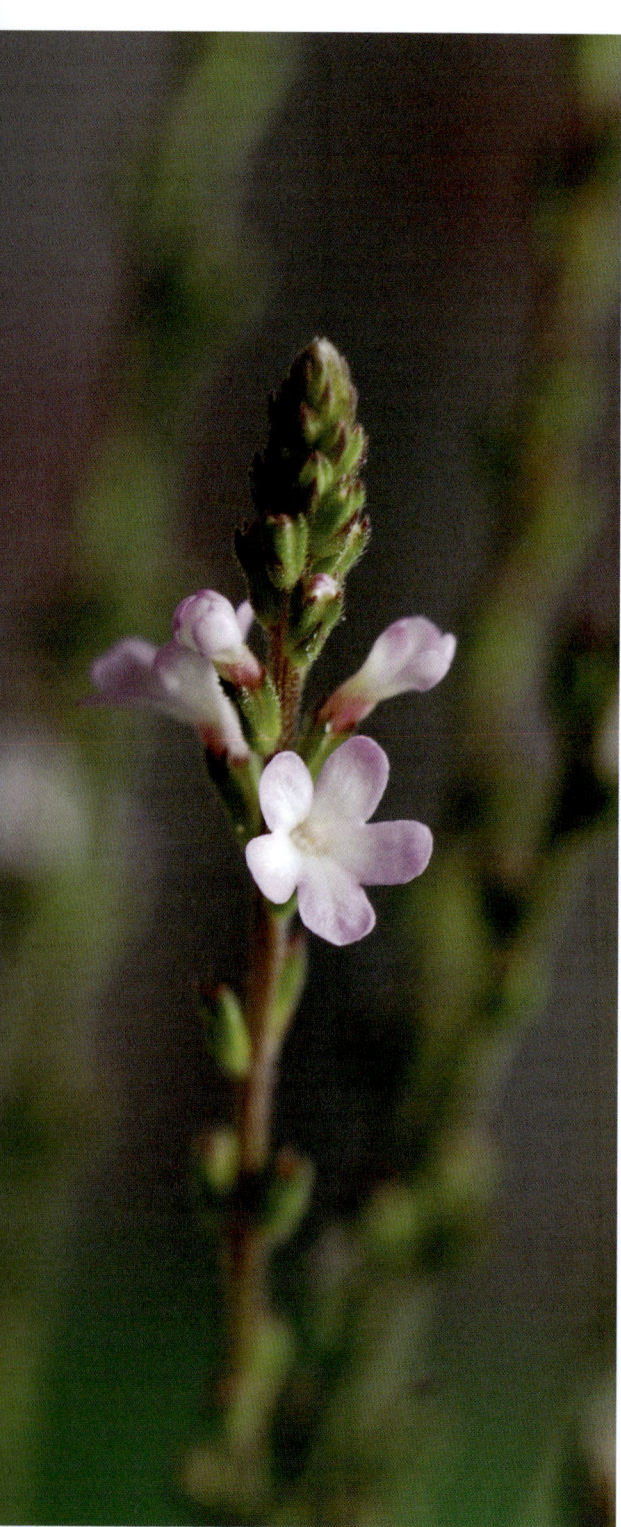

nervous exhaustion. They live on their nerves and become so keyed up they cannot relax even if they want to. Their tense, nervous natures often lead to digestive problems. As they are often intolerant and angry, they become progressively more depleted. This may inevitably culminate in a nervous breakdown.

Vervain helps these people to use their huge resources of energy in a more natural way. Dr Bach said, 'Vervain teaches us that it is by being rather than doing that great things are accomplished'.

It engenders a calm and open attitude to the ideas of others and allows their exuberance to be an inspiration to others. It helps towards a more balanced and harmonious life, treading the Middle Path.

Edible Uses
Vervain is popular in France as a bitter tisane. The flowers are also used as a garnish in cocktails and alcoholic beverages.

Growing
Vervain has pretty but small lilac-coloured flowers on slender spikes and can be grown in pots or in clumps in the garden. It looks attractive grown by marshmallow and white echinacea.

It will grow easily on most soils and likes full sun to partial shade. Propagate by sowing seeds in spring/autumn on the surface of well-drained soil in full sun. Press or water in the seeds. Grows 1–3' (30– 90cm) and flowers July – September. Self-seeds easily. Harvest leaves and flowers just as the flowers come out.

Cautions
Avoid in pregnancy. May cause contact dermatitis. Take away from mineral supplements. Avoid with anticoagulants and Warfarin. Vervain should be avoided by people with kidney disease and anaemia as it may inhibit iron absorption. The verbenalin found in the plant may irritate the kidneys if overused, causing inflammation.

Recipes

Cooling Stomach Tea
1 part Meadowsweet
1 part Marshmallow leaves and flowers
1 part Lemon balm
1 part Chamomile
½ part Vervain

Place herbs together in a teapot and pour over boiling water. Leave to infuse for 20 minutes. Mix 1 dessertspoonful of aloe vera juice per cup of tea and take a cupful 3–4 times daily before meals.

Marshmallow is a wonderfully soothing remedy for irritation and inflammation in the digestive tract. Meadowsweet is the most renowned herbal antacid while vervain and chamomile are cooling and calming, excellent for stress-related digestive disorders. The combination also has antimicrobial properties, helping to combat infection such as *Helicobacter pylori* that could be causing the problem.

Calming Tea
On a busy and stressful day, we might feel the need to sip a calming tea or soak in a relaxing bath to release muscle tension and calm our anxious thoughts. This combination of relaxing herbs tastes and smell delicious, relaxes muscles, calms the nerves and will help soothe your troubles away!

Place equal parts of skullcap, chamomile, vervain, lemon balm and holy basil in a teapot. Pour over boiling water and leave to infuse for 10–15 minutes. Drink 3–6 cupfuls a day

Relaxing Bath
Pour a double strength infusion into a relaxing bath or use the fresh herbs tied in a bag. Place one or two handfuls of the herbs in a piece of muslin or cotton. Tie a string around the top to close the opening and hang it from the hot tap of the bath. Make sure that the strings of the bag are long enough so that the bag soaks in the bath water once the bath is filled. Soak for 15–30 minutes for best effects.

Foot Bath for Tiredness and Exhaustion
Place equal parts of vervain, rosemary, skullcap, lemon balm and holy basil in a large teapot (50g per 500ml of water).

Pour over boiling water and leave to infuse for about half an hour. Pour into a bowl large enough for your feet, check the temperature is right and then soak your feet for 10–15 minutes.

These invigorating herbs will give you renewed energy if you are feeling tired, low or need to wake yourself up.

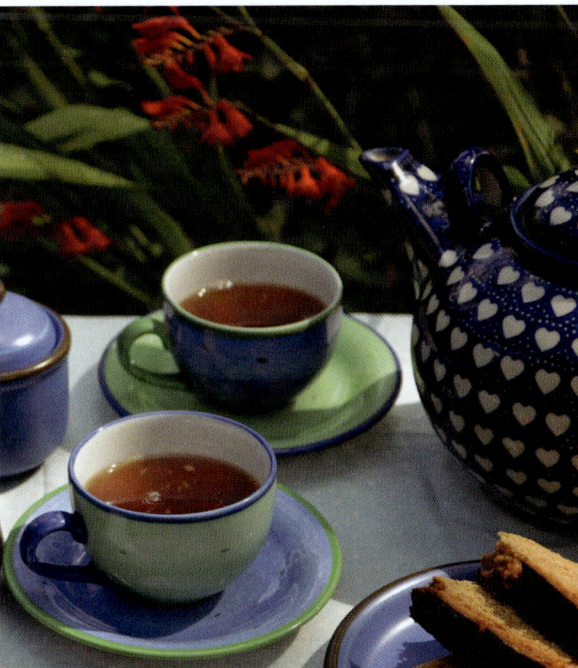

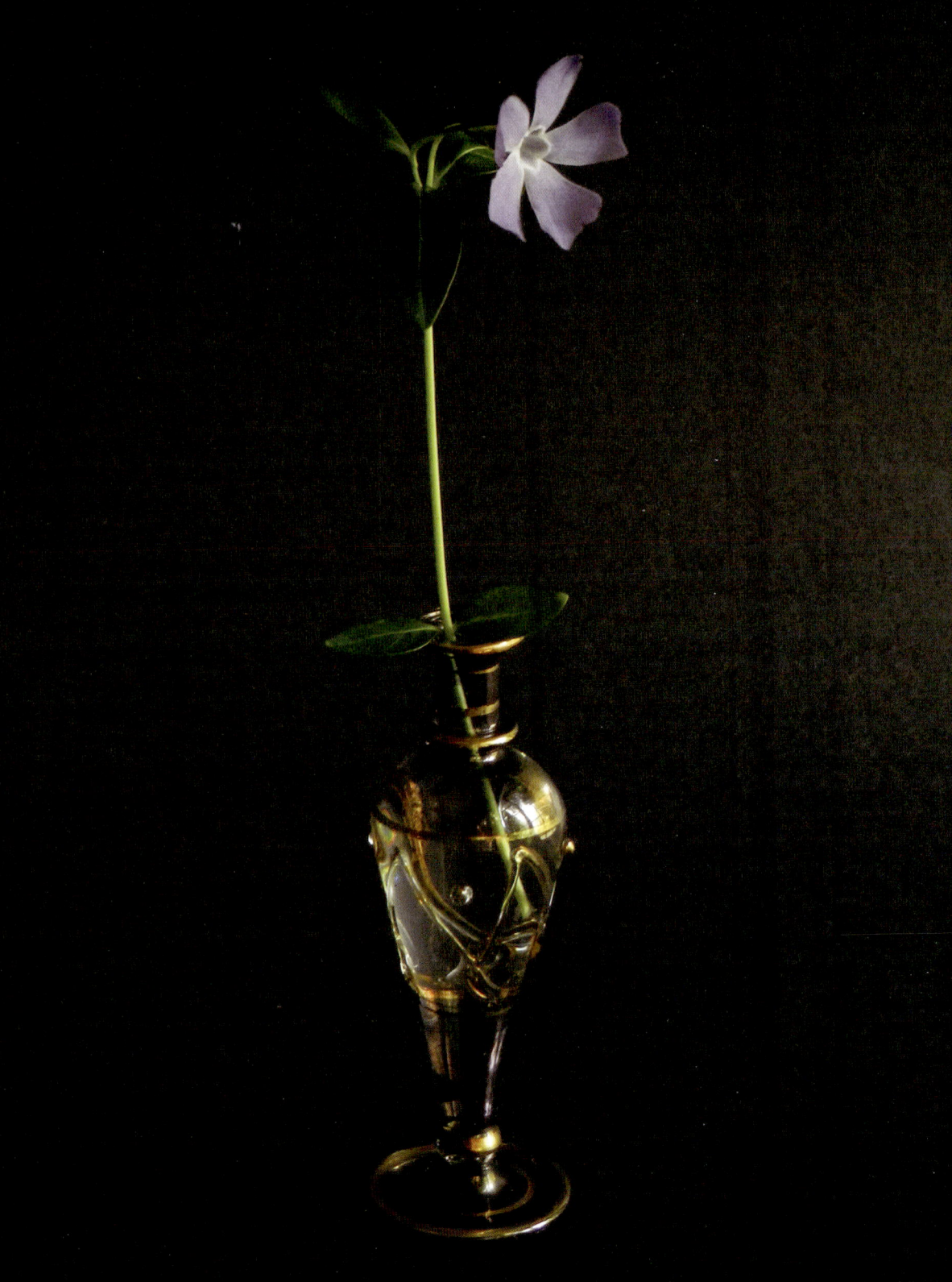

Vinca minor: Lesser Periwinkle

The Flower of Closeness

Through primrose tufts, in that green bower,
The periwinkle trailed its wreaths;
And 'tis my faith that every flower
Enjoys the air it breathes
– William Wordsworth (1770–1850)

Other Names: Blue periwinkle, joy of the ground, common periwinkle, early flowering, evergreen, myrtle, small periwinkle, Vinca pervinca, violette des morts, serpent's violet, running myrtle, blue buttons, devil's eye, sorcerer's violet, wintergreen.

Parts Used: Leaves, stems and flowers

The periwinkle with its lovely soft blue windmill-shaped flowers and shining leaves makes good ground cover in winter, earning its common name 'joy of the ground'. It is a hardy evergreen member of the Apocynaceae family, indigenous to Europe as far as the Caucasus and has been naturalised in many parts of the world. It can be found growing wild in woodlands, banks and hedgerows and is a close relative of cultivated silver-variegated form as well as the greater periwinkle *Vinca major*.

The name *periwinkle* comes from its old Latin name '*Vinca pervinca*' which came from 'pervincine' meaning to bind closely or from 'pervincere' meaning to overcome. Certainly, periwinkle has a binding nature; its long creeping stems resembling cord bind themselves together and bind to neighbouring plants and according to the doctrine of signatures, this indicated it had a binding quality. Its binding properties were also used to stop diarrhoea and dysentery and to staunch bleeding of cuts and wounds.

The ancient Greek physician Dioscorides recommended that '*the leaves be drunk in wine to lessen excessive discharges of the bowels*' (dysentery) and says that '*it cures the pain of the matrix*' (womb). Pliny (77AD) and Galen (130–210AD) recommended periwinkles for bleeding, diarrhoea, to heal wounds and as an antidote to bites by poisonous animals when taken with wine. Culpeper aptly described the medicinal virtues of periwinkle when he said it is a *"great binder and stays bleeding at the mouth and nose, if it be chewed. It is a good female medicine and may be used with advantage in hysterical and other fits."*

The binding uses of periwinkle extended further. It used to be bound to the legs to overcome cramp, to the skin to stop bleeding of cuts and wounds and when fastened around the thigh of a pregnant woman, it was believed to prevent miscarriage. It was made into a pessary or suppository to relieve the pain of the mother (uterus). It was also placed under the pillows of small children to ease cramps and teething pains. Lord Bacon testified to periwinkle's efficacy for cramp by using it successfully himself. The flowers and leaves used to be chewed to stop bleeding in the mouth and nose and to relieve toothache.

Culpeper said the periwinkle was ruled by Venus and that if the leaves were eaten by a man and woman together, it would bind them closer. The whole plant was considered a vital ingredient of love philtres and recipes to guarantee a happy marriage; the ancient sage Albertus Magnus described periwinkle as '*The most powerful flower for producing love*'. The flowers used to be strewed on the path of the bride and groom on their way to church for the wedding – the blue flowers to symbolise the virginity of the bride and the evergreen leaves for the everlasting love of the young couple. In the language of flowers, periwinkle means unbreakable friendship and tender memories. In Italy, plaited garlands of periwinkle were placed on the coffins of dead children and were known as 'flowers of death' as they symbolised immortality, eternity and tender memories of the lost loved one. This might be related to the relaxing and uplifting effect that periwinkle can have; the tea was used traditionally for grief, nervous conditions, hysteria as well as convulsions.

Periwinkle has for centuries played a part in magic practices and was commonly known as 'sorcerer's violet'. Thrown into a burning fire with other plants, it was said to cause apparitions of absent ones to form in the smoke. Periwinkle was considered the patron flower of the wicca, the wise folk of the villages and towns known for their healing skills and magic. It was said to banish all negativity and protect against evil. Apuleius in his Herbarium (printed in 1480) said of periwinkle *"This wort is of good advantage for many purposes, that is to say, first against devil sickness, and demoniacal possessions and against snakes and wild beasts and against poisons and for various wishes and for envy and for terror!"* The flowers used to be carried as amulets to bring love into one's life.

Herbal Remedy
As a herbal remedy periwinkle really does have a binding nature and stands up to its ancient reputation. It has a bitter and astringent taste and a drying and tightening quality. Its astringency is given by the tannins and its bitterness by more than 50 indole alkaloids in the leaves, flowers and root including reserpine, vincadine, vincine, vincamine, vincaminine vincristine, vinblastine, minovine and vincorine, vincamine being the most dominant. It also contains triterpenes (ursolic acid), an iridoid (loganic acid), phytosterols, phenolic acids, flavonoids, saponins, potassium and sodium salts and vitamin C. As *Vinca minor* and *major* are similar and are often used interchangeably, they are frequently classified together in publications and constituents listed are often the same. However, *Vinca minor* is the variety discussed here. The fresh flowers may have a laxative effect but lose this effect when they are dried. The root has antispasmodic effects and is used to lower blood pressure.

Periwinkle is an excellent astringent remedy used for drying excessive secretions. These could be heavy menstrual bleeding, excess mucus that accompanies respiratory infections and allergies as well as nosebleeds, diarrhoea and bleeding piles. Tannins tighten and tone tissues especially the skin and mucous membranes of the uterus and digestive tract and protect their linings from irritation, inflammation and infection.

In the digestive system, periwinkle's cooling and astringent properties can be used to reduce inflammation and stop bleeding, diarrhoea and dysentery as our ancestors knew. It makes a useful remedy for heartburn, gastritis, peptic ulcers, as well as inflammatory gut problems such as Crohn's disease and ulcerative colitis. It can help to tighten the junctions of the cell wall and regulate permeability, which is useful for treating leaky gut syndrome. In the reproductive system, the astringent tannins help to reduce excessive menstrual bleeding. They may dry up breast milk, so periwinkle should be avoided by breastfeeding mothers unless they are ready to wean.

Periwinkle had an ancient reputation as a brain tonic for nervous ailments. Today it can still be used for its benefits to the nervous system to relieve anxiety, lift depression and reduce symptoms of seasonal affective disorders (SAD). It helps to clear the mind and boost energy levels. Since the discovery of the indole alkaloid vincamine in the leaves in the 1950s, it is understood more about how periwinkle affects the brain. Vincamine increases the brain's uptake of oxygen and glucose and in this way enhances brain function and nutrition. Today it is used in pharmaceutical medicines as a cerebral stimulant and vasodilator for poor memory, behavioural disorders, speech disturbances, irritability, restlessness, dizziness and headaches.

Modern herbalists use the leaves, stems and flowers of periwinkle as a remedy similar to *Ginkgo biloba* to improve brain health. Both improve blood flow to the brain, supporting brain metabolism and improving mental acuity, memory and concentration and preventing problems arising from poor blood supply to the brain and cerebral arteriosclerosis. Periwinkle is

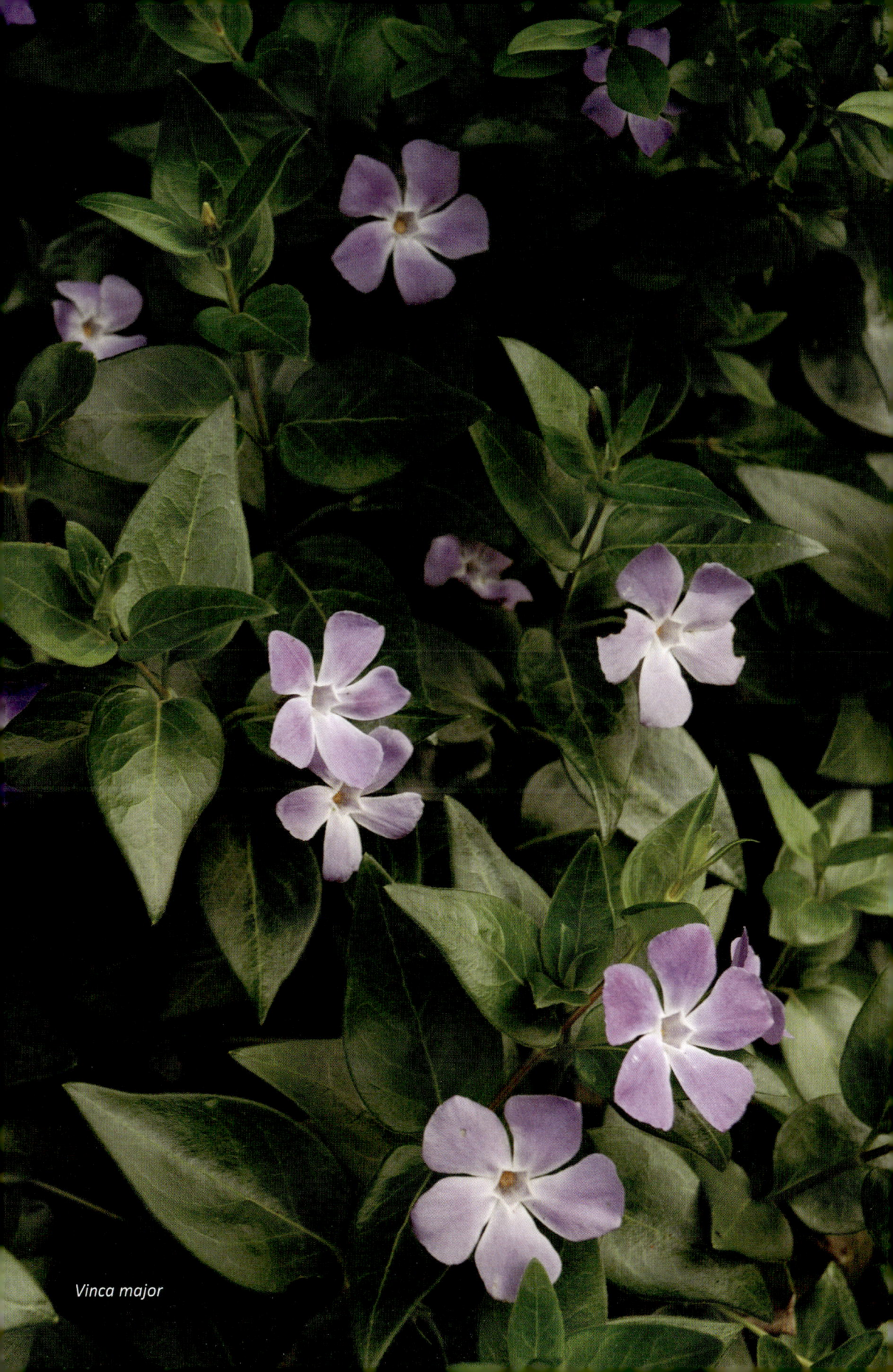

Vinca major

used to treat poor memory and concentration, tinnitus, hearing loss, impaired memory and vascular dementia, Meniere's disease, dizziness and degenerative eye problems such as glaucoma. Periwinkle is often combined with ginkgo, rosemary and gotu kola as a brain tonic for poor memory and concentration and to increase resilience to stress.

Periwinkle has neuroprotective actions, helping to prevent damage to brain tissue from free radical damage and can enhance oxygen release of haemoglobin and increase the amount available to the brain cells. It has an ability to relax and dilate blood vessels which also enhances blood supply to the brain. It is particularly good for more elderly patients as it may well prevent transient ischaemic attacks (TIAs) and other cerebrovascular accidents such as strokes if taken regularly. It can take between three to six weeks before improvements are apparent. Its antispasmodic effect, which relaxes tension in muscles including those in blood vessels, explains its old use for easing cramp.

Vinca rosea the Madagascan periwinkle (now known as *Catharanthus roseus*), a relative of the periwinkles found in Europe, was discovered in the 1920s to reduce blood sugar in diabetics and was hailed as a possible substitute for insulin. Both lesser and greater periwinkles can be used for diabetes as they have similar constituents and also reduce blood sugar.

The Madagascan periwinkle was researched in the 1950s for its anticancer effects and found to contain more than seventy different alkaloids, two of which (vinblastine and vincristine) are used extensively to treat malignant tumours, leukaemia and Hodgkin's disease.

Externally periwinkle can be used to stop bleeding. The fresh leaves can be rubbed on the skin to stop bleeding from cuts and wounds and inserted into the nose to stop nosebleeds. An infusion or dilute tincture can be used to make vaginal douches for discharges, and lotions for haemorrhoids, varicose veins and skin problems such as acne and cradle cap. The leaves can be chewed to relieve toothache, used in mouthwashes for bleeding gums and mouth ulcers and in gargles for tonsillitis and sore throats.

Homeopathic Remedy
Vinca minor prepared from the fresh leaves is used for bleeding and haemorrhage, as in uterine bleeding, heavy periods and frequent nosebleeds. It is a good remedy for scabby eruptions and itching of the skin, often on the scalp. A Vinca person tends to feel extremely weak, as if anaemic, faint, sad and fearful of dying.

Flower Essence
Periwinkle is for those who are prone to depression, nervous disorders such as anxiety, and seasonal affective disorders. It helps to clear the mind and engender a sense of inner clarity and self-knowledge which helps to dispel the depression. People who need periwinkle may feel weak and anaemic and are often prone to heavy bleeding or nosebleeds. Periwinkle helps to boost energy levels, and by healing both physical and emotional wounds from the past, it enhances regeneration.

Growing
Periwinkle is a hardy evergreen spreading perennial. Propagate by taking stem cuttings in autumn or divide roots in spring. Prefers fertile, moist soil and sun or shade. A good plant for growing along walls and fences where nothing much will grow in the shade. Grows 1–2 feet (30–60cm) long and flowers from March to August.

Cautions
Avoid in pregnancy, breastfeeding, hypotension and constipation. High doses may affect nervous system and kidneys and may decrease absorption of Digoxin. Should be avoided in those with brain tumours as it increases the cerebral circulation and may promote growth of the tumour. Avoid in high intercranial pressure.

> *Recipe*
> An ointment prepared from the leaves with olive oil and beeswax is soothing and healing and can be used for inflammatory ailments of the skin and for bleeding piles.

Viola odorata: Sweet Violet

The Flower of Shyness

Reform the errors of the Spring,
Make that tulips may have share
of sweetness, seeing they are fair,
And roses of their thorns disarm'd,
But most procure
That violets may a longer age endure
– Andrew Marvell (1621–1678)

Other names: Wood violet, English violet, banaksa, banafsha, common violet, garden violet

Parts Used: Leaf, flower, root

The heavenly-scented sweet violet with its pretty little purple or white flowers that hide beneath the heart-shaped leaves, is a symbol of shyness and modesty. It is a hardy perennial member of the Violaceae family native to Asia, North Africa and Europe that flowers, but briefly, in woods, forests and hedges in spring.

There are many myths and legends about the origins of the violet that may have given rise to such phrases as 'blushing violet' or 'shrinking violet'. One Greek myth tells how the nymph Ianthis was chased by the amorous Apollo. The frightened virgin fled to the woods and sought protection from Diana, who advised her to hide away where Apollo could not find her. Diana changed the nymph into the violet so that she could escape Apollo's importunities. Another version says that violets were created for Io, beloved of Zeus, to honour her beauty. Io's name

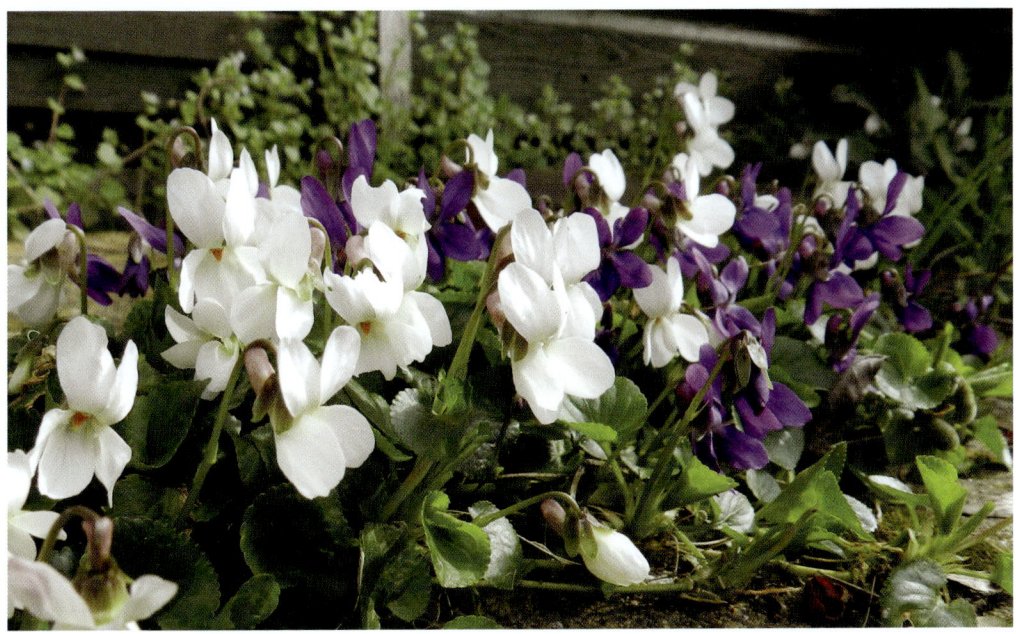

remains in the word for flower *violet* - in Greek 'io' means *violet*.

Violet is also the symbol for steadfastness and loyalty. Shakespeare was clearly fond of violet and used it as a symbol of humility and constancy in love in his writings. In medieval times violet symbolised Christ's humility. It was cultivated extensively in monastery gardens to protect against all forms of evil. Necklaces of violets were said to protect from deception and inebriation. Garlands of violets were worn by the ancient Greeks and Romans to dispel the odour of wine and spirits and prevent drunkeness. Violets were also used in love potions.

Violets have been valued as medicine at least since the time of the ancient Greeks. They were mentioned frequently by Homer and Virgil as they were used then 'to moderate anger', to procure sleep and 'to comfort and strengthen the heart'. Hippocrates recommended them for headaches, hangovers, bad eyesight, melancholia, excess bile and inflammation in the chest. Pliny said violets induced sleep, strengthened heart muscle and calmed anger. Violets were used by the Arabs for constipation, tonsillitis, insomnia and liver troubles. They were also used historically to relieve pain from cancer, to calm anxiety and lower blood pressure. The roots and seeds of sweet violet were also used, which are more purgative. The seeds are diuretic and were used for urinary problems including stones and gravel.

Herbal Remedy
Sweet violet has a combination of sweet, bitter and slightly salty tastes. Its cooling properties can be beneficial wherever there is heat and inflammation in the body. Its anti-inflammatory action is related to the presence of glycosides which include gaultherin, methyl ester and salicylic acid. The mucilage is soothing and cooling, the phenolics and flavonoids (rutin, violarutin) have anti-inflammatory and antioxidant actions and the saponins (myrosin, violin) have an expectorant effect. Other constituents include coumarins, odoratine, minerals (calcium, magnesium), tannins, triterpenoids, volatile oils, alkaloids and vitamin C. About 30 cyclotides have been identified in the aerial parts and roots. The flowers also contain anthocyanins.

The modern use of violet reflects many of the ancient claims. In the respiratory tract, the saponins and mucilage in violet make it an excellent soothing and moistening expectorant for relieving harsh irritating coughs, whooping cough, asthma and chest infections. Its anti-inflammatory effect is also helpful in sore throats, tonsillitis, laryngitis, asthma and bronchitis.

Violet is also popular in several medicinal systems including Iranian, Greco-Arab, Ayurvedic and Unani for treating whooping cough, headaches, migraine, insomnia, colds and sore throats in children and adults alike. Its antimicrobial actions may be attributed to the cyclotides that have potent activity against bacteria including *E. coli, Bacillus, Staphylococcus aureus* and *Pseudomonas aeruginosa.* This means that violet can make an effective remedy for treating bronchitis, as well as cystitis and tonsillitis. Violet syrup is a famous remedy for soothing children's coughs and other respiratory ailments.

When taken as a hot infusion, violet increases blood flow to the surface and promotes sweating, helping to bring down fevers, and relieve feverish colds and catarrhal congestion. The analgesic effect of the salicylates can relieve aches and pains that accompany respiratory infections, flu and fevers. With its anti-inflammatory and analgesic effects, violet can reduce inflammation and pain in migraine, arthritis and gout. It can also be helpful in inflammatory or infective skin problems such as abscesses and boils.

With its affinity with the heart and mind, violet is recommended for easing stress and anxiety, lifting the spirits, reducing grief and heartbreak and to improve memory and concentration. This may be explained to some extent by the antioxidant and anti-inflammatory effects of constituents including phenols and flavonoids which can improve brain function and protect from neurodegeneration that is related to free radical damage. On a more subtle level, violet is a lovely cooling remedy to cool the fire of anger, impatience, frustration and irritability as well as to relieve feelings of low self-worth and depression. With its analgesic and anti-inflammatory effects, it helps to relieve stress-related symptoms such as headaches, colic and insomnia and with its antispasmodic and nervine effects, it has been used for epilepsy, dizziness and exhaustion.

In the digestive tract, violet soothes the stomach and intestines and is very useful for cooling heartburn and indigestion, gastritis and other inflammatory gut problems. Its antimicrobial action helps to ward off infections including fungal infections such as *Candida*. Violets can be made into a syrup which makes a gentle laxative for children and they can be taken as a tincture for adults. The antioxidants in violets have a hepatoprotective effect, helping to protect the liver from damage caused by toxins, stress, alcohol and drugs.

Violet can also be used to make a soothing and antimicrobial diuretic tea to reduce fluid retention and relieve inflamed and painful conditions as well as infections in the urinary tract and kidneys. It exerts its soothing effect throughout the genito-urinary system and can ease discomfort in problems such as cystitis, vaginal infections like *Trichomonas*, urethritis, irritable bladder and urinary tract infections.

Violet can be beneficial for the immune system. In Chinese medicine, violet flowers, leaves and root are used together to resolve hot swellings, cysts and tumours. They are used in the treatment of cancer (breast, lung, digestive tract, skin, throat, tongue). Cycloviolacin O2, one of the cyclotides, has antitumour effects and may have the ability to kill abnormal cells in breast cancer. Violet has also been found to be active against *Pseudomonas aeruginosa* which is an opportunistic pathogen that is resistant to many antibiotics and causes infections in hospitalised patients such as those with extensive burn sepsis.

With its antioxidant, vasodilatory and diuretic activities, violet leaves, stems and flowers can help reduce blood pressure and lower cholesterol. In this way, violet can play a role in preventing cardiovascular disease. The leaves may affect fat metabolism through their antioxidant action and by inhibiting the synthesis and absorption of lipids, which is helpful for those wanting to lose weight.

Externally, a warm poultice of the leaves can be applied to hot swellings such as boils, abscesses or infected cysts. It can also be used to soothe and heal sore cracked nipples and inflammatory skin conditions such as eczema. Its antifungal actions make violet good in creams and lotions for fungal skin conditions and thrush. An infusion of the leaves and flowers can be used to bathe sore eyes and in conjunctivitis, and a cloth soaked in violet infusion can be applied to the back of the neck to ease headaches. It can also be used as a gargle for sore throats and a mouthwash for inflamed gums. An inhalation with steam is worth doing for coughs, colds and sore throats.

Violets have a reputation as a cancer remedy, particularly for tumours in the breast, lungs, throat and intestines. The leaves have been used as poultices in traditional systems of medicine for tumours and cysts. Combined with vinegar, the roots were traditionally used to make a liniment for arthritis and gout.

Aromatherapy Oil
Violet essential oil is delightfully fragrant. It is made from the flowers and the leaves and has many of the same virtues as when violet is used as a herbal remedy. On the skin it is soothing and cooling and has a moistening and antimicrobial effect when used in a cream. With its anti-inflammatory properties, it can be used in preparations for sensitive skins and for conditions such as acne and eczema.

Violet oil can be used in massage oils and liniments and added to the bath to ease pain and inflammation as in tense aching muscles, arthritis, gout, back, neck or shoulder pain. Applied to the temples it can ease headaches and migraine. It is particularly good for easing stress-related symptoms such as headaches and gut problems as well as anxiety and insomnia.

When used in a diffuser or as an inhalation, violet essential oil also has decongestant and expectorant properties, helping to loosen up phlegm. Its antimicrobial and anti-inflammatory

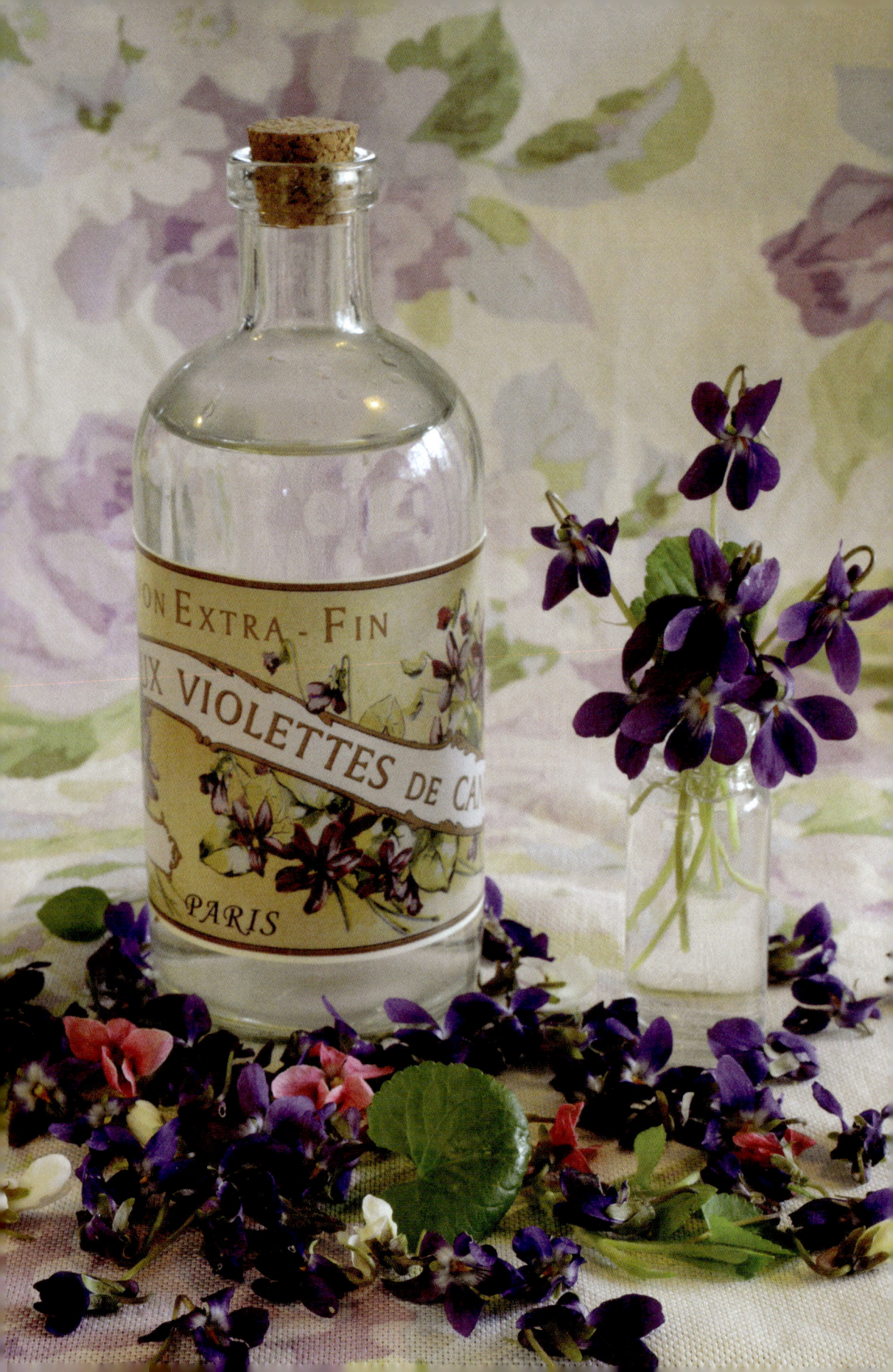

actions can be helpful in the relief of colds, coughs, flu, bronchitis and sinus congestion as well as asthma. It also makes a good insect repellent.

Homeopathic Remedy
Viola is prescribed for breathlessness and spasmodic coughs, whooping cough, and breathing problems associated with anxiety. It is also for headaches, burning of the forehead, pain above the eyebrows and vertigo. It can be used for rheumatism, and pains in the bones. A Viola odorata person easily gets tense and over-excited. The brain can be very active, and a rush of ideas can cause confusion. They are bright and perceptive, can be sad or depressed, and weep constantly without knowing why. It particularly suits thin, nervous girls.

Flower Essence
Violet is a flower remedy for profound shyness. It is for people who are delicate, sensitive, sweet and refined, who long to join in with group activities, but feel too nervous or timid. They appear reserved and aloof. Because of their shyness, they may choose jobs or lifestyles which keep them apart from others, but this can cause isolation and loneliness. Violet helps to develop trust, so that other people do not appear so threatening, and enhances the ability to join groups without the fear of losing one's identity. It engenders openness and warmth and gives support to those unassertive people with their tendency to retreat, like the violet beneath its leaves.

Edible Uses
Violets have been widely popular in perfumery, for flavouring wines and syrups and in confectionary – crystallised leaves and flowers can be used to decorate cakes and puddings. Fresh violet flowers can be used to make scented water. The flowers and young leaves can be eaten in salads, included in pesto recipes and put in sandwiches and wraps and of course look beautiful. They can be added to vinegar to give a lovely colour and fragrance and mixed into rice and porridge. The leaves can be added to soups and to stews as well as stir fries.

Growing
Propagate by sowing seeds in autumn or by planting rooted runners in autumn or spring in semi-shade in slightly acidic, moist soil. Flowers from March – April. Keep young plants well watered in dry weather. Low growing 2 to 4 inches (5 to 10cm) high. Harvest the flowers when they just come into bloom.

Cautions
Violet is considered safe if used appropriately. Do not take during pregnancy. The root in large doses has an emetic effect and could cause vomiting.

Recipes

Violet Syrup
Place violet flowers in a clean jar, cover with a layer of sugar and then place another layer of flowers, cover with sugar and so on. Leave to macerate for two weeks and then press through a sieve and discard the flowers. The syrup can be used in desserts such as ice cream or sorbet.

Violet Ointment
Melt 50g ghee in a *bain marie* and add as many flowers as you can. Leave on the heat for a few hours and then strain. When cool pour into covered pots, and use for skin conditions and problems such as bruises, aching joints, cysts and sore nipples.

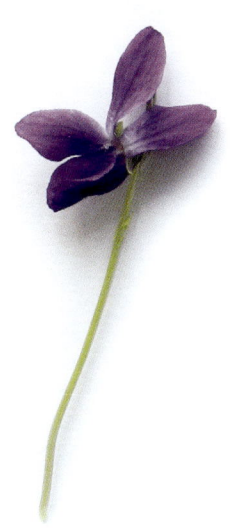

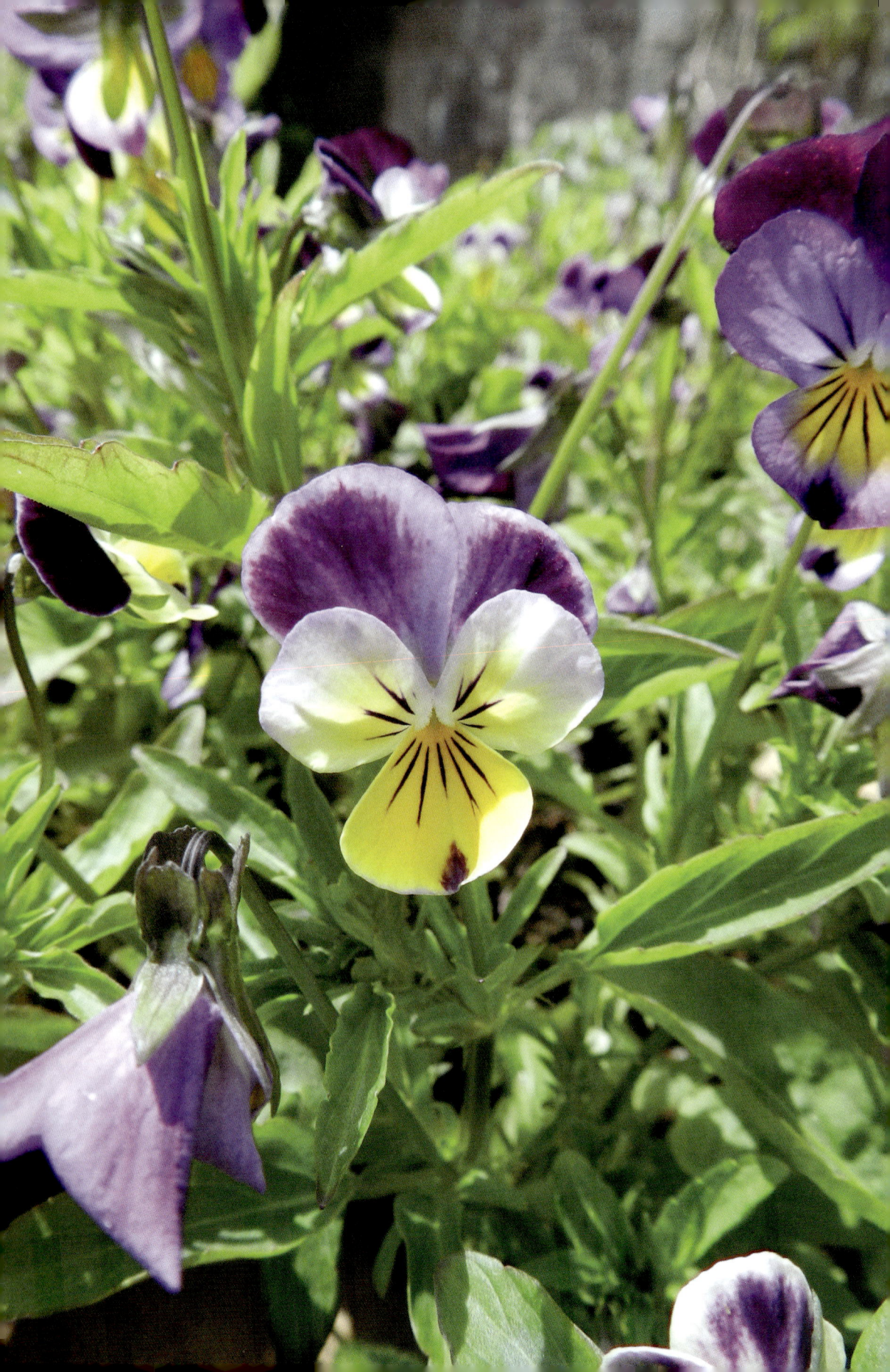

Viola tricolor: Heartsease

The Flower of Thoughts

What flowers are these?
The Pansie this;
Oh! That's for loving thoughts
 – George Chapman (1559–1634)

Other Names: Wild pansy, trinity herb, love lies bleeding, love in idleness, live in idleness, call me to you, jack jump up and kiss me, meet me in the entry, kiss her in the buttery, three faces under a hood, herb trinitatis, pink eyed John, bouncing bet, flower o'luce, bird's eye, bullweed, banwort, banewort, herb constancy, Johnny jumper

Parts Used: Leaves, stems and flowers

Wild pansy is a delightful annual member of the Violaceae family with pretty little heart-shaped flowers that can be found growing wild in cornfields and cultivated ground. It is native to or naturalised in much of Europe, the Middle East and Central Asia and flowers from spring to autumn. Wild pansy is the forerunner of cultivated pansies, which can also be used but may not have the same medicinal power.

Wild pansy is an old favourite in English gardens and in old herbals it was called 'herba trinitas' ,symbolic of the Holy Trinity because each flower has three colours, purple, white and yellow. In another legend the story is different – the pansy used to have a scent sweeter than that of its sister the violet, and the flowers' beautiful faces dotted the cornfields with colour. People picking the pretty flowers would trample down the crops leaving little grain at harvest time. The sad pansy prayed for help to the Holy Trinity and begged to lose her fragrant perfume so that people would not trample down the corn to find her. Her wish came true and since then she has been known as the *trinity herb*. Another story tells that it was Cupid's arrow that brought colour to the flower, for previously it was white.

Wild pansy or heartsease has close associations in myth and legend with affairs of the heart. It is so-called for its ability to heal the heart, soothe the pain of separation from loved ones and ease a broken heart. As far back as the days of Hippocrates, it was used as a cordial, to lift the spirits and treat heart conditions and high blood pressure.

It was used for its potency in love potions – Shakespeare had it playing an important part in *A Midsummer Night's Dream* working as a love charm on Titania and causing her to fall for an ass. Oberon sends Puck to gather 'a little western flower' that maidens call 'love-in-idleness'. The juice of the heartsease now, says Oberon, *"on sleeping eyelids laid, Will make or man or woman madly dote upon the next live creature that it sees."*

The flower's common name *pansy* comes from the French 'pensees' meaning thoughts. In Hamlet, Ophelia says, *'There is pansies – that's for thoughts'*. In the Victorian language of flowers heartsease means you are in my thoughts. People also believed that if they carried a pansy it would ensure the love of their sweetheart. Heartsease is said to be sacred to St. Valentine.

The medicinal uses of wild pansy go back at least hundreds of years. Wild pansy preparations were used during the Middle Ages, mainly as a remedy for skin ailments and were mentioned by Lonicerus (1564); Hieronimus Bock (1565) and Matthiolus (1501-1577). In 1597, John Gerard said in his *Herball* that pansy tea was helpful in curing spasms in infants. He also recommended that it could be used for treating inflammation in the chest and lungs, and also wrote about its ability to cure scabs, itching and ulcers when applied externally.

Herbal Remedy

Heartsease has a combination of sweet and bitter tastes and cooling, cleansing and anti-inflammatory properties.

The mucilage is cooling and soothing, the flavonoids (mainly rutin as well as violanthin and violaquercitrin) anthocyanins and flavone glycosides (mainly apigenin) have anti-inflammatory actions, the phenolic acids (mainly salicylic acid and its derivatives methyl salicylate and violutin) have anti-inflammatory and analgesic actions, the tannins are astringent and drying, the saponins have an expectorant action and the bitters act on the liver. In addition, heartsease contains alkaloids, carotenoids, vitamin E and C, cyclotides, polysaccharides, minerals, gums and resin.

Heartsease, as the name clearly tells us, is a remedy for affairs of the heart. It is excellent for reducing excessive or unwanted thoughts and emotional problems that cause low self-esteem, fear of failure, feeling downhearted or depressed, intolerant or impatient. It also benefits the cardiovascular system physically.

Taken regularly, it enhances the circulation and can reduce blood pressure. The bioflavonoid rutin with its antioxidant action helps prevent oxidative stress on the arteries, it strengthens blood capillaries, helps prevent bruising and nosebleeds, and is used in varicose ulcers, capillary fragility and haemorrhoids. It also helps prevent inflammation in the arteries and the build-up of atheroma, and has an antioxidant effect comparable to ginkgo.

Wild pansy is valued for its soothing and expectorant properties in the respiratory system. Taken in a hot infusion, wild pansy can clear catarrhal congestion and bring down fevers. The

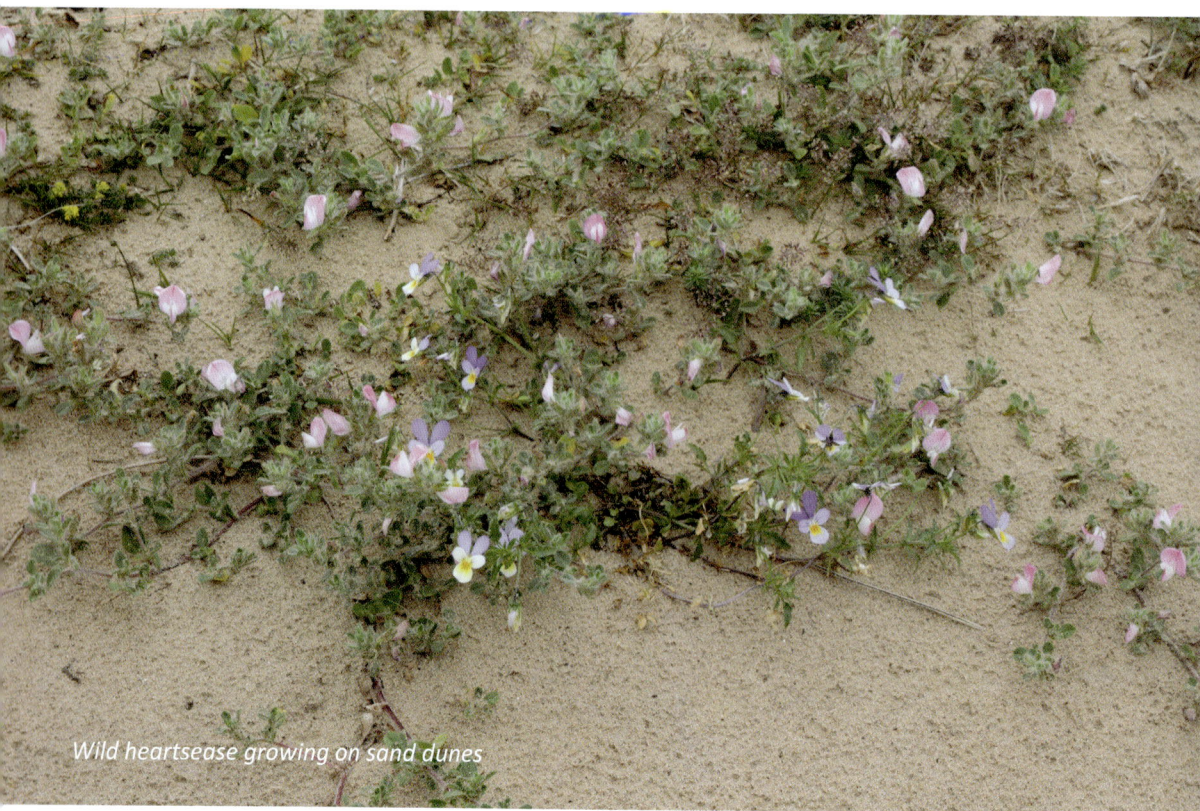

Wild heartsease growing on sand dunes

triterpenes, flavonoids and methylsalicylates have anti-inflammatory effects and liquify thick tenacious mucus, making it easier to clear. They contribute to the ability of heartsease to ease inflammatory chest problems, bronchitis, harsh irritating coughs, whooping cough, asthma, tonsillitis, laryngitis, swollen glands and croup.

The saponins account for its expectorant action, while its mucilage content soothes irritation and soreness in the chest. Heartsease can be a good remedy for treating asthma-associated anxiety. Its calming effects may be associated with the stimulation of GABA receptor by the main flavonoid, rutin.

Wild pansy also benefits the immune system. It has antimicrobial actions and helps to combat bacterial and fungal infections in the respiratory, digestive and urinary systems and on the skin. These include *Staphylococcus aureus, Bacillus cereus, Staphylococcus epidermidis, Klebsiella pneumoniae, Pseudomonas aeruginosa, Enterococcus faecalis, E. coli* and *Candida albicans*. It contains cyclotide compounds with anticancer actions and has potential in the treatment of cancers such as lymphoma, cervical and breast cancer. Together with the phenolic acids and flavonoids, the cyclotides may kill cancer cells or inhibit their growth and angiogenesis (the formation of new blood vessels to supply the tumour and support its growth). They could also inhibit the growth of lymphocytes and could be helpful in the treatment of disorders related to an overactive immune system.

In the digestive system, the antispasmodic actions of heartsease can be helpful in stress-related gut problems such as wind, bloating and colic, and the anti-inflammatory effect of the flavonoids and salicylates could be helpful in inflammatory gut problems including ulcerative colitis and Crohn's disease. The mucilage provides its soothing properties and could also be helpful in heartburn and indigestion.

The mucilage and saponin content of wild pansy makes it a soothing and cooling diuretic remedy for the urinary tract. It is used to relieve cystitis, irritable bladder and fluid retention, and through

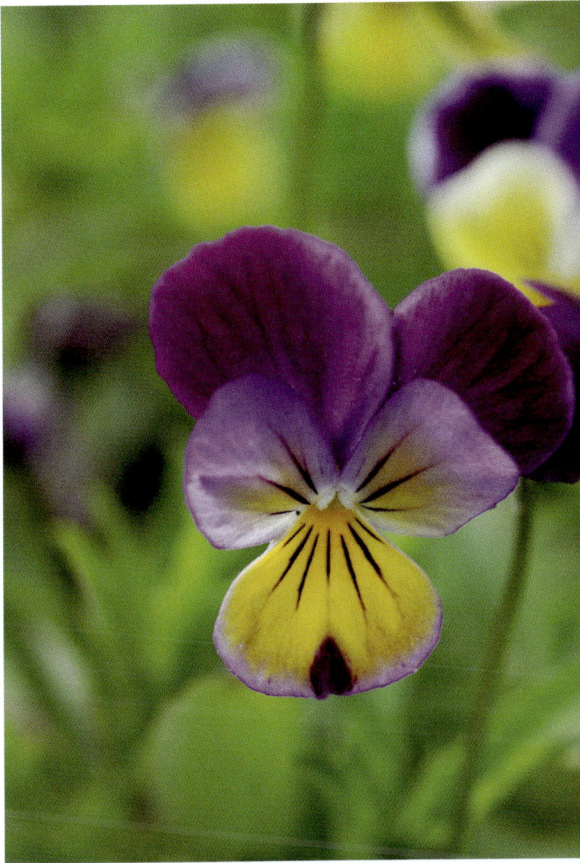

its diuretic action it helps to clear toxins from the system via the kidneys.

The salicylates are helpful for reducing pain and inflammation in arthritis and gout. Its diuretic action has a detoxifying effect and wild pansy is often prescribed to cool the system and clear inflammatory problems including skin conditions. It has traditionally been used for skin cancer, seborrheic skin disease, impetigo, pruritus vulvae, and cradle cap and eczema in babies and other crusty skin complaints. It can be used for psoriasis and acne and helps clear chronic skin disorders with purulent sticky discharge, moist eczema, and ringworm.

Externally an infusion can be used as a lotion or the herb prepared in a cream for inflammatory skin problems including seborrhoeic skin diseases, scabs, itching, ulcers, eczema, psoriasis, acne, impetigo, pruritus vulvae and cradle cap.

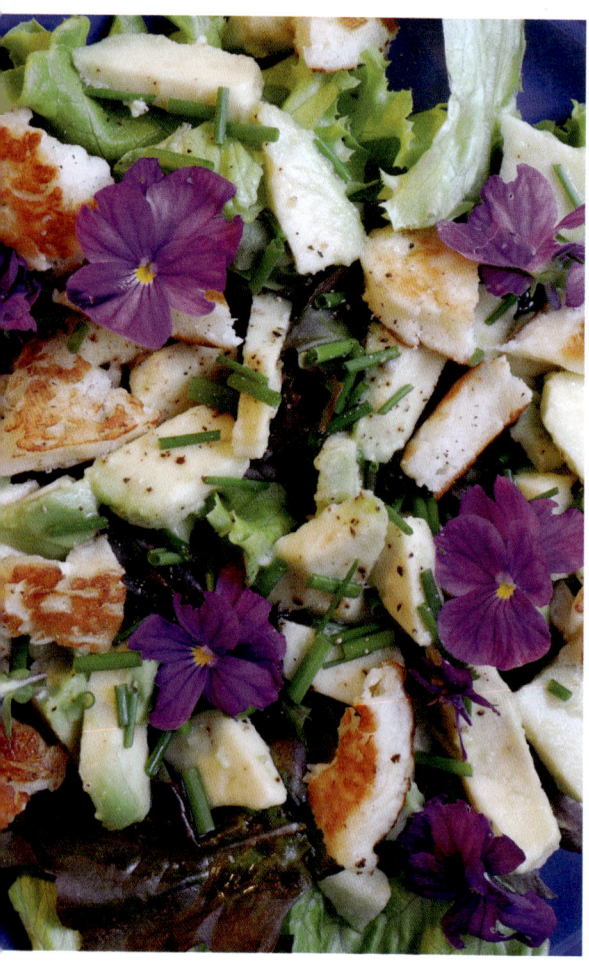

Flower Essence
Heartsease or pansy is used similarly for healing the heart. It brings comfort to those feeling hurt, rejected, lonely or broken-hearted. It is for disappointment in love, pain of separation, and when broken hearts cause symptoms in those previously happy and healthy.

Growing
Heartsease grows wild in cultivated places, mostly in disturbed garden soil and ploughed ground. Propagate by sowing seeds in spring and summer in rich, damp soil. Press seeds into the soil and leave them uncovered. The plant grows 4 to 8 inches (10 to 20cm) and flowers from spring to autumn and prefers semi-shade. It self-seeds freely. Deadhead the flowers to increase flowering and cut back leggy stems to encourage bushy growth.

Cautions
Avoid if allergic to salicylates.

Homeopathic Remedy
Heartsease is used similarly for skin problems, particularly cradle cap, eczema of the scalp, impetigo and scabby skin complaints. Symptoms tend to be worse in winter and cold air. It is indicated for people with swollen cervical glands, coughs and phlegm in the throat, for rheumatism, gout and itching eruptions around the joints. It is also prescribed for bedwetting in children who have vivid or disturbing dreams, and whose urine smells particularly strong, like a cat's. Relating back to its folk usage, it is also taken for conditions relating to the heart — anxiety about the heart and palpitations on lying down. Clarke recommended it for *'sadness respecting domestic affairs'*, and a *'tendency to shed tears'*. It is used for adults who have vivid or amorous dreams.

Recipes

Heartsease and Chamomile Infusion
With its ancient reputation for healing the heart, soothing the pain of separation from loved ones and easing a broken heart, heartsease is lovely when combined with chamomile. Chamomile also helps to ease emotional pain, to soothe anger and conflict and to release tension accumulating from inner problems that might otherwise contribute to stress-related illness and insomnia. Together they make a pleasant light, tisane, perfect for reducing anxiety or heartache and promoting inner harmony.

½ teaspoon heartsease flowers
½ teaspoon chamomile flowers
250ml boiling water
Honey to taste (optional)

Place the herbs in a small teapot and pour over boiling water. Cover and leave to infuse for 10–15 minutes before serving. Sweeten with honey if you like. 1 serving.

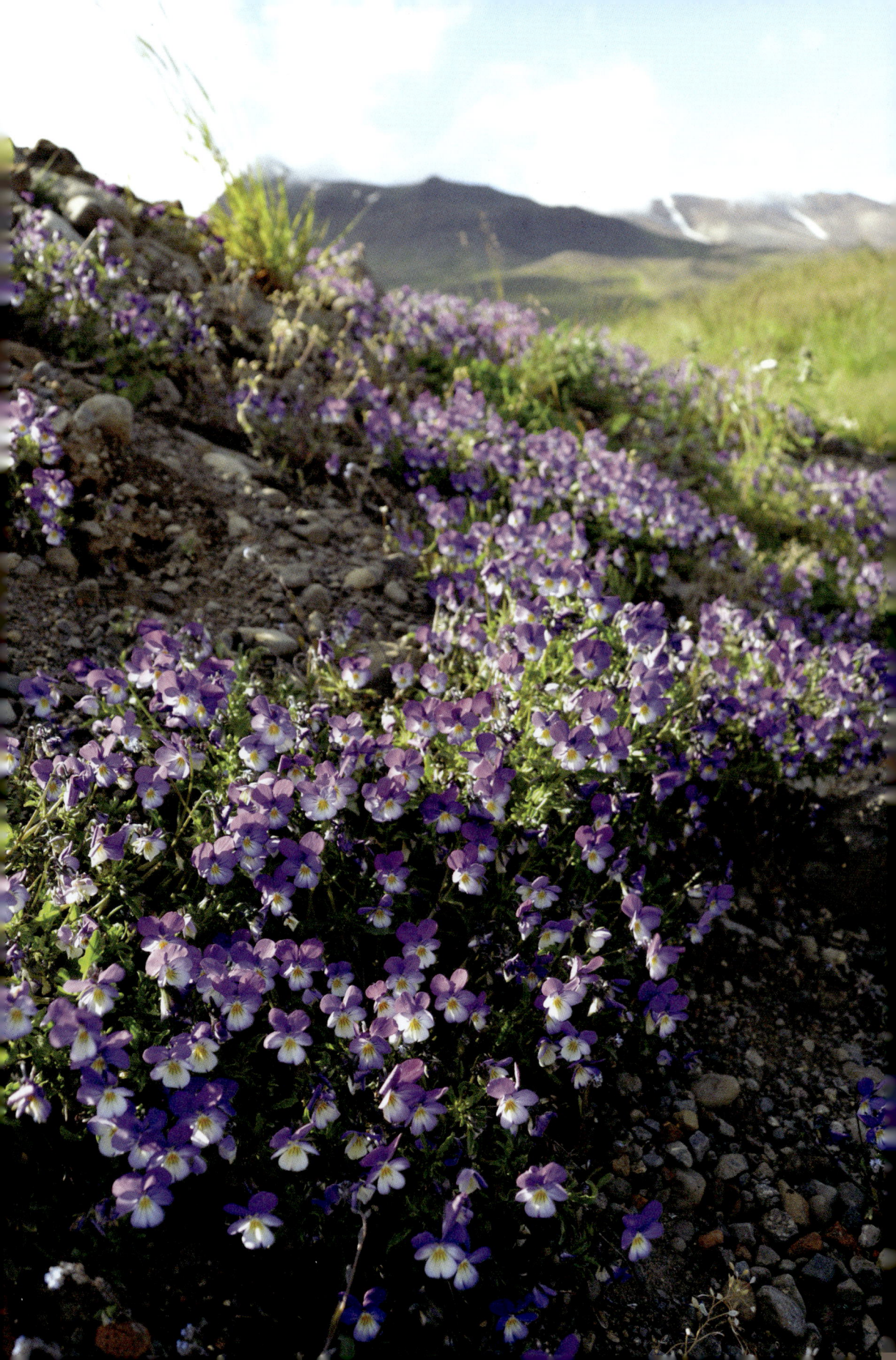

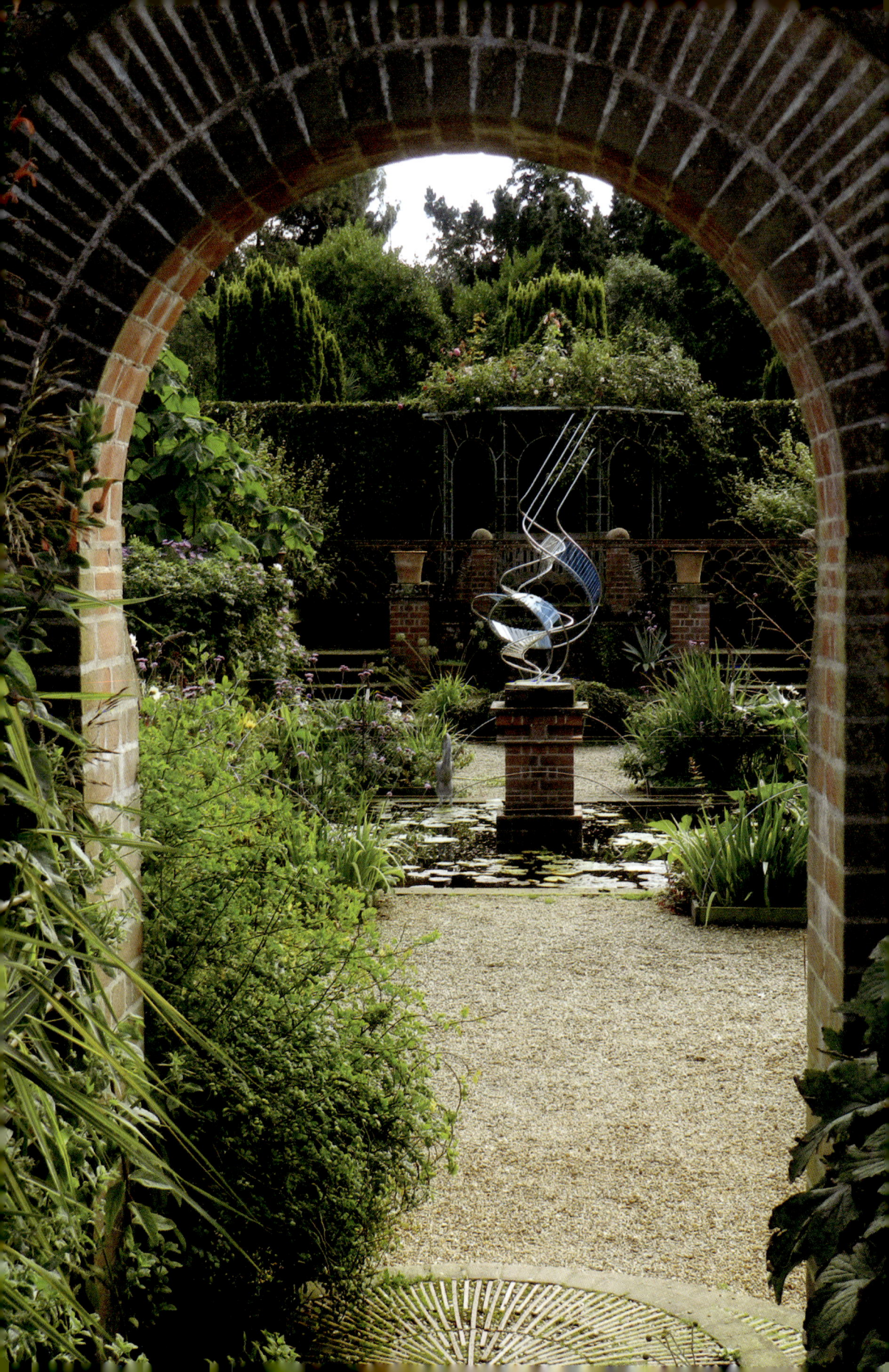

Gardening, Growing and Gathering Flowers

Flowers always make people better, happier, and more helpful;
They are sunshine, food and medicine for the soul
– Luther Burbank (1849–1926)

The best way to find the flowers you choose to use for healing is to grow them yourself and forage them from the wild. These pursuits are wonderful therapy in themselves as any gardener or forager will know. This may not be possible for town and city dwellers in which case the best advice is to find a good source of organic flowers either through your local farmers' market, herb growers, market gardeners or friends with gardens. Whenever possible plan trips to the countryside armed with walking boots and baskets for collecting, and enjoy!

Making our own medicines especially from plants around us that we have grown or gathered ourselves or sourced locally, means that we can be much more in touch with the remedies we are using than if we bought them over the counter. We are able to know their source, where they were grown, make sure they were grown well away from busy roads and contamination of pesticides and other chemicals, we can be sure of their botanical identity, that they are unadulterated, not mixed or substituted with other unwanted ingredients and not bacterially contaminated. We can also be sure that our medicines are made from the best possible quality plants as their freshness will determine the potency of the remedies we make from them. From garden and hedgerow to medicine – using the freshest plants we can make medicines with as much vital energy as possible.

Each flower has its own unique blend of many different attributes. It has myriad chemical constituents and physiological actions; it has its qualities and properties, being for example hot or cold, dry or moist, heavy or light, and with time and experience it is possible to become acquainted with each individual flower almost like a different personality. Every plant has its way of communicating its properties to us so that we can understand it and use its healing benefits. Before the days of microscopes and thin layer chromatography, we had only our senses to rely on and understandably the classification of medicinal plants according to their effect on the senses comprises the 'energetics' of the ancient wisdom traditions of medicine. Even now our senses can still serve us very well in this respect. We have taste, smell, sight and touch to interpret the messages from plants and maybe even hearing, as the wonders of the plant world may even speak to us in subtle ways. And of course, we have the mind.

Growing and gathering flowers is also the best way to learn about their healing properties and gain a deeper understanding of them that is beyond books and the rational mind.

It becomes *your* own experience of them which you will never forget. You will become intimately acquainted with each flower as you look at it, smell it and feel it as you pick it. All of your senses will engage with it – sight, touch, smell, taste and even sound as you listen to the sounds of leaves and flowers and the way they rustle in the breeze. The time it takes to pick each flower or cluster of flowers and their leaves provides a wonderful opportunity for spending quiet and contemplative time with that flower and reawakening your intuitive skills that are always there even though you may not fully realise it. It means that you can develop a more profound relationship with each flower and a knowing at a subtle level of your being that will give you an understanding beyond thoughts and words of the healing gifts of nature all around us.

A Healing Garden

A flower garden is a wonderfully healing place. If you love gardening, you will know the joy and fulfilment gained from spending hours immersed in the beauty of nature and flowering plants. Being outside, preparing the ground with your hands in the rich earth, planning and designing a planting plan, sowing seeds, nurturing seedlings, planting and tending your plants, seeing them develop in shape, form and colour can all take us into a world where the taxman never enters and the day-to-day stresses of modern life have no place. As described by many a writer and poet, "*one who plants a garden, plants happiness,*" such pursuits can calm the mind and lift the spirits. For many the garden, whatever size or form that comes in, is their sanctuary, a place of peace and refreshment. Even if you do not have enough space for a real garden, you can still create form and beauty, not forgetting wonderful scents, from herbs grown in pots and containers, either inside or out.

> *Gardening is the purest of human pleasures*
> *– Francis Bacon (1561–1626)*

The Garden as Paradise

The first gardens of western civilization were created when people started to settle in communities and needed to grow plants to provide them with food and medicines. The oldest pictures of gardens that exist are from ancient Egypt dating around 1400 BC and they were surrounded by walls or palisades to protect them from harsh desert winds and thieves. Fruit trees, nutritious and medicinal herbs and flowers were laid out in symmetrical shapes and rows interspersed with waterways to ease irrigation and despite being mostly utilitarian, they were also highly decorative.

Early gardens represented the contrast between two separate worlds, that outside the garden where untamed nature was all-powerful and potentially threatening and the sanctuary inside the enclosure away from the heat of the desert, with trees to provide cool shade and water to sustain the plants and refresh the spirit. As time went by the enclosed garden came to symbolise the joys of paradise. The early gardens of Islam were highly sophisticated and the ancient Persian name for such gardens was 'pairidaeza' from which we get the word paradise. It was taken into old Testament Hebrew as 'pardes' and into Greek as 'paradeisos' by which time it meant a royal and beautiful garden or park, and in later Hebrew it represented both the Garden of Eden from whence sprung all creation and the heavenly kingdom or celestial paradise, the home of the angels and saints and the abode of the blessed after death.

To the early Christians the enclosed garden, 'hortulus conclusus' symbolised the feminine in nature, the purity of the virgin and the womb for the conception and growth of everything that lives. The garden was the purity of the virgin bride of Solomon's Song of Songs,

> *A garden locked is my sister, my bride,*
> *A garden locked is a fountain sealed.*

Mary the Virgin was described as 'the fountain of gardens' and Dante called her *"a fountain of living things"* to wash away the sins of the world and confer grace. In medieval days Mary gardens were popular and decorated with flowers dedicated to the Virgin Mary such as lady's mantle, lavender, rosemary, chamomile, daisies, violets and marigolds. The Christian church incorporated the small enclosed garden style of the Middle East into their own round or semi-circular gardens which adjoined their monasteries and cathedrals, which were actually known as 'the paradise'. This was usually tended by the sacrist who grew plants there with religious significance for decorating the church on special occasions. The cloister garden was larger, planted with aromatic herbs and flowers which created beauty, scented the air and enhanced the tranquillity of the monks' place of study and meditation.

> *Though a life of retreat offers various joys,*
> *none, I think, will compare with the time one employs,*
> *In the study of herbs, or in striving to gain*
> *some practical knowledge of Nature's Domain.*
> *Get a garden!*
> – Walafrid Strabo (c. 808–849)

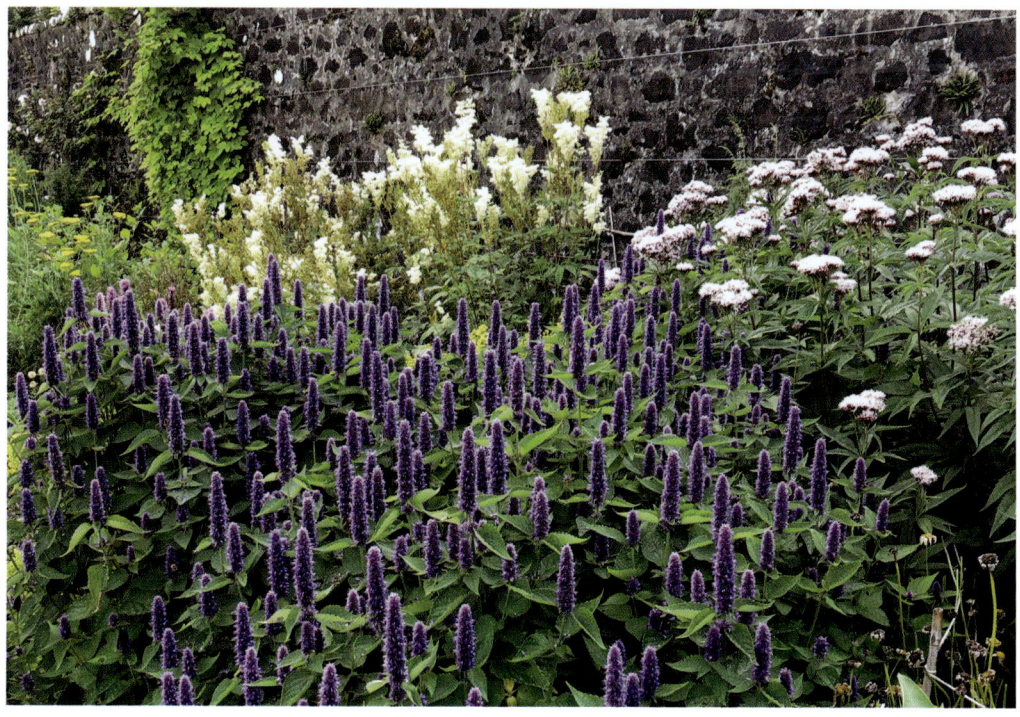

Most monasteries aimed to be self-sufficient, growing food in one area of the garden and medicinal plants to supply the infirmary in another. The oldest known plan of a medicinal herb garden designed by Abbot Walafrid Strabo in the 9th century was discovered at the Benedictine monastery of St. Gall in Switzerland. The square garden was situated by the physician's house and the infirmary and it was divided into sixteen parallel beds planted with different flowering herbs including fennel, cumin, borage, mint, rose, rosemary, sage and savoury. Although this plan may never have been actually constructed, its design was clearly echoed in gardens throughout the next few hundred years. The 12th century garden at Canterbury Cathedral apparently bears a striking resemblance to the St. Gall plan.

For over 1000 years after the Roman conquest, knowledge of medicinal herbs was kept alive predominantly within the medieval monasteries which were the principal places of learning. Texts of the classic Greek herbals were copied and recopied from ancient Greek and Latin texts often illustrated with woodcuts by the monks bearing little resemblance to the original plants. Other herbal knowledge was passed down by oral tradition from one generation to another. It was usually women who were the herb gatherers and neighbouring families relied heavily on the skills of such 'wise women' particularly if the local monastery was some distance away. The oldest surviving English herbal dates from the second half of the 9th century – the Leech Book of Bald. It was written in Anglo Saxon under the direction of a monk called Bald, a contemporary of King Alfred, and describes the monastic herb gardens of the time planted with familiar flowering herbs such as vervain, wood betony, periwinkles and violets.

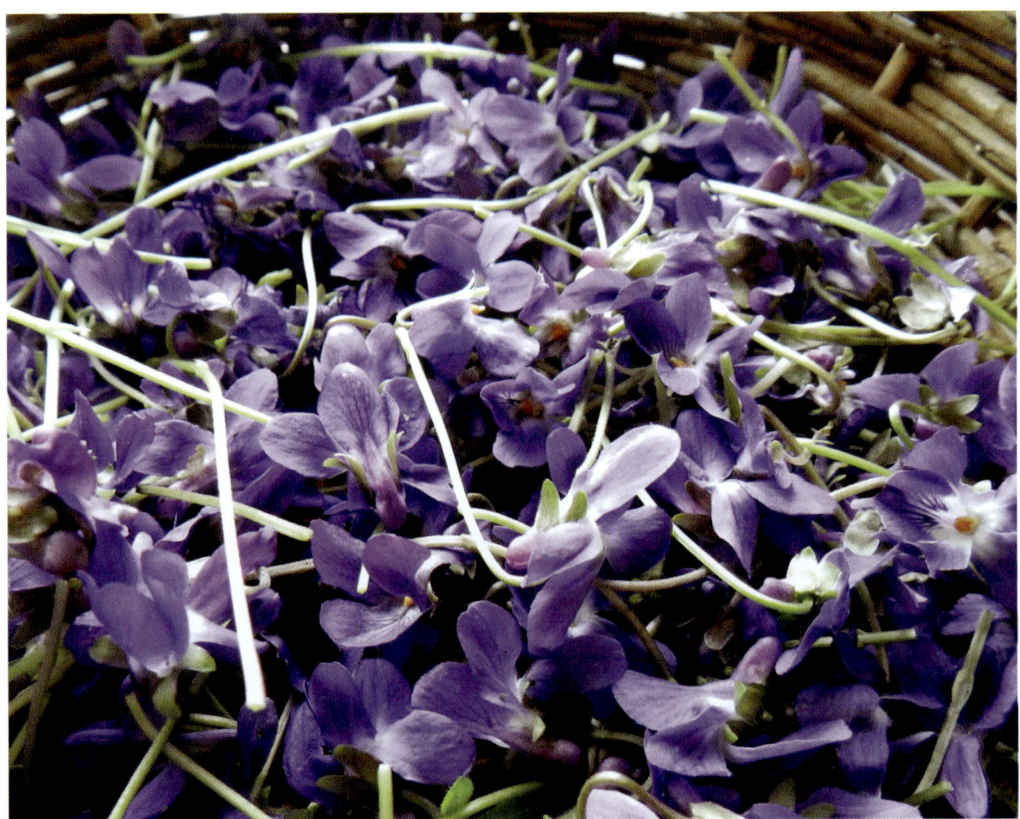

During the renaissance the invention of the printing press revolutionised the spread of herbal information. Old copied herbals were replaced by printed books which were more freely available to medical students and those studying plants. The new spirit of learning brought a new approach to the study of medicinal plants with an emphasis of observing and drawing plants from nature rather than copying more copied texts. Botany as a science was beginning to develop as a study of the plants themselves rather than a review of their efficacy as remedies for disease. A great number of new herbals began to appear around this time, notably the still popular herbals of Gerard and Culpeper. In London John Gerard, catalogued 1030 plants in his garden in 1596 and his *Herball* was published in 1597. Culpeper's *English Physician* published in 1652 related herbs and the symptoms of the body to stars and planets. John Parkinson's herbals, *Paradisi in Sole Paradisus Terrestris* (1629), a pun on his name (Park in sun's Earthly Paradise) and *Theatrum Botanicum* (1640) were among the last to bring all aspects of plant knowledge together – botany, pharmacy, horticulture and history.

Physic Gardens
At this time, plants needed by physicians and for the teaching of their students were grown together in physic gardens. The first such comprehensive collections of medicinal plants were established in Italy, first in Pisa (1543), then Padua (1545) and Florence (1550). Other countries soon followed suit in Leipzig (1580), Heidelburg (1593) and Paris (1635). In Britain the first university medicinal herb garden for studying herbs was founded in 1621 in Oxford. Edinburgh's physic garden was planted in 1656 for the teaching of surgeons and apothecaries, and doctors were appointed to lecture at universities on the healing properties of herbs. Chelsea physic garden was established in 1673 for apprentices of the Society of Apothecaries for *"the manifestation of the glory, power and wisdom of God, in the works of creation."* The garden originally ran right down to the Thames until the Embankment was built in the 1870's, as the apprentices were brought frequently by barge during their nine year's training. John Evelyn the 17th century diarist called the Chelsea physic garden *"the Apothecaries' Garden of Simples."* Nearly all the botanic gardens that still exist today started as physic gardens – the Royal Botanic Gardens at Kew were originally founded as Princess Augusta's physic garden.

In the latter Renaissance the attitude towards plants and gardens began to change considerably. Gardens became inundated with new exotic flowers and species brought almost daily by navigators and explorers from abroad, while at the same time the therapeutic properties of herbs were being re-evaluated in the new spirit of scientific analysis. Traditional rituals associated with the prescribing of herbs became highly suspect as they smacked of mysticism even sorcery, rather than the workings of the rational scientific mind. Interestingly witch hunts reached their peak during this period. Doctors were beginning to rely on other often toxic substances such as mercury and arsenic, as well as bloodletting for their treatments.

Until this time in history, herbs had not been cultivated separately from ornamental plants and flowers, for almost all plants grown possessed culinary or medicinal virtues or were used in a symbolic way, such as for protection against evil or conferring the spiritual protection of the Virgin Mary. Even the beauty of their flowers had healing effects to enhance general health and well-being by awakening the spirit and enriching the soul. By the 18th century medicinal herbs were generally grown away from the purely decorative plants and flowers in the ornamental garden. The philosophy of the day, of the separation of man and nature, mind and body, was being reflected in garden content and design. In the contemporary mechanistic theory, nature was no longer perceived as alive and inextricably linked with human life on all levels, but as an inanimate source of natural resources to be plundered for economic development. Herbalism was fast becoming obsolete and in gardens all but the culinary elite (parsley, rosemary, sage, thyme, marjoram and bay) disappeared, and these were mostly banished to the kitchen garden. A few favourite ornamental flowering herbs like lavender, violets and roses became rapidly unfashionable. Healing herbs did remain in the traditional cottage gardens where old values still stood, planted as medleys of fruit, flowers, vegetables and herbs to be used by the 'old wives' for the everyday ills of country folk.

Flower Power
It was not until the 1960s that change was in the air with the emergence of environmental consciousness and 'flower power'. Since then, as a good diet and healthy lifestyle as a basis for health has been increasingly recognised and people are feeling more able to take their health into their own hands, the role of herbs and flowers as medicines is being re-evaluated. The growing disenchantment with fast foods, artificial additives and the overuse of powerful drugs for minor ills has also served to credit natural medicines with some of their former respect. An interesting variety of culinary herbs and flowers is enhancing our increasingly cosmopolitan and adventurous cuisine, while in many homes herb and flower remedies are being used to treat common ailments and in most pharmacies a range of natural medicines is likely to be found for the asking.

Philosophically the separation of body from mind and spirit and human life from nature which accompanied the reductionist approach of modern science, is giving way to a more wholistic, almost mystic, approach to life where there is no separation between our inner selves and our bodies, and our lives and the natural world around us. Modern science is looking at this close inter-relationship, discovering that nature like humans is indeed alive, animated by the same vital force that pervades us on every level of existence. The earth and all plant, animal and human life on it, is being perceived as one vast living organism, a self-organising and self-regulating system. This old idea, clearly propounded by the British scientist James Lovelock in the 1970's as the 'Gaia hypothesis', reflects the medieval concepts of microcosm and macrocosm, the astrological approach to healing plants and the body set out by Culpeper and many before him including Hippocrates, as well as the humoral philosophy of Hippocrates and his followers.

Such philosophical shifts are being reflected in the garden. Herbs are being reinstated from their lowly position in the corner of the vegetable patch to enhance flower borders and even warrant whole gardens of their own. Many gardeners now buy plants not only for their decorative attributes but for their magical, romantic, symbolic, medicinal and historical associations. Growing these in the garden is an excellent way to acquaint yourself more fully not only with plants that are beautiful and aromatic, but also effective medicines. Your garden can actually be your instant medicine cabinet, enabling you to treat a wide range of every day minor ailments such as coughs and colds, catarrh, stomach aches, headaches, and aches and pains, and thereby reduce unnecessary visits to your doctor and the use of powerful medicines for minor self-limiting illness. As the old saying goes, *'There is no illness but there is a plant to cure it'*.

In the Garden
Tending your herb garden may stimulate your curiosity and entice you to learn more about these amazing inhabitants of your garden. You may be surprised to discover how many common garden flowers or even nuisance 'weeds' are valuable herbal remedies and have potent therapeutic compounds. Pasque flowers, violets, peonies, pansies, irises,

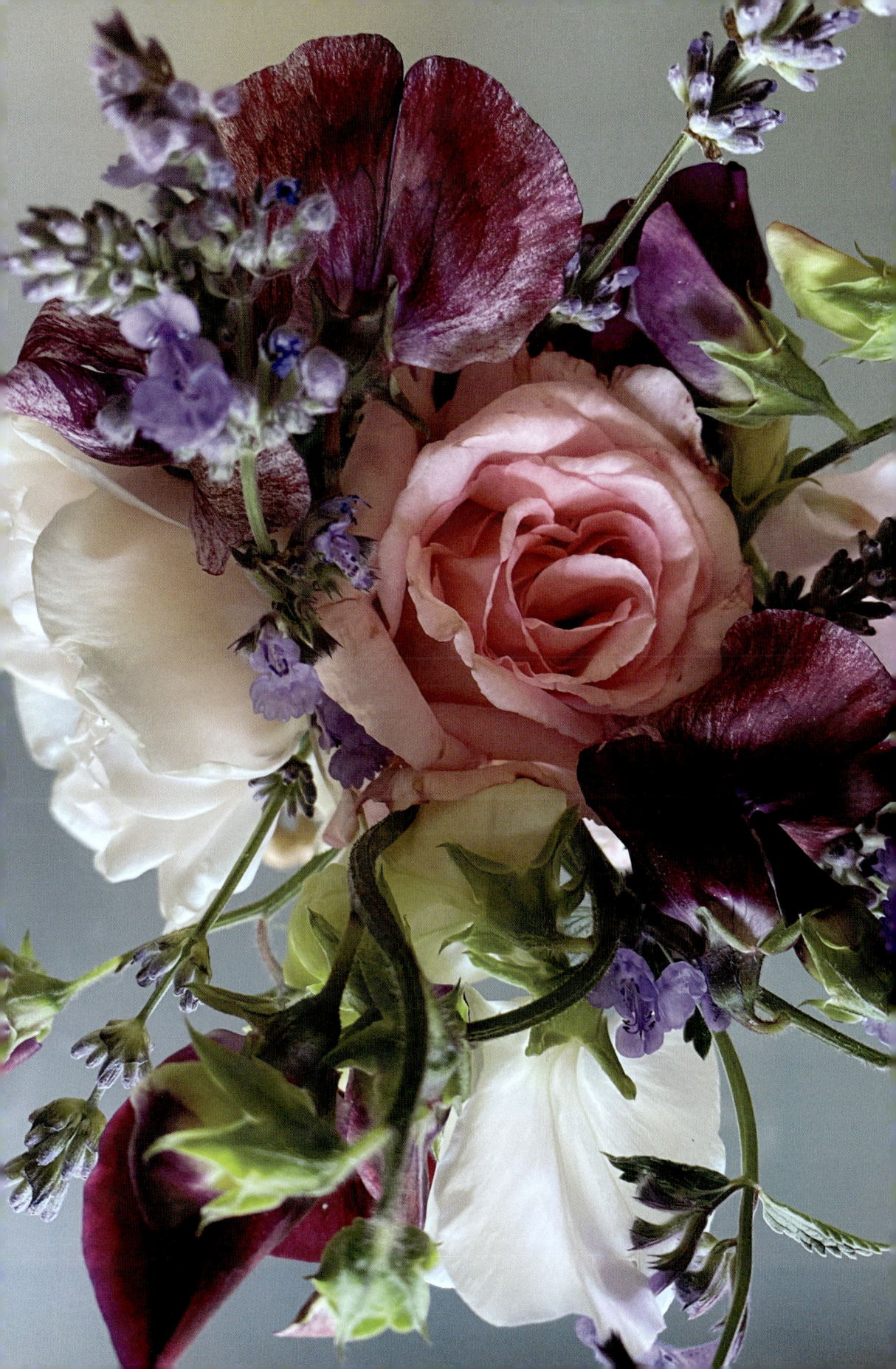

roses, dandelions and even the common daisy spring instantly to mind. Apparently simple herbs and flowers that will grow easily in most soils have warranted much time and money invested in their current research as potential answers to illness such as viral infection, immune deficiency, depression, malaria, peptic ulcers and many acute and degenerative as well as stress-related disorders. Echinacea, St John's wort, evening primrose, rosemary, oregano and periwinkle are such valuable herbs as these. A medicinal garden can include healing plants from all over the world that will grow in a temperate climate such as Chinese flowers magnolia, forsythia, peony and honeysuckle, Indian flowers such as Holy basil, and native American flowers such as skullcap, bergamot and California poppy.

*The lesson I have thoroughly learnt, and wish to pass on to others,
is to know the enduring happiness that the love of a garden gives*
– Gertrude Jekyll (1843–1932)

By creating a healing or apothecary's garden you will be following in the footsteps of many an eminent herbalist and gardener of the past, maintaining the continuity of growing medicinal plants through history. Healing flowers that have been grown by

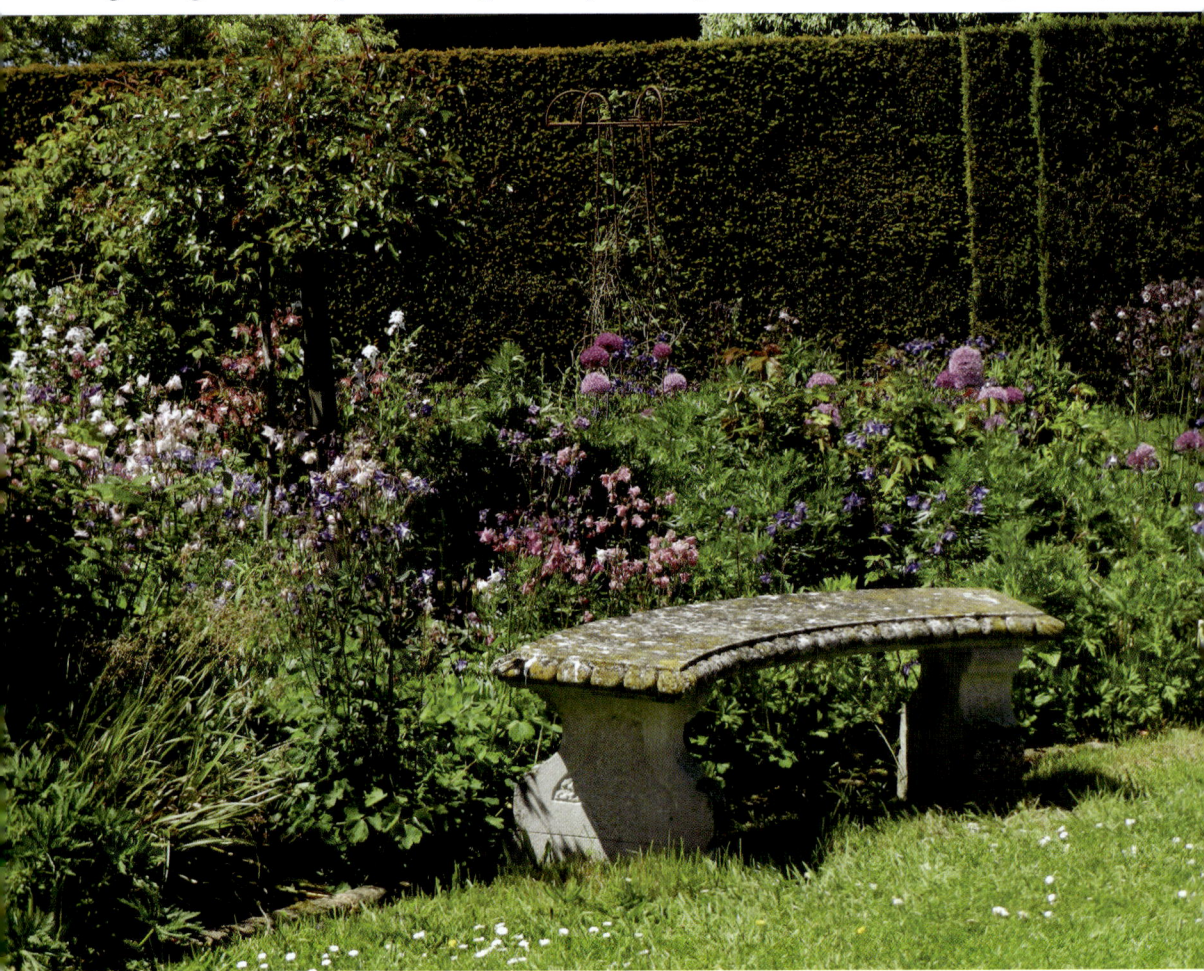

priests, physicians and apothecaries through millennia are little changed today – cowslips, periwinkles, violets and roses are popular inhabitants of gardens today as they were over 1000 years ago in medieval monastery gardens. Such plants and gardens connect us through centuries of existence to men and women who have gardened, cooked and healed with these flowers as we do now. Plants represent a living history, connecting us to a time when they were valued not only for their earthly gifts but also for their benefits in the realm of the spirit. ,

> *The glory of gardening: hands in the dirt, head in the sun, heart with nature.*
> *To nurture a garden is to feed not just on the body, but the soul*
> – Alfred Austin (1835–1913)

Creating a Healing Garden

When growing edible and healing flowers, you will have the added reward of harvesting and preparing them in a practical way, so that you have your own personal tools to enhance your health and wellbeing and to supply the kitchen. Snipping off leaves and flowers and adding them into tasty recipes – foods, tisanes, tinctures, massage oils and body creams – can bring you into a closer relationship with nature and an awareness of and respect for the amazing tools you have around you to treat the common ailments that you may fall prone to. Your garden, small or large, can actually be your instant medicine cabinet. It makes ecological and economic sense and it's surprisingly easy.

Healing and edible flowers are greatly rewarding plants to grow. Providing they have suitable soil and shelter from prevailing winds most plants grow easily in temperate climates, with no specialist knowledge or skills required. Any flowers that originate from tropical regions will take a little more care, only being put outside after the last frosts have gone and taken indoors in the autumn. A healing garden can be as large or small, as formal or informal as you like and whatever space you have available can be adapted to growing the plants you choose. Medicinal and edible flowers can be interspersed with ornamental flowers and shrubs in large or small herbaceous borders, adding interest and beauty with their flowers, attractive foliage and architectural shapes, not to mention their delicious scents. They can be planted in specially designed gardens, in corners of vegetable gardens or intermingled with the vegetables (where they can work well as companion plants to deter pests). If you have less space, you can plant healing and edible flowers in pots on a patio or on your windowsill and in window boxes. Both the planning and the practical laying out of a healing garden can bring many hours of pleasure and satisfaction.

> *Here's flow'rs for you*
> *Hot lavender, mints, savory, marjoram,*
> *The marigold, that goes to bed wi' th' sun,*
> *And with him rises weeping. these are flow'rs*
> *Of middle summer....*
> – Perdita, the Winter's Tale, William Shakespeare

Medicinal and edible flowers come from plants that are a mixture of annuals, biennials, perennials, shrubs and even trees. Annuals include dill, coriander, basil, German chamomile, borage and marigold, and these can easily be grown from seed. Once grown they may self-seed fairly freely and either left to grow where they are, or the seedlings can be transplanted to their preferred site in the garden in springtime. Biennials take two summers to come into flower, usually producing an attractive rosette of leaves in the first

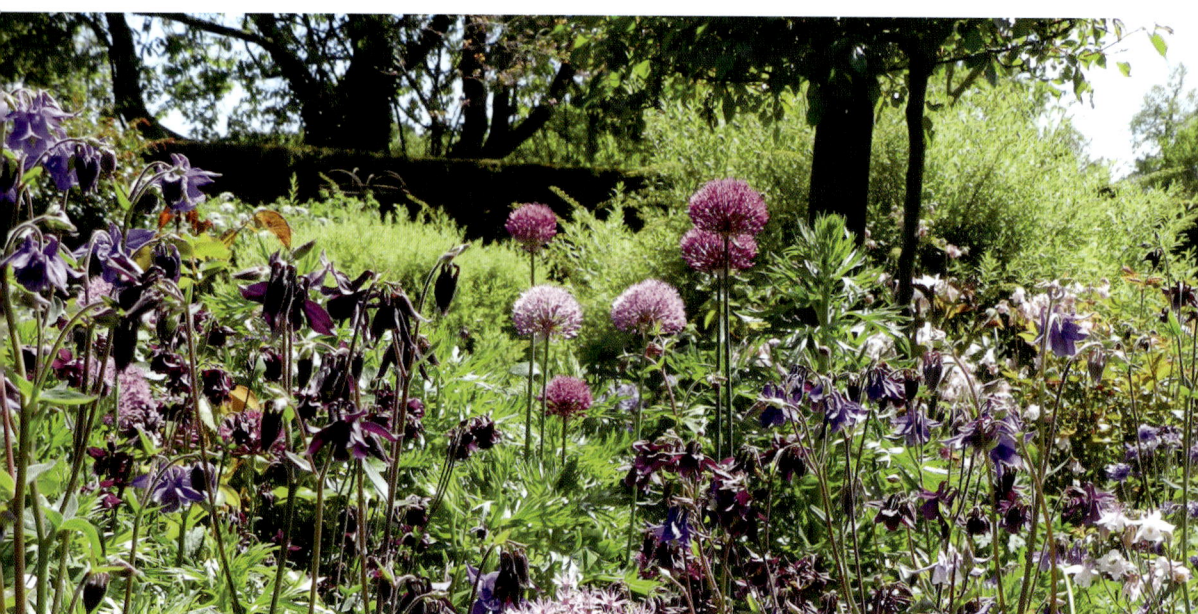

year. They include angelica, mullein and evening primrose, all of which also self-seed freely. Herbaceous perennials continue from one year to the next, dying down in autumn and reappearing in spring the following year. They can mostly be grown from seed but may be easier to grow from other methods of propagation such as root division, planting cuttings or offsets.

Many edible and medicinal flowers originate in warm climates, so to grow happily in cool temperate regions, they prefer a sheltered position. If you plant them by a hedge or fence for their protection, there will be the added advantage of allowing the delicate fragrances of the flowers to linger on warm air, rather than being blown away in a breezy open position. If your garden is warm and sheltered, there is no need to be concerned about enclosing it and plants can thrive happily in the open.

Many common plants can be bought in nurseries or garden centres and more unusual ones can be found in specialist plant nurseries. If you buy plants from a nursery, it is important to ensure that they have not been sprayed with chemicals which could be toxic if you want to harvest them to eat or use as medicines. They can be planted at most times of the year, except when the ground is frozen or covered with snow, and provided they are healthy and watered regularly they will establish themselves with very little trouble. Try to avoid planting new potted plants in dry, hot weather unless you live in a climate like this, in which case you will need to keep them well watered. Always ensure that you choose strong healthy-looking plants, free from disease or insects and avoid straggly ones and those whose roots are escaping from the bottom of the pot. Make sure the plants are clearly labelled to avoid confusion later. If you want your garden to look established quickly, buy two or three of each plant to place in groups. Some fast-growing perennials may have to be moved once they grow and need more space.

No occupation is so delightful to me as the culture of the earth,
and no culture comparable to that of the garden
– Thomas Jefferson (1743–1826)

Tips for Growing Flowers

Soil Conditions

Most of the plants described in this book are fairly easy to grow as they are generally not fussy about where they grow and will take in most situations and soils. Specific growing conditions are listed under each main flower. If your soil is deep, moist and rich, the plants will probably grow quickly with lots of lush foliage, but their flavour and smell will not be as strong as plants grown in poorer dry soil. Many of our favourite herbs such as rosemary, sage, lavender, basil and oregano are natives of the Mediterranean where it is dry and the soil is hard and stony, so they are used to withstanding fairly adverse conditions. Plants grown in such soils do not look so vibrant and lushly attractive but will taste and smell wonderful. Because they grow less fast then those grown on rich, moist soil, they cannot be harvested as frequently. The kind of soil that plants tolerate least well is heavy clay soil which in wet conditions does not drain well and can become waterlogged. Many Mediterranean herbs like lavender and thyme will rot away in such damp situations. If your soil is wet and heavy, add plenty of organic matter and sharp sand to lighten it and help drainage. If your soil is very light and sandy, dig in a small amount of organic matter to make it more water retentive and able to retain nutrients in the soil.

Sowing Seeds

You can buy flower and herb seeds from specialist suppliers or save them from the previous year. For early plants sow seeds in pots or seed trays in a greenhouse or propagator in early spring. Using fresh seedling compost, sow the seed evenly and sparingly by sprinkling them over the firmed surface of the soil or in shallow drills. Cover the seeds lightly with a thin layer of compost or fine sand and water with a fine rose on your watering can. Label the pots or trays clearly with an indelible pen so the name of the plants does not get washed away with watering. Cover the tray with a piece of glass or plastic or a sheet of newspaper. Once the seeds have germinated you can remove the newspaper, glass or plastic sheet and when the seedlings are large enough to handle, you can thin them or transplant them to individual pots to encourage their growth. In early summer, once they have become sturdy little plants, they are ready to plant outdoors. Alternatively, you can sow seeds directly into warmer soil in late spring or early summer, once all sign of winter frosts has gone. Cover the seeds with soil, the depth of which can be measured by multiplying the diameter of the seeds 2 to 3 times.

Growing plants from seed is both rewarding and fascinating, particularly if you are using seed that you have collected yourself. You may often find that your own seeds germinate more successfully than bought ones, particularly if they are fresh and sown as soon as they are ripe and ready to drop. They can be sown in trays and left in a greenhouse or cold frame covered with a piece of glass or polythene until they germinate. They may not germinate till the following spring, so you need to be fairly patient.

Many plants self-seed freely if their seed heads are left alone; elecampane, lady's mantle, chamomile, meadowsweet, coriander, self-heal, marshmallow, St John's wort, marigold and motherwort are good examples. Seeds will germinate when conditions are right and grow into strong healthy plants. If they grow where you don't want them, they can easily be moved when robust enough. Many variegated and decorative coloured plants such as variegated lemon balm, marjoram and mugwort, purple and golden sages will not come true when grown from seed and need to be propagated by other methods such as cuttings or root division.

Root Division
Plants that form good clumps are excellent candidates for root division, in fact lemon balm, marjoram, lady's mantle, mint, primrose, periwinkle, elecampane and yarrow need to be divided every 3 – 4 years into smaller clumps for best results. Root division is best done in autumn or early spring. First cut back the top growth and dig up the entire plant with a fork. Carefully divide the clump with your hands into several pieces, each retaining a good system of roots, and replant where you have chosen. If the clump is too solid to divide with your hands, you will need to use a garden fork. Dig the fork into the middle of the clump and lever it about, forcing the clump to separate.

Taking Cuttings
Taking cuttings from established plants is an easy way to propagate herbs and can be very rewarding. Softwood, semi-ripe and hardwood cuttings can be taken depending on the plant. Softwood cuttings are generally successful with most herbaceous perennials, while semi-ripe and hardwood cuttings are suitable for shrubs and small trees.

When taking cuttings, gently tear a small side-shoot off a stem so that it has a heal on it, or cut the shoot's stem just below a leaf joint using a sharp knife 2–4"/5–10cms long. Remove the lower leaves and insert into holes made with a pencil, stick or dibber around the edge of a pot of cutting compost, or a mixture of peat and sand. You may wish to dip the end into hormone rooting powder first. Firm the soil around the cuttings and water them in well. Once you detect signs of new growth at the tip, lift each cutting gently using your fingers or your dibber and plant up in individual pots, disturbing the new roots as little as possible.

Softwood Cuttings
These are best taken in spring and early summer from healthy looking plants. Once inserted around the edge of your pot or tray, spray the cuttings with water using a plant spray and cover with a plastic propagator lid, a sheet of polythene or an inflated plastic bag to retain the moisture. Roots develop quickly on softwood cuttings generally within 3–6 weeks, but it can be just a few days in warm conditions. Root development stimulates leaf growth so you will know roots are formed when you see tiny new leaves shooting at the growing tip. Once the root system has had a chance to establish itself, the cutting can be gently lifted and potted up in an individual pot or planted in a nursery bed. Generally speaking, cuttings are best kept in pots in a sheltered area, a greenhouse or plastic tunnel in cold areas during their first winter and planted out in their positions the following spring.

Semi-ripe Cuttings
These are taken in summer when stems are harder as they ripen at the base but are still flexible. Side shoots are taken off the new growth, torn away from the main stem leaving a little heal of older wood. Once inserted in pots or trays and watered in, they are also best covered with plastic or polythene to retain moisture, but it is not absolutely vital as they are more resilient than soft wood cuttings. Keep the cuttings in pots in a cold frame or a sheltered area of the garden out of direct sunlight until growth starts the following spring, as rooting of semi-ripe cuttings takes considerably longer than softwood cuttings.

Ripe Cuttings
These are taken from shrubby herbs or trees such as lilac, witch hazel, rosemary, hawthorn and cramp bark in autumn once the plant is dormant. Take a side shoot of the current year's growth up to 12"/30cm, remove the lower leaves and insert half their length in

light soil in the garden in a sheltered position. Firm the soil around the cutting and water well. Leave in position for around a year until a good root system is developed.

Root Cuttings or Offsets
This is the ideal method of propagation for plants that have running roots or that send side shoots around the main plant such as yarrow, rose, phlox, crab apple, lilac, chamomile and mint. Cut the spreading roots or runners from the parent plant at the end of summer or early autumn. Cut the root into small pieces about 2"/5cm long and put them flat on top of a compost with a little sand in a seed tray. Cover with a plastic bag or sheet of plastic and leave in a cold frame, greenhouse, plastic tunnel or sheltered part of the garden. Once new shoots appear remove the plastic bag and plant out.

Layering
Low growing and shrubby herbs such as sage, thyme, lavender and periwinkle can be propagated by layering. Take a low growing branch and fix it with a peg or a stone in contact with the soil. If you nick the underside of the branch it will root more readily. Once a root has developed you can separate the formed new plant, dig it up and replant.

Mounding
Spreading herbs such as chamomile, thyme and marjoram can be partially covered with soil in their centre, thus bringing many different parts of the plant in contact with the soil so that once rooted, lots of new plants can be separated off.

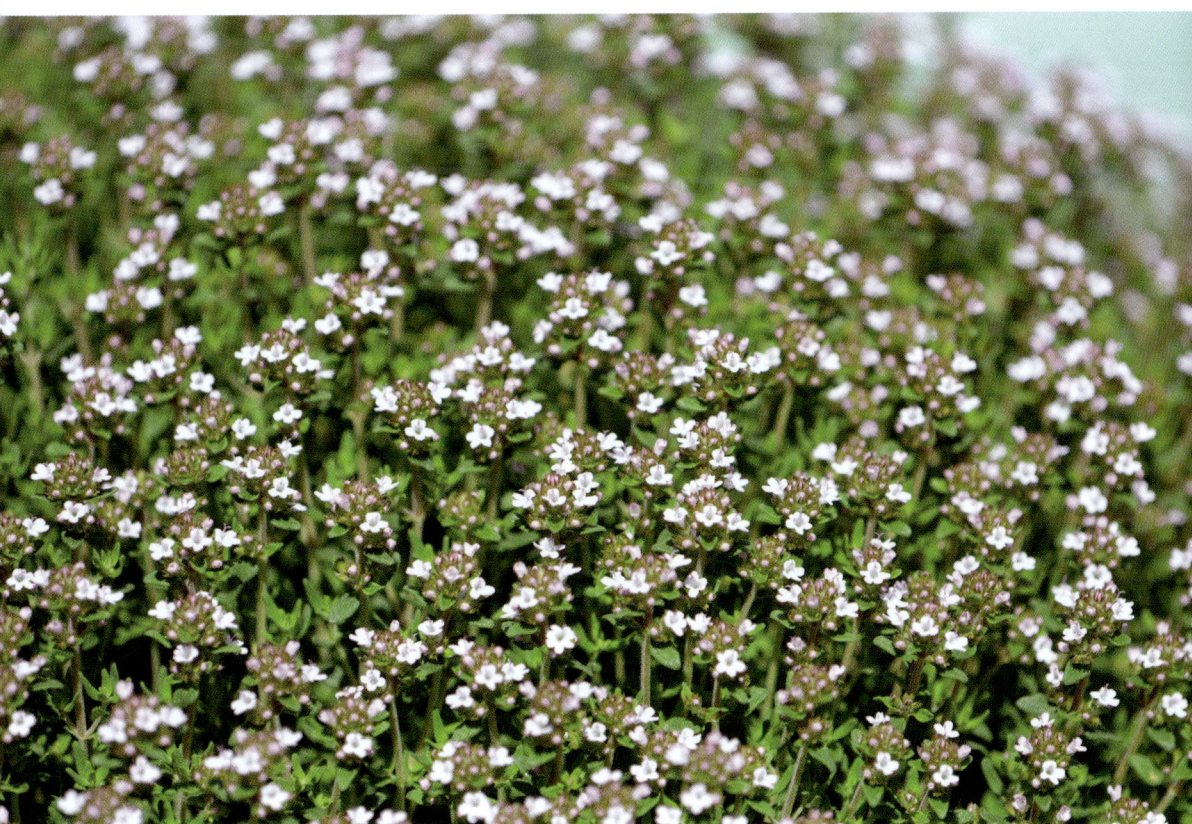

A Wildflower Garden

There are many beautiful wildflowers, both edible and medicinal, which you might like to find a space for in a wild corner in your garden if you have room. Many wildflowers that used to abound in the countryside have now disappeared due to use of chemical sprays, pollution and the destruction of natural habitats and they survive only in unsprayed, often wasteland areas on roadsides and industrial sites. By allowing them space in your garden, you will be helping the continued survival of these threatened plants.

> *To see a world in a grain of sand and heaven in a wildflower*
> *Hold infinity in the palms of your hand and eternity in an hour*
> – William Blake (1757–1827)

You could create a beautiful profusion of colour and smell with meadow flowers such as:

meadowsweet	pasque flower	violets
ground ivy	cowslips	greater celandine
yarrow	marshmallow	St John's wort
honeysuckle	evening primrose	primrose
wild dog rose	elderflowers	mullein
wild pansy	agrimony	hawthorn
cleavers	self-heal	wood betony
chickweed	dandelion	wild garlic
mugwort	chicory	centaury

An area under a deciduous tree, like a cherry or apple tree, is always a good area for a patch of wild garden. If you have a larger area, even a meadow, you could mow paths among tall grass and meadow flowers so you will be able to appreciate them better and check they are not getting lost or smothered.

> *A weed is a plant whose virtue is not yet known*
> – Ralph Waldo Emerson (1803–1882)

Planting a Wildflower Garden

You may already have several wildflowers like primroses, cowslips, daisies, dandelions, ground ivy, evening primrose, violets and honeysuckle growing happily in your garden. Others can be grown from packets of bought wildflower or meadow flower seed in seed trays. Once ready to plant out you can choose whether to grow them among your garden flowers, in the vegetable patch, in a neglected area of the garden or in an area of lawn. If planting in grass, lift a large piece of turf for each plant, dig a hole larger than is needed and fill it with plenty of good, fine-textured loam to help the plant make a good start. Water it in once planted and keep an eye on it until well established. Check that the ground does not dry out in hot weather, and that neighbouring grass does not completely smother it. By autumn of the same year resilient perennials such as agrimony, primroses, cleavers, ground ivy, daisies and dandelion should be able to cope with competition. Annuals and biennials such as wild pansy, cornflowers and mullein may self-seed, but

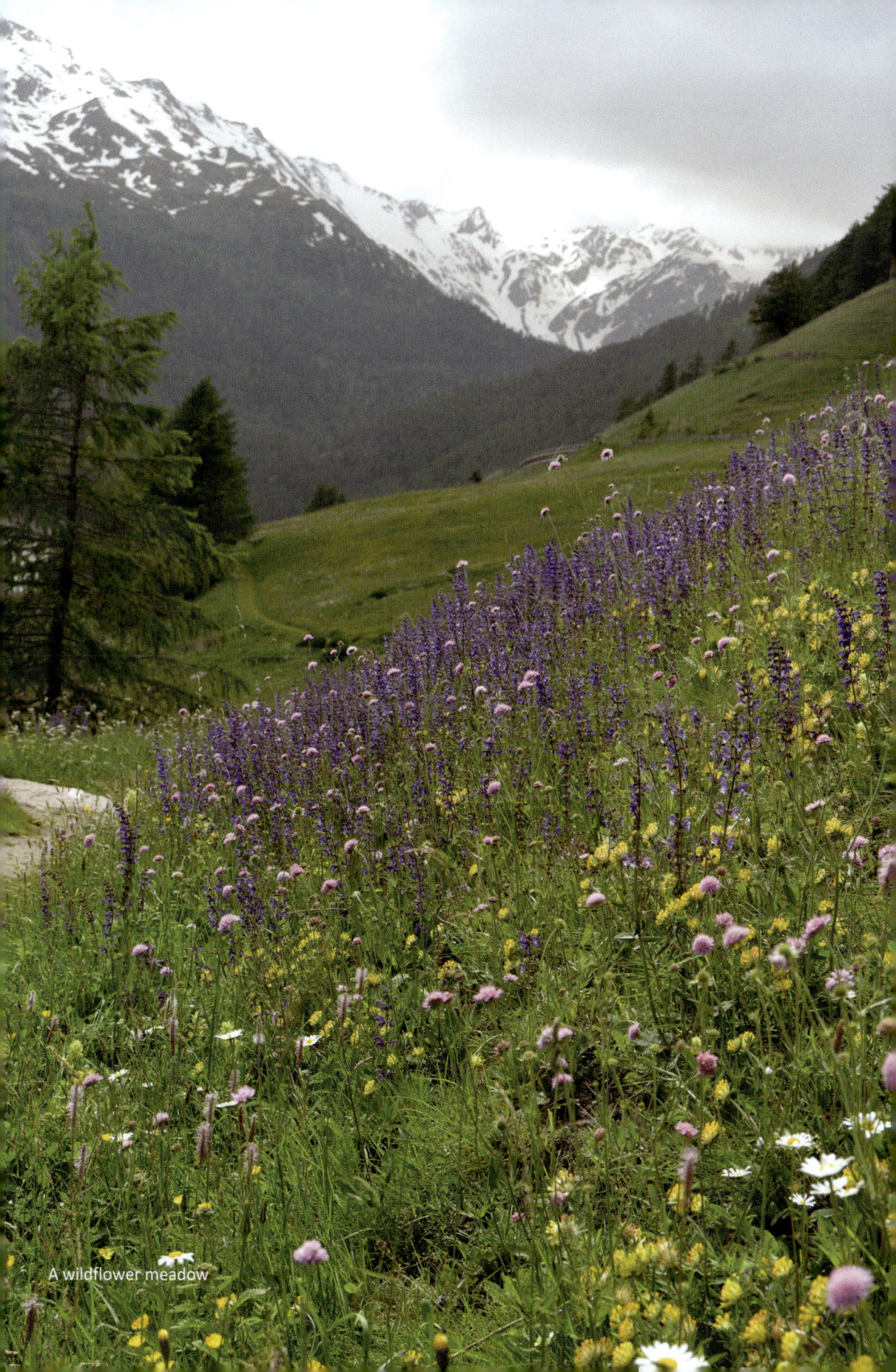
A wildflower meadow

it is worth collecting some seed just in case they do not. Less aggressive plants such as violets, cowslips, pasque flower and wood betony may need to be kept an eye on.

Another way of planting a wild area is to buy wild herb seed already mixed with grass seed or mix it yourself. Clear the ground of weeds, dig it well, level it and sow seed as you would for a lawn. Keep the area watered well in dry weather until growth is well established. The toughest plants will survive while some of the less forceful wildflowers may get lost by this method. A wild garden can look very attractive by early to mid-summer. Once all the flowers have gone over and seeds have dropped, the area can be scythed down to about 18"/25cm high.

Flowers in the Vegetable Garden
Flowers look very decorative planted in a corner here and there in the vegetable garden or in rows interspersed among the vegetables. Low growing or edging flowers like chamomile, pinks, chives, dill, marigolds, thyme, holy basil and stocks could really enhance the visual impact of your vegetable garden and give it more of a feeling of a *parterre* garden. Taller flowering plants or shrubs such as lavender, hyssop, roses (particularly *Rosa rugosa*), vervain, sweet Williams, carnations, echinacea, anise hyssop and mullein can look stunning planted in rows between vegetables or as low growing hedges for edging. Nasturtiums look striking anywhere in the vegetable garden, but need space. Aromatic, flowering plants in the vegetable garden not only look impressive but are also highly beneficial as companion plants.

Companion Planting
Since time immemorial aromatic plants have been known for their beneficial effects on the growth and health of vegetables and have been grown as border plants or in small patches in the vegetable garden. All vegetables are helped by aromatic plants in their vicinity, with the exception of fennel which can retard the growth of beans, tomatoes and kohlrabi. Borage, lavender, hyssop, sage, parsley, chervil, tarragon, thyme, marjoram, dill, chamomile and lovage are all useful; when planted near vegetables they will repel certain insects such as cabbage butterfly and deter plant diseases. Stinging nettles growing near aromatic plants increases the intensity of their fragrance by increasing their essential oil content. Yarrow acts similarly. When a mixture of plants is grown together, all plants grow more quickly and healthily than if planted singly, so they are mutually beneficial. The more variation in plants grown together the better.

Some plants make excellent companions to others; some high in essential oils such as thyme, rosemary, and hyssop give off such as strong scent that they disguise the smell of neighbouring plants and in this way protect them from predators. Others secrete substances from their roots into the soil that benefit their neighbours or have such deep roots that they bring nutrients up to the more superficial soil and they help break up heavy soil. Tall resilient plants like mullein, hollyhocks, sunflowers and marshmallow protect smaller or more delicate ones from wind, sun and cold. Many flowering plants are popular with moths, bees and other insects, bringing pollinators to the area.

Plants	Good Companions	Plants to Avoid
Apple trees:	Chives, nasturtium, chamomile coriander, dill, fennel, basil, mint, yarrow, marigold, hyssop, garlic	
Asparagus:	Basil, tomatoes, anise, coriander, dill, marigolds, nasturtiums	
Beans: Runner and French	Nasturtium, sweet peas, summer savoury	Fennel, garlic, onions, chives gladioli, sunflowers
Broad beans:	Calendula, summer savoury, dill	
Brussel sprouts:	Chamomile, coriander dill, hyssop, mint, thyme rosemary, sage, nasturtium, oregano	Garlic, rue, strawberries
Cabbage, kale:	Hyssop, chamomile, dill, celery	Strawberries, rue, garlic
Cauliflower:	Nasturtium, sage, rosemary, wormwood, rosemary, mint, thyme, southernwood, coriander	
Carrots:	Chives, spring onions, leek, coriander onions, garlic, rosemary, sage, wormwood	Dill
Celery:	Dill, onions, leeks, chives, tomatoes	
Courgettes:	Calendula	
Cucumber:	Chives, marjoram, nasturtium nettle spray	
Grapes:	Basil, hyssop, nasturtium	
Lettuce:	Calendula, onions, strawberries, calendula, French marigolds	
Onion:	Mint, chamomile, summer savoury	Peas, beans
Parsnips	Garlic, roses, chives, beans, peas	Carrots, celery, caraway
Potatoes:	Calendula, asparagus, horseradish nasturtium	Rosemary, sunflowers
Radishes:	Nasturtium, mint	Hyssop
Raspberries:	Tansy	
Roses:	Calendula, mint, thyme, chives, garlic	
Strawberries:	Borage, sage	Garlic
Tomatoes:	Basil, mint, French marigolds, calendula, chives, dill, parsley	Fennel, rosemary
Courgettes:	Nasturtium	

Insect Repellent Flowers
Certain plants make excellent companion plants because they have the ability to repel insects when several are planted in the vicinity. Basil around a rose bush for example, will keep aphids away and feverfew around a bed of carrots will deter carrot fly. They can be planted in rows between vegetables or as borders around the vegetable patch, as well as amongst flowers in herbaceous borders and rose gardens. They can also be used as plant sprays when prepared as a strong infusion.

Ants: marjoram, mint, oregano, pennyroyal, rue, chrysanthemums
Aphids: basil, chives, coriander, elder, nasturtium, garlic, petunias
Asparagus beetle: petunias,
Beetles: catnip, lavender, nasturtium, rosemary, wormwood, mint
Black fly: thyme, nettle spray
Cabbage moth: coriander, dill
Cabbage worm: chamomile, coriander
Carrot fly: coriander, rosemary, sage, wormwood, garlic, chives
Caterpillars: elder, mint
Fleas: fennel, pennyroyal, rosemary, rue, eucalyptus, lavender
Flies: basil, rue, lavender, pennyroyal, bay, lavender
Japanese beetles: garlic, chives, chrysanthemums
Mice: mint, tansy, catnip
Mosquitos: basil, elder, peppermint, feverfew, garlic, pennyroyal, lavender, French marigold, calendula
Moths: lavender, bay, chamomile, feverfew, tansy, garlic
Root maggots: garlic
Tomato worms: petunias

Chamomile and borage increase resistance to disease. Coriander hinders seed formation of fennel but attracts bees to garden when in bloom. Fennel does not grow well near wormwood.

Other Organic Gardening Hints

Nettle Plant Feed
You can make a liquid feed for your garden very easily from the nettles that pop up in the garden. Cut the nettles and fill a bucket or container with them. Cover the nettles with water, put lid on and leave to ferment for about 3 weeks, after which time it will not smell that great, but you will have a highly nutritious and free natural fertiliser as well as an effective insect repellent so it's worth it! Nettles are rich in vitamins A and C and minerals including iron, calcium, silica and potassium. Strain the water into another container and throw the nettles on the compost heap. To water your plants, use one part of nettle fertiliser to 10 parts of water in a watering can. Repeat the process throughout the growing period so that you always have a ready supply.

The Plants' Physician: Chamomile Spray
Place about three teaspoonfuls of chamomile flowers in a cup. Pour on boiling water. Cover and leave to stand for 24 hrs. Transfer to a spray bottle and use to spray on sick plants or to water seedlings to prevent damping off.

Compost Accelerators

Plants that are rich in minerals and trace-elements such as comfrey, nettle, dandelion and yarrow are rich in copper and phosphates and accelerate the fermentation of the compost heap. Elderflower trees around sites of compost help the fermentation of compost. Humus under elder trees is particularly light and fluffy and makes very good topsoil for the garden.

Growing Flowers in Small Spaces

If you do not have a large garden or even a garden at all, you can easily grow flowers and herbs in containers of various kinds – in window boxes, troughs, old sinks, urns or decorative pots including strawberry pots, but they do require a little more care than growing them in open ground. Container grown plants are prone to both waterlogging from overwatering or to drying out, particularly in dry weather when they will need lots of attention. They need to be fed regularly and the soil kept just moist all the time. You can plant up containers and put them on balconies, windowsills, porches and patios providing there is enough shelter and light; most herbs need a minimum of 5 to 6 hours of sunlight a day. Plants tend to grow better outside on balconies and windowsills than indoors as they get more light and air.

Terracotta pots and flowers make very good partners; they look decorative and attractive together. You need to make sure they are frost-proof or be prepared to take them inside for the winter. In fact, bringing potted herbs indoors in winter is a means of providing yourself with fresh edible and medicinal plants throughout the changing seasons. In a large outdoor pot, you can either use garden loam or a loam-based compost. In a smaller pot lighter peat-based compost can be used which will need to be replenished each

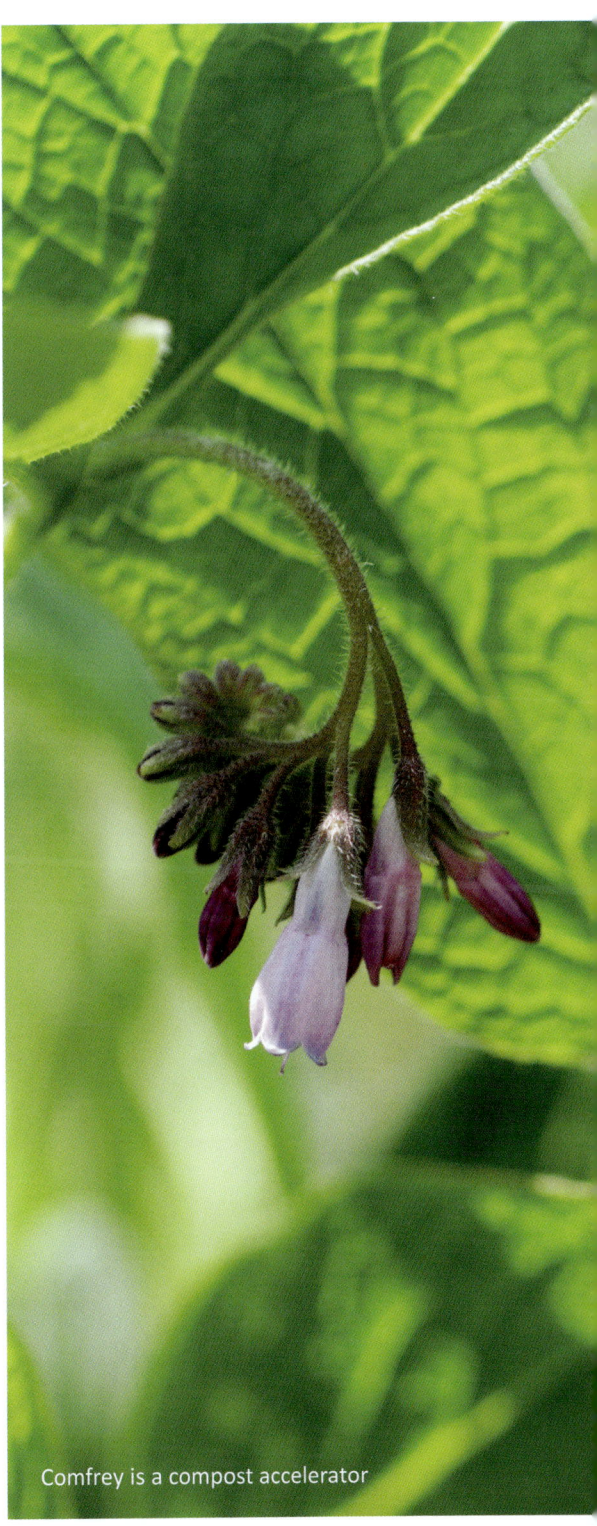

Comfrey is a compost accelerator

year. Make sure there is proper drainage in your pot before filling it with compost; there need to be holes in the base covered with crocks.

When planting up pots or window boxes, use small plants or rooted cuttings and try not to be tempted to cram too many together in one pot as they will fast outgrow their space. Avoid large vigorous growing plants such as mullein, clary sage, elecampane, angelica and marshmallow. If you want to grow rather invasive herbs like mint, yarrow, meadowsweet and lemon balm, the variegated varieties tend to be less fast-growing and so might be preferable. Strawberry pots are pots with holes in the sides and are excellent for creeping, trailing herbs such as ground ivy, creeping thyme, sweet woodruff and mint. Otherwise, invasive herbs such as mint can be planted in containers and sunk in the ground to contain them and restrict their growth, or else they can be too rampant particularly in a small garden.

When growing plants in pots you may find that from time to time they need to be replaced as they outgrow their space or begin to grow straggly and less attractive. It may be easier to leave the plant in its pot in your terracotta pot or window box, covered with compost or gravel, then it can simply be lifted out when it needs replacing.

Planting in Patios or Paving
Many flowers and herbs look attractive planted in gaps between stones in patios, paths or paving stones, between bricks or in gravel. Low creeping aromatic plants are most suitable and are delightful to walk on or by as they release their exquisite scents when bruised or brushed against. They include creeping thyme, thyme, marjoram, lawn chamomile, pinks, self-heal, chickweed, chives, Corsican mint, sweet woodruff, violets and pansies. If you are laying a path or patio you could leave gaps for plants in random places, or design a more symmetrical pattern, the easiest of which is alternate paving stones and flower beds. If your path or patio is already in place, try removing chipped or crumbling corners of stone or bricks, dig a small hole and squeeze a little fresh loam in to make space for your small plant.

A garden to walk in and immensity to dream in--what more could he ask?
A few flowers at his feet and above him the stars
– Victor Hugo (1802–1885)

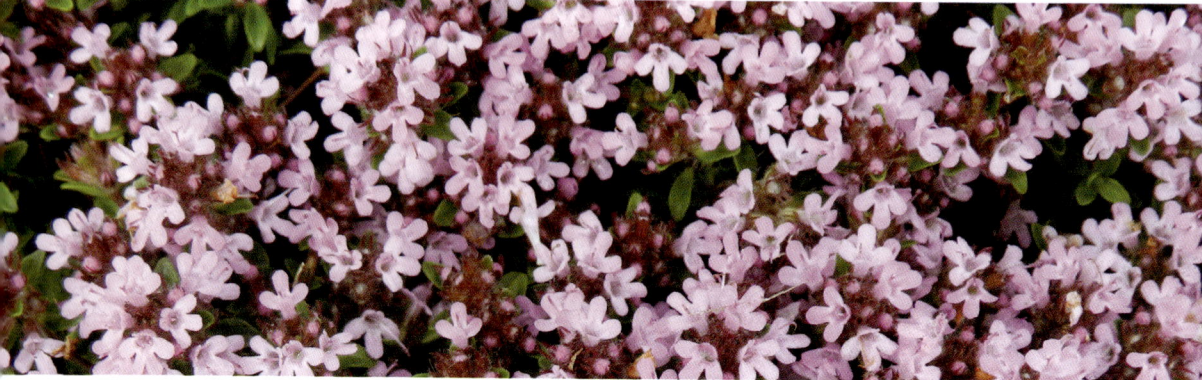

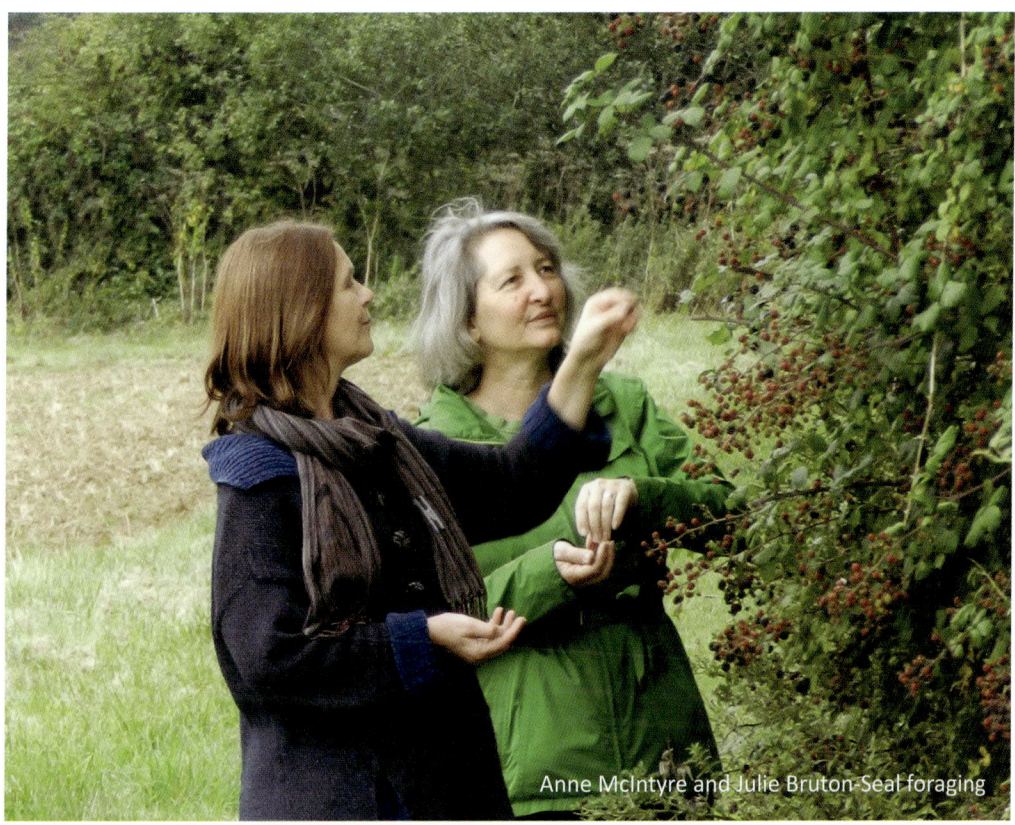
Anne McIntyre and Julie Bruton-Seal foraging

Gathering and Foraging

*And forget not that the earth delights to feel your bare feet
And the winds long to play with your hair*
– Khalil Gibran (1883–1931)

Flowers have the extraordinary power to heal us in many ways. Simply being amongst them in a garden, picking flowers and leaves for the kitchen, gathering baskets of flowers and leaves for making medicines or gathering wild herbs in a country lane is enough to experience for ourselves their wonderful effects. When gathering flowers and their leaves for healing or for the kitchen it is important to choose those looking as healthy and vibrant as possible, free from disease and infestation. Only pick the amount you need at any one time as they will easily spoil and be wasted otherwise. Harvest just a few leaves and flowers from each plant so as not to threaten the health or survival of any one plant.

When gathering plants for healing for your home medicine chest, floral pharmacy or still room, there are certain guidelines to follow to ensure your remedies are as potent as they possibly can be. Flowers and leaves of aromatic plants such as dill, coriander, basil, rosemary, thyme, sage, mint and lemon balm are best harvested when the flowers are about to open as the essential oil content is highest at that period. When gathering only

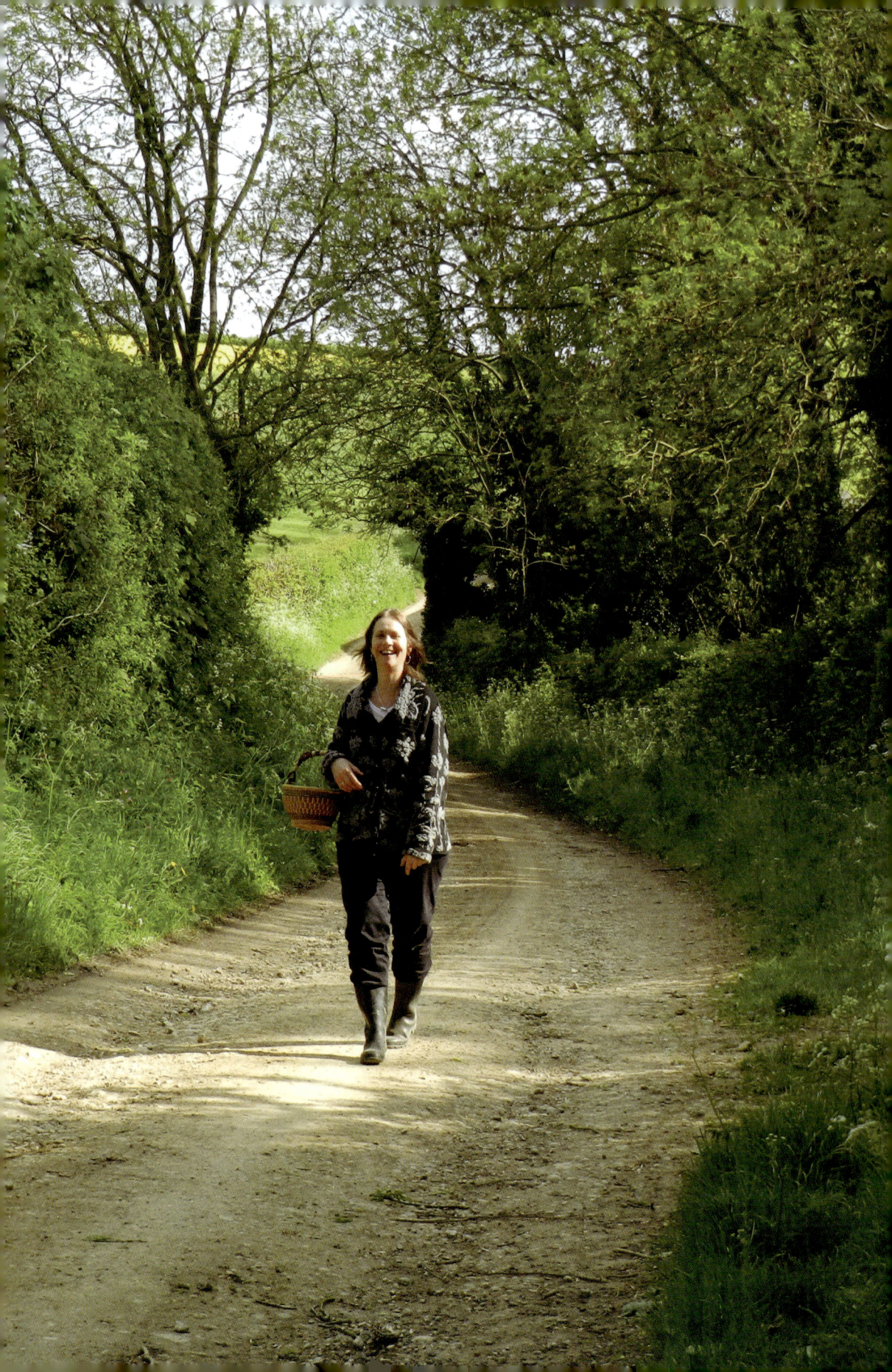

the flowers or flowering tops such as roses, lavender, St John's wort, honeysuckle, jasmine, orange flower, violets, cowslips, yarrow, skullcap and hyssop, they are best picked in their prime, just as they burst into bloom.

A flat basket is best for collecting leaves and flowers, making it easier not to bruise or crush the leaves or flowers. Gather them on a dry day, once the dew has dried, unless they are going straight into a meal in which case it is not so important. During the growing season, leaves and flowers are best gathered and used fresh, ideally straight from the garden before they have time to wilt and lose their vitality for both kitchen use and for making medicines. At the same time, it is a good harvest some extra for drying to last through the winter months, as the growing time for many flowers is relatively short.

You may want to collect seeds, either for the kitchen or for medicines or to plant for next year's garden. If so, you need to catch them when they are ripe just before they drop. You can cut off the whole flower head when harvesting them, tie it up in muslin or a paper bag with string or rubber band and hang it upside down in a well-ventilated dry room. As the flower head dries the seeds will conveniently drop into the bag. Store the seeds in envelopes, foil or small boxes with well-fitting lids, and label clearly with the herb name and collection date.

Foraging for Wildflowers

> *Nature....she will hang the night stars so that I may walk abroad in the darkness without stumbling, and send word the wind over my footprints so that none may track me to my hurt: she will cleanse me in great waters, and with bitter herbs make me whole*
> – Oscar Wilde (1854–1900)

Foraging means looking for, identifying and gathering wild foods and it is becoming an increasingly popular pastime and for many good reasons; it can give us a great sense of enjoyment as well as the satisfaction of finding food for free. It is also a lovely way to make sure we spend more time outside in the fresh air as an antidote to our busy lives, often indoors at a desk. It also helps us to keep an active lifestyle while providing opportunities for connecting more deeply with nature and getting a sense of and respect for the origins of all our food.

Though foraging as an activity and hobby has gained popularity and a somewhat fashionable status in recent years (it has even been chosen for hen dos!), it was once just a normal human way of life. From the beginning of human existence on earth maybe 200,000 years ago, our distant ancestors would spend their days in nature foraging for food and needed a profound awareness of their surrounding environment and all that it had to offer in order to sustain themselves. Living as we do today in such a convenience-led and modernised culture it is hard to imagine a way of life like this. But if nothing else, what the current global crisis is telling us is that we cannot continue as we have been and activities such as growing and foraging for foods and medicines in our local landscape may become the norm again before we know it. Hopefully becoming more connected with and interested in our local environment can teach us and the generations that follow us the importance of celebrating our precious wild lands and help us to learn more about ways to protect and look after them.

While you might love the idea of exploring the depths of the countryside to forage and it would certainly be a rewarding experience to do so, it is not a necessity. Even if you live in a city, there are likely to be ample edible and medicinal flowers growing much closer to home, in fact they can be found almost anywhere from wild parks to canal or riverside banks and pathways, from the edges of woodland areas to hedgerows and from allotments to the 'weeds' growing in your own garden.

Foraging Best Practice

Learning to identify and then recognise plants is much like getting to know a person; once you know them it becomes second nature to recognise them even if they get a new hair style or wear different clothes. As we move through the seasons the appearance of most plants is likely to change, and it is important to be mindful of this when foraging. Only pick plants you know enough about and are completely confident that you can identify. The best way to begin familiarising yourself with wild plants is to go out foraging with an expert who can teach you. Otherwise, you could pick one that you feel confident that you know, such as a nettle or dandelion, and use it to familiarise yourself with the common characteristics of plants in general before moving on to a plant you know less about. Begin by reading an easy-to-digest description of your chosen plant from whichever

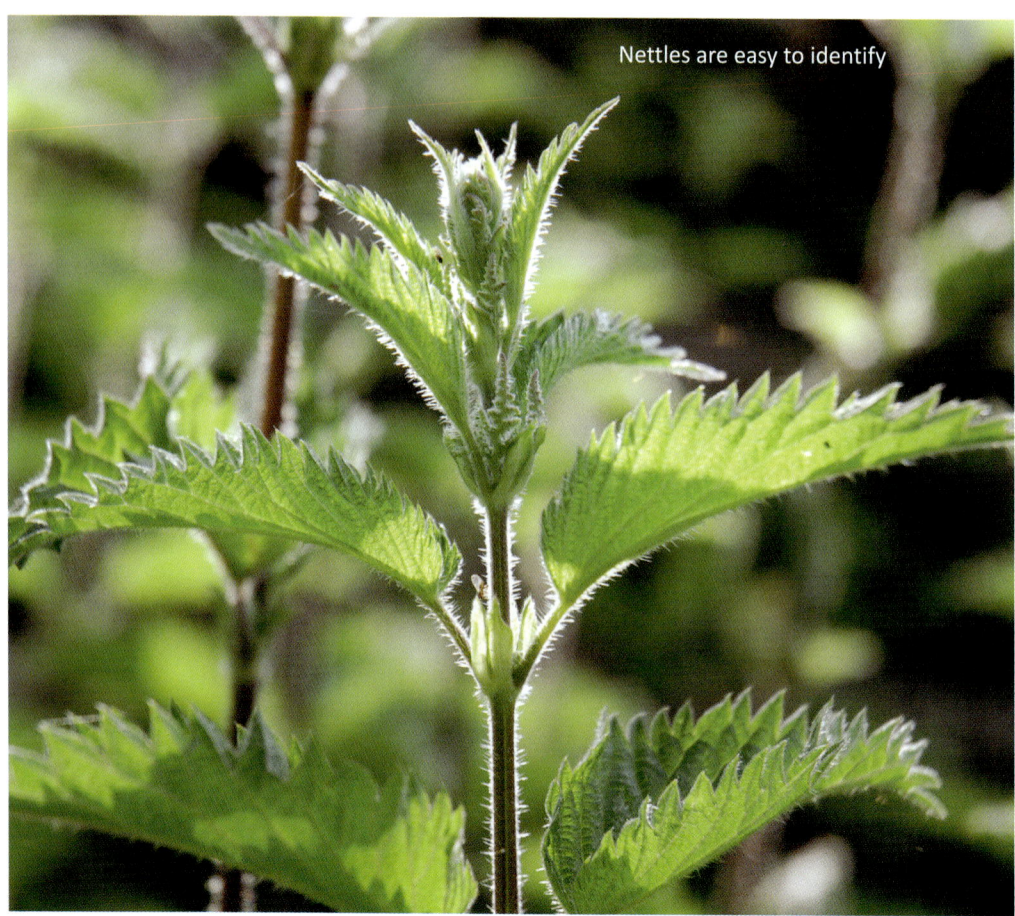

Nettles are easy to identify

source you've chosen to learn about foraging, either a book or a website. Start to notice the details in the plant in front of you; the length of the stalk, the shape of the leaf and the style of its edges, whether it has any seeds or blossoms. Once you feel confident matching the characteristics of the plants you know to their description in this way, then you can transfer the same level of attention to detail on to unfamiliar plants and start to branch out.

Foraging Safely and Responsibly
Growing our own remedies and foraging for wild ones means that we can adhere more closely to the increasing need for us all to live more sustainably. Modern medicine is expensive. The running of hospitals, surgeries, equipment and the manufacture of medicines are all reliant on energy and other resources. Plant medicine, meanwhile, uses very little. The amount of pressure that the current healthcare system is working under is not sustainable. Waiting times can be long, doctors are overworked and over-stressed and healthcare costs increasing. The use of plant medicine, particularly in preventative medicine, can help to reduce some of the pressure and strain; when people look after their own health by using simple plant remedies and dietary changes at home, it helps to reduce demands made on the doctor. The use of plant medicine may also be more sustainable for our bodies and for our health, as it generally comes without the risk of side effects and the development of iatrogenic disease. The wider use of plant medicines could mean less illness overall, less side effects, and freeing up of the resources of conventional medicine for when it is really needed, thus making the whole system more sustainable.

Of course, there are some aspects of plant medicine that are not sustainable. One of the main concerns is that some plants are over-harvested in the wild. Goldenseal, false unicorn, cowslips and some species of Echinacea are examples of this. In the latter case, it is mainly due to the huge popularity of Echinacea coupled with harvesters not properly distinguishing the different types of Echinacea, and harvesting those that are less common. If you are not able to grow or forage for your own healing plants, sourcing organically cultivated or sustainably wildcrafted herbs to use is always best. Even with local non-endangered plants, there can be a risk of over-harvesting and of damaging the local population of a particular plant. There are a set of principles it is recommended to follow when picking plants from the wild.

When foraging for wildflowers, always choose areas which are least likely to have been affected by pollution; gather as far away from roadsides or car parks as possible, from industrial sites and cultivated land that may have been sprayed with fertilisers and pesticides. When it comes to public footpaths or other similar areas, be sure to steer clear of places frequented by dog walkers which could have been contaminated.

There are a few more things to consider and make sure that we are foraging responsibly and sustainably. It is important to be mindful not to collect from places where a plant looks scarce or to over-pick in the same area. Instead forage plants in areas where they are growing in abundance and only pick what you feel you really need and will use. Never strip an area of a particular species of plant, as this could threaten the survival of that plant or of the wildlife who depend on it for their survival. With this in mind, do remember to take care not to disturb or damage the areas from which you are collecting, so as to protect the natural habitat of the wildlife living there.

While gathering flowers you have an opportunity to pause and just relish the sheer pleasure of what you are doing…collecting wildflowers, the fruits of abundant nature, to delight the senses, excite the palate, please the eye and bring you healing beyond your imagination! What a gift we are given!

Drying Plants
The object of the drying process is to eliminate the moisture in the plant quickly before it starts to die, so that it can be stored for a few months without deteriorating and retains its therapeutic properties.

When harvesting flowers and leaves for storage, make sure they are dry from rain or dew and pick them in the morning before the sun reaches its peak. Use your fingers/hands to pick, unless stalks such as agrimony or yarrow are very tough, in which case you will need scissors. Pick gently, taking care not to bruise the plant.

When lifting roots, dig them up with a garden fork, trying not to puncture the outer skin. Wash the soil off the roots and cut off any leaves left, then chop up into sections or slices to speed drying and lie them out to dry. If bark is needed, it is best to peel the bark off whole branches that have been pruned rather than shaving bark off branches on the tree, as it may not do the tree much good.

Providing that plants are dried properly, those you dry at home are often of a much higher quality than shop-bought herbs in terms of colour, flavour and healing properties. Drying needs to occur as quickly and evenly as possible. Shade, air and constant warmth are all essential.

The best place for drying is a dehydrator, which takes around 4 hours to dry most flowers and leaves, unless they are thick and a bit heavy like marshmallow when they could take a few hours longer. Put the heat on around 40 degrees C and check them regularly. When they are dry and crunchy, they are ready. They should have retained all their colour and look vibrant. If they look slightly brown, then you have the heat too high.

If you choose not to use a dehydrator, the best place to dry plants is a shaded, well-ventilated room or warm garden shed or barn, free from moisture or condensation. It is

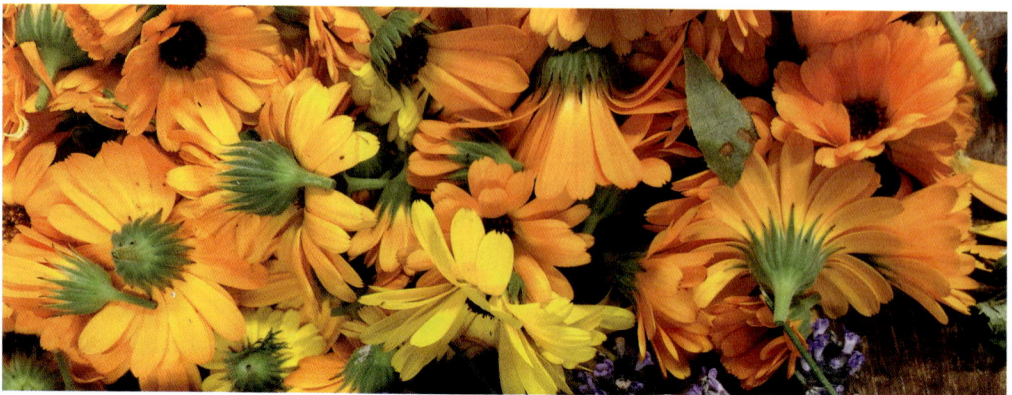

vital to avoid the kitchen, bathroom, utility room, sheds or garages if they are steamy or damp, as the plants will not dry properly and will deteriorate. You can loosely tie flowers and leaves in small bunches by their stems and hang them from a beam or a hook indoors. In warm dry climates, bunches of herbs can be hung up out of doors in the shade or from a high ceiling in a warm room with the windows open. This may be rather an unpredictable way to dry herbs as the temperature varies so much through 24 hours.

More reliable results may be obtained by spreading sprigs of flowers and leaves or pieces of bark or root or seed evenly over either a tray, wire netting, a box lid, a fruit tray, a drying frame, sheets of paper or muslin. Drying frames can be made fairly easily by stretching muslin or fine netting over a wooden frame and are excellent for drying as they allow free circulation of air. Spread out the plants so there is plenty of space between them and turn them frequently – once or twice on the first day and once daily after that. Large leaved or heavier leaves and flowers such as mullein and marshmallow will dry more quickly if you remove the leaves and flowers from their fleshy stems and discard the stems.

A steady temperature of about 90 degrees F/32 degrees C is ideal and this could be achieved in an airing cupboard, above a range such as an Aga or Rayburn, or in a low oven with the door left open to allow water to evaporate and air to circulate. If the atmosphere is too cold (below 72 degrees F/22 degrees C) the plants will reabsorb moisture from the air and take too long to dry. You will know if they have taken too long or have got damp as they will lose quite a bit of their colour or even turn slightly brown or yellow. Always dry plants separately – never mix species together.

Storing Flowers and Leaves
Dried leaves and flowers are best stored in air-tight dark containers, wooden or cardboard boxes, paper bags or jars – glass jars are ideal kept in a dark cupboard, as exposure to light will cause deterioration of medicinal constituents of the plants. Never store in plastic as it encourages condensation. Make sure to label the plants clearly with their name and date harvested. Remove stalks and twigs from aerial parts of plants, and break roots, rhizomes and barks into small pieces before storing. Store seeds in packets in the fridge or in air-tight jars. Before storing your dried plants, it is important to check that they are properly dry by seeing if they are brittle and rustle, crumble or snap easily between your fingers and thumb. If herbs are stored before they are completely dry, they will reabsorb moisture from the atmosphere and deteriorate.

Some plants (particularly those with soft leaves and flowers such as marjoram, borage, coriander, fennel, lemon balm, basil, forget-me-not and mint) are ideal for freezing. Pick the leaves or flowers, wash them and then place them in small plastic bags to freeze.

> *The many great gardens of the world, of literature and poetry,*
> *of painting and music, of religion and architecture,*
> *all make the point as clear as possible:*
> *The soul cannot thrive in the absence of a garden.*
> *If you don't want paradise, you are not human;*
> *and if you are not human, you don't have a soul*
> – Sir Thomas More (1478–1535)

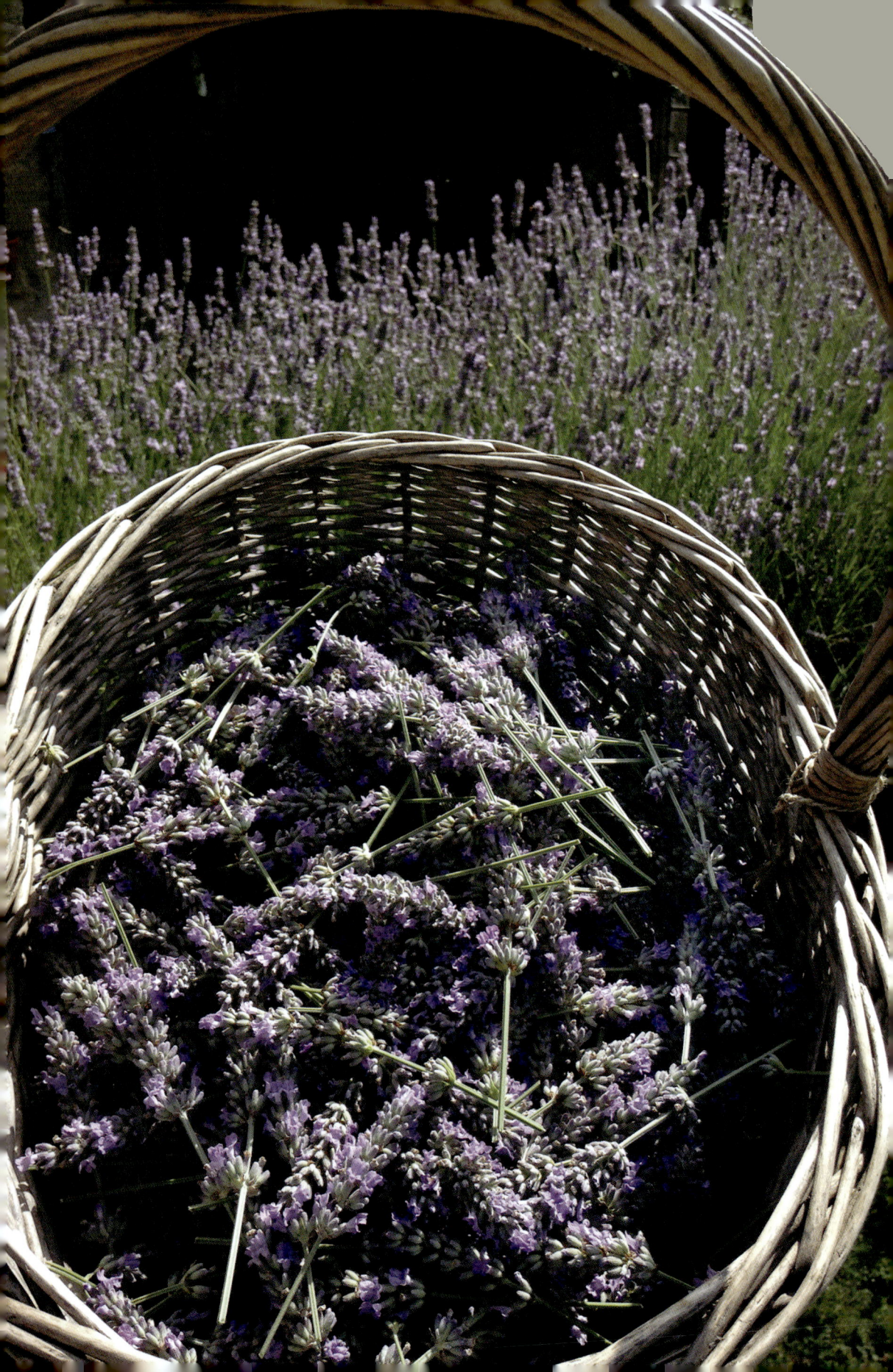

The Floral Pharmacy or Still Room

There is immense pleasure to be gained gathering flowers for making medicines and as you do, you will be following in the footsteps of traditions that go back centuries. What you can create in your own home is something akin to the 16th century still room that could be found in most large European country houses. The still room could sound like a haven for those of us who love herbs and flowers and to create foods and medicines imbued with their exquisite scents and flavours, providing healthcare for the household. In the times of our ancestors, flowers and herbs grown in the garden were gathered and brought to the still room to be made into aromatic and medicinal preparations for culinary, medicinal, cleaning and cosmetic purposes. The still room held a very important place and was presided over by the woman of the household, often supported by a still room maid. It was a hub of essential activity to support the wellbeing of the household which included the family, their servants, tenant farmers and even their animals. It held its central place in family life until the 19th century by which time physicians and apothecaries took many of their activities over. Preparations previously the province of the still room became available to buy over the counter from the local apothecary and the still room became more of an adjunct to the kitchen, dedicated more to making jams and jellies, homebrews and cakes and became the responsibility of the housekeeper or cook.

If it appeals to you to create a room or a space in the house for your floral preparations, it might help to visualise the still room. It would house a wonderful variety of plant materials with their array of hues and scents, hanging up being dried, stored in drawers, prepared as aromatic waters, beers, wines and meads for medicinal and dining purposes, tinctures, essential oils, soaps and other cleaning materials, furniture polish, candles, insect repellents, pot pourris, perfumes, cosmetics, honeys and culinary oils. Medicines were made from an array of plants from the garden that we commonly use today such as coriander, fennel, mint, rose, wood betony, angelica and hyssop. Aromatic waters were made, probably in a copper still, from lavender, roses, myrtle, orange blossom, jasmine and other fragrant plants for the kitchen and to use as medicines. Floral waters were applied to the skin and used to scent linen and clothes as well as floors and furniture. Aromatic herbs were dried and strewn on floors throughout the house to dispel bad smells as well as insects, vermin and infection. Bunches of dried plants were also hung from the rafters.

In the still room there would be found various different items used in the preparation of herbs and flowers. There would be a mortar and pestle for grinding herbs and making powders, a herb crusher for seeds and woody parts of plants, a still for distillation of flowers and herbs to make essential oils and aromatic waters, and a sieve for powdered herbs. There would be earthenware jars and glass bottles containing meads and other herbal concoctions covered with a piece of linen and sealed with wax or lard.

The lady of the house would keep a still room book like a journal or diary that was used for recording recipes prepared there and these were added to and amended as they passed down the generations of women who took care of the household. It is a very good idea to do the same and a 'still room book' today can be a repository of our experience in the 'still room' in our own lives, containing recipes we have made, notes on how they worked and recipes collected from others. It helps to know how much of certain floral preparations we actually used in a year so that we know how much we need to prepare for the next.

Although your still room may not be as large a room or laid out with the same organisation as that of a 16th century country house, the beauty of flowers and aromatic herbs means that the space you make for your floral preparations could look arty and uplifting and be a place you love to be and spend many happy hours. Bringing the plants and herbs that you have grown or gathered directly from the garden or countryside to the still room can be exciting! The deeply rewarding sense of being close to nature can be brought inside your house into the 'still room' which could be any size or shape or even just a few shelves, cupboards or surface in the kitchen or even the garden shed.

How could such sweet and wholesome hours be reckoned, but in herbs and flowers?
– Andrew Marvell (1621–1678)

Preparing Floral Medicines

The art of healing comes from nature and not from the physician.
Therefore, the physician must start from nature with an open mind
– Paracelsus (c. 1493–1541)

It is best to pick the flowers you are planning to use first thing in the morning on a fine dry day once the dew has dried, so they are as fresh as possible. Choose the healthiest looking plants, remove any soil and old leaves or flowerheads and check for insects. The sooner you make the flowers up into your preparations the better, so they don't lose any of their vibrancy and medicinal effects.

There are many ways that you can take healing flowers to benefit from their remedial effect. The easiest way to do this is in food and drink by using edible flowers and culinary herbs and herbal teas, which many people may be doing without realising their medicinal benefits.

A man may esteem himself happy when that which is his food is also his medicine
– Henry David Thoreau (1817–1862)

Salads with basil, coriander, nasturtiums and chives, vinaigrettes with garlic, fish with dill or wild garlic, new potatoes with fresh mint, casseroles with thyme and pizza with oregano are all very familiar. Once your food is absorbed from the digestive tract, the nutrients and therapeutic constituents of the plants enter the bloodstream and then circulate around the body. Your favourite culinary flowers and herbs all contain volatile oils that lend their wonderful flavours and scents. These oils have antioxidant and antimicrobial effects, helping to protect the body against stresses of all kinds and to ward off a wide variety of infections, which would have been vital for health as well as enhancing culinary skills in the days before fridges, when food may have been less than fresh.

Edible flowers don't just heighten the visual impact and the flavour of our food, they can also contribute a wide range of nutrients and medicinal compounds. Almost all of them contain vitamins A and C and mineral such as calcium, phosphorous, iron and potassium.

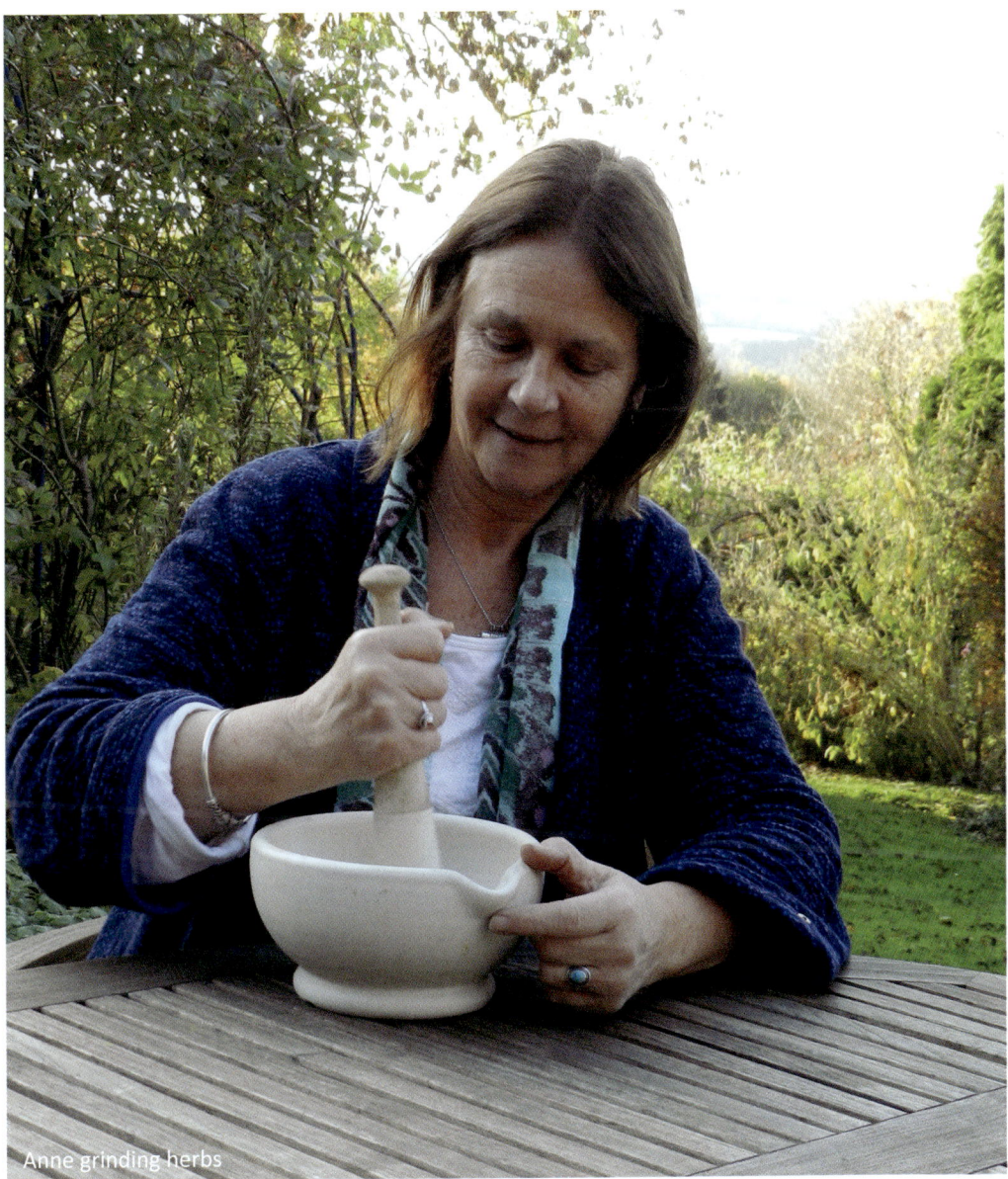

Anne grinding herbs

They are also rich in antioxidants which give the flowers and leaves their colours. Pigments that make carnations red, chrysanthemums and calendula orange for example, are rich in antioxidant polyphenols including flavonoids which protect the body against oxidative stress and may help prevent chronic diseases such as heart disease and cancer. Calendula flowers contain more flavonoids known as lutein and zeaxanthin (that help protect the eyes from age-related disorders) than cabbage, kale or spinach and nasturtiums are also rich in them. Violets are a good source of another bioflavonoid called rutin which protects the blood vessels from damage and reduces inflammation. Apparently, even though it is an ancient practice, there is a scientific name for people who eat flowers for food, it is called *floriphagia*!

> *Let your food be your medicine and your medicine be your food*
> – Hippocrates (c.460BC–c. 370BC)

Nutrients Found in our Favourite Flowers

Vitamins

Vitamin A: Dandelion, squash flowers, basil, dill, peppermint, rosemary, sage, coriander, lavender, violets

Vitamin B: Peppermint, sage, coriander, garlic, dandelion, sunflowers, feverfew, peppermint, hibiscus

Vitamin C: Echinacea, borage, nasturtium, garlic, peppermint, rosehips, dandelion, dill, rocket, rosemary, basil, sage, coriander, oregano, roses, purslane, calendula, fennel, violets

Vitamin D: Dandelion, rosehips, nasturtiums

Vitamin E: Dandelion, skullcap, sage, rose, sunflowers

Vitamin K: Basil, sage, coriander, dandelion

Minerals

Calcium: Bergamot, chamomile, fennel, marshmallow, sage, dill, peppermint, rosemary, garlic, oregano, coriander, dandelion, lavender, borage, violets, hibiscus

Iron: Peppermint, bergamot, nasturtium, begonia, French marigold, dianthus, rosemary, day lily, skullcap, peony, lavender, dill, sage, coriander, oregano, dandelion, echinacea, calendula, chamomile

Magnesium: Rosemary, day lily, wood betony, basil, dill, peppermint, sage, oregano, coriander, dandelion, dianthus, sunflowers

Manganese: Basil, dill, rosemary, peppermint, sage, chrysanthemum, coriander, garlic, oregano, dandelion

Potassium: Dandelion leaf, peony, bergamot, day lily, dianthus, fennel, rosehips, dill, rosemary, peppermint, oregano, violets, wild pansy

Zinc: Chamomile, day lily, skullcap, peony, bergamot, dandelion, marshmallow, rosemary, peppermint, sage, caraway, garlic, coriander leaf

Chromium: Coriander, hibiscus, dandelion

Copper: Skullcap, sage, day lily, fuchsia, bergamot, peony, dill, rosemary, peppermint, wild garlic, coriander, dandelion

Selenium: Garlic, coriander, fennel, basil, chamomile, St John's wort, oregano, sage, rosemary, lime flowers

You can also prepare a variety of different floral preparations including tinctures, elixirs, oxymels and honeys which are described below. Theses floral preparations can be made with single plants and then when needed you can combine several together to address the health problem you are trying to resolve or you can make ready-made combinations all in the same preparation for treating common ailments such as colds and coughs, digestive troubles, stress and insomnia when they arise. A good example of a popular and old fashioned cold and catarrh remedy is a combination of equal parts of peppermint, elderflowers and yarrow.

You can also make preparations to apply to the skin as it is very absorbent and covers a large surface area for absorption. Tiny blood capillaries under the surface of the skin take the medicinal compounds in the flowers into the bloodstream and from there they are circulated throughout the body. Infusions of flowers can be used as hand and foot baths, infused or diluted essential oils can be massaged into the skin, tincture-based rubbing lotions can be applied to the skin as can ointments and creams, compresses and poultices. In addition, fresh flowers and leaves can be applied directly such as yarrow, marigold or lavender flowers to staunch bleeding from minor cuts and abrasions and relieve minor burns.

The conjunctiva of the eye will also absorb floral extracts. A calendula, elderflower or chamomile eyebath or compress can be used to relieve sore and inflamed eyes. The nose and the nerve endings lying in it can provide another therapeutic pathway which we use when we smell a flower or use oils for inhalations. When we use a hot tea or a few drops of essential oil in hot water as an inhalation, the messages from the aromatic flowers are carried directly to the brain and are also taken into the lungs where they are absorbed with oxygen into the bloodstream and circulated throughout the body.

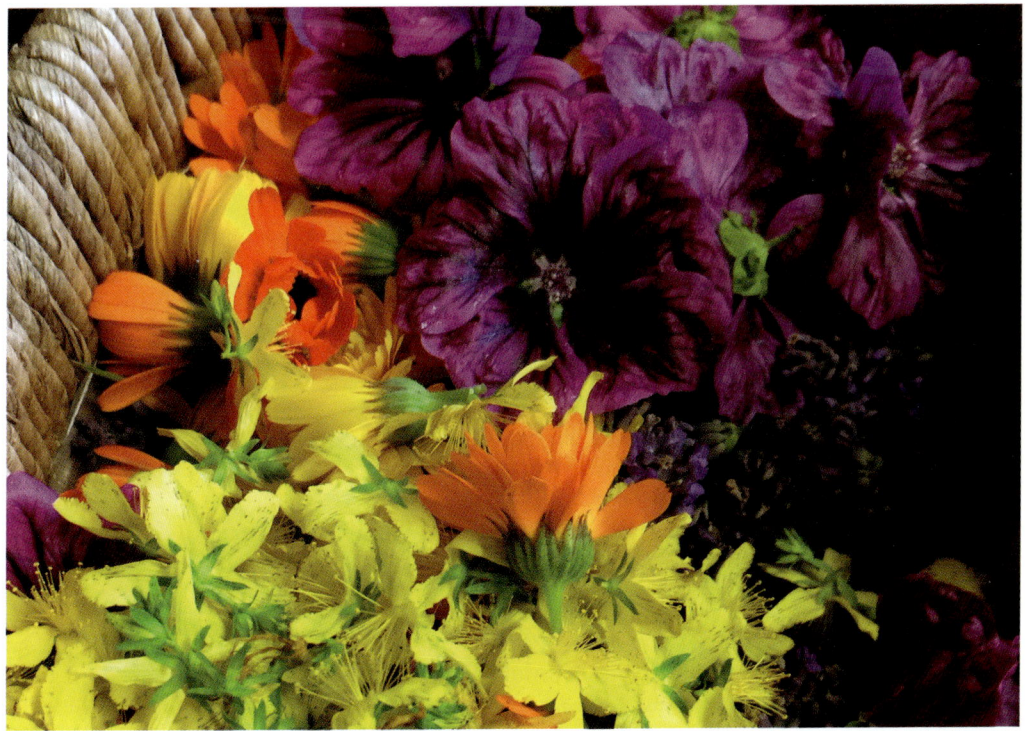

Preparations for Taking Flowers Internally

All that man needs for health and healing has been provided by God in nature, the Challenge of science is to find it
– Paracelsus (c. 1493–1541)

Infusions

Infusions, teas or tisanes are the easiest and most common way to prepare the soft parts of plants, the leaves, stems and flowers, using the same method as you would for a normal cup of tea. The hot water acts to extract certain of the constituents of the plant, if it is left to steep. You can use a favourite teapot, a cafetière or a stainless-steel infuser ball for loose herbs or if necessary, you can buy teabags. You could also make your own reusable teabags with muslin drawstring teabags, which you can buy. The usual ratio is 1 oz/25 gms of dried plant per pint/600 mls of water or a teaspoon of dried plant per cupful of water. If you are using fresh plants, you can double their amount.

When making tea in a pot, place the flowers and/or leaves in the warmed pot and pour boiling water over them. Cover immediately with the lid to prevent the volatile oils escaping into the atmosphere. Leave it to infuse for 10–15 minutes and then strain. The infusion can then be drunk immediately or stored in the fridge for up to 2 days.

The therapeutic components of some of the more soothing herbs may be destroyed by high temperatures and need to be prepared as cold infusions. These include plants that have a high proportion of mucilage such as marshmallow, mullein and hollyhock. The method of preparation and the dosage is the same, but they are covered with cold water and left to infuse for 10–12 hours before being strained.

Dosage: Floral infusions can be taken as cupfuls (200 mls) three times daily for chronic symptoms and up to six times a day for acute problems such as sore throats, flu and chest infections. Many people expect healing flowers and herbs to taste as exquisite as they smell, and accustomed as we are to sweet tasting foods and often even medicines, may find it hard initially to adjust to the rather unfamiliar flavour of some flowers. Although the bitters in some flowers such as chamomile, wood betony, rosemary, sage and dandelion may need to be tasted to be effective, the bitter taste can be hard to stomach if it is too intense. However, it is possible to combine several flowers and leaves together in an infusion to allow aromatic, pleasant tasting herbs such as peppermint, fennel, lemon balm and lavender to mask the flavour of less palatable herbs, whilst not reducing their effect. Infusions can also be sweetened with honey if you prefer, especially if you want your children to take them regularly.

Infusions are usually drunk when they are warm or hot, particularly when you are treating fevers, colds and catarrhal congestion. They are taken lukewarm or cool for problems associated with the kidneys and urinary tract, such as irritable bladder, urinary tract infections, cystitis, urethritis and bed wetting.

Decoctions

The harder, more solid or woody parts of plants have tough cell walls and need higher temperatures than flowers and leaves to break them down before their constituents can be extracted by the water. Bark, seeds, roots, rhizomes and nuts all need to be prepared as decoctions. Break the plant part up into small pieces with a pestle and mortar or, if they are particularly hard, smash them with a hammer and this will allow their constituents to be more accessible to water.

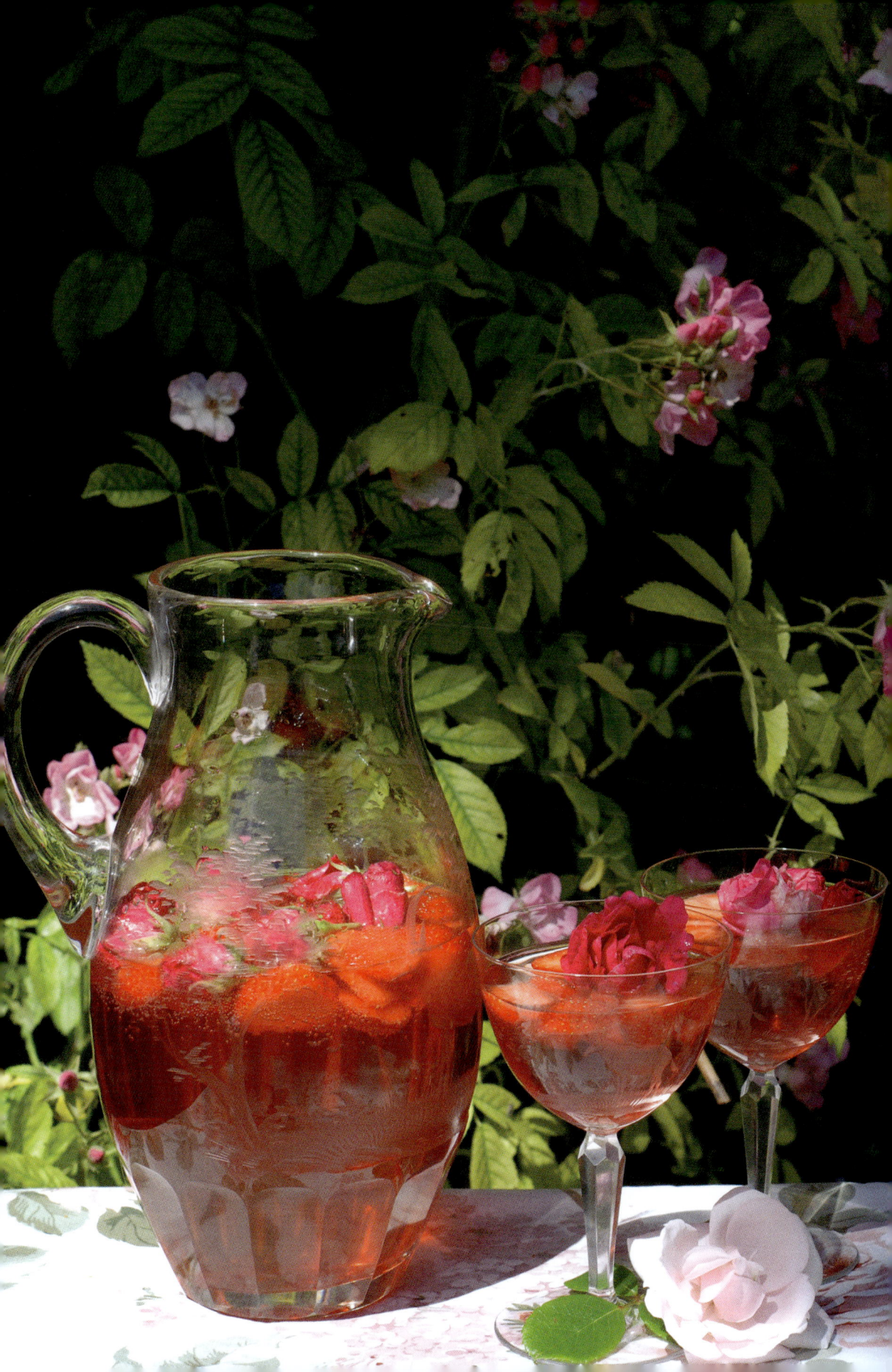

When you make decoctions, you can use the same ratio of plant to water as you do for an infusion, but add a little more water to compensate for water lost during boiling. Place the plant in a stainless-steel or enamel saucepan and cover it with water. Bring to the boil, cover and simmer for 10–15 minutes. Strain and drink as an infusion.

Tinctures and Glycerites
Tinctures are concentrated extracts of plants that involve a mixture of water and alcohol to extract the active constituents of the plants and also to act as a preservative. According to herbal pharmacopoeias, there is a correct ratio of water and alcohol to plant matter for each individual plant, depending on the constituents that you need to extract. This can range from 25% alcohol for simple glycosides and tannins as in lady's mantle, to 90% for resins and gums such as those in marigold flowers. When making tinctures at home you can easily use neat vodka, brandy or gin which are about 45% alcohol and these will act as good extractives and preservatives and might even make the medicine taste more appealing!

Flower and leaves can be used fresh or dried. Place them in a large jar and pour over the alcohol of choice. If you use dried flowers, the ratio is one part of plant to 5 parts of liquid; fresh plants are used in a ratio of 1 of part plant to 2 parts liquid. For example, to make 1 litre (1¾ pints) of chamomile tincture, take 200g (7ozs) of dried flowers and pour over 1 litre (1¾ pints) of fluid. Chamomile requires a 45% alcohol solution, so brandy or vodka would be perfectly acceptable. Pour the fluid over the plant, place an airtight lid on the jar, label it clearly with the name and the date you made it and leave it to macerate away from direct sunlight for at least a fortnight and shake the jar, once daily. Neat cider vinegar can be used to prepare tinctures as the acetic acid acts as a solvent and preservative. Raspberry vinegar, for example, is a traditional remedy for coughs and sore throats.

You can leave the tincture macerating for a few months, as long as you check regularly that the plant has not risen above the liquid in the jar (which it has a tendency to do) in which case it will turn brown and could deteriorate. The best way to prevent this is to use as much plant and liquid as it takes to fill the jar, so that there is no place for the plant to go. Then squeeze the mixture through a press, such as a wine press, or use a muslin cloth and muscle power to extract the maximum amount of fluid, throw the plant on the compost heap and transfer the tincture to a dark preferably glass bottle, label it clearly and store in a cool place.

A mixture of alcohol and glycerol can be used to make glycerites. These are ideal for more aromatic flowers such as lavender, rosemary, mint, elderflowers, rose, lemon balm and chamomile as glycerol really draws out the aromatic qualities of the plants, making them taste absolutely delicious.

Glycerites have a sweet, syrup-like taste and consistency which makes them a good medium for children's medicines. Make a mixture of 60% glycerol and 40% vodka, gin or brandy and pour it over the plant in the jar using the same proportion of plant to liquid as for alcohol tinctures. 80% glycerol is needed for more watery fresh herbs, such as marshmallow, to prevent deterioration.

As tinctures and glycerites are concentrated, only small amounts need to be taken at regular intervals throughout the day. The dose will vary from 10 drops to a teaspoonful taken in a little warm water, 3–6 times daily depending on whether the condition is chronic or acute. Tinctures and glycerites can also be added to bath water, mixed with water to

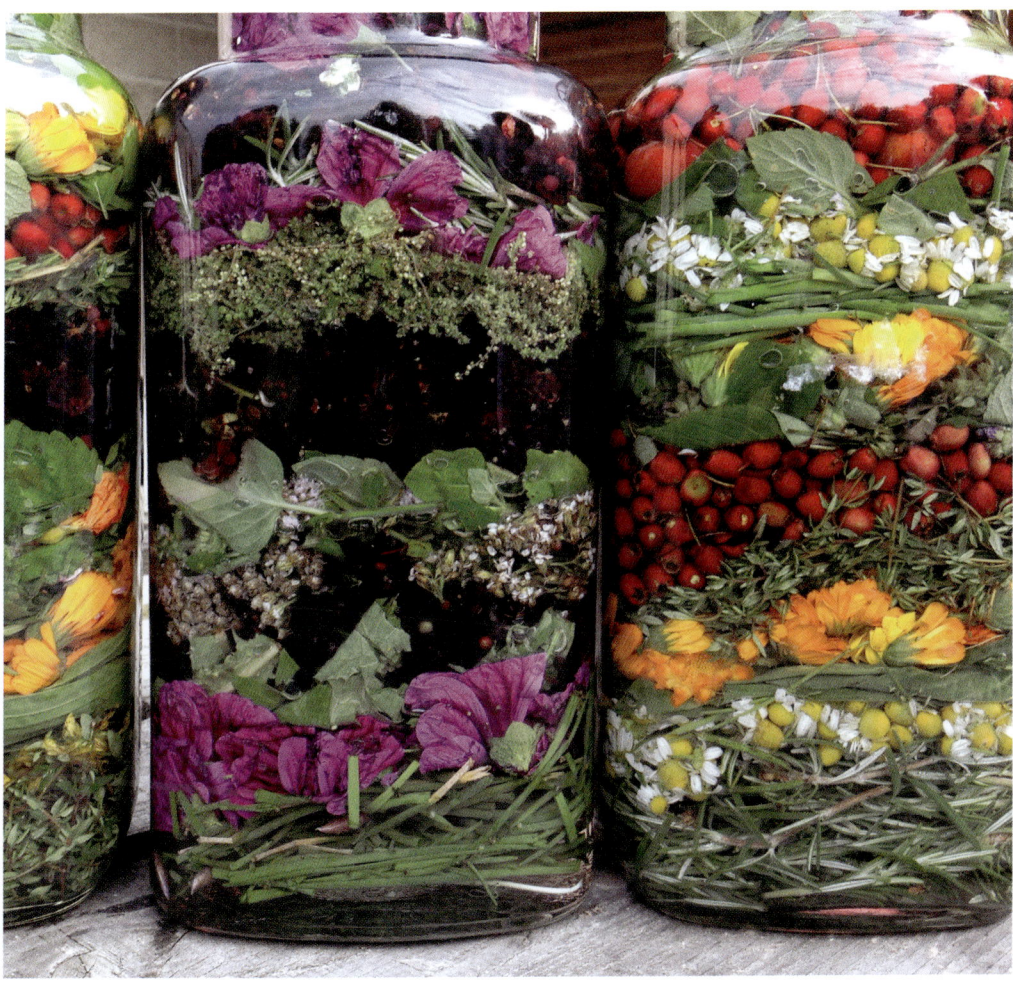

make compresses, mouthwashes or gargles, or stirred into a base to make ointments or creams. Tinctures require more preparation time than infusions or decoctions, but they do have several advantages. They are easy to store, do not deteriorate in cold or damp conditions, take up relatively little storage space and keep almost indefinitely, although they are best used within two years.

Flower Honeys – Electuaries

Floral honeys are a delicious way to take medicinal plants and are excellent way to get children to take healing flowers. Preparations using honey are also known as *electuaries* and were used by ancient herbalists such as Avicenna and Galen who used honey as a medium for administering potentially unpalatable herbs and often made electuaries which were complex mixtures of many different plants together. Galen's *Theriac electuary* was made from a combination of sixty-four ingredients, while the ancient Ayurvedic tonic called *Chayawanprash* contains up to eighty.

We lived for honey. We swallowed a spoonful in the morning to wake us up and one at night to put us to sleep. We took it with every meal to calm the mind, give us stamina, and prevent fatal disease. We swabbed ourselves in it to disinfect cuts or heal chapped lips. It went in our baths, our skin cream, our raspberry tea and biscuits. Nothing was safe from honey...honey was the ambrosia of the gods and the shampoo of the goddesses – Sue Monk Kidd, The Secret Life of Bees

Honey has been used for healing for thousands of years, at least since the time of the ancient Greeks. It is a good medium for herbal preparations, as the sweet taste of the honey brings out the exquisite aromatic flavours of the herbs and also extracts and preserves their therapeutic components. It actually increases their preservation and so extends the shelf-life of the preparation.

Honey is hydroscopic, meaning that it absorbs the water-soluble constituents and volatile oils in the flowers that are immersed in it. It has antibacterial, expectorant and wound-healing properties, so floral honeys are good for acute infections, sore throats, coughs, chest infections and asthma, and they can be used externally to heal or soothe skin problems such as cuts and grazes, burns and varicose ulcers. Honey makes an excellent medium for antimicrobial leaves and flowers such as lavender, holy basil, garlic, thyme, hyssop, oregano, sage and rosemary. It is also highly nutritive, rich in easily digestible sugars. It is energy giving and enhances immunity. It contains pollen that is rich in protein, vitamins, minerals and fatty acids and helpful in the treatment of allergies and asthma, and it also contains propolis which is a powerful antimicrobial. Thyme honey from Greece is renowned for its health-giving properties, as is Manuka honey from New Zealand, which is often used as an antibacterial for fighting off infection.

The simplest and most immediate way to use honey as a medium for flowers or leaves is to mix them (freshly chopped, dried or powdered) in a teaspoon of good organic honey and eat it off the spoon or stirred into hot water 3-6 times a day. You can also prepare flowers and leaves in honey to preserve them for longer in the following way:

Place your chosen plant material, coarsely chopped, in a clean, attractive sterilised jar of your choice. You can use a reusable tea bag or tie the herbs into a piece of muslin if you like. Cover them with runny honey and stir well. Close with an airtight lid, label clearly and leave to macerate for at least 4 weeks and then remove the plants. Store the floral honey in a cool dark place, preferably the fridge.

A faster method involves using a double boiler. Place 1 to 2 cups of the chopped flower and/or leaves of your choice in a *pyrex* or heat resistant bowl and pour over 2 cups of runny honey. Alternatively, you could place the herbs in a piece of muslin or muslin bag to contain the herbs and submerge in the honey. Place the bowl over a pan of water and place on a low heat on the stove as in a double boiler/*bain marie* for 4-5 hours and then strain it or remove the teabag and pour the honey into a clean sterilised jar. Store as above.

If you want delicately flavoured honey, you can also use aromatic flowers or leaves of roses, hyssop, holy basil, roses or lemon balm. For a stronger flavour, try lavender, thyme or even minced garlic.

To make garlic honey: use 6 to 8 cloves garlic to 1 cup of raw, organic honey. Put the honey and peeled garlic cloves in a heavy-bottomed saucepan and heat gently over medium-low heat until just before it comes to a boil. Remove it from the heat and when cool, pour it into a clean, sterilised jar and seal it with a lid. Keep it in a cool place, out of sunlight to be used as needed. The dose of floral honeys is generally one to two teaspoonfuls of honey in a little hot water or simply off the spoon. Avoid giving honeys to children under the age of one due to risk of botulism.

You can also make sweets and throat lozenges with honey. Start by rolling powdered leaves and flowers in honey to make a paste which can then be rolled into balls and then again in the powder to prevent stickiness for handling and storing. Store in a tightly fitting, well labelled tin.

Herbal Vinegars
Fill a wide mouth glass jar full of fresh or dried flowers of your choice. Cover them with good quality (preferably organic) apple cider vinegar and fill the jar to the brim. Cork or cover with a plastic lid. Keep in a cool, dark place for 6 weeks. Strain and pour into sterilised bottles and label clearly.

Vinegars have long been used as a base for preparing plant remedies and one of the most famous old recipes that is still talked about today is Four Thieves Vinegar. This is a combination of powerfully antimicrobial herbs that included lavender, rosemary, angelica, sage and mint macerated in vinegar that was thought to protect against the black death when the plague ravaged the city of Marseilles in the 17th century. According to the stories about this magical remedy, grave diggers and thieves were able to protect themselves from the plague when they buried or stole from the bodies of the dead by rubbing themselves all over with the herbal vinegar (see p209 for a recipe).

Oxymels
An oxymel is a preparation made by infusing medicinal plants in a combination of equal parts of cider vinegar and honey. Alternatively, it can be made by first infusing the plants in cider vinegar for a few weeks and then adding equal parts of raw honey. The use of oxymels originated in the Middle East and was brought to England following the Crusades, when the medicines of Avicenna were popular. Apparently knights and their ladies drank hot oxymels for breakfast as a stimulating way to start the day. Both the

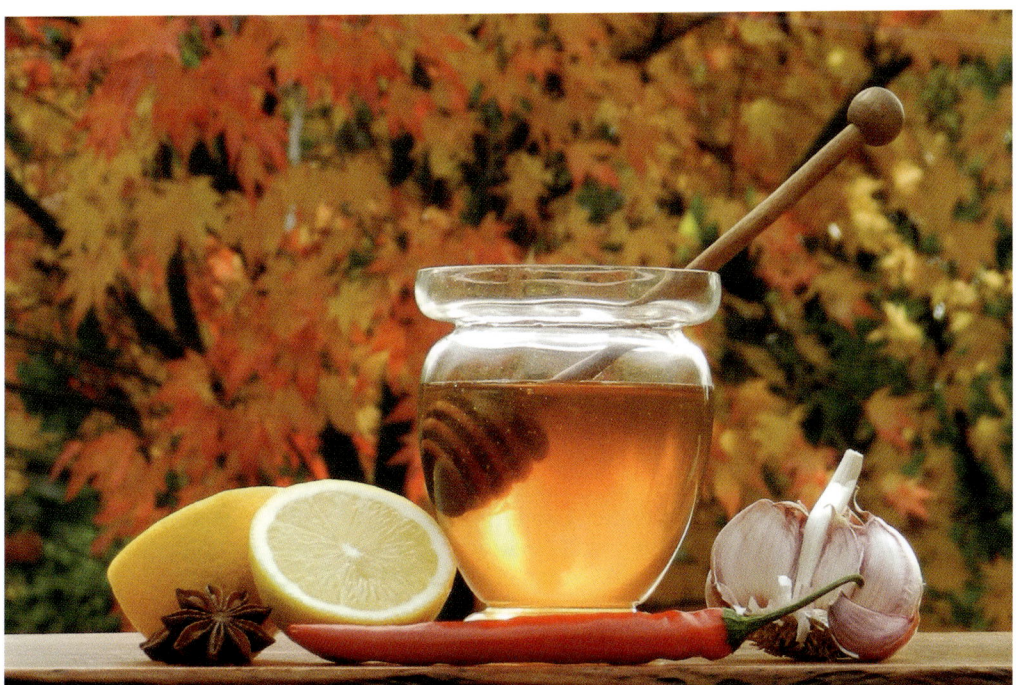

honey and the vinegar act as extractives of medicinal properties and preservatives for the plants and make a really pleasant tasting preparation.

You can make an oxymel by placing 50 grams of a herbal vinegar and 100 grams of honey into a heavy bottomed saucepan. Heat slowly and leave until the mixture has reduced by a third to 100 mls. Then strain the mixture, allow it to cool and transfer it to sterilised bottles with cork stoppers. Label it clearly. The dose is 2 tsp 3–6 times daily.

Elixirs
Honey can also be combined with brandy to make elixirs, which are an easy and delicious way to take healing flowers. The combination of honey and brandy extracts the medicinal components of the flowers and leaves and acts as a preservative. The benefit of using medicinal plants in this way is that, unlike other sweet medicines, elixirs can be taken in small doses and have a low impact on blood sugar. You can make elixirs either with single herbs or with interesting combinations that you can mix in your *still room*. The dose is half to one teaspoonful 3 times daily for chronic problems and every 2–3 hours in acute symptoms.

Floral Waters – Hydrosols
There is quite a resurgence of interest in distilling floral waters among herb lovers and practitioners and it is not surprising, as it is such a pleasurable pastime. Anyone can make floral waters. It is easy to buy copper stills in a variety of different sizes or you could put together a makeshift still in your kitchen and include distilling in your *'still room'* activities.

> *The Herbs ought to be distilled when they are in their greatest vigour,*
> *and so ought the Flowers also*
> – Nicolas Culpeper (1616–1654)

A hydrosol is made as a by-product of a steam distillation of plant matter to make essential oil. When you place flowers and/or leaves in a still, the steam passes through pipes and as it cools, the vapour condenses. The end product is the essential oil, which sits on top of the aromatic water or hydrosol.

You can make a hydrosol with either dried herbs or fresh herbs and use them singly or in combinations. Generally speaking, you use twice as much fresh plant material as you would the dried, just as you do when making tinctures, glycerites and infusions. When making floral waters you will want to choose aromatic flowers such as rose geranium, pinks, bergamot, chamomile, rosemary, rose, lavender, jasmine, orange flowers and hyssop.

If you have a copper alembic still, place the leaves and flowers of the plants you have selected in the alembic pot and half fill it with water, enough to immerse the plant. Be careful not to put too much plant matter in the still. The steam needs to be able to pass through the plants easily. Put the swan neck lid on the pot, fit the condensing unit on the swan neck and fill it with cold water. Use a mixture of flour and water or putty to seal off escaping vapours between the swan neck lid and the pot. Put the still on a low heat, which could be a range such as an AGA, an electric plate or gas burner.

Once the water starts to boil, the essential oils in the plants will be released and carried on the steam through the swan neck and then as the vapours cool in the condenser, the hydrosol will be created. You can then pour the floral water into a dark glass bottle and label it clearly before storing it. As the scent of the hydrosol being produced reduces and the amount of essential oil sitting on the top of the water disappears, you will know that your distillation has run its course and it is time to take it off the heat and finish. All alembic stills come with clear instructions and plenty of practical information is also available online and in books about how to follow this process successfully.

To Make a Makeshift Still
Place a small ramekin or heat-proof baking dish upside down on the base of a medium sized saucepan and position it in the middle. Place a medium sized *pyrex* or heat resistant bowl on top of the ramekin. Add 10 cups of fresh or 5 cups of dried flowers to the saucepan around the ramekin and add enough water to cover them. Do not put them inside the bowl, as this stays above the water and is placed so that it can be a receptacle for the steam vapour as it condenses into aromatic water. Next put the lid of the saucepan on the top but upside down, and place as much ice as you can, hopefully 2–4 cupfuls, on top of the inverted lid.

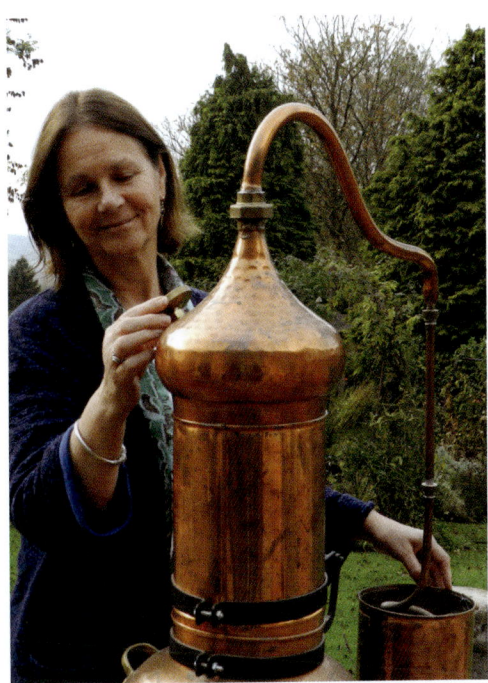

Simmer it on low heat for about half an hour, adding more ice to the top of the lid as it melts. As the steam condenses, it will collect under the inverted lid and drip into the bowl and gradually collect. This will be your hydrosol. Then remove the lid carefully and throw away the ice water and using an oven glove, take the *pyrex*/heatproof bowl out of the water in the saucepan and carefully pour it into a glass bottle using a funnel.

Floral waters will keep for a couple of years if stored in clean bottles and protected from light and heat. They are lovely for spraying directly on the skin as a toner or used as sweetly scented room sprays, body mists, linen spray, pillow sprays to aid sleep, surface cleaners, insect repellents and soothing skin lotions. Floral waters have traditionally been used in the kitchen as well, especially for drinks and desserts, cakes and biscuits. The beauty of a hydrosol is that it can replace distilled water in a lot of homemade recipes for the skin or home. Take for example a lavender hydrosol; you can use it for many different purposes such as improving sleep, soothing the skin, disinfecting a surface, refreshing pillows and scenting linen.

Powders
Plants that you gather from the garden can be dried and then powdered in batches in a coffee grinder and are a very easy and palatable way to take floral remedies. You can also buy dried herbs and powder them yourself if necessary. You can take the powders as simples with just one plant or you can mix a combination of your choice together.

Generally speaking, half to one teaspoonful of the powder is mixed in hot water, left for a few minutes to dissolve and then taken three times a day with food. Powders do not have as long a shelf life as dried herbs, tinctures or glycerites and so it is best to powder just the amount that you need and not leave it sitting around for too long before using it. Store any powders in dark glass jars, away from direct sunlight and in a dry place. Taking powders has the advantage of ingesting the whole plant and not an extract of it, as in infusions or decoctions, and so it may be more efficacious.

Tablets and Capsules
Many medicinal plants are available from herbal suppliers in tablet or capsule form and this is certainly a convenient way to take them, but the therapeutic effects may well be affected. Firstly, it is hard to know when the plants were grown and harvested, how long they have been sitting inside the tablet or capsule and how much vitality there is still left in the remedy.

In addition, only standard preparations will be available commercially, so if you want a specific combination of herbs, you will need to make them yourself. This is not hard, just time consuming, and making your own capsules means that you can use the flowers and leaves you have grown, dried and powdered yourself, so they are likely to be much better quality. Gelatine capsules or plant-based capsules are available from suppliers. These can be filled with mixtures of the appropriate dried and powdered plant matter using a capsule maker. There are two main sizes of capsule generally used; size 0 which holds 0.35 g of powder and 00 which holds about 0.5g. One or two of the size 0 capsules can be taken 3 times daily and one of the size 00 three times daily.

Suppositories
Suppositories are preparations designed to be inserted into the rectum or vagina. The advantage of this method is that the medicinal constituents of the plants can be absorbed quickly and directly into the bloodstream through the mucosa. In this way symptoms can be treated quickly and simply, avoiding the long process of swallowing unpleasant, often bitter-tasting remedies, which then have to travel through the whole digestive tract before being absorbed.

Suppositories can be made easily by mixing powdered plant material with cocoa butter. Warm cocoa butter in a double boiler until it melts, remove it from the heat and stir in powdered plants, enough to make a paste. Mix well then place in the fridge to harden. Next, roll it out until it is about ¾" thick and cut into ¾" strips which can be inserted into the rectum or vagina. Insert one suppository 2–3 times daily.

Preparations for Using Plants Externally
Most medicinal constituents of plants are absorbed readily through the skin and the following preparations are designed to enhance this pathway into the body.

Floral Baths
A wonderfully relaxing, luxurious and simple way to take absorb the benefit of healing flowers is in a fragrant hot bath. There are various ways to add aromatic flowers to bath water. Dilute essential oils (1 drop of essential oil per drop of base oil such as sesame oil) can be added. A muslin bag with fresh or dried aromatic flowers and leaves can be hung under the hot tap, or a pint (600 mls) of strong infusion (double or triple the standard dose described above) can be added to the water. Soak in the warm bath for 10–20 minutes and enjoy!

Healing begins with an aromatic bath and daily massage
– Hippocrates

When flowers are used in this way, their essential oils are absorbed via the pores of the skin that are opened up by the warmth of the water. The oils are also carried on the steam that is simultaneously inhaled via nose and mouth into the lungs and from there into the bloodstream. From the nose, messages are carried from the oils via nerve pathways to the brain.

The healing aspects of the flowers are in this way assimilated quickly and directly, bypassing the lengthy process of digestion necessary when remedies are taken by mouth. Floral baths are particularly useful for relaxing and soothing the nervous system and for easing mental and emotional strain. Lavender, basil, jasmine, rose, lemon balm, catmint and chamomile are not only wonderfully fragrant but also relaxing, calming tension and anxiety and helping to ensure restful sleep. Chamomile is excellent for fractious children, especially when they are unwell, for not only does it possess antimicrobial properties, but also helps induce sleep and is nature's best way to ward off infection and enable self-healing. Rosemary baths, whilst also relaxing, have a stimulating edge as they enhance blood flow to the head and promote greater alertness and concentration. They are good for the mornings, energising and preparing you for the day ahead.

Hand and Foot Baths
Mustard and ginger foot baths have been used for generations to relieve all afflictions associated with cold and damp climates, from colds and flu to poor circulation and arthritis. Foot baths are part of many traditions and folklore but do not have to be

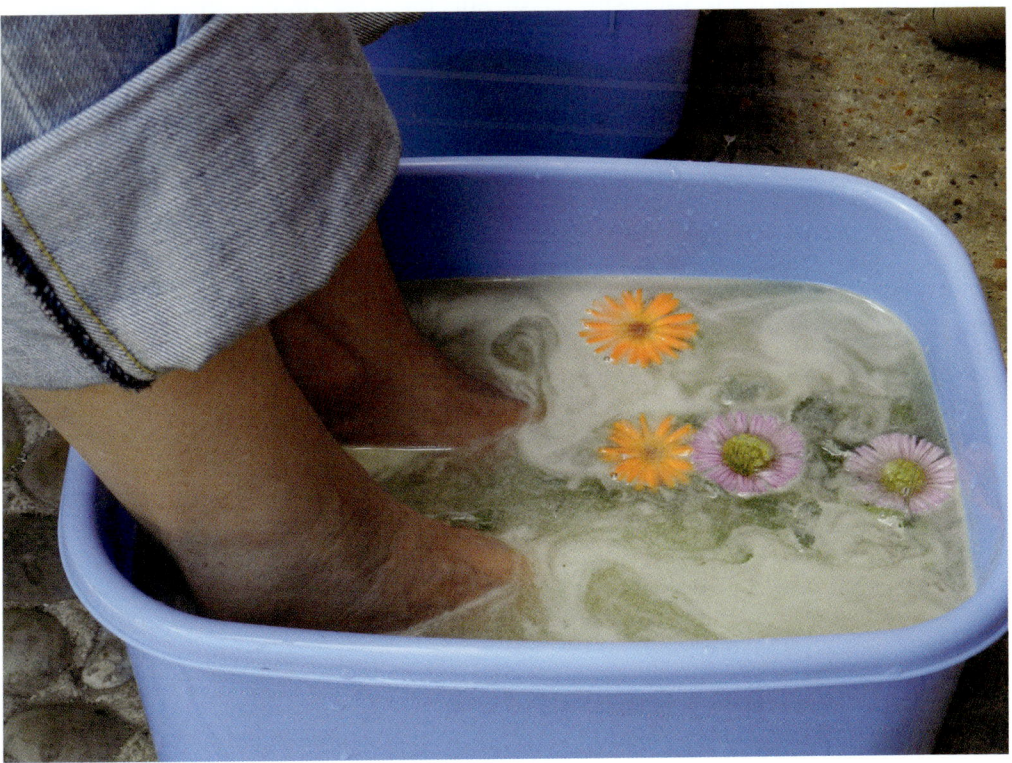

relegated to the past, as they are still a very relaxing and easy way to take floral remedies. The ancient tradition of hand and foot baths was made popular by the famous French herbalist Maurice Mességué, who has written several books on herbal therapy based simply on this form of treatment. He recommends foot baths for 8 minutes in the evening and hand baths for 8 minutes in the morning. According to Mességué, the hands and feet are highly sensitive areas of the skin, rich in nerve endings and despite some thickening of the skin from use, the plants' constituents pass easily from the skin into the body. Taking floral remedies into your body through hand and foot baths means that again the lengthy process of digestion can be avoided and the constituents of the flowers taken rapidly into the blood stream to exert their effect in mind and body.

To make hand and foot baths you can use infusions or decoctions, depending on which flowers you have chosen to use. Alternatively, you can add 2–3 tsp of powdered plants or tincture to a bowl with enough water to soak in.

Salves and Creams
Any plant fresh or dried, either singly or in combinations of your choice can be included in a salve for the skin following this simple recipe. Place as many flowers as possible in a heat resistant/*pyrex* bowl and cover with ¾ pint (450 mls) of olive oil and 2 ozs (50 g) of beeswax and leave to macerate for a few hours over a low heat in a *bain marie* (double saucepan). Once the flowers have lost much of their colour, the oil should have absorbed the constituents of the flowers and the mixture can then be pressed through a muslin bag and the plant material can be discarded. Whilst the oil is still warm, the liquid salve can be poured into ointment jars, where it will quickly solidify.

Creams can also be made up easily by stirring tinctures, double strength infusions/decoctions or a few drops of essential oil into an organic cream base. 2–3 drops of chamomile oil mixed into 2 oz (50g) of cream works well on many types of eczema. Ointments and creams can not only be applied for treatment of skin problems but also for less superficial problems such as inflamed joints and headaches.

Compresses and Fomentations
A compress is a cloth soaked in a remedial preparation and applied to the skin. A clean cloth or flannel can be soaked in a hot or cold infusion or decoction, a dilute tincture or water with a few drops of diluted essential oil. It should be wrung out and applied to the affected part. Compresses can be hot or cold depending on the symptoms that need treating. A cold compress will help reduce swelling and pain of bruises, strains and sprains or painful joints and a hot compress will reduce muscle tension and ease pain and can improve poor circulation of blood and lymph caused by cold. Compresses can help relieve symptoms such as headaches, abdominal colic, backache, boils, painful joints. A hot compress using aromatic waters or essential oils of decongesting flowers such as peppermint, thyme, catmint, ground ivy, lavender and holy basil can be helpful for colds, catarrh and coughs. The treatment needs to be repeated several times for good effect.

A fomentation is basically a hot compress generally used to treat swellings, pains, cold and flu. To prepare a fomentation, soak a towel or cloth in the desired floral infusion and apply the towel over the affected area, as hot as can be tolerated without burning. Cover the towel with a dry flannel cloth and repeat as needed.

Poultices and Plasters
A poultice is similar to a compress, but involves using the plant material itself rather than

an extract such as an infusion or tincture. It is generally used to draw toxins from the body or a specific area such as a boil, a splinter, an infection or swollen painful joint or to stimulate the circulation to the area. Some flowers and leaves are particularly suited to this method as they have the ability to draw toxins from the body, such as hollyhock and marshmallow. Other more stimulating remedies include garlic and rosemary.

Place the plant material, fresh or dried between two pieces of gauze. If you use fresh leaves, stems or flowers, they need to be chopped or bruised and softened with a little hot water before being applied. If you are using dried herbs, add a little hot water to powdered or finely chopped plant material to make a paste. Use a light cotton bandage to bind the gauze poultice to the affected part and keep it warm with a hot water bottle or cover with a hot moist towel and leave on until it cools. Repeat as often as needed using fresh herbs.

A plaster is much like a poultice, but the plant materials are placed between two pieces of cloth and applied to the affected area. When a herb such as garlic might potentially irritate the skin, this method will serve to prevent the plant from coming in direct contact with the skin.

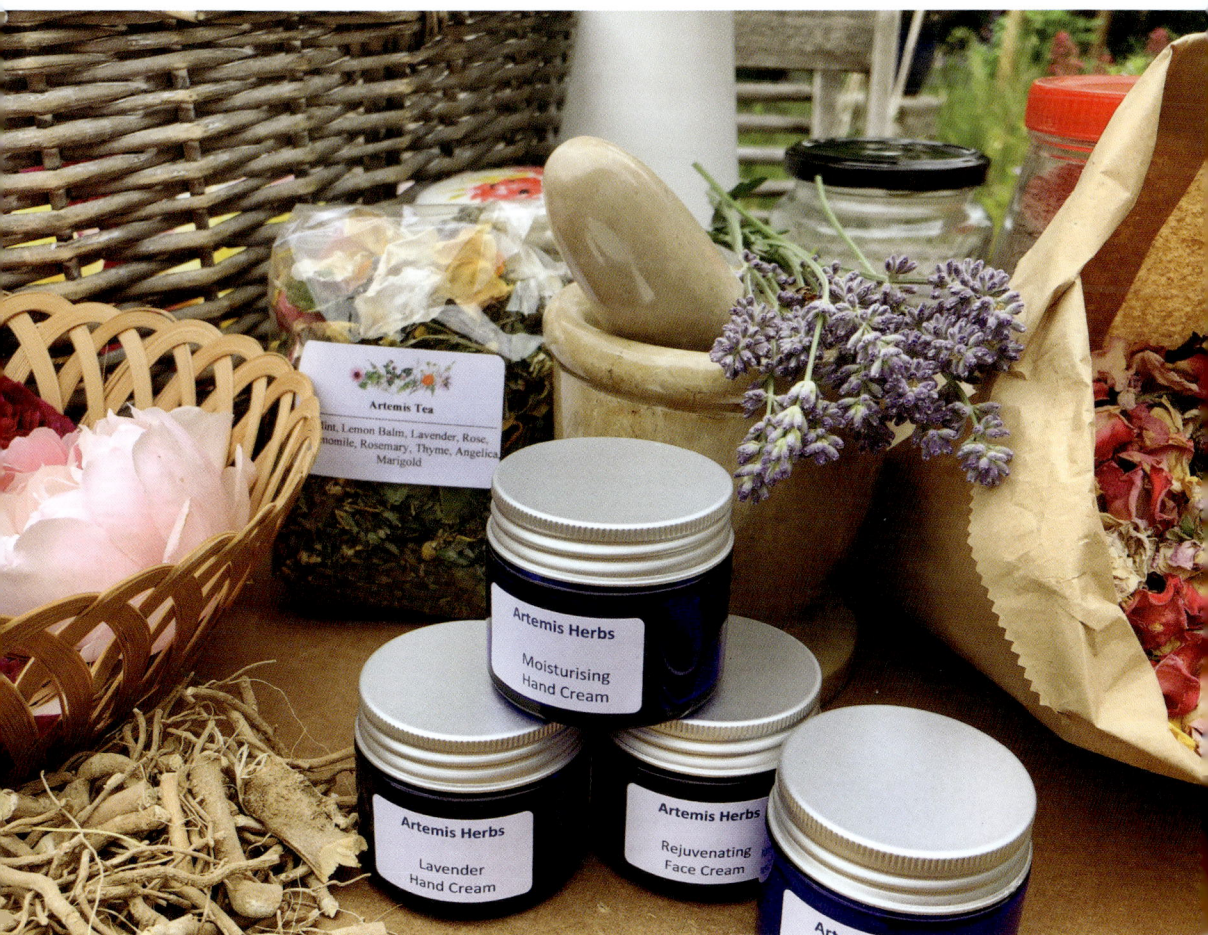

Liniments
A rubbing oil or liniment consists of plant extracts in an oil or alcohol base or a mixture of both. They are used in massage to relax or stimulate muscles and ligaments or to soothe away pain from inflammation or injury, joint pains, sprains and bruises. They need to be absorbed by the skin to reach the affected part and so they often contain a mixture of plants including small amounts of stimulating plants or essential oils such as cayenne, ginger or black pepper and are therefore not suitable for use on delicate baby skins.

An alcohol-based liniment tends to bring out the cooling qualities of a liniment, quickly evaporating and leaving the plants' properties to penetrate into the skin. An oil-based liniment will stay on the skin much longer, it is also more warming. Place your chosen plants, coarsely chopped, in a jar. Pour in alcohol such as vodka or brandy. Put a lid on the jar and store it in a warm, dark place for 7 to 10 days, shaking well at least once each day. Strain the mixture through muslin or a strainer, squeezing the plant material to get out as much of the liquid as possible. Pour it into an airtight container and label clearly.

To make an oil-based liniment, place the chopped plants in a jar and cover with sesame, jojoba or almond oil. Cover and let it stand for 3 days, shaking it well at least once each day. Add essential oils of your choice, 2 drops of essential oil per 5 mls of base oil. Follow the directions as above.

Oils
While essential oils are extracted by steam distillation from aromatic plants, infused oils can be prepared by an easier method at home in your '*still room*'. Finely chopped flowers and leaves can be placed in a jar with a tightly fitting lid, covered with oil such as olive or sesame oil, placed on a sunny windowsill and left to macerate for about two to three weeks. You will need to check the oil regularly to give it a shake and to see that no parts of the plant rise above the oil level, as they may go mouldy and cause the oil to deteriorate. The oil will slowly take up the constituents of the plant, as you can see by macerating St John's Wort in oil; within a very short space of time, the oil will turn a deep red colour. This is a very useful remedy for healing cuts and sores and when massaged over the affected area, it can relieve painful nerve conditions such as trigeminal neuralgia and shingles. After two weeks, an infused oil can be filtered off and the remainder of the oil squeezed through a muslin bag. It should be clearly labelled and stored in an airtight dark bottle to retain its therapeutic value for the maximum length of time. To prevent it from deteriorating, you can place one or two drops of essential oil on the surface or your oil.

Floral oils made in this way can be used both in the kitchen for cooking and raw in dips and vinaigrettes, as well as topically on the skin or on the hair. Aromatic oils infused in virgin olive oil or sunflower oil such as thyme, rosemary, dill, oregano, basil and rose make delicious oils for the kitchen and also lovely oils for massage to relax tense, aching muscles and ease painful joints.

> *Bread feeds the body, indeed, but flowers feed also the soul*
> – The Quran

In Your Still Room
There are so many concoctions you could make in your *still room* using these basic preparations. You can spend many happy hours creating oils and vinegars for the kitchen with any edible flower that you enjoy the taste of. You can use floral waters and infused oils in all sorts of cosmetic and beauty preparations for your skin and indulge in the

luxury of beautifully scented floral creations in the bathroom and bedroom for you as well as to give to friends and family.

You also have the best quality tools to make healing remedies for a wide range of ailments that can be safely treated at home and this way create for yourself sustainable preventative and therapeutic healthcare that could give you confidence and a sense of security and independence in this changing world. The world of flowers and their accompanying leaves and root, seeds and barks can provide a whole medicine chest of remedial tools for treating ourselves, with a quality that we can be sure about. We will be sure of the identity of our remedies, know how they were grown or where they were picked, how healthy the plants looked as we were gathering them, that they were not growing on a busy roadside or in an area that had been polluted by chemicals, that they had not been sitting around in storage for too long, so that they have little healing vitality left.

There are many other advantages of growing your own medicines, going out foraging for them, spending time harvesting them, drying them and making preparations with them. You can develop a completely different kind of relationship with the tools of your trade than you could ever do working with ready-made pills and powders you have bought. You will have access to the best way to learn about each healing flower and this is to become intimately acquainted with it – to know its natural habitat, its growing tendencies, climatic likes and dislikes, its shape, colour, taste, smell, the best harvest times and most importantly, just being with each flower gives you your own direct experience that can give you knowledge beyond the rational mind.

Ralph Waldo Emerson said, *"Many eyes go through the meadow, but few see the flowers in it."* It is far too easy to get caught up in our busy lives of pressure, stress and working through the *'to do'* list and to forget to stop and experience the sheer joy of just being alive. We can go for a country walk lost in our thoughts and not even look up! Flowers have the ability to change this, if even for a brief moment. The appearance of a new bloom in the garden or in the countryside, its shape, colour, exquisite scent and often extraordinary beauty can stop us short and we spend a moment in awe and appreciation. If we extend this moment to a few minutes of quiet time outside with these beautiful flowers, through meditation or contemplation outside in nature, we can reconnect with our ancient skills of a deeper knowing and develop our senses for better understanding of the healing properties of the flowers around us.

The earth laughs in flowers
– Ralph Waldo Emerson (1803–1882)

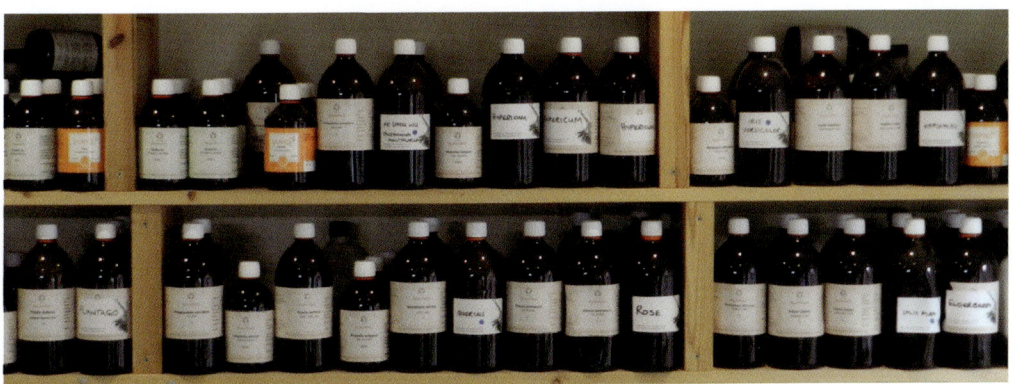

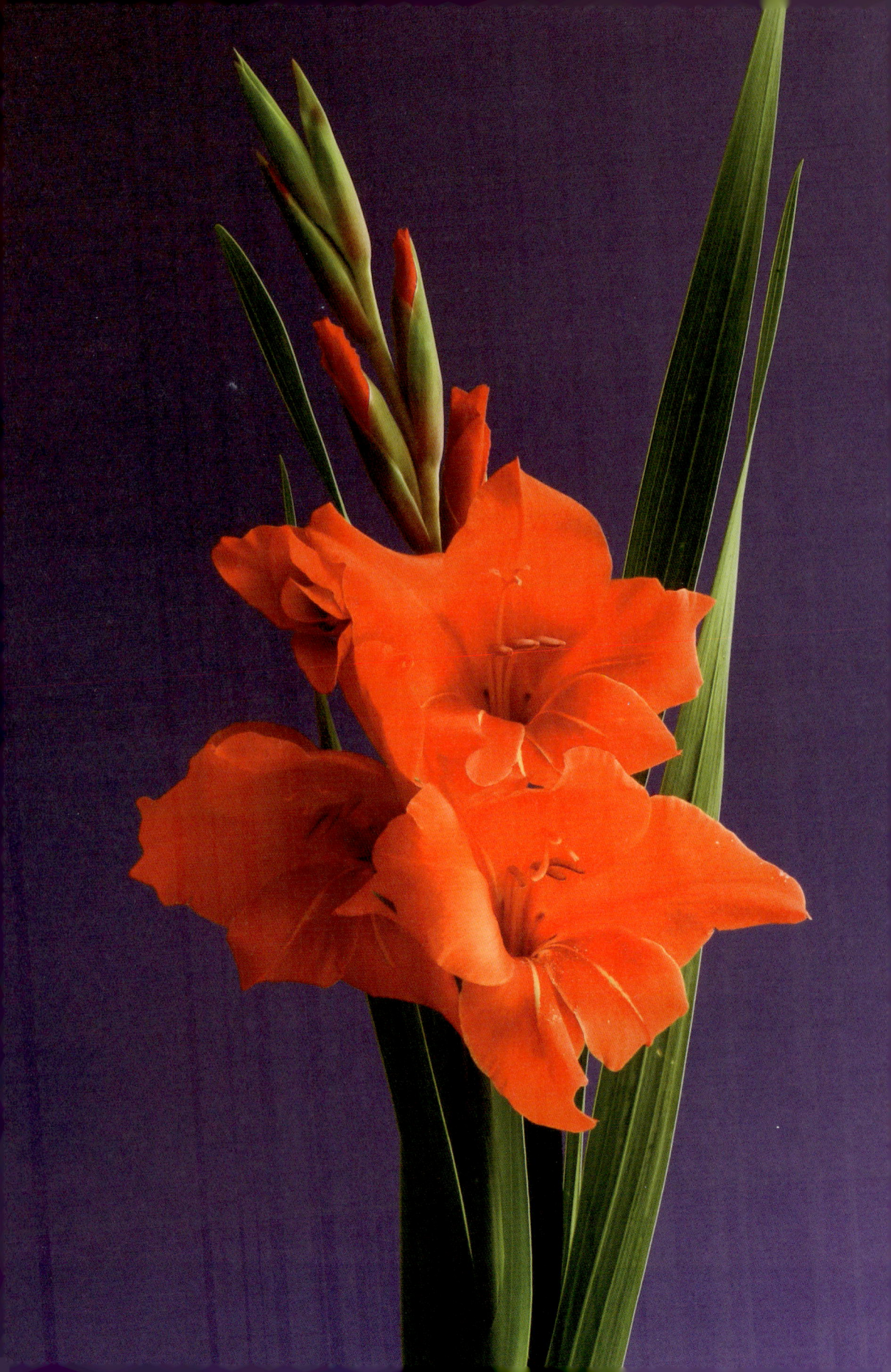

The Amazing World of Edible Flowers

Flowers are grown all over the world and admired for their beauty, their vibrant colours and their delightful fragrances. However, while in recent years Michelin-star chefs have started to cotton onto the fact that many flowers aren't just pretty faces, the vast majority of people still remain unaware of the delights of edible flowers that are readily available to us all. The edible flowers trend has begun to pick up more recently, and it is now not uncommon to see the odd nasturtium or marigold petal scattered across the top of salads, desserts or drinks in restaurants or at dinner parties hosted by innovative home-cooks, since they add that extra touch of elegance. However, people are only just beginning to tap into the range of tastes and creative experiences that are available to us from the plants that blossom in our own gardens.

Most edible flowers can be eaten raw, only requiring a quick rinse under cold water before eating. For best results when it comes to taste and appearance, the trick is usually to pick them just after they have opened and early in the morning, before they have had too much sun. If paired with the right ingredients, edible flowers can work to lift the simplest of dishes by adding a burst of colour and culinary exoticism. Each edible flower has its own unique and distinctive flavour and taste and most flowers go well with a range of dishes, whether sweet or savoury. However, it is important to remember that not every flower is edible. Some flowers are poisonous and even edible varieties may have been sprayed with pesticides, so exercise caution and do your research when selecting and picking flowers for culinary use. For the purposes of the chapter that follows, I have chosen to focus on a selection of the most popular and commonly used edible flowers, and included some thoughts on how to use them.

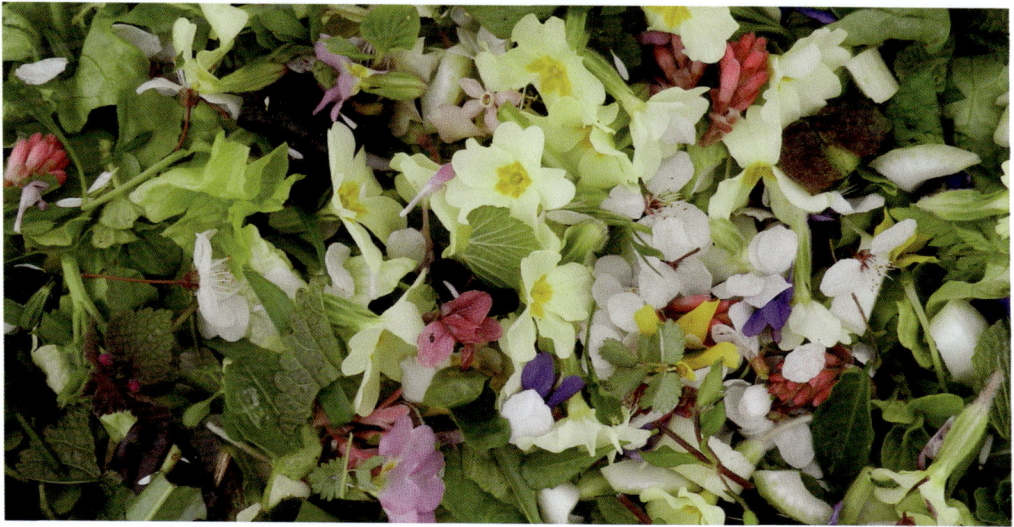

Bergamot

Otherwise known as bee balm, all aerial parts of this plant are edible, and used for flavouring in the culinary world. Though the flowers are generally red, they also come in pinks and purples. They impart their quite intense mint with subtle tones of oregano and citrus flavour to dishes they are added to. Their scent has often been likened to Earl Grey tea. The flowers are great for enhancing salads, jellies, rice, pasta and poultry dishes

Bee Balm Bread

INGREDIENTS
1 cup of warm water
1 package of dry yeast
⅓ cup warm water
3 tablespoons of butter/oil
1 teaspoon of honey
4 cups of flour
1 cup of bee balm petals
1 egg

INSTRUCTIONS
Combine the yeast, water, butter/oil and honey in a mixing bowl and stir well. Add the flour and bee balm, stirring well as you do. You will notice the dough starting to form.

Mould the dough into a ball with your hands and place it in a bowl or on a greased baking sheet. Leave it for an hour to rise then place it on a surface dusted with flour and knead for 10 minutes.

Divide the ball of dough in half and mould into two loaves. Place the two loaves on a lightly greased sheet and cover with a damp towel. Allow at least another 20 minutes to rise.

Brush the top of the bread with an egg and sprinkle with any remaining petals. Bake at 200C (400F) for 45 minutes, or until the bread is golden.

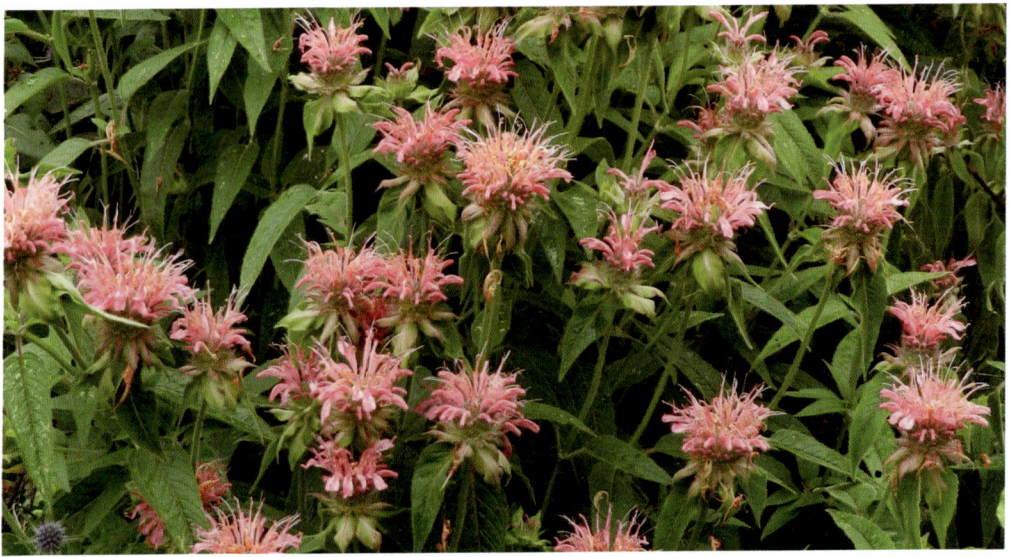

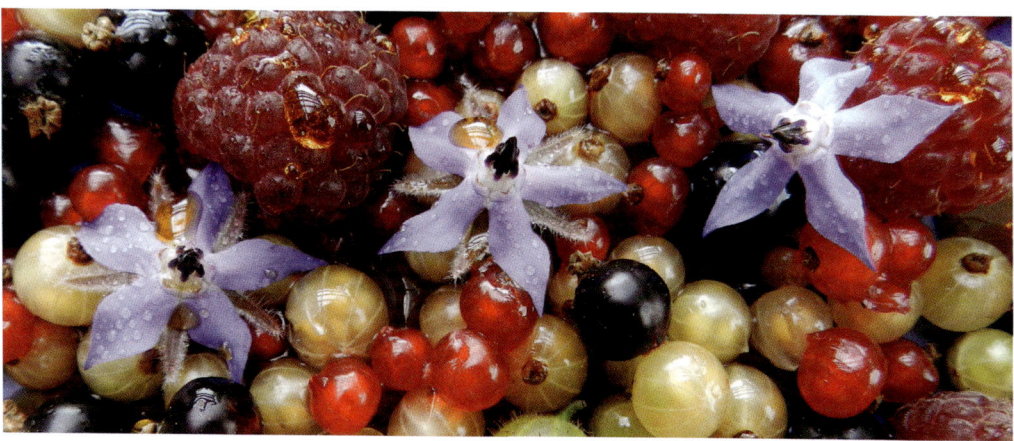

Borage

Borage is a popular medicinal herb, with edible leaves and beautiful, star-shaped blue flowers that are loved by bees. Both parts of the plant are highly nutritious being rich in potassium and calcium. Borage can be eaten both raw or cooked, since the bristles on the plant are dissolved when eaten raw and are neutralised during the cooking process. When cooked, borage plants are best served steamed rather than boiled as they can easily lose their flavour. When chopped finely, the young leaves are great for imparting their cucumber-like taste into summer salads or when mixed into coconut or dairy yoghurt as a cucumber alternative. The flowers make delightful edible decorations to garnish salads or frozen into ice cubes to brighten summer cocktails and fruit drinks. Borage flowers also look beautifully decorative when candied and used in desserts. Other ways to use this herb could be in soups, preserves, jellies and sauces.

Borage, Pea and Mint Soup

INGREDIENTS
1 tbsp olive oil
A medium sized bunch of spring onions, roughly chopped
150g borage leaves, shredded
150g peas, fresh or frozen
1 litre chicken or vegetable stock
4 large sprigs of fresh garden mint leaves
Sea salt and black pepper
A small handful of borage flowers to serve

INSTRUCTIONS
Place the oil in a large pot over a low heat and gently fry the spring onions until soft.
Stir in the peas and cook for a further minute, then stir in the shredded borage leaves.
Pour over the stock and bring to a gentle simmer, stirring occasionally.
Add the mint leaves and continue to cook for five minutes or until everything is tender, but the flavours still fresh.
Season with sea salt and black pepper, then blend until smooth.
Garnish with the fresh borage flowers and serve.

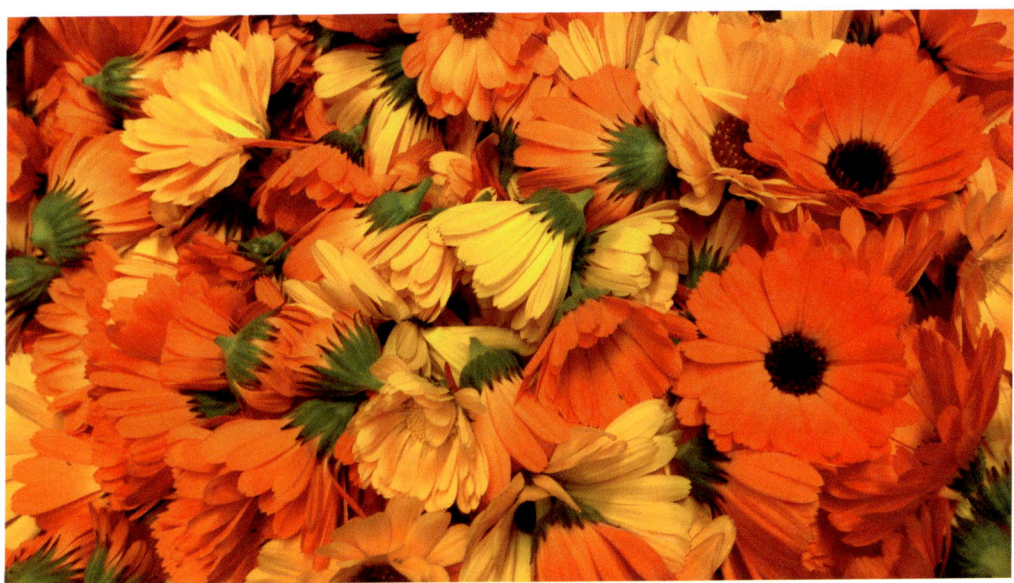

Calendula (Pot Marigold)

Calendula is a popular flower in many gardens, well known for its medicinal uses. It was once called a 'poor man's saffron' because of its yellow-orange hue that colour the dishes it is added to. Our ancestors used calendula petals for exactly this reason, to add to dishes such as soups, gravies, cheese, butters and rice.

The flowers can be used fresh or dried and impart a light and tangy taste with a subtle peppery edge to it. They make a great addition to salads, soups, dips and breads, seafood dishes and hot desserts.

Calendula and Potato Salad

INGREDIENTS
750g unpeeled small new potatoes, preferably organic, scrubbed
Coarse sea salt to taste
½ cup chives, coarsely chopped
½ cup fresh mint, finely chopped
½ cup marigold petals
Freshly ground black pepper to taste
3 tablespoons extra virgin olive oil
⅓ cup red wine/cidre vinegar

INSTRUCTIONS
Scrub and rinse the potatoes and remove any blemishes on their surface, place in a pot of cold water and bring to the boil.
Add salt. Simmer for about 20 minutes until tender. Remove, drain and rinse in cold water.

Place the potatoes in a mixing bowl and toss with all the remaining ingredients while the potatoes ares till warm. Serve immediately.

Chamomile

You may be familiar with chamomile as a well-known herbal tea to reduce anxiety and aid sleep, but chamomile is much more versatile than you might imagine. The flowers have been widely used in medicine and cooking for centuries.

Both the leaves and the flowers are edible, though they differ significantly in taste. Chamomile flowers are daisy-like and taste somewhat like apples. They can be used fresh or dried and add a sweet yet earthy flavour to dishes they are added to. They make a delicious addition to desserts, smoothies, syrups, other herbal tea infusions or smoothies. The dainty flowers can also be sprinkled onto salads or soups to garnish.

Chamomile Lemonade

INGREDIENTS
¾ cup cane or coconut sugar
2 tablespoons grated lemon zest
5 tablespoons fresh or dried chamomile flowers, or 6 chamomile tea bags
¾ cup lemon juice

INSTRUCTIONS
Combine sugar, lemon zest and 2 cups water in saucepan. Bring to a boil, stirring to dissolve sugar. Remove from heat, and add chamomile flowers. Cool.

Strain chamomile mixture into a large jug; stir in the lemon juice and 3 cups water. Serve with lemon slices, or store covered in the fridge for up to 5 days.

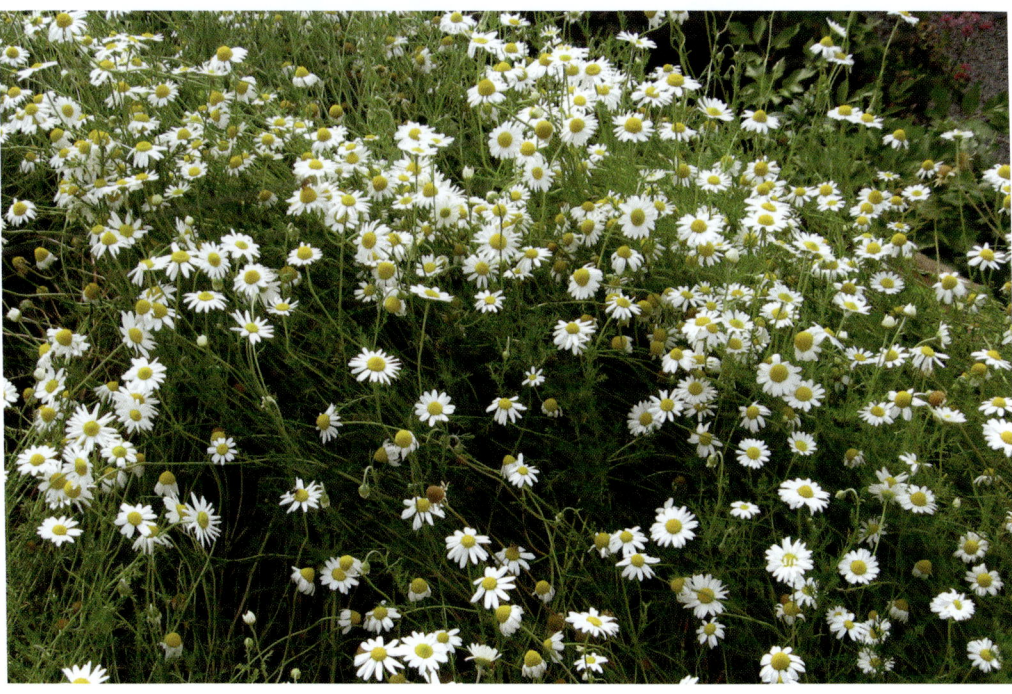

Chive Blossom

Most people will be familiar with the long, slim chive leaves that are sold fresh or dried in most supermarkets for seasoning a multitude of dishes. However, only those who grow chives in their gardens will be familiar with the delicate purple flowers that grow in ball-like clusters at the end of each scape in late spring and summer.

When separated from the flower head, the petals can be scattered on many dishes, raw or cooked, to impart their onion like flavour and add vibrant colour. You can toss them into savoury salads, or add them to pasta dishes, omelettes or scrambled eggs. They also pair perfectly with fish dishes or cheese sauces, and taste great when incorporated into soups, butter mixes or cream cheeses.

Chive Blossom Infused Vinegar

INGREDIENTS
24 chive blossoms
½ cup champagne vinegar
1 pint glass bottling jar with lid and ring, sterilised

INSTRUCTIONS
Wash the chive blossoms thoroughly. Snip or pinch off the blossoms where they meet the stem and dry them with paper towels or in a salad spinner. Pack the jar loosely with them.

Heat the vinegar in a small saucepan over medium-low heat until hot but not boiling. Pour it over the flowers in the jar, screw on the lid, and store in the fridge until you feel it has reached your desired flavour, which can take 1 to 2 weeks. Strain out the flowers and store the vinegar in a sterilised glass container.

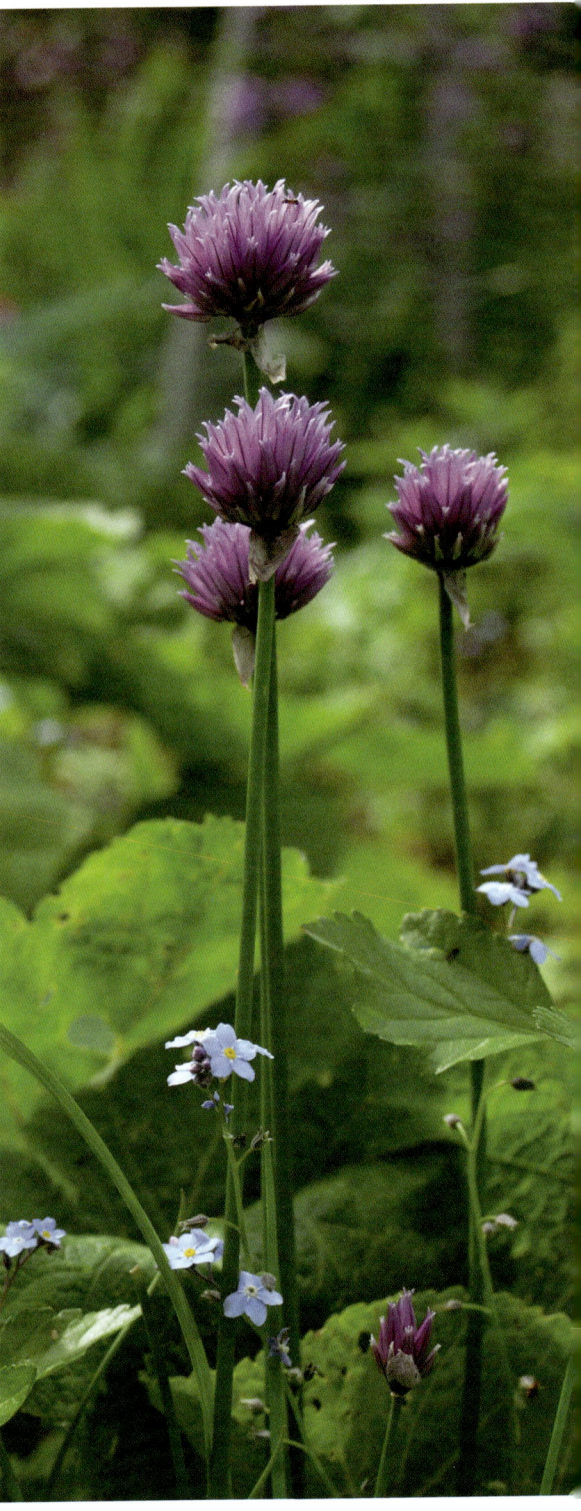

Chrysanthemum

Chrysanthemums are highly popular daisy-shaped flowers commonly grown in gardens and flowerpots. All 30+ varieties of chrysanthemum are edible. The leaves are used widely in Korean, Chinese and Japanese dishes to flavour soups, stews, hot pots, and stir-fries. Their flavour pairs well with tahini, sesame, soy sauce, lemon, garlic, nuts, rice vinegar and other leafy greens.

The flowers are also edible, though their flavours vary greatly. Ranging from a peppery to a honey-like taste, chrysanthemum flowers come in a rainbow set of colours, from red to white, yellow and orange, as well as green and purple.

Ensure the flowers are blanched before using them in the kitchen, and that only the petals are used and the bitter base discarded. For best results, lightly fry the petals in oil for a short time before adding them to soups, stir fries or salads.

The dried flowers make a delicious tea with a mild floral flavour and a deep golden colour much like chamomile tea.

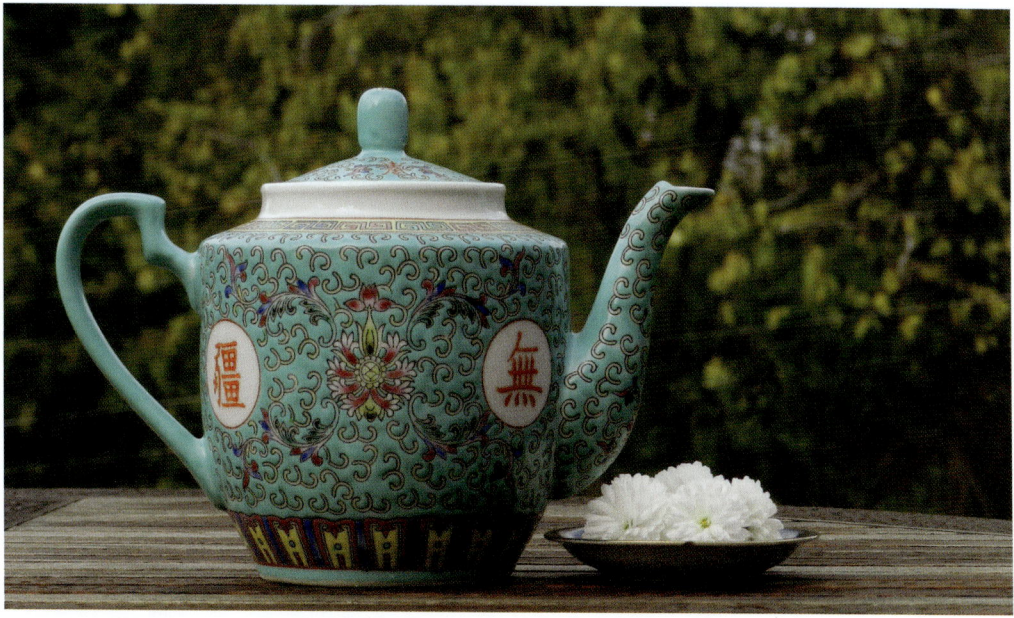

Cornflowers

Also known as *bachelors' buttons*, these flowers never fail to stand out from the crowd with their classic and vibrant cobalt-blue coloured petals. They also come in pink, white and purple variations and with delicate patterns and detail; they are great when used as a natural food dye.

Though they have no fragrance, they make an interesting and unusual garnish to some dishes since they have a somewhat spicy and clove-like flavour with a subtle sweetness to them. Sprinkle them over salads, omelettes, pasta dishes, fish dishes, canapés, cakes or summer drinks.

Daisy

You will find the ordinary daisy littering summer lawns and often being used playfully by young children to create daisy chains and necklaces. This popular little flower, often considered a weed, is in fact edible when picked from herbicide-free locations.

The leaves and flower buds or petals can be added raw to salads or featured in sandwiches, but be sure to pick young ones otherwise they can be a bit tough and bitter. When cooked, they can be used in soups, stews or omelettes. Daisies can also be used to make wine or pickled as a caper substitute.

The flowers are crunchy and when young they have a sweet honey-like flavour, though as they mature, they become slightly more bitter. Fresh or dried petals make a colourful garnish for salads or desserts, and when cooked they can be made into a delicious dandelion jam or wine. If choosing to harvest the flowers yourself, be sure to do so from an area unaffected by chemical treatments of any kind and try to separate the flower from the green stem before use as this can have a very bitter taste.

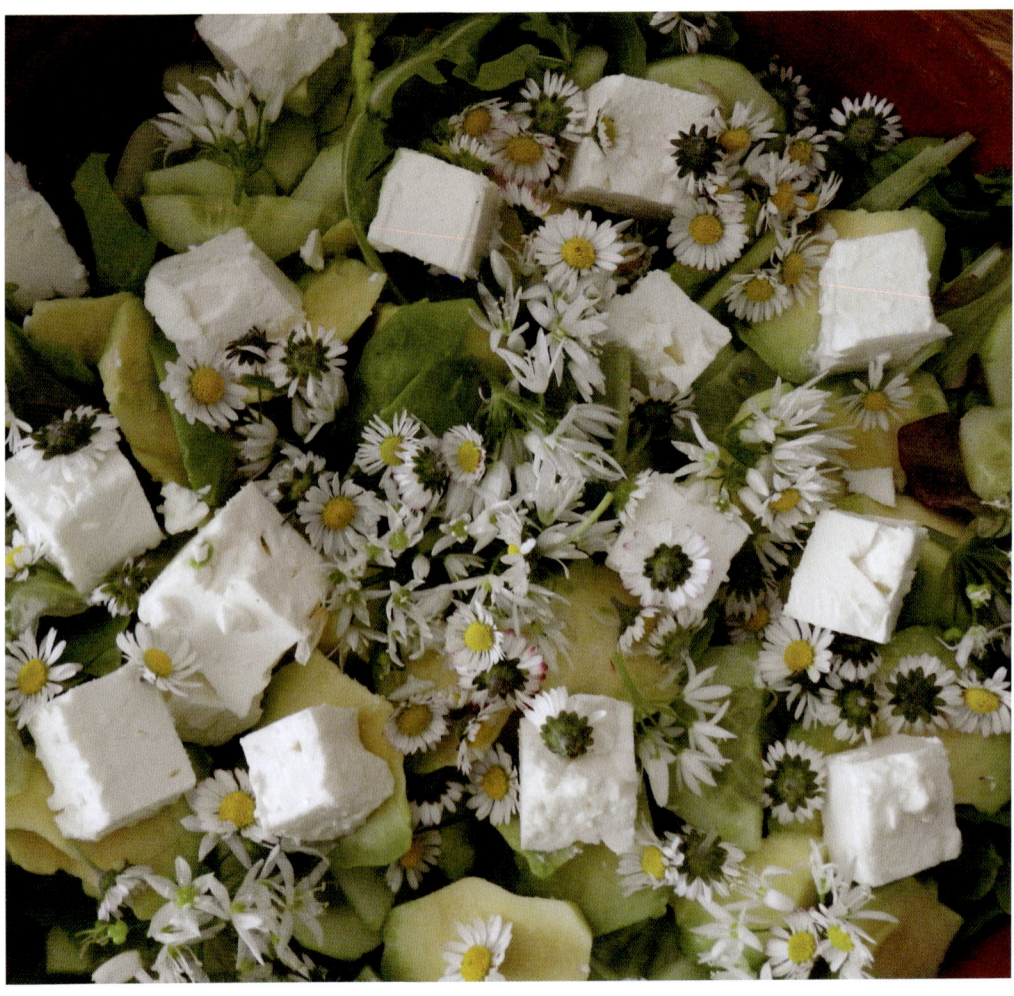

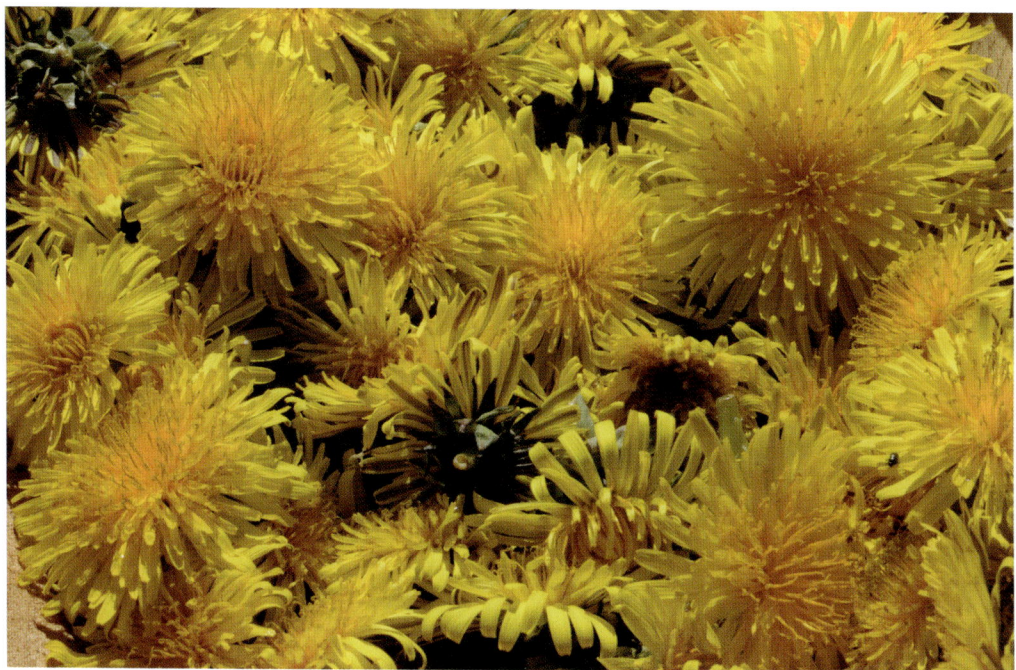

Dandelion

Come springtime, most gardens are full to the brim with wild-growing dandelions. While many homeowners will wage war against these pesky 'weeds' threatening the beauty of a picture-perfect lawn, they are actually one of the most nutrient-rich plants you can eat. The entire plant is edible; everything from the flowers to the leaves and the roots can be eaten either raw or cooked.

Dandelion Jelly

INGREDIENTS
1 quart of bright, fresh dandelion blossoms
2 tablespoons lemon juice
1 packet of powdered fruit pectin
5½ cups of sugar

INSTRUCTIONS
Rinse the dandelions quickly in cold water and snip off the stems and green collars under the blossoms. Boil the petals in 2 quarts of water for 3 minutes. Cool and strain, pressing the petals with your fingers to extract all the juice.

Measure out 3 cups of the dandelion liquid and place in a large jelly kettle. Add 2 tablespoons of lemon juice and 1 package of powdered fruit pectin (1 ¾ ounces). Bring the mixture to a boil. Add 5 ½ cups of sugar, stirring to mix well. Continue stirring and boil the mixture for 2½ minutes.

Pour into small glasses and cover when the jelly is cool.

Dandelion Risotto Cakes

INGREDIENTS
200g dandelion petals
3 tbsp olive oil
1 small onion, peeled and finely chopped
2 cloves garlic, crushed
170g Arborio rice
125ml dry white wine
½ tsp salt
500ml light vegetable stock, kept hot on a low simmer
100g vegetarian Italian-style hard cheese
Freshly ground black pepper, to taste

INSTRUCTIONS
To prepare the dandelion petals, wash the flowers under running water and shake dry. Cut off the stalk at the base of the flowers, removing and discarding all the green bits. Separate out the petals.

Heat 1 tablespoon olive oil over medium heat in a large skillet. Add the onions and sauté until softened. Add garlic and rice and stir for 2 minutes. Add wine and salt and cook, stirring until wine is nearly evaporated. Add half of the vegetable stock and stir frequently until stock has been absorbed. Continue this process until all the stock has been absorbed and the rice is soft.

Add the vegetarian Italian-style hard cheese, dandelion petals and seasoning. Transfer to a bowl and allow to chill for half an hour. To make the cakes, shape the chilled risotto into 8 small cakes, about 3cm in diameter. Heat 2 tablespoons oil over a high heat in a heavy skillet and when oil is hot, carefully place the cakes into skillet.

Turn the heat down and brown the cakes on one side, turning over to brown the other side. Serve as a starter with salad and a tomato sauce.

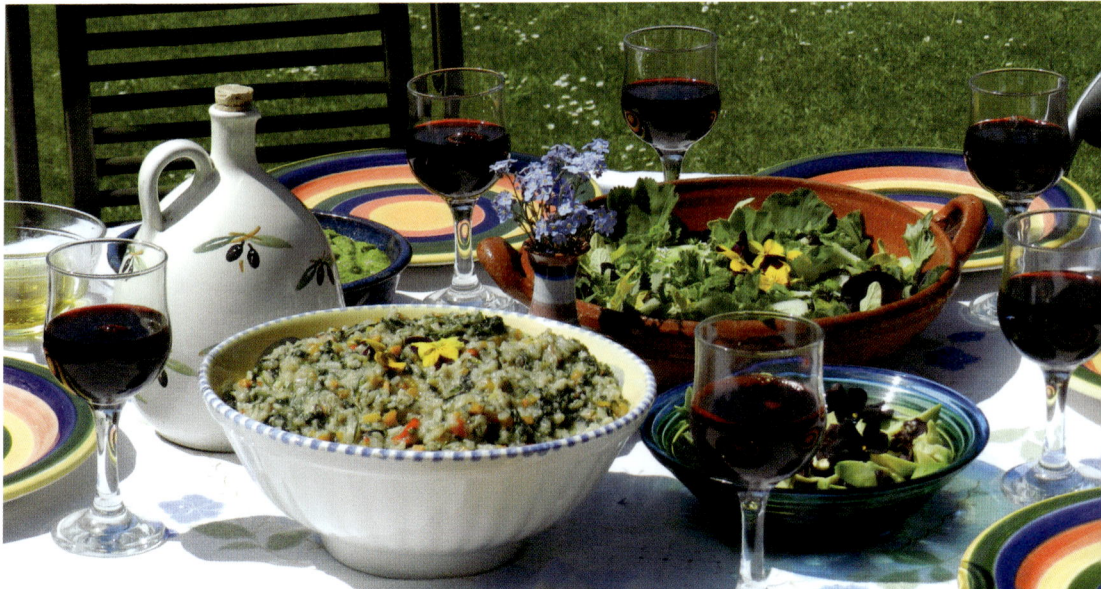

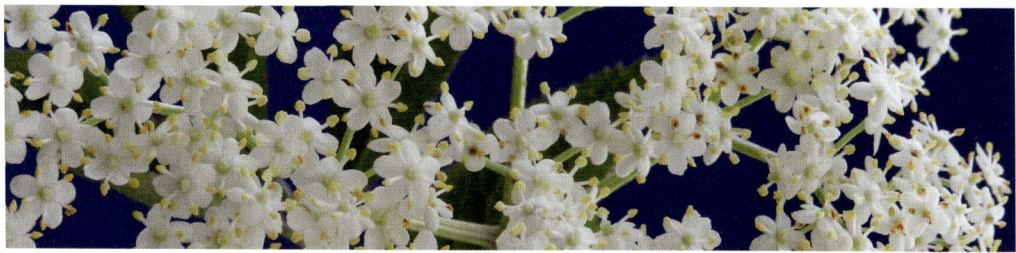

Elderflower

Elderflowers grow in abundance throughout the UK, often found in their masses in hedgerows, meadows and woodland areas, giving off their deliciously sweet and summer-like fragrance. Clusters of tiny cream-white coloured flowers will begin to appear in June, followed by elderberries in the autumn which are purple in colour.

The flowers and the berries are the only edible part of this plant, but the berries must be cooked first to neutralise their mild toxicity. Elderflowers are best picked in June when the buds are newly open, on a warm sunny day. Give them a good and thorough shake and a rinse before use as they tend to attract insects.

There are many ways of using this fragrant plant in the culinary world, but it is probably most well-known for being the centrepiece of delicious summer drinks like elderflower champagne, wine and cordial. They can also be used to flavour desserts like tarts and jellies, or deep fried to make fritters.

Elderflower Fritters

INGREDIENTS
12 elderflower heads, rinsed in cold water and shaken dry
Sunflower oil for frying
Coconut sugar to serve

To make the batter:
100g plain flour
2 tablespoons sunflower oil
175ml sparkling mineral water
1 tablespoon sugar
1 egg white

INSTRUCTIONS
Sift the flour into a basin then add 2 tablespoons of oil and the sparkling mineral water. Beat to a thick paste, and then stir in a tablespoon of sugar. Set aside for 30 minutes.

Just before frying the elderflowers, beat an egg white and fold it into the batter. Heat the oil in a pan (test the heat by dropping in a teaspoon of batter – it should bubble and start to turn golden quickly).

Dip the elderflowers one at a time into the batter and lower them into the oil. Hold them under the oil by pushing down on the stem. Fry until the batter is pale gold and crisp, then lift out and dip straight into a dish of caster sugar and give it a liberal coating.

Fennel

Fennel is grown all over the world and treasured for both its culinary and medicinal uses. Every part of the fennel plant is edible, from its highly aromatic seeds to its delicate feathery leaves.

The fennel plant produces tall umbels of elegant yellow blossoms which have an aromatic liquorice or aniseed flavour. This works wonderfully well in desserts as well as soups and salads. The flavour also combines well with many meat and fish dishes, and if the flowers or seeds are preserved in oil or vinegar, they can be used to baste the proteins before cooking.

Potato Salad with Fennel Flowers

INGREDIENTS
1 kilo (2.2lbs) of salad potatoes such as Charlottes. Peeled or unpeeled.
50g (1¾ oz) salted butter
300ml (0.6 pint) crème fraiche
Sea salt and black pepper
A handful of fennel flowers

INSTRUCTIONS
Boil the potatoes in salted water for 20 minutes or until tender. Don't over boil as they will fall apart.

Drain, place a knob of butter or drizzle some olive oil over them and let them cool. Then mix them with plenty of crème fraiche, sea salt and pepper.

Pick the little flowers off the fennel stems and mix those in too. Save some for decoration.

Mint & Fennel Flower Dip

INGREDIENTS
¼ cup Greek yoghurt
¼ cup soured cream
1 tsp chopped fresh mint leaves
A good pinch of fresh fennel flowers
Sea salt and freshly ground black pepper

INSTRUCTIONS
Stir together the yoghurt, soured cream, mint leaves and fennel flowers in a bowl. Season to taste.

Forget-me-not

Forget-me-nots are delicate and vibrantly coloured flowers, often found at springtime in gardens, fields and meadows as well as wasteland and rocky areas. While they are primarily blue in colour, some less common varieties bloom in pink, white and yellow.

The flowers are the only edible part of this plant and if you are sure the area you pick them from has not been treated with pesticides, they can be great to eat as a trail snack. Highly decorative, they are often used to brighten salads and baked goods such as cupcakes.

They can also be floated on top of cocktails, added to homemade fermented drinks and wines and made into candied blossoms. The flowers don't keep longer than about a day in the fridge, so it's best to pick them for use in the kitchen at the last possible moment.

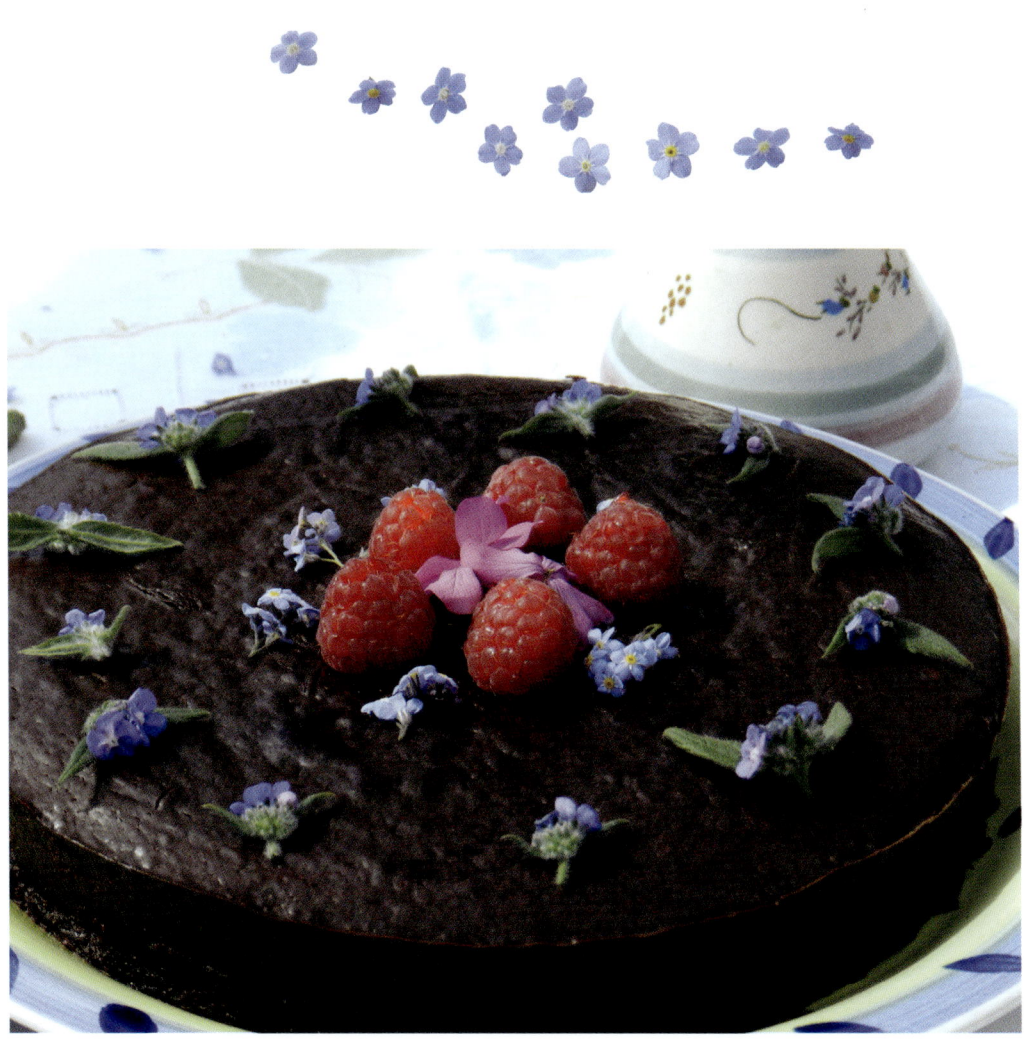

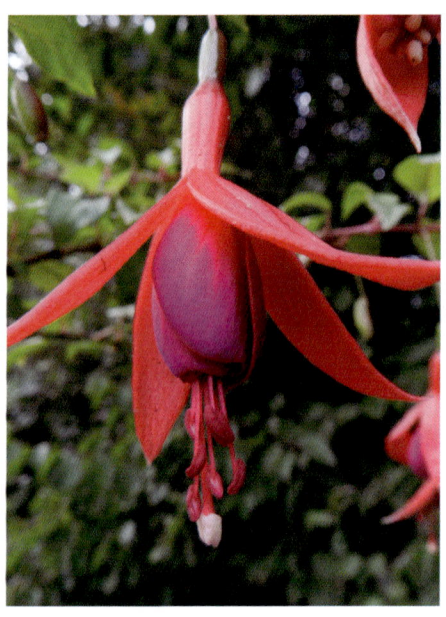

Fuchsia

The vivid colours and unusual, graceful shape of fuchsia flowers make them ideal as a garnish for dishes such as salads or fruit salads. They also look decorative once crystallised for desserts or frozen into ice cubes to brighten summer drinks.

Fuchsia blossoms have a somewhat acidic and tangy flavour, and impart the best flavour once the green and brown parts as well as the stamen have been removed.

Gladiolus

Gladiolus blossoms are colourful and blousy but somewhat bland in taste, vaguely reminiscent of the taste of lettuce. However, they do make a great base flavour for dishes such as sweet and savoury spreads or mousses, and the petals can act as a colourful addition to a salad or fruit salad. Ensure the flowers are picked fresh early in the morning before the sun dries them too much and that the anthers and the middle of the blossom have been removed before using.

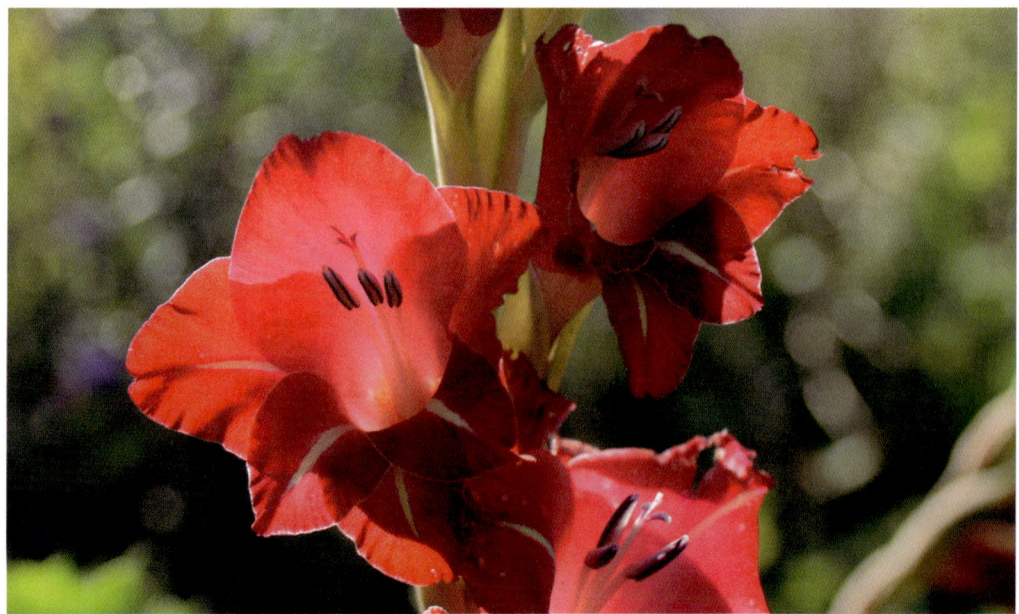

Hibiscus

There are hundreds of different species of hibiscus plant, but the most well-known and popular edible variety is known as Roselle or *Hibiscus sabdariffa*. Hibiscus plants are most common to tropical and subtropical climates, and produce large, highly decorative blossoms. Though often used for ornamental purposes, the flowers are also edible.

The flowers, leaves and fruits or 'calyces' of this plant are all edible, but the flowers have a sweeter taste than the rest of the plant. With their cranberry-like flavour and mild citrus undertones, the flowers make a great tea when infused and can be the basis for delicious jams or relishes. Since the colours are wide ranging, including red, white, yellow and pink, the vibrant hues of the petals can make them a great addition to salads or fruit salads or sprinkled on desserts.

Hibiscus Chutney

INGREDIENTS
1 litre (2 pints) fresh blackberries or 450g (1lb) frozen blackberries
8 hibiscus flowers
½ cup red onion, finely chopped
½ cup sugar
2 tablespoons minced fresh ginger
2 tablespoons Dijon mustard
Salt and pepper to taste
½ cup white wine vinegar

INSTRUCTIONS
Toss everything except the vinegar into a big pot. Cook and occasionally stir the mixture over a medium heat for about 5 minutes. Add salt and pepper if you wish.

Stir in the vinegar and let mixture simmer and thicken for about 10 minutes more. Refrigerated in an airtight container, this chutney will last for up to 6 weeks.

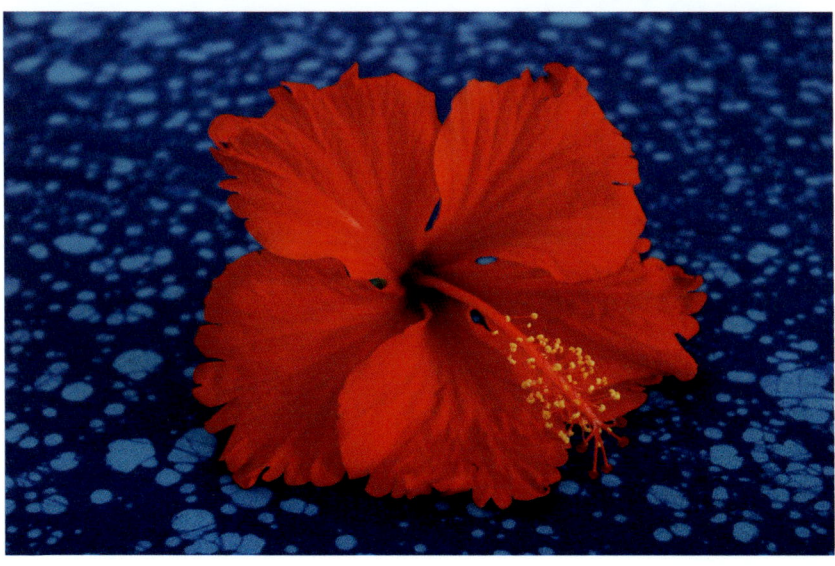

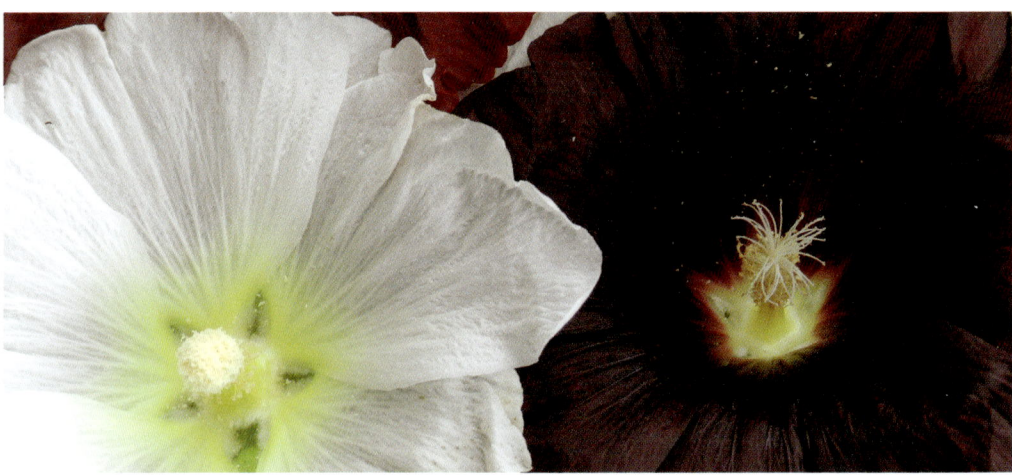

Hollyhock

Close relatives of marshmallow, these tall and impressive flowering plants are a traditional feature of British gardens. They produce delicate pink, purple, red, yellow or white blossoms, the petals of which are the only part of plant safe for culinary use. For this reason, its important to ensure that the calyx, pistill and stamens of the flowers are removed along with the bitter tasting flower base.

While vibrant in colour and great as a decorative garnish, the petals actually have a very mild taste; they are best sprinkled over salads or desserts or added to fish dishes.

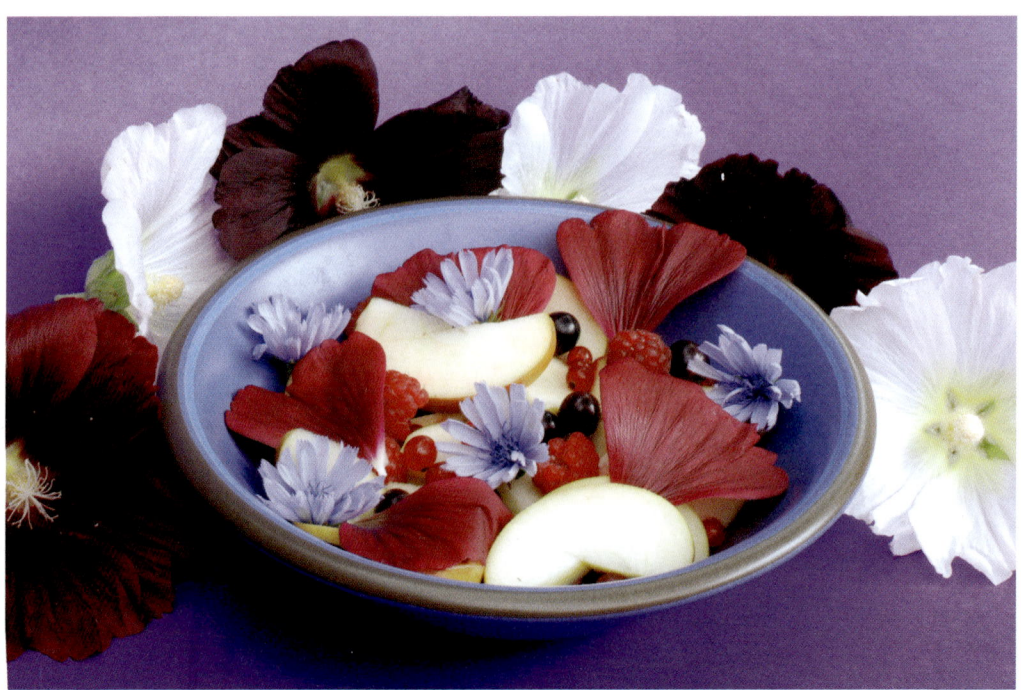

Honeysuckle

There are nearly 200 types of honeysuckle plant, but the Japanese and woodbine varieties are most commonly seen in gardens today. Honeysuckle has long been an essential ingredient in Chinese medicine on account of its myriad healing properties.

It is really no wonder that the honeysuckle plant has its name and was discovered to be edible, since its white and yellow blossoms have such a delicious and sweet, honey-like aroma and nectar and can be eaten directly from the plant.

The petals can be used to make tisanes or added into baked goods or desserts. They can also be added to drinks such as iced tea and lemonade, to replace sugar in bread making, or to flavour homemade ice creams and sorbets.

It is important to be aware that the flowers and their nectar are the only parts of the plant which are safe to eat, since the berries can be toxic.

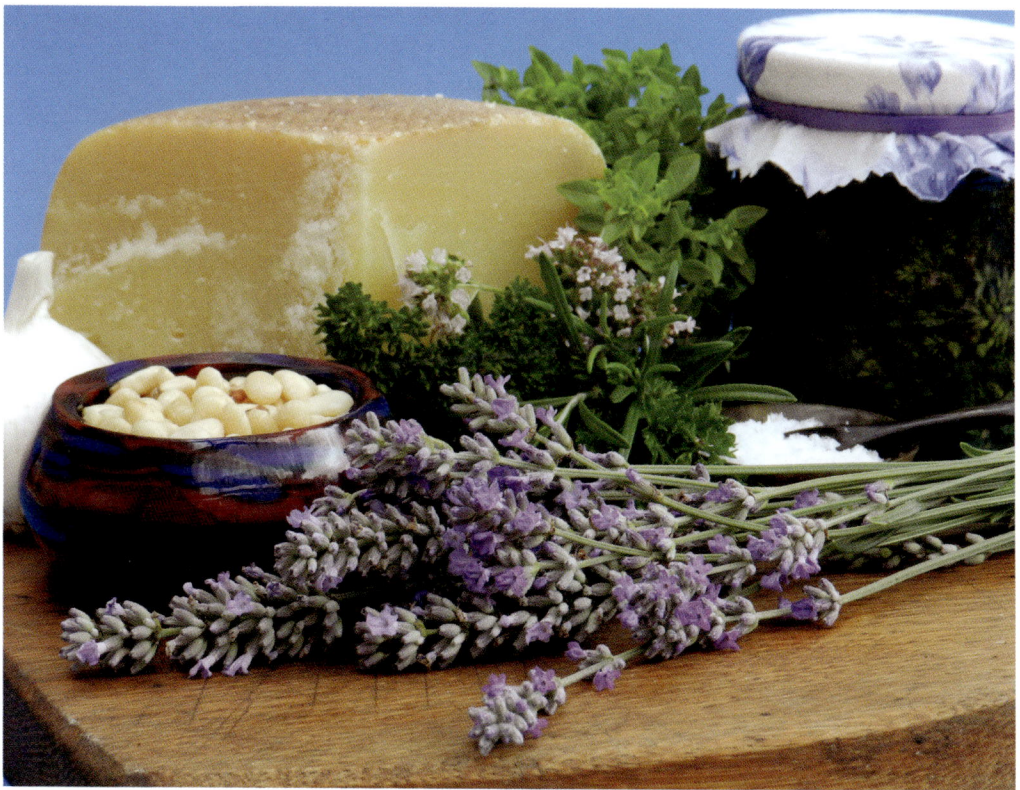

Lavender

Despite lavender often being associated with France and with its inclusion in *Herbes de Provence* and other French recipes, conjuring images of Provence in one's mind, English lavender is in fact the most commonly used in cooking.

Culinary English lavender has more of a sweet floral fragrance and taste than any other variety and its potency increases through the process of drying. To dry lavender, simply cut the stems off the plant shortly after the flowers have opened and hang them upside down or lay them flat in a dry area. Lavender is a wonderfully versatile herb to cook with, since it is seen as having an androgynous aroma and flavour which can suit both savoury and sweet dishes.

While both the leaves and stems are edible and used in cooking, the flowers are best to give dishes that subtle sweet and citrus taste; mash the lavender in a pestle and mortar or use a coffee grinder for best effects. A popular use of lavender is to infuse it with sugar and use it in baking to add a delicious and subtle flavour base. Similarly, it can be easily infused with cream, butter or chocolate for desserts such as lavender cake, shortbread biscuits or meringues. Lavender also makes a delightful garnish for sorbets or ice creams, cakes, cocktails and champagne and to add vibrant colour to salads. When it comes to savoury dishes, lavender can lend itself as a good substitute for rosemary in bread recipes, and can be added to meat based stews for that extra bit of flavour.

Lavender Granola

INGREDIENTS
3 cups rolled oats
1 cup almonds, chopped
½ cup pecans, chopped
½ cup pumpkin seeds
¼ cup culinary lavender
½ teaspoons salt
½ cup melted coconut oil
½ cup honey
1 teaspoon vanilla
¾ cup currants (or raisins)

INSTRUCTIONS
Preheat the oven to 175C/350F. Line a baking sheet with parchment paper. In a large bowl, mix together the oats, almonds, pecans, pumpkin seeds, lavender and salt.

In a small bowl, whisk together coconut oil, honey and vanilla. Stir the liquid mixture into the dry ingredients until evenly coated. Turn the granola mixture out onto a baking sheet and bake for 40 minutes, checking every 15 minutes or so to stir. Stir in currants and let the granola cool before serving (it will continue to dry out as it cools).

Lavender and Lemon Balm Tisane

INGREDIENTS
2 teaspoons lavender flowers
2 teaspoons lemon balm leaves
600ml (1 pint) boiling water
Honey to taste (optional)

INSTRUCTIONS
Place the herbs in a teapot and pour over boiling water. Cover and leave to infuse for 10–15 minutes. Drink a cupful 3 times daily or more if required. Sweeten with honey if you like.

Lilac

For many, the sweet smell of lilacs is a much-appreciated sign of spring. Though most people grow them in their gardens purely for their beauty, there is more to lilacs than first meets the eye. Much like lavender, lilac flowers have an intensely floral flavour and aroma with a hint of lemon, almost like a perfume.

The flavour of lilac pairs beautifully with yoghurt as a dip or a spread and is delicious when added to cream cheese and served with crackers. Adding the flowers into salads and summer drinks or as a garnish for cakes also looks lovely, though remember that a little goes a long way with these flowers and too many can be overpowering or produce a slightly bitter taste.

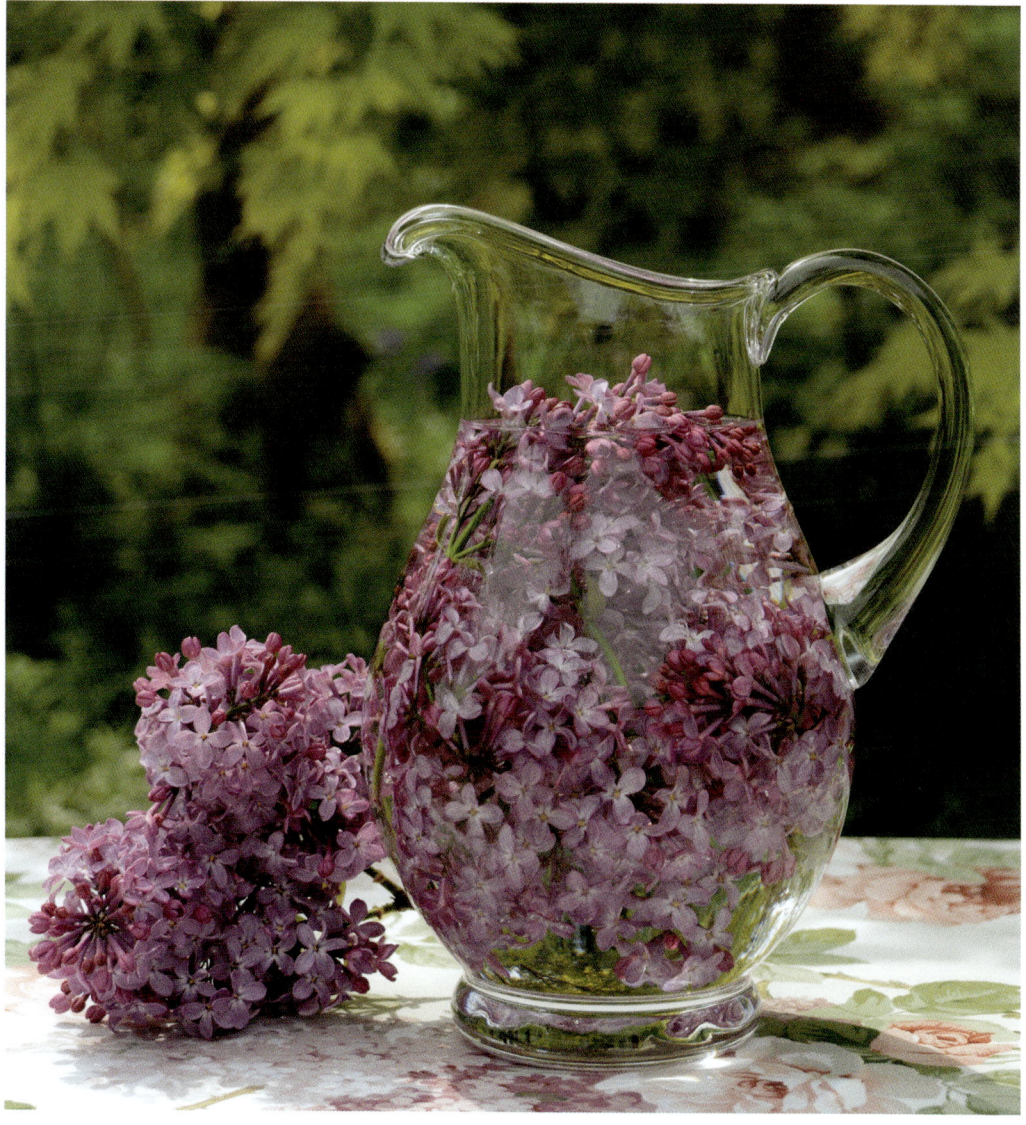

Magnolia

The flowers from the beautiful *Magnolia grandiflora* tree are certainly one of the lesser-known edible flowers, and yet their blossoms have the potential to impart a delicious and intense flavour to many dishes. Currently magnolia flower buds are used mostly in Asian cuisine; in Japan the flowers are broiled and eaten like a vegetable, and the *hoba miso* they commonly use is apparently seasoned with magnolia.

Magnolia flowers taste similar to how they smell and are generally pickled rather than eaten raw. For best results, pick them when young, pickle them and eat them on their own or incorporate them into salads. Be sure to use them sparingly though, so as not to overpower the dish with their intense flavour.

Pickled Magnolia Flowers

INGREDIENTS
1 lb/500g fresh young magnolia flowers
1½ cups rice vinegar
1 cup sugar
1 tsp salt

INSTRUCTIONS
Wash, clean and dry the magnolia flowers with paper towels and pack them fairly tightly in a sterilised jar along with the salt.

Mix the rice vinegar and sugar in a pan and bring to a boil. Pour the hot mixture of vinegar and sugar over the magnolia flowers, allow to cool, then screw a cap on the jar. They can be eaten alone or as an accompaniment to salads.

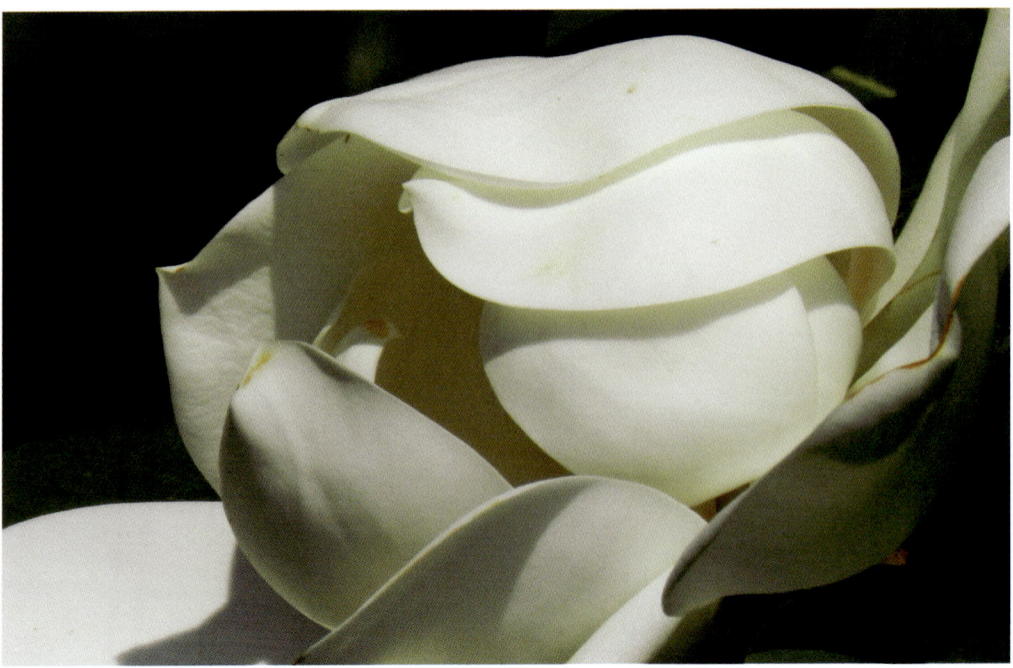

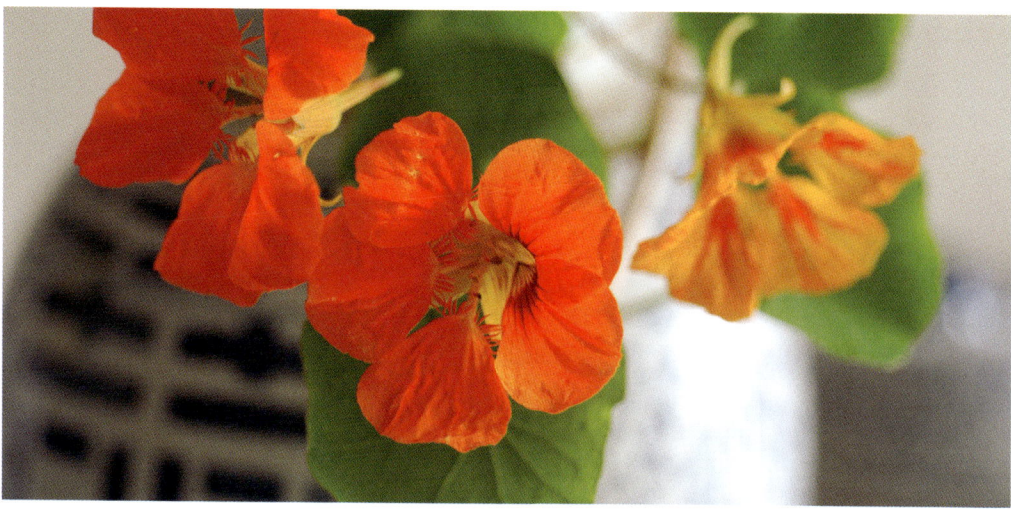

Nasturtium

Nasturtiums are a popular ornamental garden plant, a medicinal herb and a culinary favourite, owing to their brightly coloured orange, red or yellow blossoms and distinct flavour. Both the leaves and the flowers are edible and can be added to a wide range of dishes, imparting a pleasant pepper-like flavour, similar to that of watercress, though the leaves are slightly stronger in taste than the flowers. They can be enjoyed either raw or cooked. The fresh seeds can also be pickled like capers, if picked when they are in the green phase. The flowers can be used whole, but leaves, buds and petals can also be used for slightly different effects depending on the dish. They make a great addition to salads, stir fries, curries, pasta dishes and meat dishes. When it comes to sweet dishes, they make a beautiful garnish for cakes, pastries etc.

Nasturtium Pesto

INGREDIENTS
50 large nasturtium leaves or twice as many if small
¼ cup nuts of your choice
½ cup olive oil
½ cup Parmesan cheese
1 pinch pepper
salt and pepper to taste

INSTRUCTIONS
Wash the nasturtium leaves and shake them dry. Toast the nuts in a dry pan over a medium heat, stirring frequently until they start to smell good. Remove from the heat.

Fill your food processor up loosely, till ¾ full with leaves. Blend until they are chopped. Add more leaves and blend again. Continue until all the leaves are blended.

Add the nuts and blend again until they are finely chopped. Add the cheese, red pepper and half the oil and blend again. Add more oil until you reach the desired consistency. Add salt, black pepper, more nuts or cheese and blend until you are satisfied with the taste.

Pelargoniums (Scented Geraniums)

While there are many different species of pelargonium, each is characterised by a distinct fragrance of the leaves. These include hints of rose, mint, almond, hazelnut, nutmeg, cinnamon, citronella, orange, lemon, grapefruit, strawberry, peach, pineapple, coconut, celery, chocolate and many more, though the rose geranium is a common favourite.

Both the flowers and the leaves of the scented geranium plant are edible, though the flowers have a milder taste than the leaves. The use of the leaves for fragrance and flavour is a more popular choice, but the flowers are great for adding that little bit of extra flavour and the decorative colour to a dish. The key with scented geraniums is to harvest them when they first open and separate the petals from the stalks and centre.

The leaves can be added to soups, stews and sauces for their distinct flavouring. They can also be used in jellies, jams, vinegar, sorbets, ice creams and dessert mixtures. Flowers can be crystallised or frozen into ice cubes for decorative summer drinks, and rose scented geranium is often a popular and sophisticated choice to use when making a syrup or liqueur to add to cocktails.

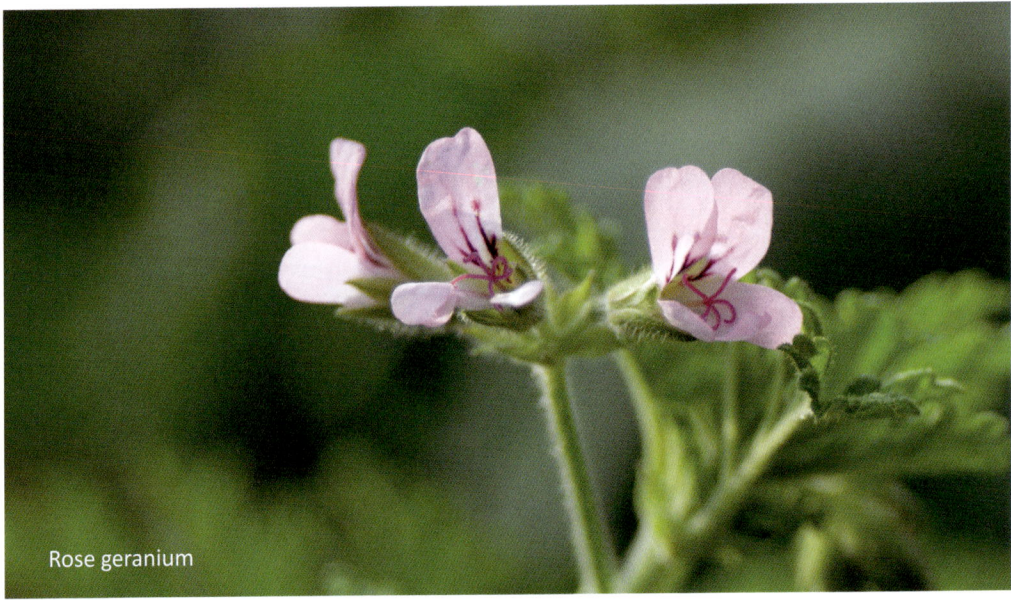
Rose geranium

Purslane

Originally native to Persia, purslane can now be found across the world having been used in cooking for thousands of years. Commonly considered a weed, this herb can often be found in cleared areas such as vegetable gardens, along lawn edges or sometimes even within the gaps of pavements.

It produces thick red stems, fleshy green leaves and bright yellow flowers, making it hard to miss. Both the leaves and the flowers are edible, raw or cooked, and work well in a variety of salads and sandwiches, or when sautéed or steamed and added to stir fries, soups and stews.

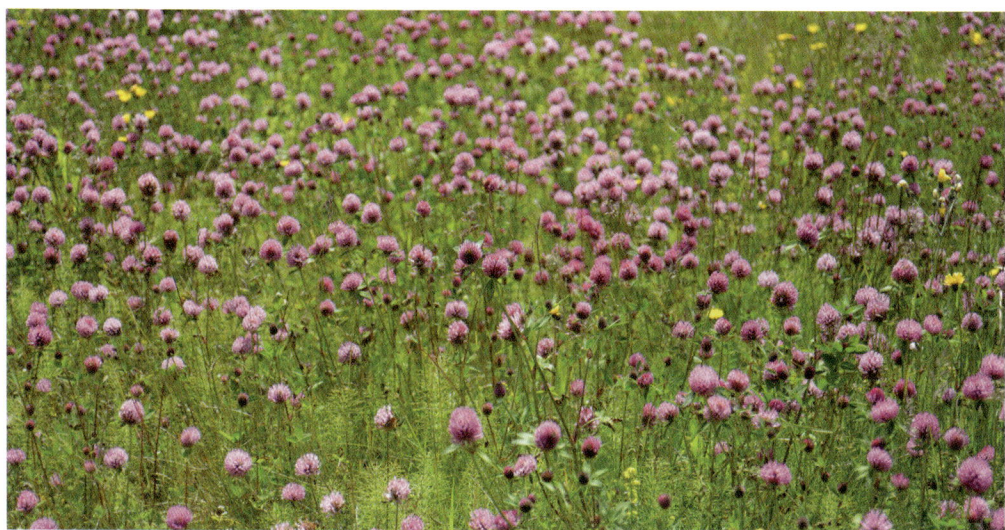

Red Clover

Clover is widely cultivated as food for cattle and for use in herbal medicine. The cheerful flowers have a sweet taste that resembles liquorice and aniseed. They can be eaten raw or cooked and make an interesting addition to a wide variety of dishes. They can be added to soups, stews and other dishes such as lasagne or tossed into salads for an attractive garnish. Whole flowers can be used to make wine.

When picking the flowers for culinary purposes, pick the flowers early in the day and choose the most vibrant in colour, as the slightly discoloured ones could have an odd bitter taste. Be sure to eat them in moderation, since eating too many may cause bloating or gas.

Red Clover Tabbouleh

INGREDIENTS
1 heaped handful of red clover leaves
Petals from 3 red clover flowerheads
Prepared couscous, 4 tablespoons
½ red pepper, chopped
½ onion, chopped finely
2 garlic cloves, chopped finely
Juice of ½ lemon
Pinch of salt
1 tablespoon olive oil

INSTRUCTIONS
Mix the garlic, lemon juice, olive oil and salt together in a bowl.
Rinse and chop the red clover leaves finely.
Place the red clover leaves, prepared couscous, red pepper and onion together in a salad bowl.
Add the garlic/lemon/salt/oil mix and stir.
Let sit for 15 minutes and serve!

Rose

While all 150+ varieties of roses are edible, you will find a stronger, more intense flavour and fragrance in darker varieties of this beautiful and quintessentially British flower.

The sweet and subtle flavour of roses is reminiscent of some common fruits, such as strawberries and green apples and can add an aromatic yet delicate flavour to your culinary dishes. For best effects, pick rose buds once they are full and just before they begin opening, by cutting them off at the base with clippers. Once harvested, lay the fresh rose buds out in single layers on a tray to dry indoors. Once dry, they can be stored in jars or bags for later use.

Rose buds make a delicious tea and are lovely to flavour and garnish dishes such as ice creams, sorbets and other desserts, salads or cereals such as granola. If you want to use fresh petals, be sure to use them within two hours of separating them from the flower before they begin to wilt.

Crystallised petals can also be used to flavour drinks and cakes or frozen into ice cubes to add a little exoticism to drinks. Petals are also a delicious addition to dishes such as honey, syrups, jellies and perfumed butters, though it is important that the small rather bitter-tasting white portion at the bottom of each petal is removed beforehand.

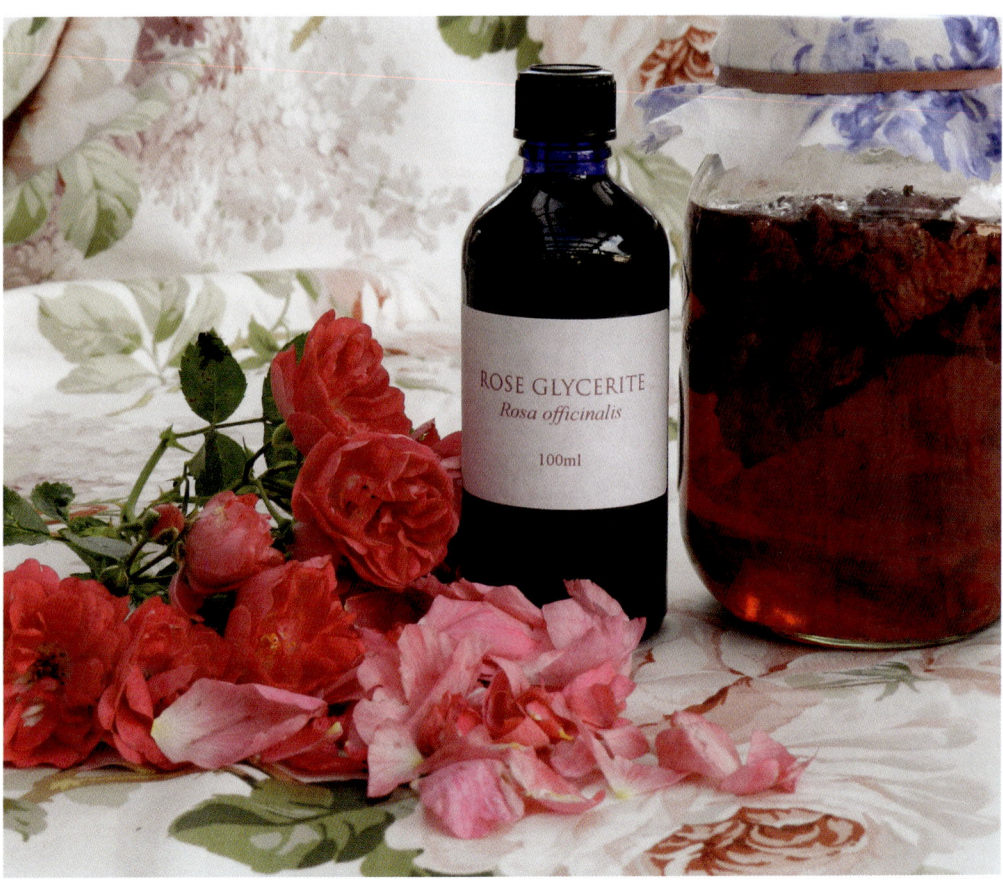

Rose Petal Harissa

INGREDIENTS
25g dried chillies (such as pequin or birds eye)
2 tablespoons dried rose petals
2 teaspoons each of caraway, coriander and cumin seeds
2 whole star anise
2 garlic cloves (peeled and sliced)
1½ teaspoons paprika to add colour and taste
2 red bell peppers
⅓ cup extra virgin olive oil
1 handful semi-dried tomatoes
4 tablespoons sundried tomato paste
2 medjool dates stoned, or 1 heaped teaspoon honey
1 teaspoon rosewater (more to taste)
2 teaspoons lemon juice

INSTRUCTIONS
Remove the seeds from the dried chillies. Place the chillies and rose petals in a small bowl and pour over enough hot water to soak. Leave for half an hour. Drain and set aside.

Toast the seeds, star anise and garlic in a pan over a low heat for about three minutes, stirring as necessary; add the paprika and heat through to release the aroma. Pulverize the toasted mix with a pestle and mortar. Stir in the soaked chillies and rose petals and blend everything together into a paste in your blender, food processor or mortar. Adjust the taste as needed, more sweet or more salt, bearing in mind that the flavour will deepen over a few days.

Spoon into sterilised jars and top with extra rose petals and enough olive oil to cover the paste. Refrigerate and use within three weeks or place small amounts into an ice tray that you don't mind staining and freeze.

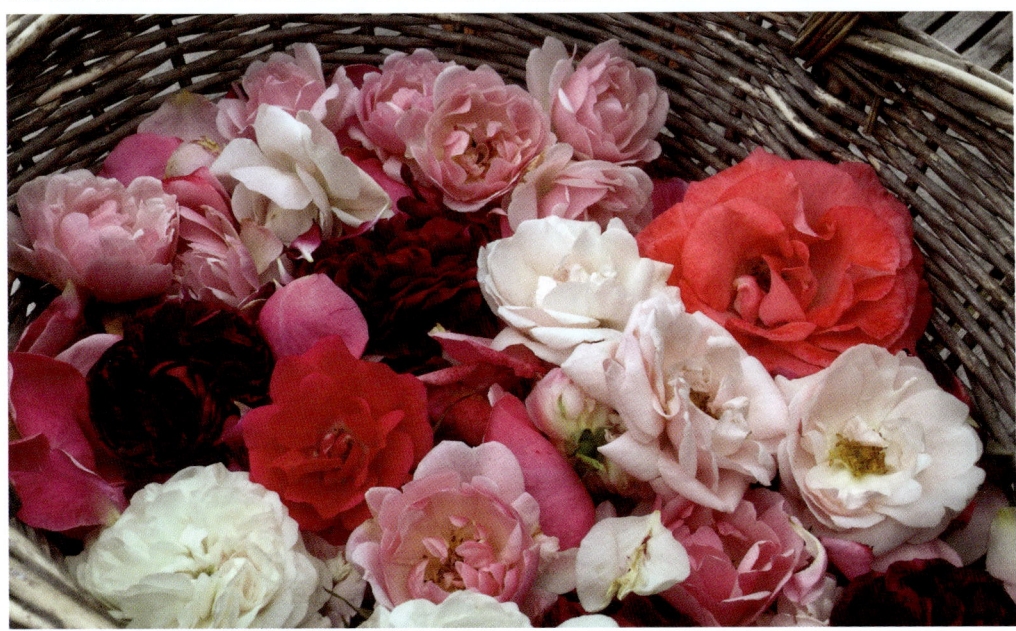

Sage

Sage flowers blossom in spring and early summer, producing clusters of deep violet-blue, pink or white flowers. Like the leaves, sage flowers are edible, though they have a slightly milder flavour.

Sage flowers make for an excellent addition to sauces such as pestos, mustards and herbed vinaigrettes and pair well with meat dishes and sautéed or stuffed mushrooms. Used fresh, they make a gorgeous garnish for salads or as cake decoration.

For best use, cut the flowers when they are partially open and first thing in the morning. Pull the flower tubes away from the stems before use.

Sage Blossom Vinegar

INGREDIENTS
1½ cup white wine vinegar
2½ cup sage blossoms

INSTRUCTIONS
Warm the vinegar in a small saucepan over low heat. Wash the sage blossoms in a bowl of cold water to remove any dirt and bugs and shake off excess water.

Fill a pint-sized jar with the blossoms and pour enough of the warm vinegar into the jar just to submerge the blossoms. Use a spoon to push the blossoms floating to the top down into the warmed vinegar.

Let the vinegar cool completely before sealing the jar. If you have a metal lid, place a square of parchment paper over the opening of the jar and screw on the top. This will prevent the acid from the vinegar from eroding the lid of your jar.

Place the jar in a cool dark place for at least two weeks to produce a vinegar with a strong sage flavour. When you are happy with the strength of your herbal blossom vinegar, strain and discard the blossoms.

Squash Blossom

Those who grow squashes at home will be aware of their beautiful blossoms, though it may come as a surprise that these flowers are just as edible as the squash itself. Both the male and female flowers of all squash, courgette and pumpkin varieties are edible, and have a mild raw squash taste.

It is best to pick only the male squash flowers for culinary purposes, as these exist solely for the purpose of fertilisation and will never actually produce a squash themselves. The male flowers have long, slender stalks, no pistils and are typically found growing around the edges of the plant, while the female flowers grow closer to the centre and have a small bulbous part at the base of the blossom where it meets the stem. After the stamens have been removed, the blossoms can be tossed into salads, sautéed, or a popular option is to fry or bake them stuffed with herbs and cheese until the petals become crispy.

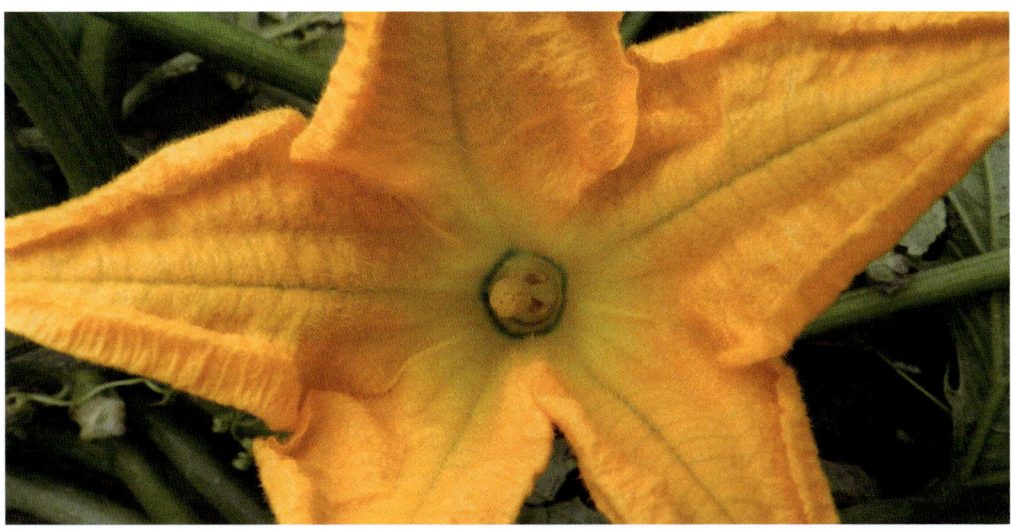

Pan-fried Courgette (zucchini) Blossoms with Ricotta and Garden Herbs

INGREDIENTS
20 large fresh courgette (zucchini) flowers
Olive oil
Sea salt to taste

For the batter
1 cup unbleached all-purpose flour
½ teaspoon fine sea salt
Freshly ground black pepper to taste
¾ cup warm water
1 extra large egg

For the stuffing
1 cup ricotta
1 shallot – skinned and finely chopped
3 tablespoons finely chopped garden herbs (parsley, basil, oregano, thyme and sage)
½ teaspoon fine sea salt
freshly ground black pepper to taste
1 extra large egg – lightly beaten

INSTRUCTIONS
For the batter
Place the flour, salt and pepper in a large bowl. Whisk until well blended. Add the water and whisk until the mixture is smooth. Set aside and let stand for 1 hour. Just before dipping the flowers into the batter, whisk in the egg.

To stuff the flowers
Place the ricotta, shallot, herbs, salt and pepper in a medium bowl and mix well. Add the egg and mix again. Make a small tear lengthwise in each flower and remove the stamen. Place a small amount of the stuffing inside each flower, at the base. Twist the petals so that the stuffing is held safely inside the flower. Place on a baking sheet. Repeat until all the flowers are stuffed.

Heat a large heavy-bottomed skillet over high heat. Add enough oil to come 5ml (1/4inch) up the sides of the pan. When the oil is hot, quickly dip each flower in the batter and add it to the pan. Sauté for 2 to 3 minutes until a deep-golden colour. Flip the flowers and continue to sauté for 1 to 2 minutes until deep-golden on the other side. Remove from the pan and drain on paper towels. Repeat until all flowers have been used, reducing the heat when the pan gets very hot so that the oil doesn't burn. Sprinkle the fritters with the sea salt and place them on a large serving platter.

Sunflower

Almost the entire sunflower plant is edible in all stages of its development, from seedling through to mature flower. For best results, pick the flower during its bud stage when its taste will resemble that of an artichoke.

Sunflower buds are delicious when steamed or sautéed and served whole with garlic and butter, but be sure to pull off the bitter green part around the bottom of the bud beforehand. Once the flower is fully open, the petals with their mild nutty taste, can be picked and used in salads, soups or stir fries.

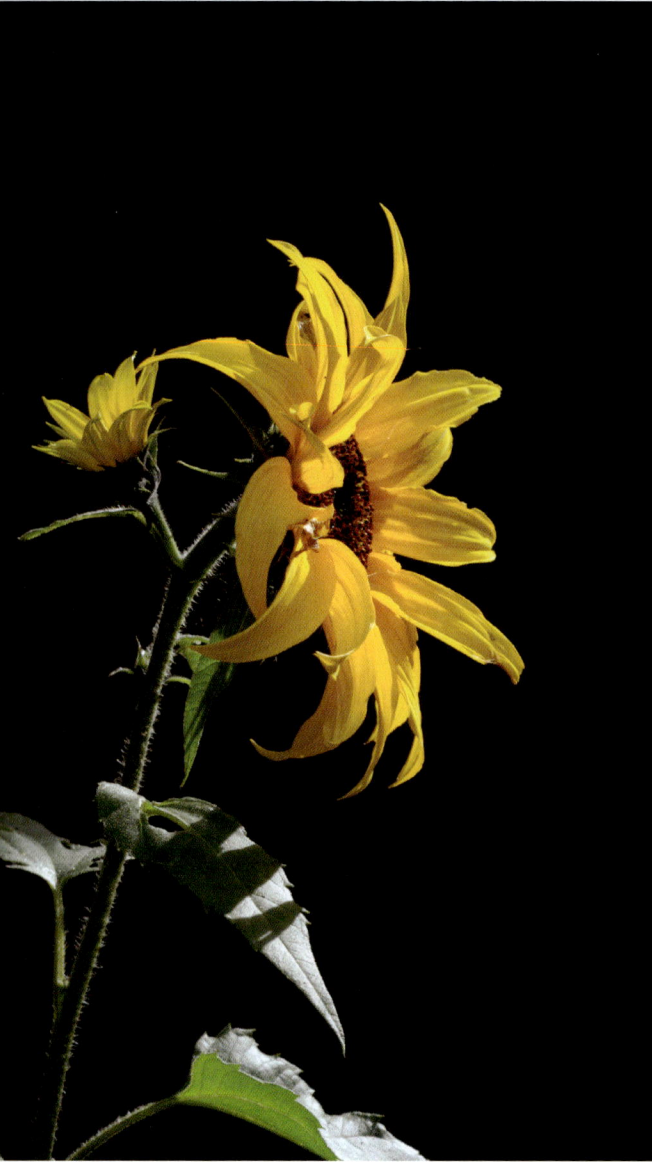

Sunflower Pesto

INGREDIENTS
¼ cup sunflower seeds
pinch of sea salt, or to taste
1 tablespoon fresh squeezed lemon juice
1 teaspoon lemon zest
2 cups sunflower petals, removed from centres, lightly packed
⅓ cup olive oil, or more to make a thinner texture

INSTRUCTIONS
Toast the sunflower seeds in a cast iron skillet on the stovetop until they are very lightly browned. Combine the sunflower seeds and salt in a mortar and pestle or food processor, and work it to a rustic paste.

Add the petals, lemon juice and zest, and olive oil, and process until the desired consistency is reached. Serve immediately on crostini or mixed into pasta or store in an airtight container in the fridge for up to 5 days.

Sweet Violet

Closely related to pansies, sweet violets tend to be found in moist and shaded areas with deep, sandy soil. They produce a range of sweet, perfumed flavours and come in a variety of colours such as white, pink, blue or lavender.

Their beautiful and delicate flowers make a fantastic garnish on both sweet and savoury dishes, such as salads, desserts or in drinks. They can also be incorporated into recipes for violet tea, violet cake and violet syrup as well as vinegars, butters, spreads and jellies. Candied violets make great toppings for cakes or soufflés.

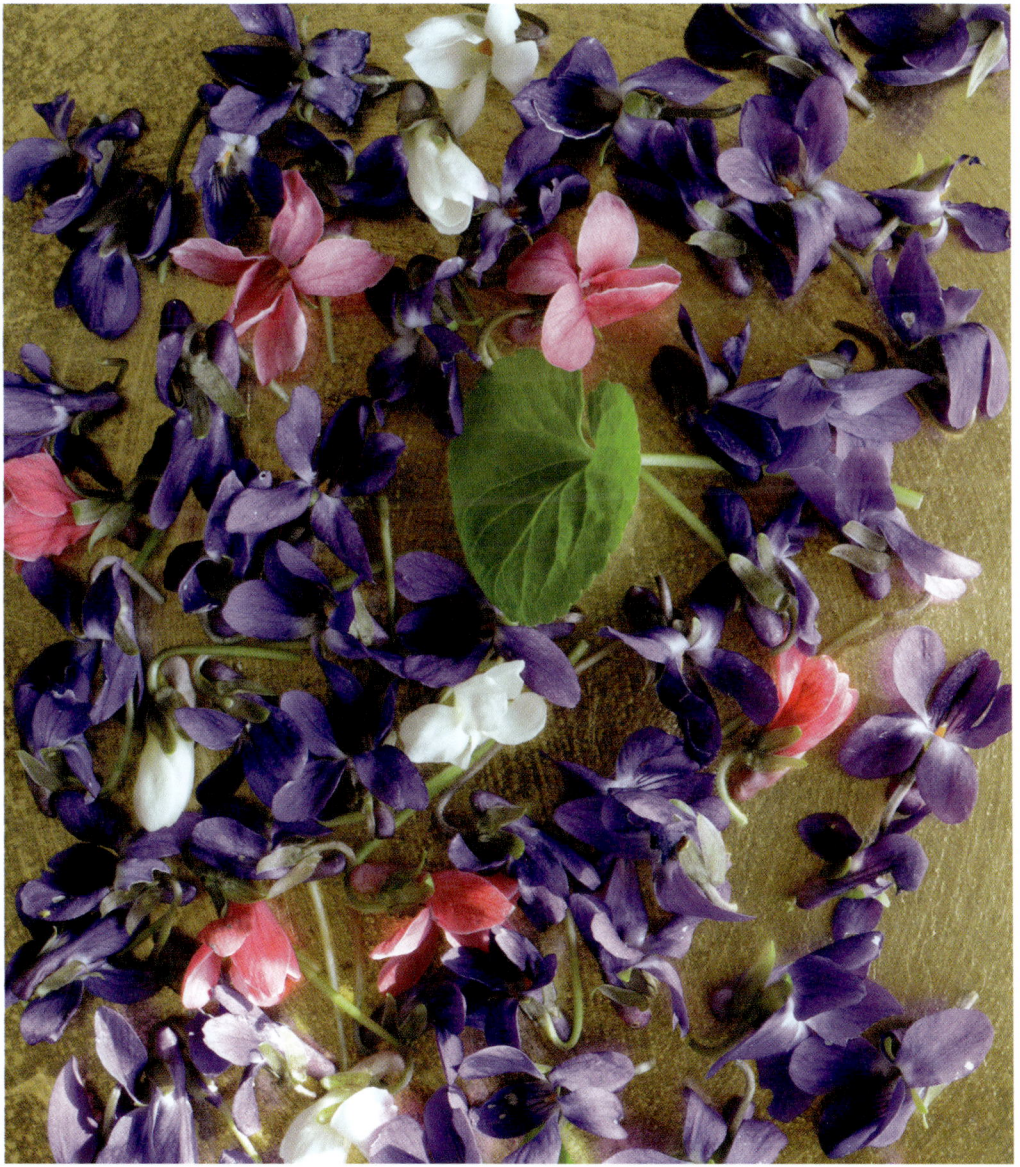

Sweet William

Despite being considered a quintessentially English summer flower, sweet Williams are in fact native to southern Europe and parts of Asia. The flowers come in clusters of small and vividly coloured flowers, which give off a delightfully sweet and spicy fragrance.

The flowers have a mild peppery and clove-like flavour, and can make a perfect addition to a salad. Sweet Williams also pair well with fish and seafood dishes, stir fries, sauces, stews and soups and are great incorporated into desserts, jams and marmalades. The petals can also add zest to sorbets, ice creams or fruit salads.

For best results when using them for garnishing, pick the flowers fresh and in the morning before the strong afternoon sunlight hits them, to keep the strong scent and freshness intact. It is best to remove the white part at the base of each flower as it can give an unwanted bitter taste.

Sweet William Bread

INGREDIENTS
2 cups flour
¼ cup ground almonds
⅛ teaspoon salt
1 cup butter/oil/coconut oil
Sugar or honey ½ cup
½ teaspoon vanilla essence
2–3 tablespoons sweet William petals

INSTRUCTIONS
Mix flour, ground almonds and salt together in a food processor. Add sugar/honey, butter/oil and vanilla essence and process for 1–2 minutes.

Gently mix the sweet William petals with your hands into the dough made in the processor. Make a log with the dough on a sheet of baking paper. Refrigerate the log for about two hours.

Preheat oven to 165C/330F and bake for about 20 minutes until golden brown around the edges. Cool on a rack and store the bread in an airtight container for up to ten days.

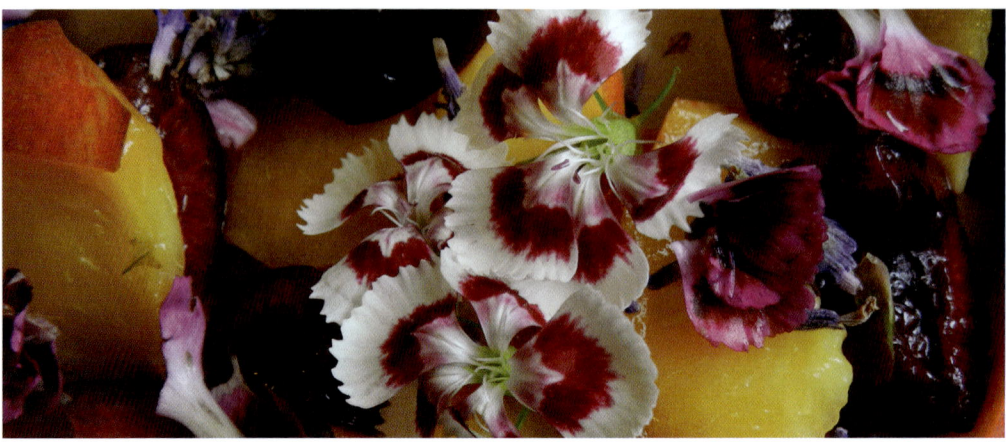

Tiger Lily

The tiger lily is a wild variety of the day lily, often found growing along roadsides and ditches like a weed in the USA and loved by gardeners in the UK. The flowers produce a strong, sweet and distinctive scent characteristic of the lily and are easy to spot, since they produce large and stunningly vivid orange flowers with large dark spots, hence the name.

Most parts of the tiger lily plant are edible, though interestingly they are toxic to cats and can cause them vomiting and kidney failure. The flower buds can be eaten raw or cooked, and have a mild, slightly sweet flavour. They make an exotically colourful feature in salads, stir fries and omelettes.

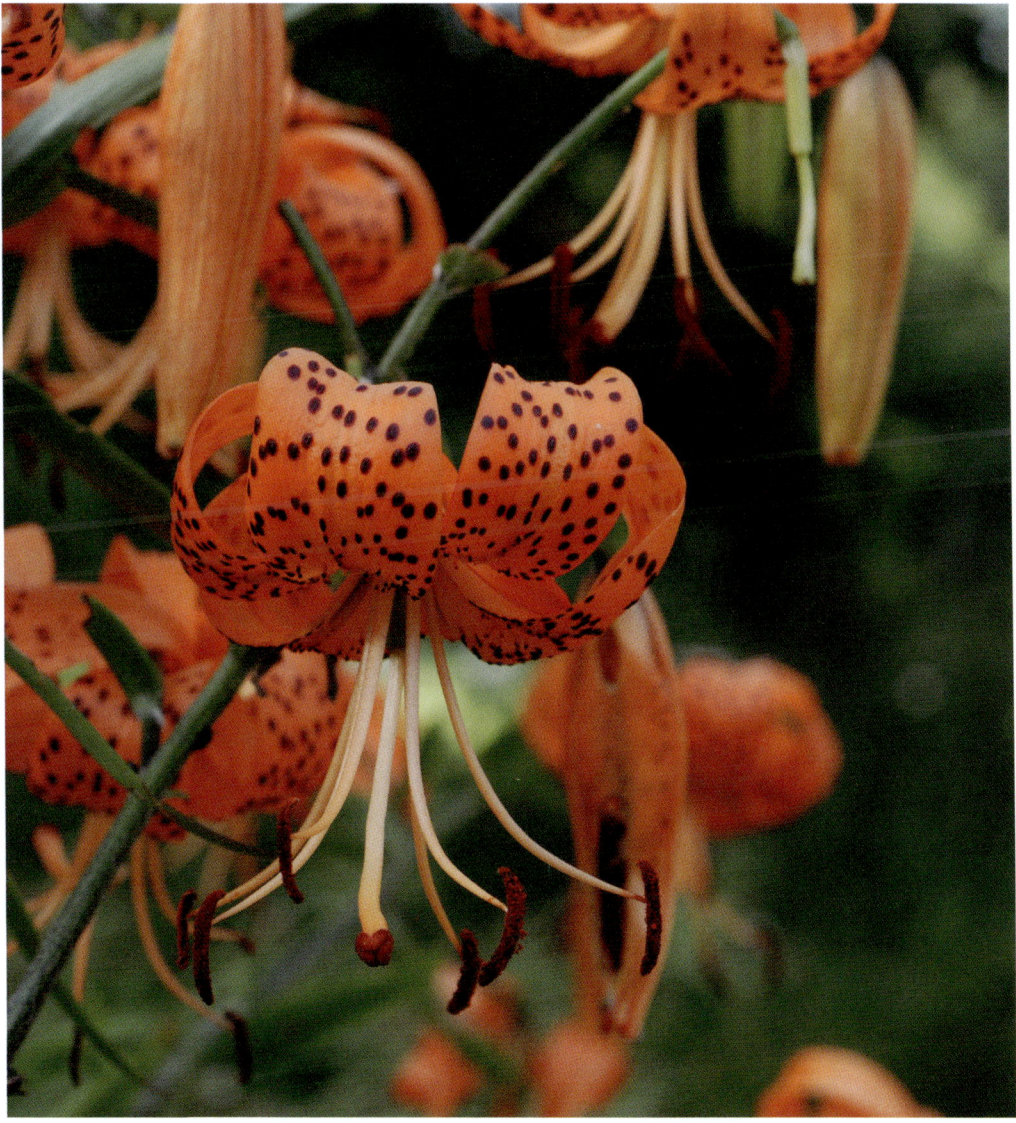

Wild Garlic

Wild garlic is widespread through shady woodland areas of Europe and Asia and has the species name *Allium ursinum* (Bear's garlic) as it is often a hibernating bear's first snack! It is also known as ramsons, wood garlic, buckrams, wild leek and hog garlic, depending on where you are. It is a member of the garlic family, alongside onions, bulb garlic, leeks and chives and, like chives, the whole plant is edible, from the stems to the leaves, seeds and flowers as well as root bulbs. For best tasting results, use the leaves when fresh and still young, before the flowers are fully out and begin to taste slightly bitter.

The flowers begin to develop between April and June, producing characteristic white blossoms grouped together in a kind of globe shape on the end of each stem. They look delightful sprinkled on top of a salad and can add a garlic punch to a savoury sandwich, but they are also delicious when incorporated into a pesto or other similar sauces.

> **Wild Garlic Pesto**
>
> My favourite way to eat wild garlic is in a delicious pesto.
>
> Simply add clean wild garlic leaves and a few flowers to a blender, along with mixed seeds, a neutral tasting oil and sea salt.
>
> You can add some nettles, chickweed, basil, or other green leaves if you wish.
>
> Pulse until blended and add more oil, lemon juice and/or seasoning until you have the consistency or flavour you are looking for.
>
> Garnish with fresh blossoms.

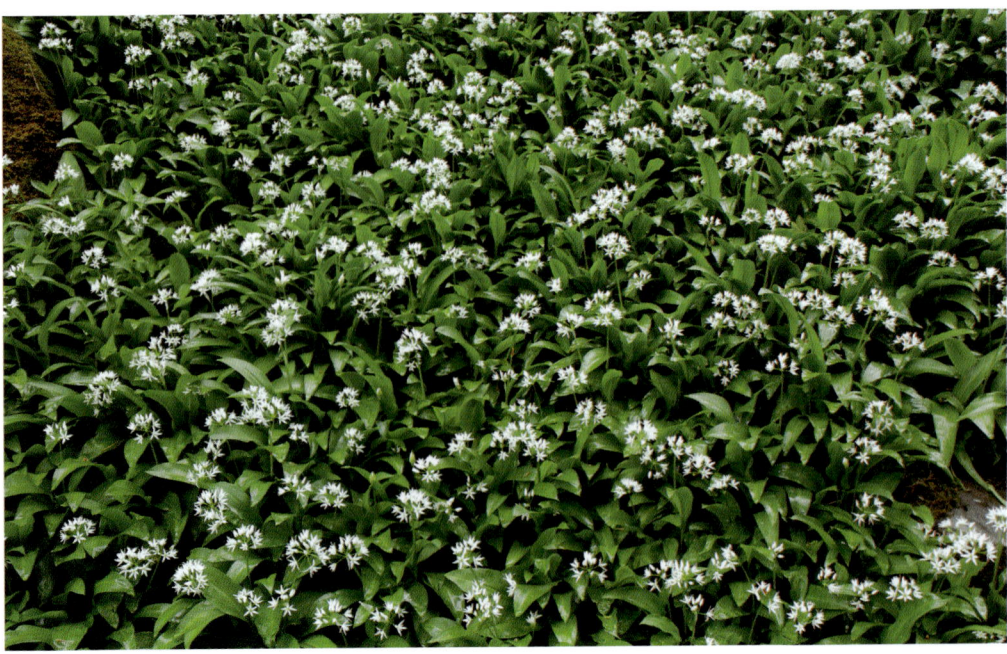

Wild Pansy

Pansies are a known gardener's favourite, as they come in a wide variety of sizes and colours (both single and combinations of colours) and are incredibly versatile. They can be used in the kitchen either whole or as individual petals, once the pistils and stamens are removed. If you eat only the petals then you will get a mild flavour, while the whole flowers have a wintergreen, grassy or lettuce type flavour and a delicate fragrance. They make a great addition to green salads, soups or cocktails. Alternatively, they can be candied and or used whole used to garnish and elegantly decorate a dessert or cake.

Purple Kale and Pansy Salad

INGREDIENTS
1 bunch kale
Fresh basil leaves, both green and purple varieties
Fresh sprigs of thyme
Fresh mint leaves
Fresh parsley
½ small red onion, halved and thinly sliced
2–3 tbsp. sunflower seeds
Pansies to garnish
Your choice of vinaigrette

INSTRUCTIONS
Wash your kale well, trim the tough stems off and remove the spines of each leaf. Chop or shred the kale and add it to a large wide salad bowl. Toss the herbs, onions and seeds in, at a ratio of about 4 to 1, greens to herbs. Use plenty of basil. Toss the salad with the dressing, and then scatter the flowers on top to garnish.

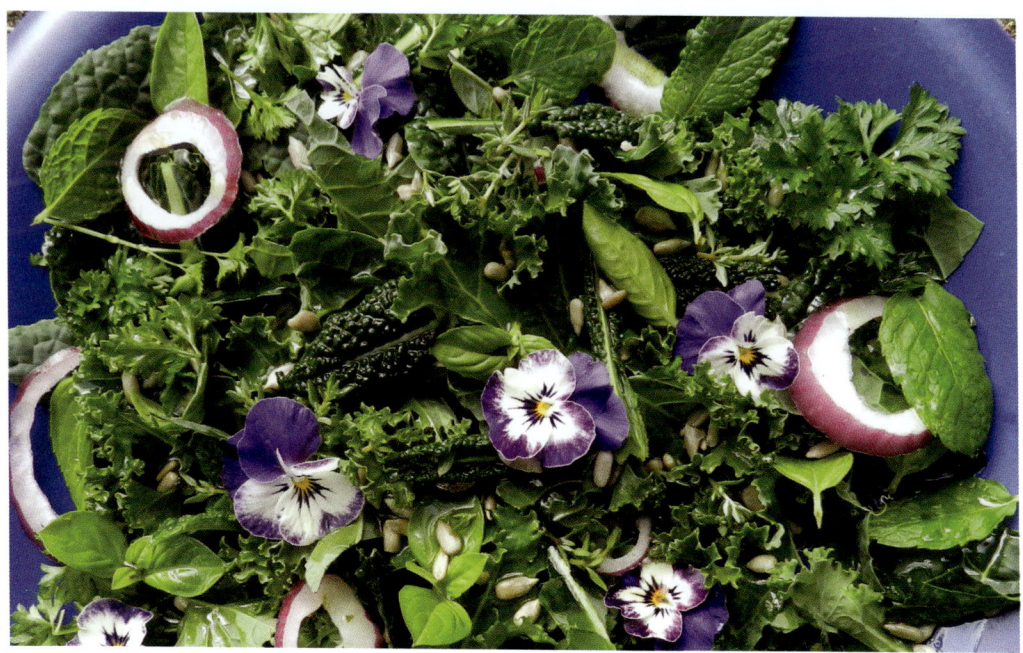

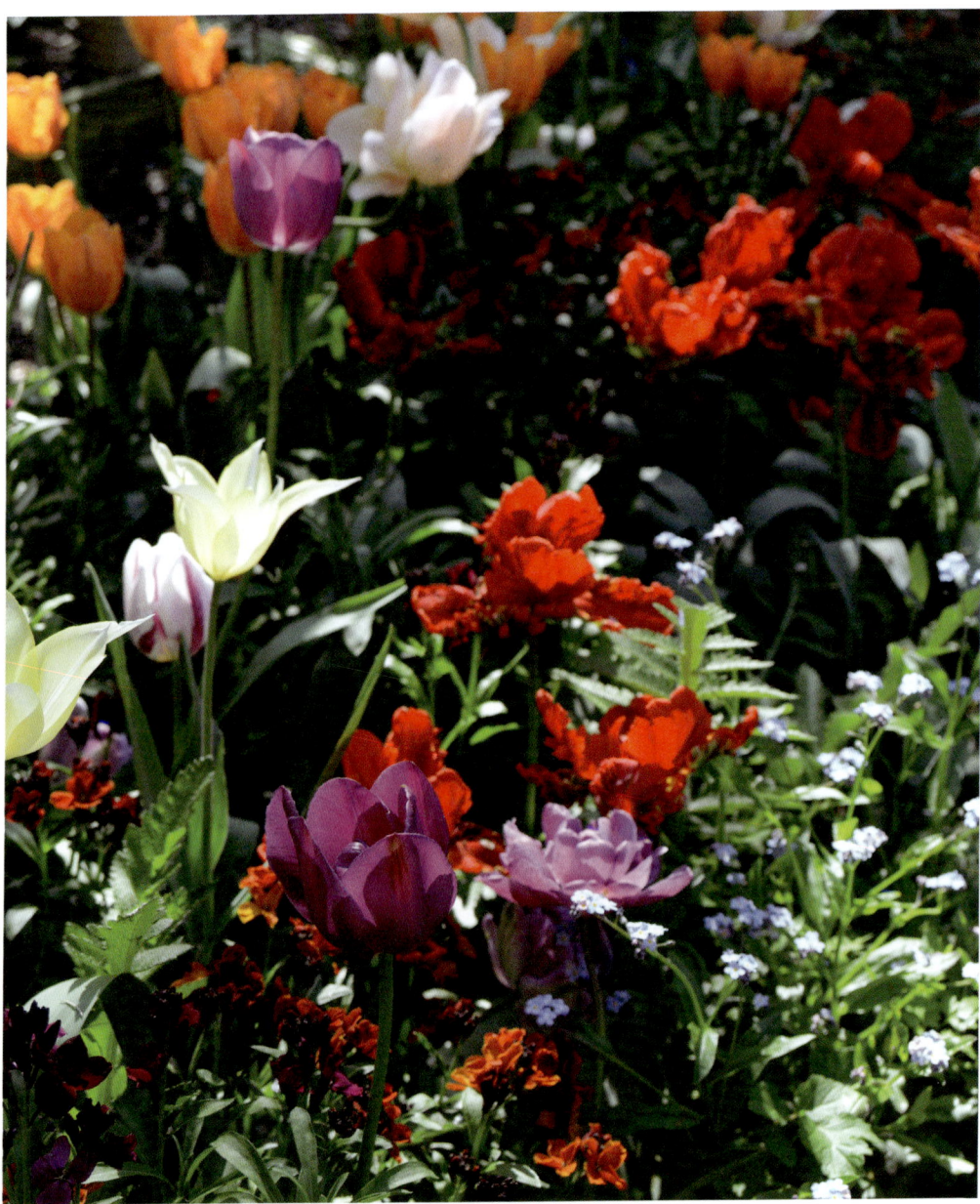

Photo credits

All photographs are by Julie Bruton-Seal except for the following:

Anne McIntyre pp. 6, 9, 75, 218, 223, 318, 332, 349, 395, 399, 418, 420, 425, 429, 437, 444, 465; André Karwath p61; Annette Meyer p164; Conger Design p116; Dave Proffer, CC BY 2.0 <https://creativecommons.org/licenses/by/2.0>, via Wikimedia Commons; Erwin Nowak p119; Gail Hampshire p86; Jen Bartlett p413; Joanjo Puertos Muñoz p135; Ghislain 118 http://www.fleurs-des-montagnes.net p320; Hardy Plant p244; Invertzoo, CC BY-SA 4.0 <https://creativecommons.org/licenses/by-sa/4.0>, via Wikimedia Commons p185; Marco Schmidt p88; Michaela Wenzler p298; R. E. Beck p249

Index

Note: Page Numbers in bold indicate herbs featured in the 'materia medica' section

acetylcholine, 302
acetyl cholinesterase (AChE), 161, 302
AChE. *See* acetyl cholinesterase
Achillea millifolium. *See* yarrow
acne, 261
ADD. *See* attention deficit disorder
ADHD. *See* attention deficit hyperactive disorder
adipocytes, 310
ageing process, 143
Agrimonia eupatoria. *See* agrimony
agrimony (*Agrimonia eupatoria*), **69**
    antimicrobial properties, 70
    cautions, 71
    flower essence, 71
    growing, 71
    herbal remedy, 69
    homeopathic remedy, 70
    toning liniment/compress, 71
Alchemilla vulgaris/mollis. *See* lady's mantle
Alexandrian school, 34
allergic
    rashes, 124, 352
    reactions, 108
Allium
    sativum. *See* garlic
    ursinum. *See* wild garlic
ALS. *See* amyotrophic lateral sclerosis
Althaea officinalis. *See* marshmallow
Alzheimer's disease, 302
American cranesbill, 177
amyotrophic lateral sclerosis (ALS), 275, 276
analgesic herbs, 222
androgenic alopecia, 356
anemone, 29. *See* wind flower
Anenome pulsatilla. *See* pasque flower
Anethum graveolens. *See* dill
angelica (*Angelica archangelica*), **97**
    cardamom, and cinnamon elixir, 100
    cautions, 100
    edible uses, 100
    flower essence, 100
    growing, 100
    herbal remedy, 98–99
    homeopathic remedy, 99

angiogenesis, 301, 389
angiosperms, 29
Anglo-Saxon healers, 37
Anthemis nobilis. *See* chamomile
anthocyanins, 227, 293
anticipatory nerves, 351
antimicrobial phenols, 242
antioxidant, 207
    flavonoids, 351
    phenols, 242
antirrhinums, 29
aromadendrene, 226
aromatherapy, 51–52. *See also* flower healing
aromatic
    flowers, 428, 432
    herbs, 31, 32, 35
    plants, 413
    waters, 421
Artemisia vulgaris. *See* mugwort
ashwaganda, 47. *See also* Ayurvedic medicine
asphodels, 13
Asteraceae family pollen, 209
atherosclerosis, 227
attention deficit disorder (ADD), 143
attention deficit hyperactive disorder (ADHD), 143, 269
Avicenna, 36
Ayurvedic medicine, 33–34. *See also* flower healing
    ashwaganda, 47
    doshas, 48
    five elements, 48

Bach, E., 52–53. *See also* flower remedies and essences
bachelors' buttons. *See* cornflowers
bacteria food poisoning, 275
Bear's garlic. *See* wild garlic
bee balm. *See* bergamot
Bellis perennis. *See* daisy
bergamot, 442. *See also* wild bergamot
biocides, 345
black cohosh, 45. *See also* healing tradition in America
blepharitis, 166
BMI. *See* body mass index
body mass index (BMI), 316
borage, 443. *See also* edible flowers

calendula (*Calendula officinalis*), **111**, 444. *See also* edible flowers
    cautions, 114
    cream, 114
    edible uses, 114
    flower essence, 113–114
    flowers, 423
    growing, 114
    herbal remedy, 112–113
    herbal tincture, 114
    homeopathic remedy, 113
    and potato salad, 444
California poppy (*Eschscholzia californica*), **163**
    cautions, 164
    flower essence, 164
    growing, 164
    herbal remedy, 163–164
    homeopathic remedy, 164
    night-time tisane, 164
capsules, 434. *See also* flower preparations for internal use
carcinogens, 255
carnation. *See* sweet William
carvacrol, 242, 347
catmint (*Nepeta cataria*), **247**
    aromatherapy oil, 249
    cautions, 249
    edible uses, 249
    flower essence, 249
    growing, 249
    herbal remedy, 248–249
    homeopathic remedy, 249
    relaxant effects, 248
catnip. *See* catmint
centaury (*Erythraea entaurium*), **159**. *See also* flower remedies and essences
    cautions, 161
    essence, 53
    flower essence, 161
    gentiopicrin, 160
    growing, 161
    herbal remedy, 159–161
chamomile (*Chamomilla recutita/Matricaria chamomilla/Anthemis nobilis*), **115**, 445. *See also* edible flowers; organic gardening
    aromatherapy oil, 117–120
    cautions, 120
    cooling stomach tea, 121
    for eyewash, 121
    eye wrap, 121
    flower essence, 120
    growing, 120
    healing salve for eczema, 121
    herbal remedy, 117–120
    homeopathic remedy, 120
    lemonade, 445
    rosemary, St John's wort and chamomile oil, 121
    spray, 410
Chayawanprash, 429
Chelidonium majus. *See* greater celandine
cherry blossom time, 25
chickweed (*Stellaria media*), **329**
    cautions, 331
    chickweed pesto, 331
    cooling properties, 329–330
    edible uses, 331
    flower essence, 331
    growing, 331
    herbal remedy, 330
    homeopathic remedy, 330–331
chicory (*Cichorium intybus*), **127**
    antifungal properties, 128–129
    cautions, 129
    edible uses, 129
    flower essence, 129
    growing, 129
    herbal remedy, 127–129
    homeopathic remedy, 129
Chinese medicine, 48. *See also* flower healing
    five elements, 50
    ginseng, 49
    indicators of health and disease, 51
    qi, 49
    'Yin' and 'yang', 49
Chinese parsley, 138
chive blossom, 446. *See also* edible flowers
chive blossom infused vinegar, 446
Chloris, 11
chlorogenic acid, 340
Christ consciousness, 271
chrysanthemum, 447. *See also* edible flowers
Chrysanthemum parthenium. *See* feverfew
Cichorium intybus. *See* chicory
cilia, 293
circulatory disorders, 351
Citrus aurantium. *See* orange blossom
cleavers (*Galium aparine*), **173**
    cautions, 175
    cleavers juice, 175
    edible uses, 175
    flower essence, 175
    growing, 175
    herbal remedy, 174
    homeopathic remedy, 174–175
    related plants, 175
    spring tonic, 175
climbing plants, 20

clove pink. *See* sweet William
CNS depressants, 145, 194, 223, 323
comfrey, 411. *See also* organic gardening
common ailments, 425
companion planting, 408, 409. *See also* wildflower garden
compost accelerators, 411. *See also* organic gardening
compresses, 436. *See also* plant preparations for external use
Constantine '*the African*', 36
cooling herbs, 33. *See also* Greek and Roman medicine, ancient
coriander (*Coriandrum sativumum*), **137**
    aromatherapy oil, 139
    cautions, 140
    cold coriander seed infusion, 140
    cooling effects, 139
    edible uses, 139–140
    flower essence, 139
    growing, 140
    herbal remedy, 138–139
cornflowers, 447. *See also* edible flowers
cortisol, 253
courtship and marriage, 19
cowslip (*Primula veris*), **279**
    cautions, 282
    edible uses, 282
    flower essence, 282
    growing, 282
    herbal remedy, 280–282
    homeopathic remedy, 282
    and primroses, 281
Crataegus monogyna, C. laevigata. *See* hawthorn
creams, 436. *See also* plant preparations for external use
culinary elite, 398
Culpeper, N., 40, 377
cuttings. *See also* flowers, growing
    ripe cuttings, 404–405
    root cuttings or offsets, 405
    semi-ripe cuttings, 404
    softwood cuttings, 404
    taking, 404
cycle of life, 13–15
cycloviolacin O2, 383
cystitis, 360

daisy (*Bellis perennis*), **107**, 448. *See also* edible flowers
    cautions, 108
    edible uses, 108
    flower essence, 108
    herbal remedy, 108–109
    homeopathic remedy, 109
    kaemferol, 108
dandelion (*Taraxacum officinale*), **337**, 449–450. *See also* edible flowers
    cautions, 342
    cold infusion, 342
    cure for warts, 342
    edible uses, 341
    flower essence, 341
    flower salve, 342
    growing, 342
    herbal remedy, 338–340
    homeopathic remedy, 340–341
    infused oil, 342
    jelly, 449
    risotto, 450
Daphne, 13
decoctions, 426–428. *See also* flower preparations for internal use
decongesting flowers, 436
degenerative problems, 339
dehydrator, 418. *See also* organic gardening
De Materia Medica, 35
Descartes, R., 41–42
Dianthus. *See* sweet William
    caryophyllus, 149–151
    chinensis, 151
digestive herb, 346, 370
dill (*Anethum graveolens*), **92**
    cautions, 95
    edible uses, 95
    flower essence, 94
    gripe water, 95
    growing, 95
    herbal remedy, 92–94
Dioscorides, P., 35, 63, 159, 173, 377. *See also* Greek and Roman medicine, ancient
distilled waters, 132, 432–433. *See also* flower preparations for internal use
Doctrine of Signatures, 39–40, 60, 127, 196, 354. *See also* flower healing
doshas, 48. *See also* Ayurvedic medicine
dreams, 17
drying. *See also* organic gardening
    herbs, 33
    plants, 418–419

earth as Gaia, 27–28. *See also* flower healing
Echinacea angustifolia, pallida and purpurea. *See* purple coneflower
Eclectics, 46. *See also* healing tradition in America

edible flowers, 441
- bergamot, 442
- borage, 443
- calendula, 444
- chamomile, 445
- chive blossom, 446
- chrysanthemum, 447
- cornflowers, 447
- daisy, 448
- dandelion, 449–450
- elderflower, 451
- fennel, 452
- forget-me-not, 453
- fuchsia, 454
- gladiolus, 454
- hibiscus, 455
- hollyhock, 456
- honeysuckle, 457
- lavender, 457–458
- lilac, 459
- magnolia, 460
- nasturtium, 461
- pelargoniums, 462
- purslane, 462
- red clover, 463
- rose, 464–465
- sage, 466
- squash blossom, 466–467
- sunflower, 468
- sweet violet, 469
- sweet William, 470
- tiger lily, 471
- wild garlic, 472
- wild pansy, 473

elder (*Sambucus nigra*), **313**. *See also* edible flowers
- aromatherapy oil, 317
- cautions, 319
- cordial, 319
- edible uses, 318–319
- elderflower, 451
- elderflower fritters, 451
- flower essence, 318
- growing, 319
- herbal remedy, 315–317
- homeopathic remedy, 317–318

elecampane (*Inula helenium*), **205**
- active ingredients in, 207
- cautions, 209
- edible uses, 208
- flower essence, 208
- four thieves vinegar, 209
- growing, 208–209
- herbal remedy, 206–208
- homeopathic remedy, 208
- inulin, 206
- pollination, 207

electuaries, 429–431. *See also* flower preparations for internal use

elixirs, 432. *See also* flower preparations for internal use

endometriosis, 149

endorphins, 323

energy vibrations of mind, 28

English Physician, 397

Enquiry into Plants, 34

Enterococcus faecalis, 301

epidermis, 260

eruptive childhood infections, 65

erysipelas, 138

Erythraea entaurium. *See* centaury

Eschscholtz, J. F., 163

Eschscholzia californica. *See* California poppy

ESCOP. *See* European Scientific Cooperative on Phytotherapy

essential oils, 51, 438

Euphrasia officinalis. *See* eyebright

European Scientific Cooperative on Phytotherapy (ESCOP), 271

Evelyn, J., 315

evening primrose (*Oenothera biennis*), **259**
- cautions, 262
- edible uses, 262
- flower essence, 262
- gamma linoleic acid, 260
- growing, 262
- herbal remedy, 260–262
- homeopathic remedy, 262
- nourishing body oil, 262

evergreens, 15

expectorants, 108

eyebright (*Euphrasia officinalis*), **165**
- flower essence, 167
- growing, 167
- herbal remedy, 166–167

fennel, 452. *See also* edible flowers

feverfew (*Tanacetum parthenium* (*Chrysanthemum parthenium*)), **333**
- anti-inflammatory tisane, 334, 335
- cautions, 335
- edible uses, 335
- flower essence, 335
- footbath, 335
- growing, 335
- herbal remedy, 334
- homeopathic remedy, 334–335

pain-relieving tisane, 335
Filipendula ulmaria. *See* meadowsweet
flavonoids, 169, 315, 320, 351, 423
floral. *See also* flower healing; plant preparations for external use
    baths, 434–435
    healing history, 31–32
    honeys, 429
    pharmacy. *See* still room
    waters, 421, 432–433
floral medicines, 422. *See also* still room
    nutrients found in flowers, 424–425
floriphagia, 423
flower healing, 27
    ancient Greek and Roman medicine, 32–36
    Anglo-Saxon healers, 37
    aromatherapy, 51–52
    Avicenna, 36
    Ayurvedic medicine, 33–34, 47–48
    in China, 32
    Chinese medicine, 48–51
    Constantine '*the African*', 36
    dawning of scientific age, 40–42
    deeper significance of flowers, 56–58
    Doctrine of Signatures, 39–40
    earth as Gaia, 27–28
    flower remedies and essences, 52–56
    flowers with spirituality, 27
    foxgloves, 44
    Greek and Arab traditions, 36
    hallucinatory and mind-altering plants, 31
    healers, 31
    healing tradition in America, 45–46
    heartsease, 30
    herbalists, 31
    herbal medicine in Egypt, 31–32
    Hildegard von Bingen, 38
    history of, 31–32
    homeopathy, 42–44
    Hyssop, 35
    John Gerard, 40
    John Parkinson, 40
    lilium regale, 38
    medieval monasteries, 37–39
    in modern times, 46–47
    Neanderthal man, 31
    Nicolas Culpeper, 40
    Rene Gattefosse, 52
    role of flowering plants, 29–31
    shamans, 31
    unity of all things, 27
    vital green energy, 38
    William Turner, 40
    wood betony, 37
flowering
    herbs, 37
    plants, 29–31
flower preparations for internal use, 426. *See also* still room
    decoctions, 426–428
    elixirs, 432
    floral waters, 432–433
    flower honeys, 429–431
    garlic honey, 430
    herbal pharmacopoeias, 428
    herbal vinegars, 431
    honey, 430
    infusions, 426
    makeshift still, 433
    oxymels, 431–432
    powders, 433–434
    suppositories, 434
    tablets and capsules, 434
    tinctures and glycerites, 428–429
flower remedies and essences, 52–56. *See also* flower healing
    centaury essence, 53
    Edward Bach, 52–53
    mountain devil essence, 54
    nosodes, 53
    sun method, 54
flowers, 7. *See also* flower preparations for internal use
    anemone, 1
    arrangement, 25
    cherry blossom time, 25
    courtship and marriage, 19
    and cycle of life, 13–15
    and dreams, 17
    flower-viewing, 25
    forget-me-not, 19
    funereal, 14
    garden, 394
    garden and religion, 23–25
    Greek myths, 11–13
    growing and gathering, 393
    growth and ephemeral, 17
    honeys from, 429–431
    and humankind, 7
    Hyacinthus, 19
    iris, 17
    jasmine, 17, 20
    Lady Mary Wortley, 21
    language of, 20–21
    and life of spirit, 15–17
    lotus, 15–17

and love, 18–20
luck bringing, 17
Madonna lily, 17
mugwort, 57
orange flowers, 20
orchids, 19–20
pansies, 20
posy, 19
power, 398
rose, 18, 20
significance of, 11, 56–58
snowdrop, 14
and soul, 23–26
with spirituality, 27
trefoil or shamrock, 17
tuberose, 26
tulip, 19
vervain, 20
Victorian language of, 21–22
vital force of subtle energy, 56
to ward off intrusion by inharmonious spirits, 23
writing and poetry, 56
yarrow, 57
flowers, growing, 403
layering, 405
mounding, 405
ripe cuttings, 404–405
root cuttings, 405
root division, 404
semi-ripe cuttings, 404
softwood cuttings, 404
soil conditions, 403
sowing seeds, 403
taking cuttings, 404
flower-viewing, 25
fomentations, 436. See also plant preparations for external use
foraging, 413–415. See also organic gardening
best practice, 416–417
safely and responsibly, 417–418
for wildflowers, 415–416
forget-me-not, 19, 453. See also edible flowers
foxgloves, 44
fuchsia, 454. See also edible flowers
funereal flowers, 14
furanocoumarins, 98

GABA. See gamma-amino butyric acid
Gaia, 28
hypothesis, 398
Galen, 34–35, 377, 429. See also Greek and Roman medicine, ancient

Galium aparine. See cleavers
gamma-amino butyric acid (GABA), 269, 321
gamma linoleic acid (GLA), 260
garden, 23, 398
culinary elite, 398
healing garden, 394
monasteries, 396
as paradise, 394–397
physic gardens, 397–398
and religion, 23–25
tending herb garden, 398–401
garlic (*Allium sativum*), **77**
cautions, 82
edible uses, 81–82
flower essence, 81
garlic syrup, 82
growing, 82
herbal remedy, 78–81
homeopathic remedy, 81
honey, 430
probiotic breakfast, 82
wild garlic pesto, 82
Gattefosse, R., 52
Geranium robertianum. See herb Robert
Gerard, J., 40, 264, 293, 344, 397
ginseng, 49. See also Chinese medicine
GLA. See gamma linoleic acid
gladiolus, 454. See also edible flowers
Glechoma hederacea. See ground Ivy
glycerites, 428–429. See also flower preparations for internal use
greater celandine (*Chelidonium majus*), **123**
antitumor properties, 125
cautions, 125
flower essence, 125
growing, 125
herbal remedy, 124–125
homeopathic remedy, 125
Greek. See also flower healing
and Arab flower healing, 36
myths, 11–13
physicians, 11
Greek and Roman medicine, ancient, 32. See also flower healing
cooling herbs, 33
Galen, 34–35
Hippocrates, 33
humours, 33
Metrodora, 34
moistening herbs, 33
Pedanius Dioscorides, 35
Pliny the Elder, 36
Theophrastus, 34
warming and drying herbs, 33

ground Ivy (*Glechoma hederacea*), **181**
    cautions, 184
    edible uses, 184
    flower essence, 184
    ground ivy oil, 184
    growing, 184
    herbal remedy, 182–184
    homeopathic remedy, 184
gut problems, 322
gymnosperms, 29
gynaecological problems, 70, 104, 294

Hahnemann, S., 42. *See also* homeopathy
hallucinatory and mind-altering plants, 31
hand and foot baths, 435–436. *See also* plant preparations for external use
harmine, 269
hawthorn (*Crataegus monogyna*, *C. laevigata*), **141**
    cautions, 145
    edible uses, 145
    flower essence, 144
    growing, 145
    herbal remedy, 143–144
    homeopathic remedy, 144
    Mayday, 141
    maypole ceremony, 141
HDLs. *See* high-density lipoproteins
healers, 31
healing flowers, 59
    Doctrine of Signatures, 60
    getting acquainted with, 60
    pharmacological approach, 61
    plant language, 60
healing garden, 394
    creating, 401–402
    English Physician, 397
    Leech Book of Bald, 396
    medicinal herbs, 396
    Paradisi in Sole Paradisus Terrestris, 397
    tending herb garden, 398–401
    Theatrum Botanicum, 397
healing plants, 8
healing tradition in America, 45. *See also* flower healing
    black cohosh, 45
    Eclectics, 46
    homoeostasis, 46
    National Institute of Medical Herbalists, 45
    Native American medicine, 45
    Physiomedicalism, 46
    physiomedicalists, 45
    Samuel Thomson, 46

heartsease (*Viola tricolor*), 30, **387**
    cautions, 390
    and chamomile infusion, 390
    flower essence, 390
    growing, 388, 390
    herbal remedy, 388–390
    homeopathic remedy, 390
hedge thorn. *See* hawthorn
Henbane, 32
herbalists, 31
Herball, The, 40
herbal medicine in Egypt, 31–32
herbal pharmacopoeias, 428. *See also* flower preparations for internal use
herbal vinegars, 431. *See also* flower preparations for internal use
herb Robert (*Geranium robertianum*), **177**
    cautions, 180
    edible uses, 180
    flower essence, 180
    growing, 180
    herbal remedy, 178–180
    homeopathic remedy, 180
herbs
    analgesic, 222
    aromatic, 31, 32, 35
    cooling, 33
    drying, 33
    flowering, 37
    hormone balancing, 322
    invasive, 412
    medicinal, 396
    moistening, 33
    pleasant tasting, 426
    relaxing, 46
    shrubby, 405
    spreading, 405
    trailing, 412
    warming, 33
    watery fresh, 428
hermaphrodite, 145
hibiscus (*Hibiscus sabdariffa*), **185**, 455. *See also* edible flowers
    aromatherapy oil, 189
    cautions, 189
    edible uses, 189
    flower essence, 189
    growing, 189
    herbal remedy, 187–189
    hibiscus chutney, 455
high-density lipoproteins (HDLs), 188, 355
highly pathogenic avian IV (HPAIV), 156
Hill, J., 280, 333
Hippocrates, 33. *See also* Greek and Roman

medicine, ancient
hollyhock, 456. *See also* edible flowers
holy basil. *See* tulsi
homeopathy, 42. *See also* flower healing
    Mandrake, 42
    miasms, 43
    Organon of Rational Medicine, The, 43
    Samuel Hahnemann, 42
    succession, 43
    symptom picture, 43
homoeostasis, 46. *See also* healing tradition in America
honey, 430. *See also* flower preparations for internal use
honeysuckle (*Lonicera japonica, L. caprifolium, L. periclymenum*), **225**, 457. *See also* edible flowers
    aromadendrene, 226
    aromatherapy oil, 228
    cautions, 229
    cleaning agent, 229
    edible uses, 228
    flower remedy, 228
    growing, 229
    herbal remedy, 226–228
    homeopathic remedy, 228
    oil hair conditioner, 228
    related plants, 229
hops (*Humulus lupulus*), **191**
    aromatherapy oil, 193
    cautions, 194
    flower essence, 193
    growing, 194
    herbal remedy, 191–193
    homeopathic remedy, 193
    humulone, 192
    infused oil, 194
    sleep pillow, 194
    tea, 194
    xanthohumol, 192
hormone balancing herbs, 322
Hortulus, 38
hot inflammatory problems, 330
HPAIV. *See* highly pathogenic avian IV
humours, 33. *See also* Greek and Roman medicine, ancient
Humulus lupulus. *See* hops
hyacinth, 61
Hyacinthus, 19
hyaluronidase, 155
hydrosols. *See* distilled waters
hydroxycinnamic acids, 232
Hypericum perforatum. *See* St John's wort
hyssop (*Hyssopus officinalis*), 35, **201**
    aromatherapy oil, 203
    cautions, 203
    edible uses, 203
    flower essence, 203
    growing, 203
    herbal remedy, 201–203
    hyssop cough syrup, 203
    tisane, 203
Hyssopus officinalis. *See* hyssop

indole alkaloids, 269
inflammation, 330
    of digestive tract, 134
    problems, 65, 70, 129, 188, 193
infused oils, 438
infusions, 426. *See also* flower preparations for internal use
inositol, 227
insect repellent flowers, 408–410. *See also* wildflower garden
Inula helenium. *See* elecampane
inulin, 206
invasive herbs, 412
iridoid glycosides, 166
iris, 17
isoflavone phytoestrogens, 354
isoquinoline alkaloids, 124, 163

jasmine (*Jasminum officinale, J. grandiflorum*), 17, 20, **211**
    aromatherapy oil, 213
    cautions, 213
    edible uses, 213
    flower essence, 213
    growing, 213
    herbal remedy, 212–213
    homeopathic remedy, 213

Lady Mary Wortley Montagu, 21
lady's mantle (*Alchemilla vulgaris / mollis*), **73**
    astringent properties, 74
    benefits for women, 73–74
    cautions, 76
    flower essence, 76
    growing, 76
    hepato-protective effect, 76
    herbal remedy, 74
language of flowers, 20–21
laurel tree, 13
lavender (*Lavandula angustifolia*), **215**, 457–458. *See also* edible flowers
    antiseptic oils, 217
    aromatherapy oil, 216–218
    aromatic toilet vinegar, 218

cautions, 218
flower essence, 218
granola, 458
growing, 218
healing salve for eczema, 218
herbal remedy, 216
and lemon balm tisane, 458
water, 218
layering, 405. *See also* flowers, growing
LDL. *See* low-density lipoprotein
Leech Book of Bald, 37, 396
lemon balm (*Melissa officinalis*), **231**
aromatherapy oil, 235
cautions, 235
edible uses, 235
flower essence, 235
growing, 235
herbal remedy, 232–235
infused oil, 235
Leonurus cardiaca. *See* motherwort
lesser periwinkle (*Vinca minor*), **377**
cautions, 380
flower essence, 380
growing, 380
herbal remedy, 378
homeopathic remedy, 380
ointment, 380
Vinca major, 379
Vinca rosea, 380
life of spirit, 15–17
'like curing like' method of healing, 41. *See also* flower healing
lilac, 459. *See also* edible flowers
lilium regale, 38
lime. *See* linden
linden (*Tilia europaea/T. cordata*), **349**
aromatherapy oil, 352
cautions, 352
edible uses, 352
flower essence, 352
harvesting, 352
herbal remedy, 350–352
homeopathic remedy, 352
liniments, 438. *See also* plant preparations for external use
Linnaeus, C., 259
linoleic acid, 260
Lonicera japonica, L. caprifolium, L. periclymenum. *See* honeysuckle
lotus, 15–17
love, 18–20
Lovelock, J., 398
low-density lipoprotein (LDL), 188, 355
luck bringing flowers, 17

lutein, 360

macrophages, 156, 174
Madonna lily, 17
magnolia, 460. *See also* edible flowers
makeshift still, 433. *See also* flower preparations for internal use
Mandrake, 42
marigold. *See* calendula
marshmallow (*Althaea officinalis*), **83**
antimicrobial and immune-enhancing actions, 85, 86
cautions, 87
cough syrup, 87
edible uses, 87
flower essence, 87
growing, 87
herbal remedy, 84–87
strengthening tonic, 87
tea, 87
Matricaria chamomilla. *See* chamomile
Mayday, 141
maypole ceremony, 141
meadow flowers, 406
meadowsweet (*Filipendula ulmaria*), **169**
cautions, 170
edible uses, 170
flower essence, 170
growing, 170
herbal remedy, 169–170
homeopathic remedy, 170
tisane for painful joints, 171
medicinal herbs, 396
medieval monasteries, 37–39
Melissa officinalis. *See* lemon balm
Mentha piperita. *See* peppermint
methicillinresistant *Staphylococcus aureus* (MRSA), 192, 301
Metrodora, 34. *See also* Greek and Roman medicine, ancient
Meyer, H. C. F., 155
miasms, 43. *See also* homeopathy
mind-altering plants, 31, 45
mint & fennel flower dip, 452. *See also* fennel
moistening herbs, 33. *See also* Greek and Roman medicine, ancient
Monarda fistulosa. *See* wild bergamot
motherwort (*Leonurus cardiaca*), **219**
cautions, 223
edible uses, 223
flower essence, 223
growing, 223
herbal remedy, 220–223

mounding, 405. See also flowers, growing
mountain devil essence, 54. See also flower remedies and essences
moxibustion, 105
MRSA. See methicillinresistant *Staphylococcus aureus*
mugwort (*Artemisia vulgaris*), 57, **101**
    cautions, 105
    edible uses, 105
    flower essence, 105
    growing, 105
    herbal remedy, 102–105
    homeopathic remedy, 105
    nervine properties, 104
mullein (*Verbascum thapsus*), **363**
    cautions, 367
    edible uses, 367
    flower and garlic oil for earache, 367
    flower essence, 366–367
    growing, 367
    herbal remedy, 364–365
    homeopathic remedy, 366
multidrug-resistant bacteria, 301, 346

Narcissus, 12
nasturtium (*Tropaeolum majus*), **359**, 461. See also edible flowers
    edible uses, 361
    essential oils, 360
    flower essence, 360–361
    growing, 361
    herbal remedy, 359–360
    homeopathic remedy, 360
    pesto, 461
National Institute of Medical Herbalists, 45. See also healing tradition in America
Native American medicine, 45. See also healing tradition in America
Neanderthal man, 31
Nepeta cataria. See catmint
nervous symptoms, 275
nettle, 416. See also organic gardening
neurodegenerative diseases, 275
neurological disorders, 321
NF-κB. See Nuclear Factor-KappaB
Nuclear Factor-KappaB (NF-κB), 182

Ocimum tenuiflorum/sanctum. See tulsi
Oenothera biennis. See evening primrose
oestrogen-dependent tumours, 76
offsets. See also root cuttings
oils, 438. See also plant preparations for external use

orange blossom (*Citrus aurantium*), **131**
    aromatherapy oil, 133–135
    cautions, 135
    distillation process, 132–133
    edible uses, 135
    flower essence, 135
    flowers, 20
    growing, 135
    herbal remedy, 133–135
    homeopathic remedy,
    Neroli essential oil, 132
orchids, 19–20
organic gardening, 410
    chamomile spray, 410
    comfrey, 411
    compost accelerators, 411
    dehydrator, 418
    drying plants, 418–419
    foraging best practice, 416–417
    foraging for wildflowers, 415–416
    foraging safely and responsibly, 417–418
    gathering and foraging, 413–415
    growing flowers in small spaces, 411–412
    nettle plant feed, 410
    nettles, 416
    planting in patios or paving, 412
    plant medicine, 417
    storing flowers and leaves, 419–420
organoleptics, 60
Organon of Rational Medicine, The, 43. See also homeopathy
Origanum majorana. See sweet marjoram
osteoclast, 355
over the counter (OTC), 270
oxymels, 431–432. See also flower preparations for internal use

pan-fried courgette (zucchini) blossoms, 467
pansies. See wild pansy
Paracelsus, 40–41, 97
Paradisi in sole Paradisus Terrestris, 40, 397
Parkinson, J., 40, 291
pasque flower (*Anenome pulsatilla*), **89**
    cautions, 91
    flower essence, 90–91
    growing, 91
    herbal remedy, 89–90
    homeopathic remedy, 90
passionflower (*Passiflora incarnata*), **267**
    cautions, 271
    Christ consciousness, 271

edible uses, 271
  flower essence, 271
  growing, 271
  harmine, 269
  herbal remedy, 269–271
  homeopathic remedy, 271
  passiflora and vervain tea, 270
PCOS. *See* polycystic ovarian syndrome
Pelargonium graveolens. *See* rose geranium
pelargoniums, 462. *See also* edible flowers
peppermint (*Mentha piperita*), **237**
  aromatherapy oil, 237–239
  cautions, 239
  flower essence, 239
  growing, 239
  herbal remedy, 237–239
  homeopathic remedy, 239
  recipes, 239
PG2. *See* prostaglandin 2
phagocytosis, 84, 156
phenolic compounds, 108
physic gardens, 397–398
physiomedicalism, 46. *See also* healing tradition in America
physiomedicalists, 45. *See also* healing tradition in America
pickled magnolia flowers, 460
pityriasis versicolor (PV), 276
plant. *See also* organic gardening; wildflower garden
  language, 60
  medicine, 417
  sprays, 410
plant feed, nettle, 410
planting in patios or paving, 412. *See also* organic gardening
plant preparations for external use, 434. *See also* still room
  compresses and fomentations, 436
  floral baths, 434–435
  hand and foot baths, 435–436
  liniments, 438
  oils, 438
  poultices and plasters, 436–437
  salves and creams, 436
plasters, 436–437. *See also* plant preparations for external use
pleasant tasting herbs, 426
Pliny the Elder, 36, 377. *See also* Greek and Roman medicine, ancient
8-PN. *See* 8-prenylnaringenin
pollinators, 29
polycystic ovarian syndrome (PCOS), 227, 326
poppies, 12

postherpetic neuralgia, 276
posy, 19
potato salad with fennel flowers, 452. *See also* fennel
pot marigold. *See* calendula
poultices, 436–437. *See also* plant preparations for external use
powders, 433–434. *See also* flower preparations for internal use
8-prenylnaringenin (8-PN), 192
Primula veris. *See* cowslip
prostaglandin 2 (PG2), 192
prostaglandin E1, 260
Prunella vulgaris. *See* self-heal
Pseudomonas aeruginosa, 383
purple coneflower (*Echinacea angustifolia, pallida and purpurea*), **155**
  cautions, 157
  Echinacea tincture, 157
  edible uses, 157
  flower essence, 156
  growing, 157
  herbal remedy, 155–156
  homeopathic remedy, 156
purslane, 462. *See also* edible flowers
PV. *See* pityriasis versicolor

qi, 49, 286. *See also* Chinese medicine

red clover (*Trifolium pratense*), **353**, 463. *See also* edible flowers
  cautions, 357
  drying, 354
  edible uses, 357
  flower essence, 356–357
  growing, 357
  herbal remedy, 354–356
  homeopathic remedy, 356
  lemonade, 357
  ointment, 357
  syrup, 357
  tabbouleh, 463
  tincture, 357
relaxing herbs, 46
resistant strains, 301, 346
respiratory ailments, 248
respiratory syncytial (RS), 192
Roman medicine. *See* Greek and Roman medicine, ancient
root cuttings, 405. *See also* flowers, growing
root division, 404. *See also* flowers, growing
Rosa spp.. *See* rose
rose (*Rosa* spp.), 18, 20, **291**, 464–465. *See also*

edible flowers
- antioxidant effects, 294
- aromatherapy oil, 293–296
- cautions, 296
- flower essence, 296
- growing, 296
- herbal remedy, 293–296
- Indian rose syrup and coconut milk, 296
- notable medicinal roses, 296
- petal harissa, 465
- soaps, 295

rose geranium (*Pelargonium graveolens*), **273**
- aromatherapy oil, 276–277
- cautions, 277
- edible uses, 277
- flower essence, 277
- in gardens, 274
- growing, 277
- herbal remedy, 274–276
- infused rose geranium oil, 277
- infusion, 276

rosella hemp, 189

rosemary (*Salvia rosmarinus*; *Rosmarinus officinalis*), **307**
- antibacterial effects, 309
- antioxidant effect, 308–309
- aromatherapy oil, 312
- cautions, 312
- edible uses, 312
- flower essence, 312
- growing, 312
- herbal remedy, 308–312
- and lemon syrup, 311
- mouthwash, 311
- salt, 311
- tea, 311

rosmarinic acid, 265

Rosmarinus officinalis. *See* rosemary

RS. *See* respiratory syncytial

rubbing oil, 438

rutin, 423

SAD. *See* seasonal affective disorder

sage (*Salvia officinalis*), **299**, 466. *See also* edible flowers
- antimicrobial actions, 301
- antiseptic mouthwash, 305
- aromatherapy oil, 302–303
- blossom vinegar, 466
- cautions, 303, 305
- cayenne, honey and cider vinegar gargle, 305
- edible uses, 303
- flower essence, 303
- growing, 303
- herbal remedy, 300–302
- homeopathic remedy, 303
- sore throat compress, 305
- tannins, 301

salves, 436. *See also* plant preparations for external use

Salvia
- *officinalis*. *See* sage
- *rosmarinus*. *See* rosemary

Sambucus nigra. *See* elder

sattvic medhya herb, 212

scented geraniums. *See* pelargoniums

Scutellaria. *See also* skullcap
- *baicalensis*, 320
- *lateriflora*, 321, 322

seasonal affective disorder (SAD), 196, 244, 377

self-heal (*Prunella vulgaris*), **285**
- cautions, 289
- edible uses, 289
- flower essence, 288, 289
- growing, 289
- herbal remedy, 285–287
- homeopathic remedy, 287–288
- relaxant properties, 286
- self-heal salve, 289

sex hormone binding globulin (SHBG), 227

shamans, 31

shamrock, 17

SHBG. *See* sex hormone binding globulin

Shennong Bencao Jing, 285

shrubby herbs, 405

skin infections, 208

skullcap (*Scutellaria* spp.), **320**
- and California poppy tea, 323
- cautions, 323
- flower essence, 323
- growing, 323
- herbal remedy, 320–323
- homeopathic remedy, 323
- *Scutellaria baicalensis*, 320
- *Scutellaria lateriflora*, 321, 322

snowdrop, 14

soil conditions, 403. *See also* flowers, growing

S-OIV. *See* swine origin IV

soul, 23–26

sowing seeds, 403. *See also* flowers, growing

spreading herbs, 405

squash blossom, 466–467. *See also* edible flowers

Stachys betonica. *See* wood betony

Stellaria media. *See* chickweed

still room, 421, 438–439

antioxidants, 423
floral waters, 421
floriphagia, 423
flower preparations for internal use, 426–434
methods to take healing flowers, 422
nutrients and medicinal compounds, 422–423
plant preparations for external use, 434–438
preparing floral medicines, 422–425
St John's wort (*Hypericum perforatum*), **195**
antiviral activity, 196, 198
cautions, 198
flower essence, 198
growing, 198
heart of Jesus oil, 199
herbal remedy, 196–198
homeopathic remedy, 198
storing flowers and leaves, 419–420. *See also* organic gardening
Strabo, W., 38
stress-related
digestive disorders, 138
gut problems, 134, 389
problems, 235, 256, 266, 275, 280, 370
symptoms, 355, 383
styptic action, 275
sunflower, 468. *See also* edible flowers
sunflower pesto, 468
sun method, 54. *See also* flower remedies and essences
suppositories, 434. *See also* flower preparations for internal use
sweet marjoram (*Origanum majorana*), **263**
anti-inflammatory tisane, 266
aromatherapy oil, 265–266
cautions, 266
edible uses, 266
flower essence, 266
growing, 266
herbal remedy, 265–266
homeopathic remedy, 266
related plants, 266
sweet violet (*Viola odorata*), **381**, 469. *See also* edible flowers
aromatherapy oil, 383–385
cautions, 385
edible uses, 385
flower essence, 385
growing, 385
herbal remedy, 382–383
homeopathic remedy, 385
violet ointment, 385

violet syrup, 385
sweet William (*Dianthus*), **145**, 470. *See also* edible flowers
aromatherapy oil, 151–152
bread, 470
cautions, 153
Dianthus caryophyllus, 149–151
Dianthus chinensis, 151
edible uses, 153
flower essence, 152–153
growing, 153
herbal remedy, 149–151
in myth, 145–146
varieties, 145
swine origin IV (S-OIV), 156

tablets, 434. *See also* flower preparations for internal use
taller flowering plants or shrubs, 408
Tanacetum parthenium. *See* feverfew
tannins, 301
Taraxacum officinale. *See* dandelion
taraxasterol, 339
TCM. *See* Traditional Chinese Medicine
Theatrum Botanicum, 40, 397
Theophrastus, 34, 299. *See also* Greek and Roman medicine, ancient
Theriac electuary, 429
Thomson, S., 46. *See also* healing tradition in America
thyme (*Thymus vulgaris*), **343**
and apple jelly, 347
aromatherapy oil, 347
cautions, 348
edible uses, 348
flower essence, 348
growing, 348
herbal remedy, 345–347
homeopathic remedy, 348
honey, 430
infusion or tincture, 346–347
syrup, 348
TIAs. *See* transient ischaemic attacks
tiger lily, 471. *See also* edible flowers
Tilia europaea/T. cordata. *See* linden
tinctures, 428–429. *See also* flower preparations for internal use
toning plants, 46
Traditional Chinese Medicine (TCM), 151, 285, 338
trailing herbs, 412
transient ischaemic attacks (TIAs), 380
trefoil, 17

Trifolium pratense. *See* red clover
triterpenes, 220
Tropaeolum majus. *See* nasturtium
tuberose, 26
tulip, 19
tulsi (*Ocimum tenuiflorum/sanctum*), **251**
    antimicrobial activity, 254–255
    aromatherapy oil, 256
    cautions, 257
    edible uses, 256
    flower essence, 256
    growing, 256–257
    herbal remedy, 252–256
    homeopathic remedy, 256
    tulsi tea, 257
Turner, W., 40

uric acid levels, 317

vascular problems, 184
Verbascum thapsus. *See* mullein
verbenalin, 370
vervain (*Verbena officinalis*), 20, **369**
    aromatherapy oil, 372
    calming tea, 375
    cautions, 374
    cooling stomach tea, 375
    edible uses, 374
    flower essence, 372, 373
    foot bath, 375
    growing, 374
    herbal remedy, 370372
    homeopathic remedy, 372
    relaxing bath, 375
    Verbena hastata, 373
    verbenalin, 370
Victorian language of flowers, 21–22
vigorous growing plants, 412
Vinca
    major, 379
    minor. *See* lesser periwinkle
    rosea, 380
Viola
    odorata. *See* sweet violet
    tricolor. *See* heartsease
violets, 423. *See also* sweet violet
vital force of subtle energy, 56
vital green energy, 38
volatile oils, 98, 102, 104, 216, 232, 238, 308, 321
von Bingen, H., 38
von Chamisso, A., 163

warming herbs, 33. *See also* Greek and Roman

medicine, ancient
watery fresh herbs, 428
white myrtle flower, 13
wild bergamot (*Monarda fistulosa*), **241**, 442. *See also* edible flowers
    aromatherapy oil, 244–245
    bee balm bread, 442
    calming and decongestant tea, 245
    cautions, 245
    edible uses, 245
    garden varieties of bergamot, 243
    growing, 245
    herbal remedy, 242–244
    -infused honey, 245
    tincture, 245
wildflower garden, 406
    companion planting, 408, 409
    flowers in vegetable garden, 408
    insect repellent flowers, 408–410
    planting wildflower garden, 406–408
    plant sprays, 410
    wildflower meadow, 407
wild garlic, 472. *See also* edible flowers; garlic
wild garlic pesto, 472
wild pansy, 20. *See also* edible flowers
    purple kale and pansy salad, 473
wind flower, 1
winter ailments, 347
wood betony (*Stachys betonica*), 37, **325**
    cautions, 327
    flower essence, 327
    growing, 327
    headache relief tea, 327
    herbal remedy, 326–327
    homeopathic remedy, 327
    wood betony nerve tonic, 327

yarrow (*Achillea millifolium*), 57, **63**
    antihistamine effect, 65
    aromatherapy oil, 66
    astringent tannins, 65
    cautions, 67
    cyaniding, 64
    edible uses, 66
    flower essence, 66
    growing, 67
    herbal remedy, 63–66
    homeopathic remedy, 66
    mint, and elderflower tea, 66
'Yin' and 'yang', 49. *See also* Chinese medicine